Seventh Edition

Medical Terminology

A LIVING LANGUAGE

Seventh Edition

Medical Terminology
A LIVING LANGUAGE

Bonnie F. Fremgen, PhD
Former Associate Dean
Allied Health Program
Robert Morris College
Chicago, IL

Suzanne S. Frucht, PhD
Associate Professor Emeritus
Northwest Missouri State University
Maryville, MO

330 Hudson Street, New York, NY 10013

Vice President, Portfolio Management: Julie Levin Alexander
Director of Portfolio Management: Marlene McHugh Pratt
Portfolio Manager: John Goucher
Content Producer: Melissa Bashe
Portfolio Management Assistant: Lisa Narine
Development Editor: Danielle Doller
Vice President, Content Production and Digital Studio: Paul DeLuca
Vice President, Product Marketing: David Gesell
Field Marketing Manager: Brittany Hammond
Product Marketing Manager: Rachele Strober
Operations Specialist: MaryAnn Gloriande
Cover Design: Studio Montage
Interior Designer: Pam Verros
Creative Digital Lead: Mary Siener
Cover Art: Sebastian Kaulitzki/Shutterstock
Director, Digital Studio, Health Science: Amy Peltier
Digital Studio Producer, e-text 2.0: Ellen Viganola and Allison Longley
Full-Service Project Management: Joanna Stein, SPi Global
Composition: SPi Global
Editorial Project Manager: Meghan DeMaio, SPi Global
Digital Content Team Lead: Brian Prybella
Digital Content Project Lead: William Johnson
Printer/Binder: LSC Communications, Inc.
Cover Printer: Phoenix Color/Hagerstown
Text Font: Meridien Com 11/13

DEDICATION

To my husband for his love and encouragement.

Bonnie Fremgen

To my granddaughter, Adrienne, who every day brings a smile to my face.

To Danielle Doller, whose incredible editing skills (and friendship) have made each edition of this text better.

I would like to extend a special thank you to Garnet Tomich who added to her normal workload by taking on the immense task of double-checking the pronunciations of every term in this edition and updating them as needed to ensure consistency.

Suzanne Frucht

Credits and acknowledgments for content borrowed from other sources and reproduced, with permission, in this textbook appear on appropriate page within text.

Notice: The author and the publisher of this book have taken care to make certain that the information given is correct and compatible with the standards generally accepted at the time of publication. Nevertheless, as new information becomes available, changes in treatment and in the use of equipment and procedures become necessary. The reader is advised to carefully consult the instruction and information material included in each piece of equipment or device before administration. Students are warned that the use of any techniques must be authorized by their medical advisor, where appropriate, in accordance with local laws and regulations. The publisher disclaims any liability, loss, injury, or damage incurred as a consequence, directly or indirectly, of the use and application of any of the contents of this book.

Many of the designations by manufacturers and sellers to distinguish their products are claimed as trademarks. Where those designations appear in this book, and the publisher was aware of a trademark claim, the designations have been printed in initial caps or all caps.

Library of Congress Cataloging-in-Publication Data

Names: Fremgen, Bonnie F., author. | Frucht, Suzanne S., author.
Title: Medical terminology : a living language / Bonnie F. Fremgen, Suzanne S. Frucht.
Description: Seventh edition. | Hoboken, New Jersey : Pearson Education, 2017. | Includes bibliographical references and index.
Identifiers: LCCN 2017041703 | ISBN 9780134701202 | ISBN 0134701208
Subjects: | MESH: Medicine | Terminology
Classification: LCC R123 | NLM W 15 | DDC 610.1/4--dc23
LC record available at https://lccn.loc.gov/2017041703

1 17

ISBN-10: 0-13-470120-8
ISBN-13: 978-013-470120-2

Welcome!

Welcome to the fascinating study of Medical Terminology: A Living Language—a vital part of your preparation for a career as a health professional. We are glad that you have joined us. Throughout your career, in a variety of settings, you will use medical terminology to communicate with coworkers and patients. Employing a carefully constructed learning system, **Medical Terminology: A Living Language** has helped thousands of readers gain a successful grasp of Medical Terminology: A Living Language within a real-world context.

In developing this book we had seven goals in mind:

1. To provide you with a clear introduction to the basic rules of using word parts to form medical terms.
2. To use phonetic pronunciations that will help you easily pronounce terms by spelling out the word part according to the way it sounds.
3. To help you understand medical terminology within the context of the human body systems. Realizing that this book is designed for a terminology course and not an anatomy and physiology course, we have aimed to stick to only the basics.
4. To help you develop a full range of Latin and Greek word parts used to build medical terms so that you will be able to interpret unfamiliar terms you encounter in the future.

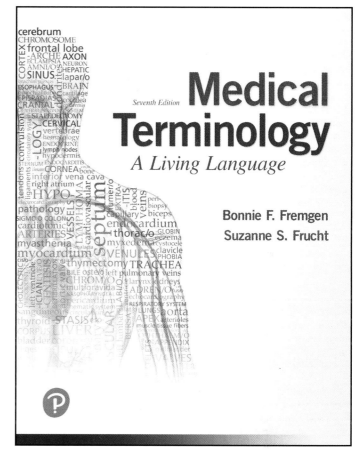

5. To help you visualize Medical Terminology: A Living Language with an abundance of real-life photographs and accurate illustrations.
6. To provide you with a wealth of practice applications throughout and at the end of each chapter to help you review and master the content as you go along.
7. To create rich multimedia practice opportunities for you by way of MyLab Medical Terminology.

Please turn the page to get a visual glimpse of what makes this book an ideal guide to your exploration of medical terminology.

A Guide to What Makes This Book Special

Streamlined Content

Thirteen chapters and only the most essential anatomy and physiology coverage make this book a perfect midsized fit for a one-term course.

Chapter-Opening Page Spreads

"At a Glance" and "Illustrated" pages begin each chapter, providing a quick, visual snapshot of what's covered.

Anatomy & Physiology

Prior to being introduced to terms associated with an organ system, the anatomy and physiology of that body system is described in concise and easy to understand language. Information coverage begins with the overall function and the organs that comprise the system. Then each organ is addressed with its structure and how it contributes to the function of that system. Having a grasp of this basic level of information before being introduced to terms associated with each system makes it easier for students to understand the pathologic, diagnostic, and therapeutic terms.

Key Terms

Every subsection starts with a list of key terms that will be covered in that section. This sets the stage for comprehension and mastery.

EXPANDED! Pronunciations

Every chapter includes sound-it-out pronunciations to help students say medical terms accurately.

Color-Coded Word Parts

Red combining forms, blue suffixes, and gold prefixes allow for quick recognition throughout the book.

Informative and Interesting Sidebars

- The popular **Med Term Tip** feature offers tidbits of noteworthy information about medical terms that engage learners.
- **Word Watch** points out words that have a similar sound or similar spelling, and also alerts students about abbreviations that have more than one meaning.
- **What's In A Name?** reinforces the breakdown of terms into word parts.

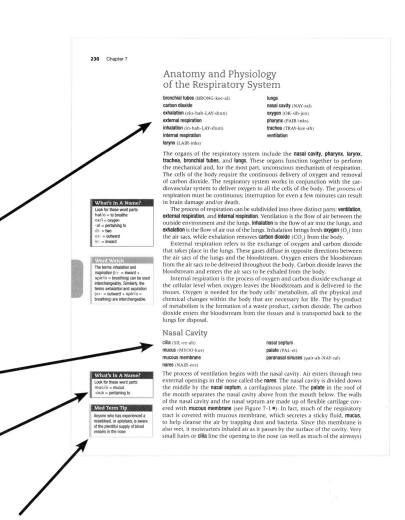

230 Chapter 7

Anatomy and Physiology of the Respiratory System

bronchial tubes (BRONG-kee-al)	lungs
carbon dioxide	nasal cavity (NAY-zal)
exhalation (eks-hah-LAY-shun)	oxygen (OK-sih-jen)
external respiration	pharynx (FAIR-inks)
inhalation (in-hah-LAY-shun)	trachea (TRAY-kee-ah)
internal respiration	ventilation
larynx (LAIR-inks)	

What's In A Name?
Look for these word parts:
hal/o = to breathe
ox/i = oxygen
-al = pertaining to
di- = two
ex- = outward
in- = inward

Word Watch
The terms *inhalation* and *inspiration* (in- = inward + spir/o = breathing) can be used interchangeably. Similarly, the terms *exhalation* and *expiration* (ex- = outward + spir/o = breathing) are interchangeable.

The organs of the respiratory system include the **nasal cavity, pharynx, larynx, trachea, bronchial tubes,** and **lungs.** These organs function together to perform the mechanical and, for the most part, unconscious mechanism of respiration. The cells of the body require the continuous delivery of oxygen and removal of carbon dioxide. The respiratory system works in conjunction with the cardiovascular system to deliver oxygen to all the cells of the body. The process of respiration must be continuous; interruption for even a few minutes can result in brain damage and/or death.

The process of respiration can be subdivided into three distinct parts: **ventilation, external respiration,** and **internal respiration.** Ventilation is the flow of air between the outside environment and the lungs. **Inhalation** is the flow of air into the lungs, and **exhalation** is the flow of air out of the lungs. Inhalation brings fresh **oxygen** (O_2) into the air sacs, while exhalation removes **carbon dioxide** (CO_2) from the body.

External respiration refers to the exchange of oxygen and carbon dioxide that takes place in the lungs. These gases diffuse in opposite directions between the air sacs of the lungs and the bloodstream. Oxygen enters the bloodstream from the air sacs to be delivered throughout the body. Carbon dioxide leaves the bloodstream and enters the air sacs to be exhaled from the body.

Internal respiration is the process of oxygen and carbon dioxide exchange at the cellular level when oxygen leaves the bloodstream and is delivered to the tissues. Oxygen is needed for the body cells' metabolism, all the physical and chemical changes within the body that are necessary for life. The by-product of metabolism is the formation of a waste product, carbon dioxide. The carbon dioxide enters the bloodstream from the tissues and is transported back to the lungs for disposal.

Nasal Cavity

cilia (SIL-ee-ah)	nasal septum
mucus (MYOO-kus)	palate (PAL-et)
mucous membrane	paranasal sinuses (pair-ah-NAY-zal)
nares (NAIR-eez)	

What's In A Name?
Look for these word parts:
muc/o = mucus
-ous = pertaining to

Med Term Tip
Anyone who has experienced a nosebleed, or *epistaxis*, is aware of the plentiful supply of blood vessels in the nose.

The process of ventilation begins with the nasal cavity. Air enters through two external openings in the nose called the **nares.** The nasal cavity is divided down the middle by the **nasal septum,** a cartilaginous plate. The **palate** in the roof of the mouth separates the nasal cavity above from the mouth below. The walls of the nasal cavity and the nasal septum are made up of flexible cartilage covered with **mucous membrane** (see Figure 7-1 ■). In fact, much of the respiratory tract is covered with mucous membrane, which secretes a sticky fluid, **mucus,** to help cleanse the air by trapping dust and bacteria. Since this membrane is also wet, it moisturizes inhaled air as it passes by the surface of the cavity. Very small hairs or **cilia** line the opening to the nose (as well as much of the airways)

Medically Accurate Illustrations

Concepts come to life with vibrant, clear, and scientifically precise images.

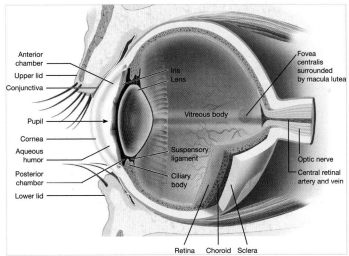

Terminology Tables

Terms are categorized and presented in a clear, logical, color-coded format that eases the learning process. The major categories include Pathology, Adjective Forms, Diagnostic Procedures, Therapeutic Procedures, Pharmacology, and Abbreviations. Each major category table is further subdivided into smaller subsections of related terms, thereby making learning easier. Also, the three-column format of the tables allows for the term (with pronunciation and/or abbreviation), word parts (if appropriate), and definitions to be displayed. The Pharmacology table also includes drug name examples in a fourth column.

Terminology

Word Parts Used to Build Eye Terms

The following lists contain the combining forms, suffixes, and prefixes used to build terms in the remaining sections of this chapter.

Combining Forms

aden/o	gland	emmetr/o	correct, proper	opt/o	eye, vision
ambly/o	dull, dim	esthesi/o	sensation, feeling	optic/o	eye, vision
angi/o	vessel	glauc/o	gray	papill/o	optic disk
bi/o	life	ir/o	iris	phac/o	lens
blast/o	immature	irid/o	iris	phot/o	light
blephar/o	eyelid	kerat/o	cornea	pneum/o	air
chromat/o	color	lacrim/o	tears	presby/o	old age
conjunctiv/o	conjunctiva	macul/o	macula lutea	pupill/o	pupil
corne/o	cornea	mi/o	lessening	retin/o	retina
cry/o	cold	myc/o	fungus	scler/o	sclera
cycl/o	ciliary body	mydr/i	widening	stigmat/o	point
cyst/o	sac	nyctal/o	night	ton/o	tone
dacry/o	tears	ocul/o	eye	uve/o	choroid
dipl/o	double	ophthalm/o	eye	xer/o	dry

Suffixes

-al	pertaining to	-logy	study of	-pexy	surgical fixation
-algia	pain	-malacia	abnormal softening	-phobia	fear
-ar	pertaining to	-meter	instrument to measure	-plasty	surgical repair
-ary	pertaining to	-metrist	specialist in measuring	-plegia	paralysis
-atic	pertaining to	-metry	process of measuring	-ptosis	drooping
-ectomy	surgical removal			-rrhagia	abnormal flow condition
-edema	swelling	-oma	tumor; mass		
-graphy	process of recording	-opia	vision condition	-scope	instrument for viewing
-ia	condition	-opsia	vision condition	-scopy	process of visually examining
-ic	pertaining to	-osis	abnormal condition		
-ician	specialist	-otomy	cutting into	-tic	pertaining to
-ism	state of	-pathy	disease	-tropia	turned condition
-itis	inflammation				

Prefixes

a-	without	exo-	outward	intra-	within
an-	without	extra-	outside of	micro-	small
anti-	against	hemi-	half	mono-	one
de-	without	hyper-	excessive	myo-	to shut
eso-	inward				

Pharmacology

Vocabulary

Term	Word Parts	Definition
cumulative action		Action that occurs in body when drug is allowed to accumulate or stay in body
prophylaxis (proh-fih-LAK-sis)	pro- = before -phylaxis = protection	Prevention of disease; for example, antibiotic can be used to prevent occurrence of bacterial infection

Drugs

Classification	Word Parts	Action	Examples
antibiotic (an-tih-bye-AW-tik)	anti- = against bi/o = life -tic = pertaining to	Kills bacteria causing respiratory infections	ampicillin; amoxicillin, Amoxil; ciprofloxacin, Cipro
		Med Term Tip There are three accepted pronunciations for the prefix anti-, "an-tih," "an-tee," and "an-tye."	
antihistamine (an-tih-HIST-ah-meen)	anti- = against	Blocks effects of histamine released by body during allergy attack	fexofenadine, Allegra; loratadine, Claritin; diphenhydramine, Benadryl
antitussive (an-tih-TUSS-iv)	anti- = without tuss/o = cough	Relieves urge to cough	hydrocodon, Hycodan; dextromethorphan, Vicks Formula 44
bronchodilator (BRONG-koh-dye-lay-ter)	bronch/o = bronchus	Relaxes muscle spasms in bronchial tubes; used to treat asthma	albuterol, Proventil, Ventolin; salmeterol, Serevent
corticosteroids (kor-tih-koh-STAIR-oydz)	cortic/o = outer layer, cortex	Reduces inflammation and swelling in respiratory tract	fluticasone, Flonase; mometasone, Nasonex; triamcinolone, Azmacort
decongestant (dee-kon-JES-tant)	de- = without	Reduces stuffiness and congestion throughout respiratory system	oxymetazoline, Afrin, Dristan, Sinex; pseudoephedrine, Drixoral, Sudafed

Abbreviations

#	number	ii	two
BCC	basal cell carcinoma	iii	three
bid	two times a day	MM	malignant melanoma
BX, bx	biopsy	oint	ointment
C&S	culture and sensitivity	qid	four times a day
decub	decubitus ulcer	SCC	squamous cell carcinoma
Derm, derm	dermatology	SG	skin graft
FS	frozen section	SLE	systemic lupus erythematosus
I&D	incision and drainage	STSG	split-thickness skin graft
i	one	Subc, Subq	subcutaneous
ID	intradermal	tid	three times a day
		UV	ultraviolet
		x	times

Word Watch
Be careful when using the abbreviation ID meaning intradermal and I&D meaning incision and drainage.

Pathology (continued)

Term	Word Parts	Definition
		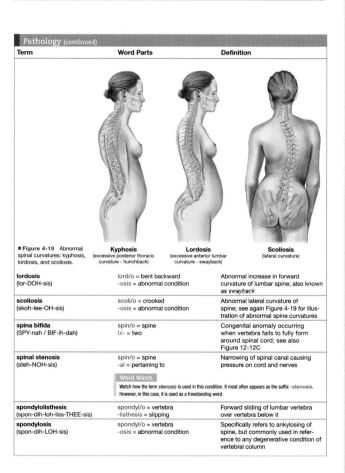

■ Figure 4-19 Abnormal spinal curvatures: kyphosis, lordosis, and scoliosis.

Kyphosis (excessive posterior thoracic curvature - hunchback) **Lordosis** (excessive anterior lumbar curvature - swayback) **Scoliosis** (lateral curvature)

Term	Word Parts	Definition
lordosis (lor-DOH-sis)	lord/o = bent backward -osis = abnormal condition	Abnormal increase in forward curvature of lumbar spine; also known as swayback
scoliosis (skoh-lee-OH-sis)	scoli/o = crooked -osis = abnormal condition	Abnormal lateral curvature of spine; see again Figure 4-19 for illustration of abnormal spine curvatures
spina bifida (SPY-nah / BIF-ih-dah)	spin/o = spine bi- = two	Congenital anomaly occurring when vertebra fails to fully form around spinal cord; see also Figure 12-12C
spinal stenosis (steh-NOH-sis)	spin/o = spine -al = pertaining to	Narrowing of spinal canal causing pressure on cord and nerves
		Word Watch Watch how the term stenosis is used in this condition. It most often appears as the suffix -stenosis. However, in this case, it is used as a freestanding word.
spondylolisthesis (spon-dih-loh-liss-THEE-sis)	spondyl/o = vertebra -listhesis = slipping	Forward sliding of lumbar vertebra over vertebra below it
spondylosis (spon-dih-LOH-sis)	spondyl/o = vertebra -osis = abnormal condition	Specifically refers to ankylosing of spine, but commonly used in reference to any degenerative condition of vertebral column

Therapeutic Procedures

Term	Word Parts	Definition
Medical Procedures		
autologous transfusion (aw-TALL-oh-gus / trans-FYOO-zhun)	auto- = self	Procedure for collecting and storing patient's own blood several weeks prior to actual need; can then be used to replace blood lost during surgical procedure
blood transfusion (trans-FYOO-zhun)	trans- = across fus/o = pouring -ion = action	Artificial transfer of blood into bloodstream
		Med Term Tip Before a patient receives a blood transfusion, the laboratory performs a **type and cross-match**. This test first double-checks the blood type of both the donor's and recipient's blood. Then a cross-match is performed. This process mixes together small samples of both bloods and observes the mixture for adverse reactions.
bone marrow transplant (BMT)		Patient receives red bone marrow from donor after patient's own bone marrow has been destroyed by radiation or chemotherapy
homologous transfusion (hoh-MALL-oh-gus / trans-FYOO-zhun)	homo- = same	Replacement of blood by transfusion of blood received from another person
packed red cells		Transfusion in which most of plasma, leukocytes, and platelets have been removed, leaving only erythrocytes
plasmapheresis (plaz-mah-fah-REE-sis)	-apheresis = removal, carry away	Method of removing plasma from body without depleting formed elements; whole blood is removed and cells and plasma are separated; cells are returned to patient along with donor plasma transfusion
whole blood		Transfusion of a mixture of both plasma and formed elements

Diagnostic Procedures (continued)

Term	Word Parts	Definition
Pap (Papanicolaou) smear (pap-ah-NIK-oh-lao)		Test for early detection of cancer of the cervix named after developer of test, George Papanicolaou, a Greek physician; a scraping of cells is removed from the cervix for examination under microscope
pregnancy test (PREG-nan-see)		Chemical test that can determine pregnancy during first few weeks; can be performed in physician's office or with home-testing kit
vaginal smear wet mount (VAJ-in-al)	vagin/o = vagina -al = pertaining to	Microscopic examination of cells obtained by swabbing vaginal wall; used to diagnose candidiasis
Diagnostic Imaging		
hysterosalpingography (HSG) (hiss-ter-oh-sal-pin-GOG-rah-fee)	hyster/o = uterus salping/o = uterine tube -graphy = process of recording	Taking of X-ray after injecting radiopaque material into uterus and uterine tubes
mammogram (MAM-oh-gram)	mamm/o = breast -gram = record	X-ray record of the breast
mammography (mam-OG-rah-fee)	mamm/o = breast -graphy = process of recording	X-ray to diagnose breast disease, especially breast cancer
pelvic ultrasonography (PEL-vik / ul-trah-son-OG-rah-fee)	pelv/o = pelvis -ic = pertaining to ultra- = beyond son/o = sound -graphy = process of recording	Use of high-frequency sound waves to produce image or photograph of an organ, such as uterus, ovaries, or fetus

Adjective Forms of Anatomical Terms

Term	Word Parts	Definition
conjunctival (kon-junk-TYE-val)	conjunctiv/o = conjunctiva -al = pertaining to	Pertaining to conjunctiva
corneal (KOR-nee-al)	corne/o = cornea -al = pertaining to	Pertaining to cornea
	Word Watch Be careful using the combining forms core/o meaning *pupil* and corne/o meaning *cornea*.	
extraocular (eks-trah-OK-yoo-lar)	extra- = outside of ocul/o = eye -ar = pertaining to	Pertaining to being outside the eyeball; for example, the extraocular eye muscles
intraocular (in-trah-OK-yoo-lar)	intra- = within ocul/o = eye -ar = pertaining to	Pertaining to within eye
iridal (IR-id-al)	irid/o = iris -al = pertaining to	Pertaining to iris
lacrimal (LAK-rim-al)	lacrim/o = tears -al = pertaining to	Pertaining to tears
macular (MAK-yoo-lar)	macul/o = macula lutea -ar = pertaining to	Pertaining to macula lutea
ocular (OK-yoo-lar)	ocul/o = eye -ar = pertaining to	Pertaining to eye
ophthalmic (off-THAL-mik)	ophthalm/o = eye -ic = pertaining to	Pertaining to eye
optic (OP-tik)	opt/o = eye, vision -ic = pertaining to	Pertaining to eye or vision
optical (OP-tih-kal)	optic/o = eye, vision -al = pertaining to	Pertaining to eye or vision
pupillary (PYOO-pih-lair-ee)	pupill/o = pupil -ary = pertaining to	Pertaining to pupil
retinal (RET-ih-nal)	retin/o = retina -al = pertaining to	Pertaining to retina
scleral (SKLAIR-al)	scler/o = sclera -al = pertaining to	Pertaining to sclera
uveal (YOO-vee-al)	uve/o = choroid -al = pertaining to	Pertaining to choroid layer of eye

UPDATED! Practice As You Go

An assortment of exercises is peppered throughout the chapters to assess students' understanding of the material discussed.

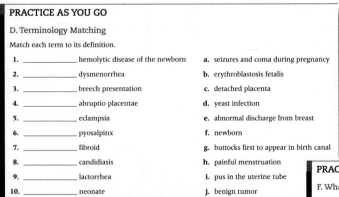

PRACTICE AS YOU GO

D. Terminology Matching

Match each term to its definition.

1. _____ hemolytic disease of the newborn
2. _____ dysmenorrhea
3. _____ breech presentation
4. _____ abruptio placentae
5. _____ eclampsia
6. _____ pyosalpinx
7. _____ fibroid
8. _____ candidiasis
9. _____ lactorrhea
10. _____ neonate

a. seizures and coma during pregnancy
b. erythroblastosis fetalis
c. detached placenta
d. yeast infection
e. abnormal discharge from breast
f. newborn
g. buttocks first to appear in birth canal
h. painful menstruation
i. pus in the uterine tube
j. benign tumor

PRACTICE AS YOU GO

F. What's the Abbreviation?

1. first pregnancy _____
2. artificial insemination _____
3. uterine contractions _____
4. full-term normal delivery _____
5. intrauterine device _____
6. dilation and curettage _____
7. hormone replacement therapy _____
8. gynecology _____
9. abortion _____
10. oral contraceptive pills _____

Chapter Review

Real-World Applications—Three critical thinking activities allow students to apply their medical knowledge to true-to-life scenarios:

1) Medical Record Analysis

Exercises that challenge students to read examples of real medical records and then to apply their medical terminology knowledge in answering related questions.

2) Chart Note Transcription

Slice-of-real-life exercise that asks students to replace lay terms in a medical chart with the proper medical term.

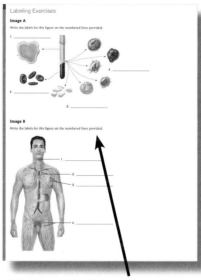

Additionally, **Labeling Exercises** provide a visual challenge to reinforce students' grasp of anatomy and physiology concepts.

3) Case Study

Scenarios that use critical thinking questions to help students develop a firmer understanding of the terminology in context.

Practice Exercises—A wide array of updated workbook exercises at the end of each chapter serve as a fun and challenging study review. A larger variety of question types leads to a more engaging assessment of student understanding of concepts like spelling, adjective formation, and anatomy and physiology.

MyLab Medical Terminology™

What is MyLab Medical Terminology?

MyLab Medical Terminology is a comprehensive online program that gives you, the student, the opportunity to test your understanding of information, concepts and medical language to see how well you know the material. From the test results, MyLab Medical Terminology builds a self-paced, personalized study plan unique to your needs. Remediation in the form of etext pages, illustrations, exercises, audio segments, and video clips is provided for those areas in which you may need additional instruction, review, or reinforcement. You can then work through the program until your study plan is complete and you have mastered the content. MyLab Medical Terminology is available as a standalone program or with an embedded etext.

MyLab Medical Terminology is organized to follow the chapters and learning outcomes in *Medical Terminology: A Living Language*. With MyLab Medical Terminology, you can track your own progress through your entire med term course.

How do Students Benefit?

Here's how MyLab Medical Terminology helps you.

- Keep up with information presented in the text and lectures.
- Save time by focusing study and review just the content you need.
- Increase understanding of difficult concepts with study material for different learning styles.
- Remediate in areas in which you need additional review.

Key Features of MyLab Medical Terminology

Pre-Tests and Post-Tests. Using questions aligned to the learning outcomes in *Medical Terminology: A Living Language*, multiple tests measure your understanding of topics.

Personalized Study Material. Based on the topic pretest results, you receive a personalized study plan, highlighting areas where you may need improvement. It includes these study tools

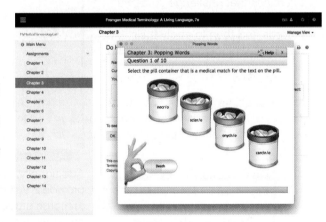

- Links to specific pages in the etext
- Images for review
- Interactive exercises
- Animations and video clips
- Audio glossary
- Access to full Personalized Study Material

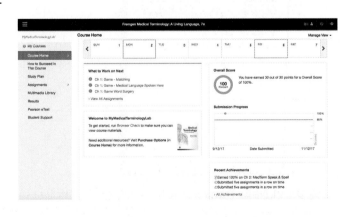

How do Instructors Benefit?

- Save time by providing students with a comprehensive, media-rich study program.
- Track student understanding of course content in the program gradebook.
- Monitor student activity with viewable student assignments.

Preface

Since the first edition of ***Medical Terminology: A Living Language*** was published it has been noted for its "clean" and logical format that promotes learning. In this revised edition, we have built upon this strength by enhancing many features to make this text an ideal choice for semester- or quarter-length courses.

Features of this Edition

This new seventh edition contains features that facilitate student mastery, while maintaining the best aspects of previous editions. Each chapter is arranged in a similar format and the content is organized with an emphasis on maintaining consistency and accuracy.

We have revised ***Medical Terminology: A Living Language*** so that it provides for an even more valuable teaching and learning experience. Here are the enhancements we have made:

- Based on market feedback, we have taken the content that appeared in the special topics chapter in previous editions, and have now broken it up and interspersed this material throughout the book to better correspond with the body systems organization of the text. We hope this change will make incorporating this information easier into your course.

- All of the phonetic pronunciations have been reviewed and revised as needed to ensure consistency and to provide the most commonly used pronunciation.

- The beginning of the Terminology section in each chapter includes an even more comprehensive list of all combining forms, suffixes, and prefixes used to build terms in the remaining sections of the chapter.

- For this seventh edition, every term presented in the book has been evaluated for its currency and additional terms have been added throughout to reflect the newest technologies and procedures.

- **Practice As You Go**, our popular "speed bump" feature scattered throughout the chapters, has been expanded to appear more frequently throughout each chapter to allow the reader to get a quick check on their grasp of the content presented by using a combination of short-answer exercises. Answers are provided at the back of the book.

- End-of-Chapter Practice Exercises have been revamped to better emphasize terminology usage rather than simple recall of word parts. In addition to the rewriting of many standard question types, new exercises have been added to the end of each chapter to provide students an engaging opportunity to assess their skills in:
  - spelling
  - building medical terms
  - using abbreviations
  - defining medical terms
  - understanding true-to-life scenarios
  - labeling drawings of human anatomy

Organization of the Book

Introductory Chapters

Chapter 1 contains information necessary for an understanding of how medical terms are formed. This includes learning about word roots, combining forms, prefixes, and suffixes, and general rules for building medical terms. Readers will learn about terminology for medical records, the different healthcare settings, and about Pharmacology and the elements of a prescription. Chapter 2 presents terminology relating to the body organization, including organs and body systems. Here readers will first encounter word-building tables, a feature found in each remaining chapter that lists medical terms and their respective word parts. Chapter 2 also includes a discussion about the routes used to introduce drugs into the body.

Body Systems Chapters

Chapters 3–13 are organized by body system. Each chapter begins with the System At a Glance feature, which lists combining forms, prefixes, and/or suffixes with their meanings and is followed by a System Illustrated overview of the organs in the system. The anatomy and physiology section is divided into the various components of the system, and each subsection begins with a list of key medical terms accompanied by a phonetic pronunciation guide. Key terms are boldfaced the first time they appear in the narrative for easy recognition. The Terminology section of each chapter begins with a list of all word parts used within the chapter. For ease of learning, the medical terms are divided into five separate sections: adjective forms of anatomical terms, pathology, diagnostic procedures, therapeutic procedures, and pharmacology. The word parts used to build terms are highlighted within each table. An abbreviations section then follows to complete each chapter.

Appendices

The appendices contain helpful reference lists of word parts and definitions provided in the text. This information is intended for quick access and includes three appendices: Word Parts Arranged Alphabetically and Defined, Word Parts Arranged Alphabetically by Definition, and Abbreviations.

Answer Keys

A comprehensive listing of answers is provided in the back of the book for all of the Practice As You Go exercises, as well as the Chapter Review section's Real-World Applications activities, Practice Exercises, and Labeling Exercises. Students should use these answer keys to check their answers as they complete each chapter to better assess any areas that may need additional study.

Glossary/Index

Lastly, all of the key terms in the book appear again in the combination glossary/index at the end of the text. In addition to providing a page reference for each entry, complete definitions of key terms are also presented for quick access.

About the Authors

Bonnie F. Fremgen

Bonnie F. Fremgen, PhD, is a former Associate Dean of the Allied Health Program at Robert Morris College and was vice president of a hospital in suburban Chicago. She was also director of continuing education at three Chicago area hospitals. She has taught medical law and ethics courses as well as clinical and administrative topics. In addition, Dr. Fremgen has served as an advisor for students' career planning. She has broad interests and experiences in the healthcare field, including hospitals, nursing homes, and physicians' offices as well as responsibility for departments of social services, home health care, discharge planning, quality assurance, and hospital-wide education. She currently has two patents on a unique circulation-assisting wheelchair.

Dr. Fremgen holds a nursing degree as well as a master's in healthcare administration. She received her PhD from the College of Education at the University of Illinois. Dr. Fremgen has performed postdoctoral studies in Medical Law at Loyola University Law School in Chicago. She has authored five textbooks with Pearson. Dr. Fremgen has also taught ethics at the University of Notre Dame, South Bend, Indiana; University of Detroit, Detroit, Michigan; and Saint Xavier University, Chicago, Illinois.

Suzanne S. Frucht

Suzanne S. Frucht is an Associate Professor Emeritus of Anatomy and Physiology at Northwest Missouri State University (NWMSU). She holds baccalaureate degrees in biological sciences and physical therapy from Indiana University, an MS in biological sciences at NWMSU, and a PhD in molecular biology and biochemistry from the University of Missouri–Kansas City.

For 14 years Dr. Frucht worked full time as a physical therapist in various healthcare settings, including acute care hospitals, extended care facilities, and home health. Based on her educational and clinical experience she was invited to teach medical terminology part time in 1988 and became a full-time faculty member three years later as she discovered her love for the challenge of teaching. Dr. Frucht has taught a variety of courses including medical terminology, human anatomy, human physiology, and animal anatomy and physiology. She received the Governor's Award for Excellence in Teaching in 2003. After retiring from teaching in 2008, she continues to be active in student learning through teaching medical terminology as an online course and writing medical terminology texts and anatomy and physiology laboratory manuals.

About the Illustrators

Marcelo Oliver is president and founder of Body Scientific International LLC. He holds an MFA degree in Medical and Biological Illustration from the University of Michigan. For the past 15 years, his passion has been to condense complex anatomical information into visual education tools for students, patients, and medical professionals. For seven years Oliver worked as a medical illustrator and creative director developing anatomical charts used for student and patient education. In the years that followed, he created educational and marketing tools for medical device companies prior to founding Body Scientific International, LLC.

Body Scientific's lead artists in this publication were medical illustrators Liana Bauman and Katie Burgess. Both hold a Master of Science degree in Biomedical Visualization from the University of Illinois at Chicago. Their contribution to the publication was key in the creation and editing of artwork throughout.

Our Development Team

We would like to express deep gratitude to the over 120 colleagues from schools across the country who have provided us with many hours of their time over the years to help us tailor this book to suit the dynamic needs of instructors and students. These individuals have reviewed manuscript chapters and illustrations for content, accuracy, level, and utility. We sincerely thank them and feel that *Medical Terminology: A Living Language* has benefited immeasurably from their efforts, insights, encouragement, and selfless willingness to share their expertise as educators.

Reviewers of the Seventh Edition

Pamela A. Dobbins, MS
Shelton State Community
College
Natural Sciences-Biology
Tuscaloosa, Alabama

**Pamela J. Edwards, MA,
CCMA, CBCS, NRCMA**
Lone Star College System
Business and Social Sciences
Division
Conroe, Texas

Gerry Gordon, BA, CPC, CPB
Daytona College
Medical Billing and Coding,
Adjunct Faculty
Ormond Beach, Florida

Marleshia D. Hall, PhD
Shelton State Community
College
Department of Natural
Sciences
Tuscaloosa, Alabama

Timothy J. Jones, BA, MA
Oklahoma City Community
College
Health Professions
Oklahoma City, Oklahoma

Tammie Petersen RNC-OB, BSN
Austin Community College
Health Sciences
Austin, Texas

Amy Bolinger Snow, MS
Greenville Technical College
Biological Sciences
Department
Greenville, South Carolina

Reviewers of Earlier Editions

Yvonne Alles, MBA, RMT
Davenport University
Grand Rapids, Michigan

**Rachael C. Alstatter, Program
Director**
Southern Ohio College
Fairfield, Ohio

Steve Arinder, BS, MPH
Meridian Community College
Meridian, Mississippi

K. William Avery, BSMT, JD, PhD
City College
Gainesville, Florida

Beverly A. Baker, DA, CST
Western Iowa Technical
Community College
Sioux City, Iowa

Michael Battaglia, MS
Greenville Technical College
Taylors, South Carolina

**Nancy Ridinger Bean, Health
Assistant Instructor**
Wythe County Vocational School
Wytheville, Virginia

Deborah J. Bedford, CMA, AAS
North Seattle Community
College
Seattle, Washington

Barbara J Behrens, PTA, MS
Mercer County Community
College
Trenton, New Jersey

Pam Besser, PhD
Jefferson Community and
Technical College
Louisville, Kentucky

Norma J. Bird, MEd, BS, CMA
Idaho State University College
of Technology
Pocatello, Idaho

Trina Blaschko, RHIT
Chippewa Valley Technical
College
Eau Claire, Wisconsin

Richard T. Boan, PhD
Midlands Technical College
Columbia, South Carolina

**Susan W. Boggs, RN, BSN,
CNOR**
Piedmont Technical College
Greenwood, South Carolina

Bradley S. Bowden, PhD
Alfred University
Alfred, New York

Jeannie Bower, BS, NRCAMA
Central Penn College
Summerdale, Pennsylvania

Joan Walker Brittingham
Sussex Tech Adult Division
Georgetown, Delaware

**Phyills J. Broughton,
Curriculum Coordinator**
Pitt Community College
Greenville, North Carolina

Barbara Bussard, Instructor
Southwestern Michigan College
Dowagiac, Michigan

Toni Cade, MBA, RHIA, CCS
University of Louisiana at
Lafayette
Lafayette, Louisiana

Nicole Claussen, MS, CST, FAST
Rolla Technical Institute
Rolla, Missouri

Gloria H. Coats, RN, MSN
Modesto Junior College
Modesto, California

Linda A. Costarella, ND
Lake Washington Institute of
Technology
Kirkland, Washington

Lyndal M. Curry, MA, RP
University of South Alabama
Mobile, Alabama

Nancy Dancs, PT
Waukesha County Technical
College
Pewaukee, Wisconsin

**Theresa H. deBeche, RN, MN,
CNS**
Louisiana State University at
Eunice
Eunice, Louisiana

Bonnie Deister, MS, BSN, CMA-C
Broome Community College
Binghamton, New York

**Antoinette Deshaies, RN,
BSPA**
Glendale Community College
Glendale, Arizona

Pamela Dobbins, MS, BS, AAS
Shelton State Community
College
Tuscaloosa, Alabama

Carole DuBose, LPN, CST
Choffin School of Surgical
Technology
Youngstown, Ohio

Carol Eckert, RN, MSN
Southwestern Illinois College
Belleville, Illinois

**Pamela Edwards, MA,
NRCMA**
Lone Star College System
The Woodlands, Texas

Jamie Erskine, PhD, RD
University of Northern Colorado
Greeley, Colorado

Robert Fanger, MS
Del Mar College
Corpus Christi, Texas

**Mildred K. Fuller, PhD, MT
(ASCP), CLS(NCA)**
Norfolk State University
Norfolk, Virginia

Deborah Galanski-Maciak
Davenport University
Grand Rapids, Michigan

Debra Getting, Practical
Nursing Instructor
Northwest Iowa Community
College
Sheldon, Iowa

Ann Queen Giles, MHS, CMA
Western Piedmont Community
College
Morganton, North Carolina

Brenda L. Gleason, MSN
Iowa Central Community
College
Fort Dodge, Iowa

Steven B. Goldschmidt, DC,
CCFC
North Hennepin Community
College
Brooklyn Park, Minnesota

Linda S. Gott, RN, MS
Pensacola High School
Pensacola, Florida

Martha Grove, Staff Educator
Mercy Regional Health System
Cincinnati, Ohio

Kathryn Gruber
Globe College
Oakdale, Minnesota

Karen R. Hardney, MSEd
Chicago State University
Chicago, Illinois

Mary Hartman, MS, OTR/L
Genesee Community College
Batavia, New York

Joyce B. Harvey, PhD, RHIA
Norfolk State University
Norfolk, Virginia

Beulah A. Hofmann, RN, BSN,
MSN, CMA
Ivy Tech Community College of
Indiana
Greencastle, Indiana

Kimberley Hontz, RN
Antonelli Medical and
Professional Institute
Pottstown, Pennsylvania

Dolly Horton, CMA (AAMA), EdD
Asheville Buncombe Technical
Community College
Asheville, North Carolina

Pamela S. Huber, MS, MT
(ASCP)
Erie Community College
Williamsville, New York

Eva I. Irwin
Ivy Tech State College
Indianapolis, Indiana

Susan Jackson, EdS
Valdosta Technical College
Valdosta, Georgia

Mark Jaffe, DPM, MHSA
Nova Southeastern University
Ft. Lauderdale, Florida

Carol Lee Jarrell, MLT, AHI
Brown Mackie College
Merrillville, Indiana

Holly Jodon, MPAS, PA-C
Gannon University
Erie, Pennsylvania

Virginia J. Johnson, CMA
Lakeland Academy
Minneapolis, Minnesota

Marcie C. Jones, BS, CMA
Gwinnett Technical Institute
Lawrenceville, Georgia

Robin Jones, RHIA
Meridian Community College
Meridian, Mississippi

Rebecca Keith, PT, MSHS
Arkansas State University
Jonesboro, Arkansas

Gertrude A. Kenny, BSN, RN,
CMA
Baker College of Muskegon
Muskegon, Michigan

Dianne K. Kuiti, RN
Duluth Business University
Duluth, Minnesota

Andrew La Marca, EMT-P
Mobile Life Support Services
Middletown, New York

Francesca L. Langlow, BS
Delgado Community College
New Orleans, Louisiana

Julie A. Leu, CPC
Creighton University
Omaha, Nebraska

Norma Longoria, BS, COI
South Texas Community
College
McAllen, Texas

Jeanne W. Lovelock, RN, MSN
Piedmont Virginia Community
College
Charlottesville, Virginia

Jan Martin, RT(R)
Ogeechee Tech College
Statesboro, Georgia

Leslie M. Mazzola, MA
Cuyahoga Community College
Parma, Ohio

Michelle C. McCranie, CPhT
Ogeechee Technical College
Statesboro, Georgia

Lola McGourty, MSN, RN
Bossier Parish Community
College
Bossier City, Louisiana

Patricia Moody, RN
Athens Technical College
Athens, Georgia

Bridgit R. Moore, EdD, MT
(ASCP), CPC
McLennan Community
College
Waco, Texas

Christine J. Moore, MEd
Armstrong Atlantic State
University
Savannah, Georgia

Catherine Moran, PhD
Breyer State University
Birmingham, Alabama

Connie Morgan
Ivy Tech State College
Kokomo, Indiana

Katrina B. Myricks
Holmes Community College
Ridgeland, Mississippi

Pam Ncu, CMA
International Business College
Fort Wayne, Indiana

Judy Ortiz MHS, MS, PA-C
Pacific University
Hillsboro, Oregon

Tina M. Peer, BSN, RN
College of Southern Idaho
Twin Falls, ID

Dave Peruski, RN, MSA,
MSN
Delta College
University Center, Michigan

Lisa J. Pierce, MSA, RRT
Augusta Technical College
Augusta, Georgia

Sister Marguerite Polcyn, OSF,
PhD
Lourdes College
Sylvania, Ohio

Vicki Prater, CMA, RMA,
RAHA
Concorde Career Institute
San Bernardino, California

Carolyn Ragsdale CST, BS
Parkland College
Champaign, Illinois

LuAnn Reicks, RNC, BS, MSN
Iowa Central Community
College
Fort Dodge, Iowa

Linda Reigel
Glenville State College
Glenville, West Virginia

Shiela Rojas, MBA
Santa Barbara Business College
Santa Barbara, California

Ellen Rosen, RN, MN
Glendale Community College
Glendale, California

Georgette Rosenfeld, PhD,
RRT, RN
Indian River State College
Fort Pierce, Florida

Brian L. Rutledge, MHSA
Hinds Community College
Jackson, Mississippi

Sue Shibley, MEd, CMT,
CCS-P, CPC
North Idaho College
Coeur d'Alene, Idaho

Misty Shuler, RHIA
Asheville Buncombe Technical
Community College
Asheville, North Carolina

Patricia A. Slachta, PhD, RN,
ACNS-BC, CWOCN
Technical College of the
Lowcountry
Beaufort, South Carolina

Donna J. Slovensky, PhD,
RHIA, FAHIMA
University of Alabama at
Birmingham
Birmingham, Alabama

Connie Smith, RPh
University of Louisiana at
Monroe School of Pharmacy
Monroe, Louisiana

Karen Snipe, CPhT, ASBA,
MAEd
Trident Technical College
Charleston, South Carolina

Janet Stehling, RHIA
McLennan College
Lorena, Texas

Karen Stenback, MFA, CHHC
Antelope Valley College
Lancaster, California

Donna Stern
University of California San
Diego
La Jolla, California

Jodi Taylor, AAS, LPN, RMA
Terra State Community College
Fremont, Ohio

Annmary Thomas, MEd, NREMT-P
Community College of Philadelphia
Philadelphia, Pennsylvania

Lenette Thompson, CST, AS
Piedmont Technical College
Greenwood, South Carolina

Scott Throneberry, BS, NREMTP
Calhoun Community College
Decatur, Alabama

Maureen Tubbiola, MS, PhD
St. Cloud State University
St. Cloud, Minnesota

Marilyn Turner, RN, CMA
Ogeechee Technical College
Statesboro, Georgia

Marianne Van Deursen, MS, Ed, CMA (AAMA), MLT
Warren County Community College
Washington, New Jersey

Joan Ann Verderame, RN, MA
Bergen Community College
Paramus, New Jersey

Twila Wallace, MEd
Central Community College
Columbus, Nebraska

Kathy Wallington
Phillips Junior College
Campbell, California

Linda Walter, RN, MSN
Northwestern Michigan College
Traverse City, Michigan

Jean Watson, PhD
Clark College
Vancouver, Washington

Twila Weiszbrod, MPA
College of the Sequoias
Visalia, California

Sara J. Wellman, RHIT
Indiana University Northwest
Gary, Indiana

Leesa Whicker, BA, CMA
Central Piedmont Community College
Charlotte, NC

Lynn C. Wimett, RN, ANP, EdD
Regis University
Denver, Colorado

Kathy Zaiken, PharmD
Massachusetts College of Pharmacy and Health Sciences
Boston, Massachusetts

Judith Zappala, MT, ASCP, MBA
Middlesex Community College
Lowell, Massachusetts

Carole A. Zeglin, MSEd, BS, MT, RMA (AMT)
Westmoreland County Community College
Youngwood, Pennsylvania

A Commitment to Accuracy

As a student embarking on a career in healthcare you probably already know how critically important it is to be precise in your work. Patients and coworkers will be counting on you to avoid errors on a daily basis. Likewise, we owe it to you—the reader—to ensure accuracy in this book. We have gone to great lengths to verify that the information provided in *Medical Terminology: A Living Language* is complete and correct. To this end, here are the steps we have taken:

1. **Editorial Review**—We have assembled a large team of developmental consultants (listed on the preceding pages) to critique every word and every image in this book. Multiple content experts have read each chapter for accuracy.

2. **Medical Illustrations**—A team of medically trained illustrators was hired to prepare many of the pieces of art that grace the pages of this book. These illustrators have a higher level of scientific education than the artists for most textbooks, and they worked directly with the authors and members of our development team to make sure that their work was clear, correct, and consistent with what is described in the text.

3. **Accurate Ancillaries**—Realizing that the teaching and learning ancillaries are often as vital to instruction as the book itself, we took extra steps to ensure accuracy and consistency within these components. We assigned some members of our development team to specifically focus on critiquing every bit of content that comprises the instructional ancillary resources to confirm accuracy.

While our intent and actions have been directed at creating an error-free text, we have established a process for correcting any mistakes that may have slipped past our editors. Pearson takes this issue seriously and therefore welcomes any and all feedback that you can provide along the lines of helping us enhance the accuracy of this text. If you identify any errors that need to be corrected in a subsequent printing, please notify us. Thank you for helping Pearson to reach its goal of providing the most accurate medical terminology textbooks available. Any corrections can be sent to us through your institution's Pearson representative or please mail them to:

Pearson Health Science Editorial
Medical Terminology Corrections
211 River Street
4th Floor
Hoboken, NJ 07030

Contents

1 Introduction to Medical Terminology 1

2 Body Organization 25

3 Integumentary System 55

10 Reproductive System 345

11 Endocrine System 393

Chapter 1

Introduction to Medical Terminology

 Learning Objectives

Upon completion of this chapter, you will be able to

1. Discuss the four parts of medical terms.
2. Recognize word roots and combining forms.
3. Identify the most common prefixes and suffixes.
4. Define word building and describe a strategy for translating medical terms.
5. State the importance of correct spelling of medical terms.
6. State the rules for determining singular and plural endings.
7. Discuss the importance of using caution with abbreviations.
8. Recognize the documents found in a medical record.
9. Recognize the different healthcare settings.
10. Understand the importance of confidentiality.
11. Describe how drugs are named and classified.
12. Read and understand all abbreviations and notations in a written prescription.

(Pearson Education, Inc.)

MEDICAL TERMINOLOGY

AT A GLANCE

Learning medical terminology can initially seem like studying a strange new language. However, once you understand some of the basic rules about how medical terms are formed using word building, it will become much like piecing together a puzzle. This chapter discusses the general guidelines for forming words; an understanding of word roots, combining forms, prefixes, and suffixes; pronunciation; and spelling. Chapter 2 introduces you to terms that are used to describe the body as a whole. Chapters 3–13 each focus on a specific body system and present new combining forms, prefixes, and suffixes, as well as exercises to help you gain experience building new medical terms. Additionally, sprinkled throughout all chapters are "Med Term Tips" to assist in clarifying some of the material, "Word Watch" boxes to point out terms that may be particularly confusing, and "What's In A Name?" boxes to highlight the word parts found in the text. Key terms (with their pronunciations) are listed at the beginning of the section in which they are discussed, and each chapter contains numerous pathological, diagnostic, treatment, and surgical terms. Use these lists as an additional study tool for pre-viewing and reviewing terms.

Understanding medical terms requires being able to put words together or build words from their parts. It is impossible to memorize thousands of medical terms; however, once you understand the basics, you can distinguish the meaning of medical terms by analyzing their prefixes, suffixes, and word roots. Remember that there will always be some exceptions to every rule, and medical terminology is no different. We attempt to point out these exceptions where they exist. Most medical terms, however, do follow the general rule that there is a **word root** (indicated by a red color) or fundamental meaning for the word, a **prefix** (indicated by a gold color) and a **suffix** (indicated by a blue color) that modify the meaning of the word root, and sometimes a **combining vowel** to connect other word parts. You will be amazed at the seemingly difficult words you will be able to build and understand when you follow the simple steps in word building (see Figure 1-1 ■).

■ **Figure 1-1** Nurse completing a patient report. Healthcare workers use medical terminology in order to accurately and efficiently communicate patient information to each other.
(Monkey Business Images/Shutterstock)

Building Medical Terms From Word Parts

Med Term Tip
Medical terms are built from word parts:

Word Part	Example (Meaning)
Word root	**cardi** *(heart)*
Prefix	**peri-** *(around)*
Suffix	**-itis** *(inflammation)*

When these components are put together, the word *pericarditis* is formed, meaning *inflammation around the heart.*

Four different word parts or elements can be used to construct medical terms:

1. The **word root** is the foundation of the word.

   cardi ogram = *record of the heart*

2. A **prefix** is at the beginning of the word.

   peri cardium = *around the heart*

3. A **suffix** is at the end of the word.

   card **itis** = *inflammation of the heart*

4. The **combining vowel** is a vowel (usually *o*) that links the word root to another word root or a suffix.

   cardi **o** my **o** pathy = *disease of the heart muscle*

The following sections on word roots, combining vowels and forms, prefixes, and suffixes consider each of these word parts in more detail and present examples of some of those most commonly used.

PRACTICE AS YOU GO

A. Complete the Statement

1. The four components of a medical term are _____, _____, _____, and _____.

2. The combination of a word root and the combining vowel is called a(n) _____.

3. The vowel that connects two word roots or a suffix with a word root is usually a(n) _____.

4. A word part used at the end of a word root to change the meaning of the word is called a(n) _____.

5. A(n) _____ is used at the beginning of a word to indicate number, location, or time.

Word Roots

The word root is the foundation of a medical term and provides the general meaning of the word. The word root often indicates the body system or part of the body being discussed, such as **cardi** for *heart*. At other times, the word root may be an action. For example, the word root **cis** means *to cut* (as in incision).

A term may have more than one word root. For example, **osteoarthritis** (oss-tee-oh-ar-THRY-tis) combines the word root **oste** meaning *bone* and **arthr** meaning *joint*. When the suffix **-itis**, meaning *inflammation,* is added, we have the entire word, meaning an *inflammation involving bone at a joint.*

Combining Vowel/Form

A combining vowel makes it possible to pronounce long medical terms with ease and to combine several word parts. This is most often the vowel *o*. Combining vowels are utilized in two places: between a word root and a suffix or between two word roots.

To decide whether or not to use a combining vowel between a word root and a suffix, first look at the suffix. If it begins with a vowel, do not use the combining vowel. If, however, the suffix begins with a consonant, then use a combining vowel. For example: To combine **arthr** with **-scope** will require a combining vowel: **arthroscope** (AR-throh-skohp). But to combine **arthr** with **-itis** does not require a combining vowel: **arthritis** (ar-THRY-tis).

The combining vowel is typically kept between two word roots, even if the second word root begins with a vowel. For example, in forming the term **gastroenteritis** (gas-troh-en-ter-EYE-tis), the combining vowel is kept between the two word roots **gastr** and **enter** (gastrenteritis is incorrect). As you can tell from pronouncing these two terms, the combining vowel makes the pronunciation easier.

When writing a word root by itself, its **combining form** is typically used. This consists of the word root and its combining vowel written in a word root/vowel form, for example, **cardi/o.** Since it is often simpler to pronounce word roots when they appear in their combining form, this format is used throughout this book.

Common Combining Forms

What follows are some commonly used word roots in their combining form, their meaning, and examples of their use. Review the examples to observe when a combining vowel was kept and when it was dropped according to the rules presented above.

COMBINING FORM	MEANING	EXAMPLE (DEFINITION)
bi/o	life	biology (study of life)
carcin/o	cancer	carcinoma (cancerous tumor)
cardi/o	heart	cardiac (pertaining to the heart)
chem/o	chemical	chemotherapy (treatment with chemicals)
cis/o	to cut	incision (process of cutting into)
dermat/o	skin	dermatology (study of the skin)
enter/o	small intestine	enteric (pertaining to the small intestine)
gastr/o	stomach	gastric (pertaining to the stomach)
gynec/o	female	gynecology (study of females)
hemat/o	blood	hematic (pertaining to the blood)
immun/o	protection	immunology (study of protection)
laryng/o	larynx	laryngeal (pertaining to the voice box)
nephr/o	kidney	nephromegaly (enlarged kidney)
neur/o	nerve	neural (pertaining to a nerve)
ophthalm/o	eye	ophthalmic (pertaining to the eye)
ot/o	ear	otic (pertaining to the ear)
path/o	disease	pathology (study of disease)
pulmon/o	lung	pulmonary (pertaining to the lungs)
rhin/o	nose	rhinoplasty (surgical repair of the nose)

Med Term Tip

Remember to break down every word into its components (prefix, word root/combining form, and suffix) when learning medical terminology. Do not try to memorize every medical term. Instead, figure out how the word is formed from its components. In a short time you will be able to do this automatically when seeing a new term.

PRACTICE AS YOU GO

B. Name That Term

Use the suffix **-logy** to write a term for each medical specialty.

1. heart   _____

2. stomach   _____

3. skin   _____

4. eye   _____

5. immunity _____

6. kidney   _____

7. blood   _____

8. female   _____

9. nerve   _____

10. disease   _____

Prefixes

Adding a prefix to the front of a term forms a new medical word. Prefixes frequently provide information about the location of an organ, the number of parts, or time (frequency). For example, the prefix **bi-** stands for two of something, such as **bilateral** (bye-LAT-er-al), meaning *to have two sides*. However, not every term will have a prefix.

Common Prefixes

What follows are some of the more common prefixes, their meanings, and examples of their use. When written by themselves, prefixes are followed by a hyphen.

PREFIX	MEANING	EXAMPLE (DEFINITION)
a-	without	aphasia (without speech)
an-	without	anoxia (without oxygen)
anti-	against	antibiotic (against life)
auto-	self	autograft (a graft from one's own body)
brady-	slow	bradycardia (slow heartbeat)
de-	without	depigmentation (without pigment)
dys-	painful; difficult; abnormal	dysuria (painful urination); dyspnea (difficulty breathing); dystrophy (abnormal development)

PREFIX	MEANING	EXAMPLE (DEFINITION)
endo-	within; inner	endoscope (instrument to view within); endocardium (inner lining of heart)
epi-	above	epigastric (above the stomach)
eu-	normal	eupnea (normal breathing)
ex-	outward	exostosis (condition of outward, or projecting, bone)
extra-	outside of	extracorporeal (outside of the body)
hetero-	different	heterograft (graft [like a skin graft] from another species)
homo-	same	homograft (graft [like a skin graft] from the same species)
hyper-	excessive	hypertrophy (excessive development)
hypo-	below; insufficient	hypodermic (below the skin); hypoglycemia (insufficient blood sugar)
in-	not; inward	infertility (not fertile); inhalation (to breathe in)
inter-	between	intervertebral (between the vertebrae)
intra-	within	intravenous (within a vein)
macro-	large	macrotia (having large ears)
micro-	small	microtia (having small ears)
neo-	new	neonatology (study of the newborn)
para-	beside; abnormal; two like parts of a pair	paranasal (beside the nose); paresthesia (abnormal sensation); paraplegia (paralysis of two like parts of a pair [the legs])
per-	through	percutaneous (through the skin)
peri-	around	pericardial (around the heart)
post-	after	postpartum (after birth)
pre-	before	preoperative (before a surgical operation)
pro-	before	prolactin (before milk)
pseudo-	false	pseudocyesis (false pregnancy)
re-	again	reinfection (to infect again)
retro-	backward; behind	retrograde (to move backward); retroperitoneal (behind the peritoneum)
sub-	under	subcutaneous (under the skin)
tachy-	fast	tachycardia (fast heartbeat)
trans-	across	transurethral (across the urethra)
ultra-	beyond	ultrasound (beyond sound [high-frequency sound waves])
un-	not	unconscious (not conscious)

Word Watch

Be extremely careful with prefixes; many have similar spellings but very different meanings. For example:
inter- means *between;* intra- means *inside*
per- means *through;* peri- means *around*
re- means *again;* retro- means *behind*

Number Prefixes

What follows are some common prefixes pertaining to the number of items or measurement, their meanings, and examples of their use.

PREFIX	MEANING	EXAMPLE (DEFINITION)
bi-	two	bilateral (two sides)
hemi-	half	hemiplegia (paralysis of one side/half of the body)
mono-	one	monoplegia (paralysis of one extremity)
multi-	many	multigravida (woman with many [two or more] pregnancies)
nulli-	none	nulligravida (woman with no pregnancies)
pan-	all	pansinusitis (inflammation of all the sinuses)
poly-	many	polymyositis (inflammation of many muscles)
quadri-	four	quadriplegia (paralysis of all four limbs)
semi-	partial	semiconscious (partially conscious)
tetra-	four	tetraplegia (paralysis of all four limbs)
tri-	three	triceps (muscle with three heads)

PRACTICE AS YOU GO

C. Prefix Practice

Circle the prefixes in the following terms and then define them in the spaces provided.

1. tachycardia _____

2. pseudocyesis _____

3. hypoglycemia _____

4. intercostal _____

5. eupnea _____

6. postoperative _____

7. monoplegia _____

8. subcutaneous _____

Suffixes

A suffix is attached to the end of a word to add meaning, such as a condition, disease, or procedure. For example, the suffix **-itis**, meaning *inflammation,* when added to **cardi** forms the new word **carditis** (kar-DYE-tis), meaning *inflammation of the heart.* Every medical term *must* have a suffix. Most often the suffix is added to a word root, as in carditis above; however, terms can also be built from a suffix added directly to a prefix, without a word root. For example, the term **dystrophy** (DIS-troh-fee), meaning *abnormal development*, is built from the prefix **dys-** (meaning *abnormal*) and the suffix **-trophy** (meaning *development*).

Common Suffixes

What follows are some common suffixes, their meanings, and examples of their use. When written by themselves, suffixes are preceded by a hyphen.

SUFFIX	MEANING	EXAMPLE (DEFINITION)
-algia	pain	gastralgia (stomach pain)
-cele	protrusion	cystocele (protrusion of the bladder)
-cyte	cell	erythrocyte (red cell)
-dynia	pain	cardiodynia (heart pain)
-ectasis	dilation	bronchiectasis (dilated bronchi)
-gen	that which produces	pathogen (that which produces disease)
-genic	producing	carcinogenic (cancer producing)
-ia	condition	bradycardia (condition of slow heart)
-iasis	abnormal condition	lithiasis (abnormal condition of stones)
-ism	state of	hypothyroidism (state of low thyroid)
-itis	inflammation	dermatitis (inflammation of skin)
-logist	one who studies	cardiologist (one who studies the heart)
-logy	study of	cardiology (study of the heart)
-lytic	destruction	thrombolytic (clot destruction)
-malacia	abnormal softening	chondromalacia (abnormal cartilage softening)
-megaly	enlarged	cardiomegaly (enlarged heart)
-oma	tumor, mass	carcinoma (cancerous tumor)
		hematoma (mass of blood)
-opsy	view of	biopsy (view of life)
-osis	abnormal condition	cyanosis (abnormal condition of being blue)
-pathy	disease	myopathy (muscle disease)
-plasm	formation	neoplasm (new formation)
-plegia	paralysis	laryngoplegia (paralysis of larynx)
-ptosis	drooping	blepharoptosis (drooping eyelid)
-rrhage	abnormal flow	hemorrhage (abnormal flow of blood)
-rrhagia	abnormal flow condition	cystorrhagia (abnormal flow from the bladder)
-rrhea	discharge	rhinorrhea (discharge from the nose)
-rrhexis	rupture	hysterorrhexis (ruptured uterus)

SUFFIX	MEANING	EXAMPLE (DEFINITION)
-sclerosis	hardening	arteriosclerosis (hardening of an artery)
-stenosis	narrowing	angiostenosis (narrowing of a vessel)
-therapy	treatment	chemotherapy (treatment with chemicals)
-trophy	development	hypertrophy (excessive development)

Adjective Suffixes

The following suffixes are used to convert a word root into an adjective. Each of these suffixes is usually translated as *pertaining to*.

SUFFIX	MEANING	EXAMPLE (DEFINITION)
-ac	pertaining to	cardiac (pertaining to the heart)
-al	pertaining to	duodenal (pertaining to the duodenum)
-an	pertaining to	ovarian (pertaining to the ovary)
-ar	pertaining to	ventricular (pertaining to a ventricle)
-ary	pertaining to	pulmonary (pertaining to the lungs)
-atic	pertaining to	lymphatic (pertaining to lymph)
-eal	pertaining to	esophageal (pertaining to the esophagus)
-iac	pertaining to	chondriac (pertaining to cartilage)
-ic	pertaining to	gastric (pertaining to the stomach)
-ical	pertaining to	chemical (pertaining to a chemical)
-ile	pertaining to	penile (pertaining to the penis)
-ine	pertaining to	uterine (pertaining to the uterus)
-ior	pertaining to	superior (pertaining to above)
-nic	pertaining to	embryonic (pertaining to an embryo)
-ory	pertaining to	auditory (pertaining to hearing)
-ose	pertaining to	adipose (pertaining to fat)
-ous	pertaining to	intravenous (pertaining to within a vein)
-tic	pertaining to	acoustic (pertaining to hearing)

Surgical Suffixes

The following suffixes indicate surgical procedures.

SUFFIX	MEANING	EXAMPLE (DEFINITION)
-centesis	puncture to withdraw fluid	arthrocentesis (puncture to withdraw fluid from a joint)
-ectomy	surgical removal	gastrectomy (surgical removal of the stomach)
-ostomy	surgically create an opening	colostomy (surgically create an opening for the colon [through the abdominal wall])
-otomy	cutting into	thoracotomy (cutting into the chest)

> **Med Term Tip**
>
> Surgical suffixes have very specific meanings:
> -otomy means *to cut into*
> -ostomy means *to surgically create an opening*
> -ectomy means *to cut out* or *remove*

SUFFIX	MEANING	EXAMPLE (DEFINITION)
-pexy	surgical fixation	nephropexy (surgical fixation of a kidney)
-plasty	surgical repair	dermatoplasty (surgical repair of the skin)
-rrhaphy	to suture	myorrhaphy (suture together muscle)
-tome	instrument to cut	dermatome (instrument to cut skin)

Procedural Suffixes

The following suffixes indicate procedural processes or instruments.

SUFFIX	MEANING	EXAMPLE (DEFINITION)
-gram	record	electrocardiogram (record of heart's electricity)
-graphy	process of recording	electrocardiography (process of recording the heart's electrical activity)
-meter	instrument for measuring	audiometer (instrument for measuring hearing)
-metry	process of measuring	audiometry (process of measuring hearing)
-scope	instrument for viewing	gastroscope (instrument for viewing stomach)
-scopic	pertaining to visually examining	endoscopic (pertaining to visually examining within)
-scopy	process of visually examining	gastroscopy (process of visually examining the stomach)

PRACTICE AS YOU GO

D. Combining Form and Suffix Practice

Join a combining form and a suffix to build words with the following meanings.

1. study of lungs _____

2. nose discharge _____

3. abnormal softening of a kidney _____

4. enlarged heart _____

5. cutting into the stomach _____

6. inflammation of the skin _____

7. surgical removal of the voice box _____

8. surgical repair of a joint _____

Word Building

Word building consists of putting together two or more word elements to form a variety of terms. Prefixes and suffixes may be added to a combining form to create a new descriptive term. For example, adding the prefix **hypo-** (meaning *below*) and the suffix **-ic** (meaning *pertaining to*) to the combining form **derm/o** (meaning *skin*) forms **hypodermic** (high-poh-DER-mik), which means *pertaining to below the skin*.

Interpreting Medical Terms

The following strategy is a reliable method for puzzling out the meaning of an unfamiliar medical term.

STEP	EXAMPLE
1. Divide the term into its word parts.	gastr/o/enter/o/logy
2. Define each word part.	**gastr** = stomach
	o = combining vowel, no meaning
	enter = small intestine
	o = combining vowel, no meaning
	-logy = study of
3. Combine the meaning of the word parts.	stomach, small intestine, study of

> **Med Term Tip**
>
> To gain a quick understanding of a term, it may be helpful to you to read from the end of the word (or the suffix) back to the beginning (the prefix), and then pick up the word root. For example, *pericarditis* reads inflammation (**-itis**) around (**peri-**) the heart (**cardi/o**).

Pronunciation

You may hear different pronunciations for the same terms depending on where a person was born or educated. As long as it is clear which term people are discussing, differing pronunciations are acceptable. Some people are difficult to understand over the telephone or on a transcription tape. If you have any doubt about a term being discussed, ask for the term to be spelled. For example, it is often difficult to hear the difference between the terms **abduction** and **adduction**. However, since the terms refer to opposite directions of movement, it is very important to double-check if there is any question about which term is being used.

Each new term in this book is introduced in boldface type, with the phonetic or "sounds like" pronunciation in parentheses immediately following. The part of the word that should receive the greatest emphasis during pronunciation appears in capital letters, for example, **pericarditis** (pair-ih-kar-DYE-tis). Each term presented in this book is also pronounced on the accompanying MyLab Medical Terminology website (*www.mymedicalterminologylab.com*). Listen to each word, then pronounce it silently to yourself or out loud.

Spelling

Although you may hear differing pronunciations of the same term, there is only one correct spelling. If you have any doubt about the spelling of a term or of its meaning, always look it up in a medical dictionary. If only one letter of the word is changed, it can make a critical difference for the patient. For example, imagine the problem that could arise if you note for insurance purposes that a portion of a patient's **ileum**, or small intestine, was removed when in reality he had surgery for removal of a piece of his **ilium**, or hipbone.

> **Med Term Tip**
>
> If you have any doubt about the meaning or spelling of a word, look it up in a medical dictionary. Even experienced medical personnel still need to look up a few words. It is never acceptable to "make up" your own spelling for a term.

Some words have the same beginning sounds but are spelled differently. Examples include:

Sounds like *si*

psy   **psychiatry** (sigh-KIGH-ah-tree)

cy   **cytology** (sigh-TALL-oh-jee)

Sounds like *dis*

dys   **dyspepsia** (dis-PEP-see-ah)

dis   **dislocation** (dis-loh-KAY-shun)

Singular and Plural Endings

Many medical terms originate from Greek and Latin words. The rules for forming the singular and plural forms of some words follow the rules of these languages rather than English. For example, the heart has a left atrium and a right atrium for a total of two *atria*, not two *atriums*. Other words, such as *virus* and *viruses*, are changed from singular to plural by following English rules. Each medical term needs to be considered individually when changing from the singular to the plural form. The following examples illustrate how terms that follow Greek and Latin rules are pluralized. Throughout the book, unusual or unexpected plural forms will be included with the term definition.

WORDS ENDING IN	SINGULAR	PLURAL
-a	vertebra	vertebrae
-ax	thorax	thoraces
-ex or -ix	appendix	appendices
-is	metastasis	metastases
	epididymis	epididymides
-ma	sarcoma	sarcomata
-nx	phalanx	phalanges
-on	ganglion	ganglia
-um	ovum	ova
-us	nucleus	nuclei
-y	biopsy	biopsies

PRACTICE AS YOU GO

E. Make It Plural

Change the following singular terms to plural terms.

1. metastasis _____

2. ovum _____

3. nucleus _____

4. phalanx _____

5. appendix _____

6. vertebra _____

Abbreviations

Abbreviations are commonly used in the medical profession as a way of saving time. However, some abbreviations can be confusing, such as *SM* for simple mastectomy and *sm* for small. Using incorrect abbreviations can result in problems for a patient, as well as with insurance records and processing. If you have any concern that you will confuse someone by using an abbreviation, spell out the word instead. It is never acceptable to use made-up abbreviations. All types of healthcare facilities will have a list of approved abbreviations, and it is extremely important that you become familiar with this list and follow it closely. Throughout this book abbreviations are included, when possible, immediately following terms. Additionally, a list of common abbreviations for each body system is provided in each chapter. Finally, Appendix III offers a complete alphabetical listing of all the abbreviations used in this text.

The Medical Record

The **medical record** or chart documents the details of a patient's hospital stay. Each healthcare professional that has contact with the patient in any capacity completes the appropriate report of that contact and adds it to the medical chart. This results in a permanent physical record of the patient's day-to-day condition, when and what services he or she received, and the response to treatment. Each institution adopts a specific format for each document and its location within the chart. This is necessary because each healthcare professional must be able to locate quickly and efficiently the information he or she needs in order to provide proper care for the patient. The medical record is also a legal document. Therefore, it is essential that all chart components be completely filled out and signed. Each page must contain the proper patient identification information: the patient's name, age, gender, physician, admission date, and identification number.

While the patient is still in the hospital, a unit clerk is usually responsible for placing documents in the proper place. After discharge, the medical records department ensures that all documents are present, complete, signed, and in the correct order. If a person is readmitted, especially for the same diagnosis, parts of this previous chart can be pulled and added to the current chart for reference (see Figure 1-2 ■). Physicians' offices and other outpatient care providers such as clinics and therapists also maintain a medical record detailing each patient's visit to their facility.

■ **Figure 1-2** Health information professionals maintain accurate, orderly, and permanent patient records. Medical records are stored securely and available for future reference. *(B. Franklin/Shutterstock)*

The digital revolution has also impacted healthcare with the increasing use of the **Electronic Medical Record** (EMR). A software program allows for entering of patient information via a computer or tablet, which then organizes and stores the data. Information is entered either at a centralized workstation or by using mobile devices at the point of care. Once digitally stored, the information may be analyzed and monitored to detect and prevent potential errors. Since the records are digitally stored, they can be accessed and shared between healthcare providers easily, which reduces unnecessary repetition of tests and inadvertent medication errors. Table 1-1 ■ includes the most common elements of a paper chart with a brief description.

■ **TABLE 1-1   Elements of the Medical Record**

Component	Description
History and Physical	Written or dictated by admitting physician; details patient's history, results of physician's examination, initial diagnoses, and physician's plan of treatment
Physician's Orders	Complete list of care, medications, tests, and treatments physician orders for patient
Nurse's Notes	Record of patient's care throughout the day; includes vital signs, treatment specifics, patient's response to treatment, and patient's condition
Physician's Progress Notes	Physician's daily record of patient's condition, results of physician's examinations, summary of test results, updated assessment and diagnoses, and further plans for patient's care
Consultation Reports	Reports given by specialists whom physician has asked to evaluate patient
Ancillary Reports	Reports from various treatments and therapies patient has received, such as rehabilitation, social services, or respiratory therapy
Diagnostic Reports	Results of diagnostic tests performed on patient, principally from clinical lab (e.g., blood tests) and medical imaging (e.g., X-rays and ultrasound)
Informed Consent	Document voluntarily signed by patient or a responsible party that clearly describes purpose, methods, procedures, benefits, and risks of a diagnostic or treatment procedure
Operative Report	Report from surgeon detailing an operation; includes pre- and postoperative diagnosis, specific details of surgical procedure itself, and how patient tolerated procedure
Anesthesiologist's Report	Relates details regarding substances (such as medications and fluids) given to patient, patient's response to anesthesia, and vital signs during surgery
Pathologist's Report	Report given by pathologist who studies tissue removed from patient (e.g., bone marrow, blood, or tissue biopsy)
Discharge Summary	Comprehensive outline of patient's entire hospital stay; includes condition at time of admission, admitting diagnosis, test results, treatments and patient's response, final diagnosis, and follow-up plans

PRACTICE AS YOU GO

F. Medical Records Matching

Match each definition to its medical record element.

_____ 1. physician's orders

_____ 2. discharge summary

_____ 3. ancillary reports

_____ 4. consultation reports

_____ 5. nurse's notes

a. written after patient care is completed

b. includes vital signs

c. lists medications to be given to patient

d. written by specialists

e. location of rehabilitation reports

Healthcare Settings

The use of medical terminology is widespread. It provides healthcare profession-als with a precise and efficient method of communicating very specific patient information to one another, regardless of whether they are in the same type of facility (see Figure 1-3 ■). See Table 1-2 ■ for descriptions of the different types of settings where medical terminology is used.

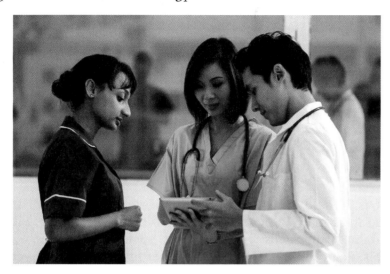

■ **Figure 1-3**   Medical team reviewing patient's medical record on a tablet. *(Stuart Jenner/ Shutterstock)*

■ **TABLE 1-2**   **Healthcare Settings**

Healthcare Setting	Description
Acute Care or General Hospitals	Provide services to diagnose (laboratory, diagnostic imaging) and treat (surgery, medications, therapy) diseases for a short period of time; in addition, they usually provide emergency and obstetrical care
Specialty Care Hospitals	Provide care for very specific types of diseases (e.g., psychiatric hospital)
Nursing Homes or Long-Term Care Facilities	Provide long-term care for patients needing extra time to recover from illness or injury before returning home or for persons who can no longer care for themselves
Ambulatory Care Centers, Surgical Centers, or Outpatient Clinics	Provide services not requiring overnight hospitalization; services range from simple surgeries to diagnostic testing or therapy
Physicians' Offices	Provide diagnostic and treatment services in a private office setting
Health Maintenance Organization (HMO)	Provides wide range of services by a group of primary-care physicians, specialists, and other healthcare professionals in a prepaid system
Home Health Care	Provides nursing, therapy, personal care, or housekeeping services in patient's own home
Rehabilitation Centers	Provide intensive physical and occupational therapy; includes inpatient and outpatient treatment
Hospices	Provide supportive treatment to terminally ill patients and their families

PRACTICE AS YOU GO

G. Healthcare Settings

Match each setting listed on the left with a setting listed on the right that provides similar services.

_____ **1.** long-term care facility   **a.** ambulatory care center

_____ **2.** outpatient clinic   **b.** general hospital

_____ **3.** acute care hospital   **c.** nursing home

Confidentiality

Anyone working with medical terminology and involved in the medical profession must have a firm understanding of confidentiality. Any information or record relating to a patient must be considered privileged. This means that there is a moral and legal responsibility to keep all information about the patient confidential. If there is a request to supply documentation relating to a patient, the proper authorization form must be signed by that patient. Give only the specific information that the patient has authorized. The Health Insurance Portability and Accountability Act of 1996 (HIPAA) set federal standards providing patients with more protection of their medical records and health information, better access to their own records, and greater control over how their health information is used and to whom it is disclosed.

Pharmacology

pharmacology (far-mah-KALL-oh-jee)

Pharmacology is the study of the origin, characteristics, and effects of drugs. Drugs are obtained from many different sources. Some drugs, such as vitamins, are found naturally in the foods we eat. Others, such as hormones, are obtained from animals. Penicillin and some of the other antibiotics are developed from mold, which is a fungus. Plants have long since been used for medicinal healing purposes and continue to be a source of many of today's modern medicines. Many drugs, such as those used in chemotherapy, are synthetic, meaning they are developed by artificial means in a laboratory.

Drug Names

brand name	**pharmaceutical** (far-mah-SOO-tih-kal)
chemical name	**pharmacist** (FAR-mah-sist)
generic name	proprietary name
nonproprietary name	(proh-PRYE-ah-tair-ee)
(non-proh-PRYE-ah-tair-ee)	**trademark**

All drugs are chemicals. The **chemical name** describes the chemical formula or molecular structure of a particular drug. For example, the chemical name for ibuprofen, an over-the-counter pain medication, is 2-*p*-isobutylphenyl propionic acid. Just as in this case, chemical names are usually very long, so a shorter name is given to the drug. This name is the **generic** or **nonproprietary name**, and it is recognized and accepted as the official name for a drug.

Each drug has only one generic name, such as ibuprofen, and this name is not subject to copyright protection, so any **pharmaceutical** manufacturer may use it. However, the pharmaceutical company that originally developed the drug has exclusive rights to produce it for 20 years. After that time, any manufacturer may produce and sell the drug. When a company manufactures a drug for sale, it must choose a **brand name**, or **proprietary name**, for its product. This is the company's **trademark** for the drug. For example, ibuprofen is known by several brand names, including Motrin™, Advil™, and Nuprin™. All three contain the same ibuprofen; they are just marketed by different pharmaceutical companies. (See Table 1-3 ■ for examples of different drug names.)

Generic drugs are usually priced lower than brand name drugs. A physician can indicate on a prescription if the **pharmacist** may substitute a generic drug for

■ **TABLE 1-3** Examples of Different Drug Names

Chemical Name	Generic Name	Brand Names
2-*p*-isobutylphenyl propionic acid	Ibuprofen	Motrin™
		Advil™
		Nuprin™
Acetylsalicylic acid	Aspirin	Anacin™
		Bufferin™
		Excedrin™
S-2-[1-(methylamino) ethyl] benzenemethanol hydrochloride	Pseudoephedrine hydrochloride	Sudafed™
		Actifed™
		Nucofed™

a brand name. The physician may prefer that a particular brand name drug be used if he or she believes it to be more effective than the generic drug.

Legal Classification of Drugs

controlled substances
Drug Enforcement Administration
over-the-counter drug

prescription (prih-SKRIP-shun)
prescription drug (prih-SKRIP-shun)

A **prescription drug** can only be ordered by licensed healthcare practitioners such as physicians, dentists, or physician assistants. These drugs must include the words "Caution: Federal law prohibits dispensing without prescription" on their labels. Antibiotics, such as penicillin, and heart medications, such as digoxin, are available only by prescription. A **prescription** is the written explanation to the pharmacist regarding the name of the medication, the dosage, and the times of administration. A licensed practitioner can also submit a prescription order electronically (if it is not a controlled substance) or orally to a pharmacist.

A drug that does not require a prescription is referred to as an **over-the-counter** (OTC) **drug**. Many medications or drugs can be purchased without a prescription, for example, aspirin, antacids, and antidiarrheal medications. However, taking aspirin along with an anticoagulant, such as coumadin, can cause internal bleeding in some people, and OTC antacids interfere with the absorption of the prescription drug tetracycline into the body. It is better for the physician or pharmacist to advise the patient on the proper OTC drugs to use with prescription drugs.

Certain drugs are classified as **controlled substances** if they have a potential for being addictive (habit forming) or can be abused. The **Drug Enforcement Administration** (DEA) enforces the control of these drugs. Some of the more commonly prescribed controlled substances are:

- butabarbital
- chloral hydrate
- codeine
- diazepam

- oxycontin
- morphine
- phenobarbital
- secobarbital

Controlled drugs are classified as Schedule I through Schedule V, indicating their potential for abuse with I being most addictive and V being the least addictive drugs. The differences between each schedule are listed in Table 1-4 ■.

Med Term Tip

It is critical that patients receive the correct drug, but it is not possible to list or remember all the drug names. You must acquire the habit of looking up any drug name you do not recognize in the *Physician's Desk Reference (PDR)*. Every medical office or medical facility should have either an electronic or hard copy of this book.

■ TABLE 1-4 Schedule for Controlled Substances

Classification	Meaning
Schedule I	Drugs with the highest potential for addiction and abuse; they are not accepted for medical use; examples are heroin and LSD
Schedule II	Drugs with a high potential for addiction and abuse accepted for medical use in the United States; examples are codeine, cocaine, morphine, opium, and secobarbital
Schedule III	Drugs with a moderate to low potential for addiction and abuse; examples are butabarbital, anabolic steroids, and acetaminophen with codeine
Schedule IV	Drugs with a lower potential for addiction and abuse than Schedule III drugs; examples are chloral hydrate, phenobarbital, and diazepam
Schedule V	Drugs with a low potential for addiction and abuse; an example is low-strength codeine combined with other drugs to suppress coughing

PRACTICE AS YOU GO

H. True or False

_____ **1.** The nonproprietary name is also called the generic name.

_____ **2.** A drug's chemical name is the company's trademark for its product.

_____ **3.** Controlled substances have a potential for being addictive.

_____ **4.** A drug may have many generic names, but only one brand name.

_____ **5.** OTC drugs do not require a prescription.

Med Term Tip

Many abbreviations have multiple meanings, such as od, which can mean overdose (od) or right eye (OD), depending on whether the letters are lowercase or uppercase. Care must be taken when reading abbreviations since some may be written too quickly, making them difficult to decipher. Never create your own abbreviations. When in doubt, confirm with the prescriber.

How to Read a Prescription

A prescription is not difficult to read once you understand the symbols that are used. Symbols and abbreviations based on Latin and Greek words are used to save time for the physician. For example, the abbreviation po, meaning *to be taken by mouth*, comes from the Latin term *per os*, which means *by mouth*.

See Figure 1-4 ■ for an example of a prescription. In this sample, the prescribed drug (Rx) is Tagamet (a medication to reduce stomach acid) in the 800 milligram (mg) size. The instructions on the label are to say (Sig) to take 1 (ī) by mouth (po) three times a day (tid). The pharmacist is to dispense (disp) 30 tablets (#30). The prescription concludes by informing the pharmacist to refill the prescription two times, and he or she may substitute with another medication. Each prescription must contain the date, physician's name, address, and Drug Enforcement Administration number as well as the patient's name and date of birth. The physician must also sign his or her name at the bottom of the prescription. A blank prescription cannot be handed to a patient.

The physician's instruction to the patient will be placed on the label. The pharmacist will also include instructions about the medication and alert the patient to side effects that may need to be reported to the physician. Additionally, any special instructions regarding the medication (i.e., take with meals, do not take along with dairy products, etc.) are supplied by the pharmacist.

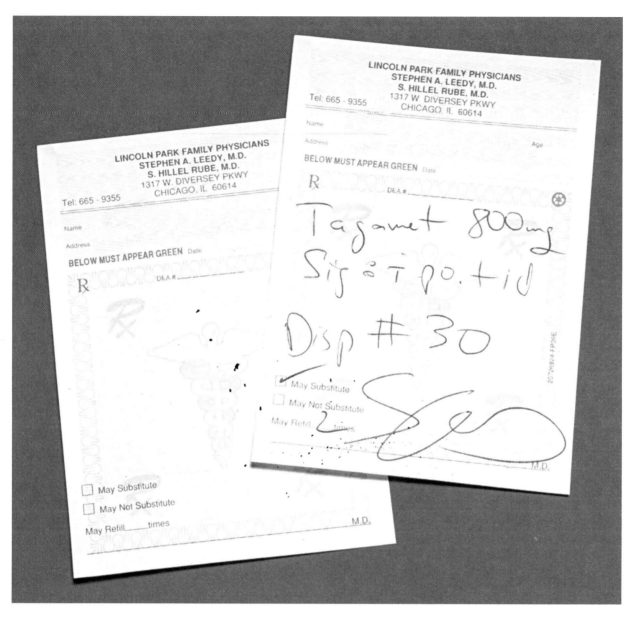

■ **Figure 1-4** A sample prescription written by a physician. *(Michal Heron/Pearson Education, Inc.)*

PRACTICE AS YOU GO

I. Prescription Abbreviation Matching

_____ **1.** milligram   **a.** disp

_____ **2.** by mouth   **b.** ī

_____ **3.** three times a day   **c.** Sig

_____ **4.** dispense   **d.** po

_____ **5.** label instructions   **e.** mg

_____ **6.** one   **f.** tid

Chapter Review

Practice Exercises

A. Terminology Matching

Match each definition to its term.

1. _____ Provides services for a short period of time
2. _____ Complete outline of a patient's entire hospital stay
3. _____ Describes purpose, methods, benefits, and risks of procedure
4. _____ Contains updated assessment, diagnoses, and further plans for care
5. _____ Provides supportive care to terminally ill patients and families
6. _____ Written by the admitting physician
7. _____ Reports results from study of tissue removed from the patient
8. _____ Written by the surgeon
9. _____ Provides services not requiring overnight hospital stay
10. _____ Report given by a specialist
11. _____ Record of a patient's care throughout the day
12. _____ Clinical lab and medical imaging reports
13. _____ Provides intensive physical and occupational therapy
14. _____ Report of treatment/therapy the patient received
15. _____ Provides care for patients who need more time to recover

a. rehabilitation center
b. nurse's notes
c. ancillary report
d. hospice
e. discharge summary
f. physician's progress notes
g. ambulatory care center
h. diagnostic report
i. long-term care facility
j. informed consent
k. history and physical
l. acute care hospital
m. pathologist's report
n. consultation report
o. operative report

B. Prefix Practice

The prefix has been underlined in each term below. Fill in the blank in the term's definition with the meaning of that prefix.

Term	Definition
1. <u>a</u>phasia	_____ speech
2. <u>brady</u>cardia	_____ heartbeat
3. <u>an</u>oxia	_____ oxygen
4. <u>eu</u>pnea	_____ breathing
5. <u>hyper</u>trophy	_____ development
6. <u>inter</u>vertebral	pertaining to _____ the vertebrae
7. <u>pre</u>operative	_____ an operation
8. <u>sub</u>cutaneous	pertaining to _____ the skin

Term	Definition
9. <u>un</u>conscious	_____ conscious
10. <u>poly</u>myositis	inflammation of _____ muscles
11. <u>intra</u>venous	pertaining to _____ a vein
12. <u>extra</u>corporeal	pertaining to _____ of the body
13. <u>bi</u>lateral	pertaining to _____ sides
14. <u>pan</u>sinusitis	inflammation of _____ the sinuses
15. <u>epi</u>gastric	pertaining to _____ the stomach
16. <u>anti</u>biotic	pertaining to _____ life
17. <u>tachy</u>cardia	_____ heartbeat
18. <u>hypo</u>glycemia	_____ blood sugar
19. <u>per</u>cutaneous	pertaining to _____ the skin
20. <u>peri</u>cardial	pertaining to _____ the heart

C. Suffix Practice

The suffix has been underlined in each term below. Fill in the blank in the term's definition with the meaning of that suffix.

Term	Definition
1. cardio<u>logy</u>	_____ the heart
2. laryngo<u>plegia</u>	_____ of the larynx
3. rhino<u>rrhea</u>	_____ from the nose
4. angio<u>stenosis</u>	_____ of a vessel
5. chemo<u>therapy</u>	_____ with chemicals
6. duoden<u>al</u>	_____ the duodenum
7. patho<u>gen</u>	_____ disease
8. thrombo<u>lytic</u>	clot _____
9. bi<u>opsy</u>	_____ life
10. gastr<u>ectomy</u>	_____ of the stomach
11. arterio<u>sclerosis</u>	_____ of an artery
12. uter<u>ine</u>	_____ the uterus
13. gastr<u>algia</u>	stomach _____
14. nephro<u>pexy</u>	_____ of a kidney
15. audio<u>metry</u>	_____ hearing
16. acous<u>tic</u>	_____ hearing
17. dermato<u>plasty</u>	_____ of the skin
18. thoraco<u>tomy</u>	_____ the chest
19. gastro<u>scope</u>	_____ the stomach
20. cardi<u>ac</u>	_____ the heart

D. Building Medical Terms

Build a medical term by combining the word parts requested in each question.

For example, use the combining form for *spleen* with the suffix meaning *enlargement* to form a word meaning *enlargement of the spleen* (answer: *splenomegaly*).

1. combining form for *heart* _____
   suffix meaning *abnormal softening* _____
   term meaning *abnormal softening of the heart* _____

2. word root form for *stomach* _____
   suffix meaning *to surgically create an opening* _____
   term meaning *surgically creating an opening into the stomach* _____

3. combining form for *nose* _____
   suffix meaning *surgical repair* _____
   term meaning *surgical repair of the nose* _____

4. prefix meaning *excessive* _____
   suffix meaning *development* _____
   term meaning *excessive development* _____

5. combining form meaning *disease* _____
   suffix meaning *the study of* _____
   term meaning *the study of disease* _____

6. word root meaning *nerve* _____
   suffix for *tumor/mass* _____
   term meaning *nerve tumor* _____

7. combining form meaning *stomach* _____
   combining form meaning *small intestine* _____
   suffix meaning *study of* _____
   term meaning *study of stomach and small intestine* _____

8. word root meaning *ear* _____
   suffix meaning *inflammation* _____
   term meaning *ear inflammation* _____

9. prefix meaning *chemical* _____
   suffix meaning *treatment* _____
   term meaning *chemical treatment* _____

10. combining form meaning *cancer* _____
    suffix meaning *that which produces* _____
    term meaning *that which produces cancer* _____

E. Define the Combining Form

1. **bi/o** _____

2. **carcin/o** _____

3. **cardi/o** _____

4. **chem/o** _____

5. **cis/o** _____

6. **dermat/o** _____

7. **enter/o** _____

8. **gastr/o** _____

9. **gynec/o** _____

10. **hemat/o** _____

11. **immun/o** _____

12. **laryng/o** _____

13. **nephr/o** _____

14. **neur/o** _____

15. **ophthalm/o** _____

16. **ot/o** _____

17. **path/o** _____

18. **pulmon/o** _____

19. **rhin/o** _____

F. Making Plurals

For each singular term below, write the plural form.

1. diagnosis _____

2. diverticulum _____

3. bursa _____

4. bronchus _____

5. artery _____

G. Complete the Statement

1. The reference book containing important information regarding medications is the _____.

2. A person specializing in the dispensing of medications is a _____.

3. The accepted official name for a drug is the _____ name.

4. The trade name for a drug is the _____ name.

5. The chemical name represents _____.

6. The federal agency that enforces controls over the use of drugs causing dependency is the _____.

H. Prescription Practice

Write out the following prescription instructions in the space provided. Some of the abbreviations were introduced in this chapter. Refer to Appendix III for unfamiliar abbreviations.

1. Pravachol, 20 mg, Sig. ī q noc, #30, refill 3x, no sub.

_____

2. Lanoxin, 0.125 mg, Sig. īīī stat, then īī q am, #100, refills prn.

_____

3. Synthroid, 0.075 mg, Sig. ī daily, #100, refill x4.

_____

4. Norvasc, 5 mg, Sig. ī q am, #60, 0 refills.

_____

MyLab Medical Terminology™

MyLab Medical Terminology is a premium online homework management system that includes a host of features to help you study. Registered users will find:

- A multitude of activities and assignments built within the MyLab platform
- Powerful tools that track and analyze your results—allowing you to create a personalized learning experience
- Videos and audio pronunciations to help enrich your progress
- Streaming lesson presentations (Guided Lectures) and self-paced learning modules
- A space where you and your instructors can check your progress and manage your assignments

Chapter 2

Body Organization

Learning Objectives

Upon completion of this chapter, you will be able to

1. Recognize the combining forms introduced in this chapter.
2. Correctly spell and pronounce medical terms and anatomical structures relating to body structure.
3. Discuss the organization of the body in terms of cells, tissues, organs, and systems.
4. Describe the common features of cells.
5. Define the four types of tissues.
6. List the major organs found in the 12 organ systems and their related medical specialties.
7. Describe the anatomical position.
8. Define the body planes.
9. Identify regions of the body.
10. List the body cavities and their contents.
11. Locate and describe the nine anatomical and four clinical divisions of the abdomen.
12. Define directional terms.
13. Build body organization medical terms from word parts.
14. Describe routes used to introduce drugs into the body.
15. Interpret abbreviations associated with body organization.

AT A GLANCE

Arrangement
The body is organized into levels; each is built from the one below it. In other words, the body as a whole is composed of systems, a system is composed of organs, an organ is composed of tissues, and tissues are composed of cells.

Levels
The major body structural levels from smallest to largest are:

cells   tissues   organs   systems   body

Word Parts
Presented here are some of the more common combining forms used to build body organizational terms.

Combining Forms

abdomin/o	abdomen	hal/o	to breathe
adip/o	fat	hemat/o	blood
aer/o	air	hist/o	tissue
anter/o	front	immun/o	protection
brachi/o	arm	infer/o	below
bucc/o	cheek	inguin/o	groin
cardi/o	heart	laryng/o	larynx
caud/o	tail	later/o	side
cephal/o	head	lingu/o	tongue
cervic/o	neck	lumb/o	loin (low back)
chondr/o	cartilage	lymph/o	lymph
crani/o	skull	medi/o	middle
crin/o	to secrete	muscul/o	muscle
crur/o	leg	nephr/o	kidney
cutane/o	skin	neur/o	nerve
cyt/o	cell	ophthalm/o	eye
derm/o	skin	orth/o	straight
dermat/o	skin	or/o	mouth
dist/o	away from	ot/o	ear
dors/o	back	pariet/o	cavity wall
enter/o	small intestine	ped/o	foot
epitheli/o	epithelium	pelv/o	pelvis
gastr/o	stomach	peritone/o	peritoneum
glute/o	buttock	pleur/o	pleura
gynec/o	female		

(continued on page 28)

Body Organization Illustrated

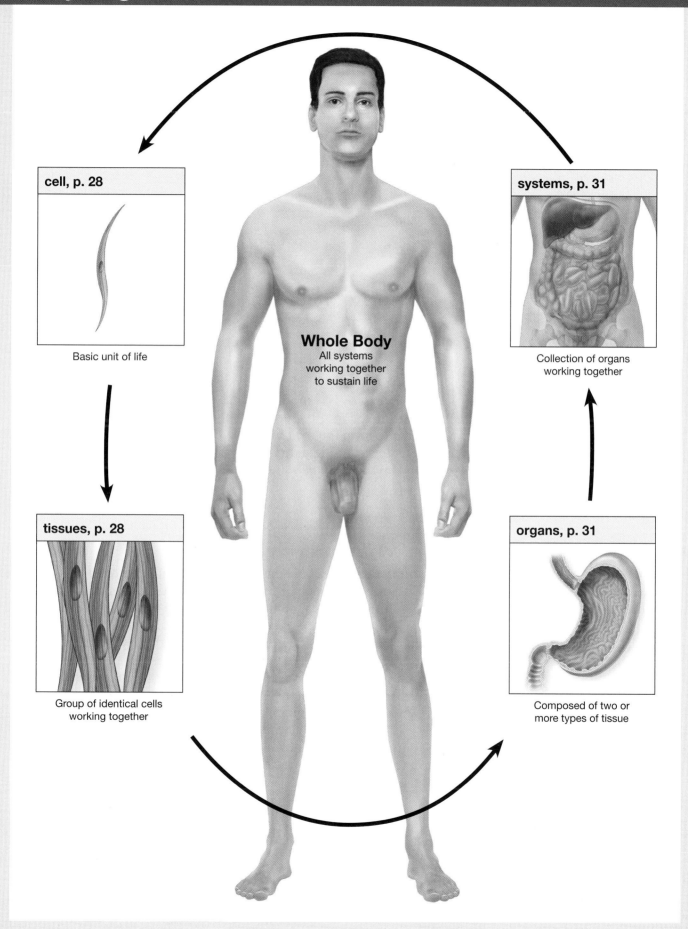

cell, p. 28

Basic unit of life

tissues, p. 28

Group of identical cells working together

Whole Body
All systems working together to sustain life

systems, p. 31

Collection of organs working together

organs, p. 31

Composed of two or more types of tissue

(continued from page 26)

poster/o	back	**thorac/o**	chest
proct/o	rectum and anus	**topic/o**	a specific area
proxim/o	near to	**ur/o**	urine
pub/o	genital region	**urin/o**	urine
pulmon/o	lung	**vagin/o**	vagina
rect/o	rectum	**vascul/o**	blood vessel
rhin/o	nose	**ven/o**	vein
spin/o	spine	**ventr/o**	belly
super/o	above	**vertebr/o**	vertebra
thec/o	sheath (meninges)	**viscer/o**	internal organ

Levels of Body Organization

body	**organs**	**tissues**
cells	**systems**	

Before taking a look at the whole human body, we need to examine its component parts. The human **body** is composed of **cells**, **tissues**, **organs**, and **systems**. These components are arranged in a hierarchical manner. That is, parts from a lower level come together to form the next higher level. In that way, cells come together to form tissues, tissues come together to form organs, organs come together to form systems, and all the systems come together to form the whole body.

Cells

cell membrane	**cytoplasm** (SIGH-toh-plazm)
cytology (sigh-TALL-oh-jee)	**nucleus**

The cell is the fundamental unit of all living things. That is to say, it is the smallest structure of a body that has all the properties of being alive: responding to stimuli, engaging in metabolic activities, and reproducing itself. All the tissues and organs in the body are composed of cells. Individual cells perform functions for the body such as reproduction, hormone secretion, energy production, and excretion. Special cells are also able to carry out very specific functions, such as contraction by muscle cells and electrical impulse transmission by nerve cells. The study of cells and their functions is called **cytology**. No matter the difference in their shape and function, at some point during their life cycle, all cells have **cytoplasm**, a **nucleus**, and a **cell membrane** (see Figure 2-1 ■). The cell membrane is the outermost boundary of a cell. It encloses the cytoplasm, the watery internal environment of the cell, and the nucleus, which contains the cell's DNA.

Tissues

connective tissue	**muscular tissue**
epithelial tissue (ep-ih-THEE-lee-al)	**nervous tissue**
histology (hiss-TALL-oh-jee)	

Histology is the study of tissue. When like cells group together and function together to perform a specific activity, they form tissue. The body has four types of tissue: **muscular tissue**, **epithelial tissue**, **connective tissue**, and **nervous tissue** (see Figure 2-2 ■).

What's In A Name?

Look for these word parts:
cyt/o = cell
-logy = study of
-plasm = formation

Med Term Tip

Cells were first seen by Robert Hooke over 300 years ago. To him, the rectangular shapes looked like prison cells, so he named them cells. It was a common practice for early anatomists to name an organ solely on its appearance.

What's In A Name?

Look for these word parts:
epitheli/o = epithelium
hist/o = tissue
muscul/o = muscle
-al = pertaining to
-ar = pertaining to
-logy = study of
-ous = pertaining to

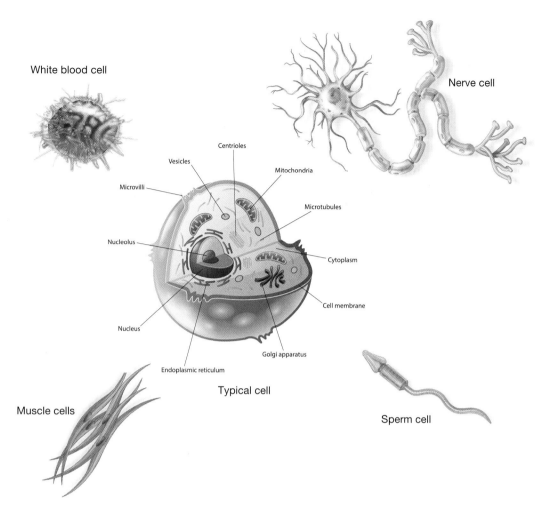

White blood cell

Nerve cell

Centrioles

Vesicles

Mitochondria

Microvilli

Microtubules

Nucleolus

Cytoplasm

Cell membrane

Nucleus

Golgi apparatus

Endoplasmic reticulum

Typical cell

Muscle cells

Sperm cell

■ **Figure 2-1** Typical cell (in center) illustrates three main cellular structures: cell membrane, nucleus, and cytoplasm. Examples of four cells with very different shapes are located around the typical cell. Although each cell has a cell membrane, nucleus, and cytoplasm, each has a unique shape depending on its location and function. *(La Gorda/Shutterstock)*

Muscular Tissue

cardiac muscle   muscle fibers
smooth muscle   skeletal muscle

Muscular tissue produces movement in the body through contraction, or shortening in length, and is composed of individual muscle cells called **muscle fibers**. Muscle tissue forms one of three basic types of muscles: **skeletal muscle**, **smooth muscle**, or **cardiac muscle**. Skeletal muscle attaches to bone. Internal organs, such as the intestine, uterus, and blood vessels, contain smooth muscle. Only the heart contains cardiac muscle.

> **What's In A Name?**
>
> Look for these word parts:
> **cardi/o** = heart
> **-ac** = pertaining to
> **-al** = pertaining to

Epithelial Tissue

epithelium (ep-ih-THEE-lee-um)

Epithelial tissue, or **epithelium**, is found throughout the body and is composed of close-packed cells that form the covering for and lining of body structures. For example, both the top layer of skin and the lining of the stomach are epithelial tissue (see Figure 2-2). In addition to forming a protective barrier, specialized epithelial tissues absorb substances (such as nutrients from the intestine), secrete substances (such as sweat glands), or excrete wastes (such as the kidney tubules).

> **Med Term Tip**
>
> The term *epithelium* comes from the prefix **epi-** meaning *on top of* and the combining form **theli/o** meaning *nipple* (referring to any projection from the surface).

■ **Figure 2-2** The appearance of different types of tissues—muscle, epithelial, nervous, connective—and their location within the body.

Nervous Tissue
Brain

Epithelial Tissue
Epidermis layer of skin

Muscle Tissue
Skeletal muscle of deltoid

Connective Tissue
Adipose layer of skin

Muscle Tissue
Cardiac muscle of heart

Epithelial Tissue
Lining of colon

Muscle Tissue
Smooth muscle of stomach

Connective Tissue
Tendon

Connective Tissue
Cartilage

Connective Tissue
Bone

Connective Tissue

adipose (AD-ih-pohs)   cartilage (KAR-tih-lij)
bone   tendons

Connective tissue is the supporting and protecting tissue in body structures. Because connective tissue performs different functions depending on its location, it appears in several forms so that each is able to perform the task required at that location. For example, **bone** provides structural support for the whole body. **Cartilage** is the shock absorber in joints. **Tendons** tightly connect skeletal muscles to bones. **Adipose** provides protective padding around body structures (see Figure 2-2).

> **What's In A Name?**
> Look for these word parts:
> **adip/o** = fat
> **-ose** = pertaining to

Nervous Tissue

brain   neurons
nerves   spinal cord

Nervous tissue is made up of cells called **neurons** (see Figure 2-2). This tissue forms the **brain**, **spinal cord**, and a network of **nerves** throughout the entire body, allowing for the conduction of electrical impulses to send information between the brain and the rest of the body.

> **What's In A Name?**
> Look for these word parts:
> **neur/o** = nerve
> **spin/o** = spine
> **-al** = pertaining to

PRACTICE AS YOU GO

A. Complete the Statement

1. The levels of organization of the body in order from smallest to largest are: _____,

   _____, _____, _____, _____.

2. No matter its shape, all cells have _____, a _____, and a _____.

3. _____ tissue lines internal organs and serves as a covering for the skin.

4. _____ muscle is located in the heart, _____ muscle is attached

   to bones, and _____ muscle is found in internal organs.

5. Cartilage and tendons are examples of _____ tissue.

6. Nervous tissue is composed of _____.

Organs and Systems

Organs are composed of several different types of tissue that work as a unit to perform special functions. For example, the stomach contains smooth muscle tissue, nervous tissue, and epithelial tissue that allow it to contract to mix food with digestive juices.

Several organs working in a coordinated manner to perform a complex function or functions comprise a system. To continue with our example, the stomach plus the other digestive system organs—the oral cavity, pharynx, esophagus, liver, gallbladder, pancreas, small intestine, and large intestine—work together to ingest, digest, and absorb food.

Table 2-1 ■ presents the organ systems this book discusses, along with the major organs found in each system, the system functions, and the medical specialties that treat conditions of that system.

■ **TABLE 2-1** Organ Systems of the Human Body

System and Medical Specialty	Word Parts	Structures		Functions
Integumentary System (in-teg-yoo-MEN-tah-ree) **dermatology** (der-mah-TALL-oh-jee) **plastic surgery** (PLAS-tik)	**-ary** = pertaining to **dermat/o** = skin **-logy** = study of	• Skin • Hair • Nails • Sweat glands • Sebaceous glands		Forms protective two-way barrier; aids in temperature regulation
Musculoskeletal System (MS) (mus-kyoo-loh-SKEL-eh-tal) **orthopedics** (or-thoh-PEE-diks) **orthopedic surgery** (or-thoh-PEE-dik) **rheumatology** (roo-mah-TALL-oh-jee)	**muscul/o** = muscle **-al** = pertaining to **orth/o** = straight **ped/o** = foot **-ic** = pertaining to **-logy** = study of	• Bones • Joints • Muscles		Skeleton supports and protects body, forms blood cells, and stores minerals; muscles produce movement
Cardiovascular System (CV) (kar-dee-oh-VAS-kyoo-lar) **cardiology** (kar-dee-ALL-oh-jee)	**cardi/o** = heart **vascul/o** = blood vessel **-ar** = pertaining to **-logy** = study of	• Heart • Arteries • Veins		Pumps blood throughout entire body to transport nutrients, oxygen, and wastes

■ TABLE 2-1   Organ Systems of the Human Body (continued)

System and Medical Specialty	Word Parts	Structures		Functions
Blood (Hematic System) (hee-MAT-ik)	**hemat/o** = blood	• Plasma		Transports oxygen, protects against pathogens, and controls bleeding
hematology (hee-mah-TALL-oh-jee)	**-ic** = pertaining to	• Erythrocytes		
	-logy = study of	• Leukocytes		
		• Platelets		
Lymphatic System (lim-FAT-ik)	**lymph/o** = lymph	• Lymph nodes		Protects body from disease and invasion from pathogens
immunology (im-yoo-NALL-oh-jee)	**-atic** = pertaining to	• Lymphatic vessels		
	immun/o = protection	• Spleen		
	-logy = study of	• Thymus gland		
		• Tonsils		
Respiratory System	**-ory** = pertaining to	• Nasal cavity		Obtains oxygen from the environment and removes carbon dioxide from the body
otorhinolaryngology (ENT) (oh-toh-rye-noh-lair-in-GALL-oh-jee)	**ot/o** = ear	• Pharynx		
	rhin/o = nose	• Larynx		
pulmonology (pull-moh-NALL-oh-jee)	**laryng/o** = larynx	• Trachea		
	pulmon/o = lung	• Bronchial tubes		
thoracic surgery (tho-RASS-ik)	**thorac/o** = chest	• Lungs		
	-ic = pertaining to			
	-logy = study of			

■ **TABLE 2-1**   Organ Systems of the Human Body (continued)

System and Medical Specialty	Word Parts	Structures		Functions

Digestive or **Gastrointestinal (GI) System**
 	
  gastroenterology
  (gas-troh-en-ter-ALL-oh-jee)
 	
  proctology
  (prok-TALL-oh-jee)
	gastr/o = stomach
	
	enter/o = small intestine
	
	proct/o = rectum and anus
	
	-al = pertaining to
	
	-logy = study of
		• Oral cavity
		• Pharynx
		• Esophagus
		• Stomach
		• Small intestine
		• Large intestine
		• Liver
		• Gallbladder
		• Pancreas
		• Salivary glands
				Ingests, digests, and absorbs nutrients for the body

Urinary System
(YOO-rih-nair-ee)
 	
  nephrology
  (neh-FROL-oh-jee)
 	
  urology
  (yoo-RALL-oh-jee)
	urin/o = urine
	
	-ary = pertaining to
	
	nephr/o = kidney
	
	ur/o = urine
	
	-logy = study of
		• Kidneys
		• Ureters
		• Urinary bladder
		• Urethra
			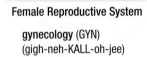	Filters waste products out of blood and removes them from body

Female Reproductive System
 	
  gynecology (GYN)
  (gigh-neh-KALL-oh-jee)
 	
  obstetrics (OB)
  (ob-STET-riks)
	gynec/o = female
	
	-logy = study of
		• Ovaries
		• Fallopian tubes
		• Uterus
		• Vagina
		• Vulva
		• Breasts
				Produces eggs for reproduction, provides place for growing baby, and nourishes infant

■ **TABLE 2-1**   **Organ Systems of the Human Body (continued)**

System and Medical Specialty	Word Parts	Structures		Functions
Male Reproductive System **urology** (yoo-RALL-oh-jee)	**ur/o** = urine **-logy** = study of	• Testes • Epididymis • Vas deferens • Penis • Seminal vesicles • Prostate gland • Bulbourethral gland		Produces sperm for reproduction
Endocrine System (EN-doh-krin) **endocrinology** (en-doh-krin-ALL-oh-jee)	**endo-** = within **crin/o** = to secrete **-ine** = pertaining to **-logy** = study of	• Pituitary gland • Pineal gland • Thyroid gland • Parathyroid glands • Thymus gland • Adrenal glands • Pancreas • Ovaries • Testes		Regulates metabolic activities of the body
Nervous System **neurology** (noo-RALL-oh-jee) **neurosurgery** (noo-roh-SER-jer-ee)	**-ous** = pertaining to **neur/o** = nerve **-logy** = study of	• Brain • Spinal cord • Nerves		Receives sensory information and coordinates body's response

■ TABLE 2-1   Organ Systems of the Human Body (continued)

System and Medical Specialty	Word Parts	Structures	Functions
Special Senses ophthalmology (off-thal-MALL-oh-jee)	ophthalm/o = eye -logy = study of	• Eyes	Sensory organ that converts light into electrical impulses allowing for vision
otorhinolaryngology (ENT) (oh-toh-rye-noh-lair-in-GALL-oh-jee)	ot/o = ear rhin/o = nose laryng/o = larynx -logy = study of	• Ears	Sensory organ with dual purpose: converts sound waves into electrical impulses allowing for hearing, and maintains body's sense of balance

PRACTICE AS YOU GO

B. Organ System and Function Challenge

For each organ listed below, identify the name of the system to which it belongs and then match it to its function.

Organ	System	Function
1. _____ skin	_____	a. supports the body
2. _____ heart	_____	b. provides place for growing baby
3. _____ stomach	_____	c. filters waste products from blood
4. _____ uterus	_____	d. provides two-way barrier
5. _____ bones	_____	e. produces movement
6. _____ lungs	_____	f. produces sperm
7. _____ kidney	_____	g. ingests, digests, and absorbs nutrients
8. _____ testes	_____	h. coordinates body's response
9. _____ brain	_____	i. pumps blood through blood vessels
10. _____ muscles	_____	j. obtains oxygen

Body

anatomical position

As shown in the previous sections, the body is the sum of all its systems, organs, tissues, and cells. It is important to learn the anatomical terminology that applies to the body as a whole in order to correctly identify specific locations and directions when dealing with patients. The **anatomical position** is used when describing the positions and relationships of structures in the human body. A body in the anatomical

What's In A Name?
Look for this word part:
-al = pertaining to

position is standing erect with the arms at the sides of the body, the palms of the hands facing forward, and the eyes looking straight ahead. In addition, the legs are parallel with the feet, and the toes are pointing forward (see Figure 2-3 ■). For descriptive purposes, the assumption is always that the person is in the anatomical position even if the body or parts of the body are in any other position.

Body Planes

coronal plane (koh-ROH-nal)	median plane
coronal section	midsagittal plane (mid-SAJ-ih-tal)
cross-section	sagittal plane (SAJ-ih-tal)
frontal plane	sagittal section
frontal section	transverse plane
horizontal plane	transverse section
longitudinal section	

Use terminology for body planes to assist medical personnel in describing the body and its parts. To understand body planes, imagine cuts slicing through the body at various angles. This imaginary slicing allows for use of more specific language when describing parts of the body. These body planes, illustrated in Figure 2-4 ■, include the following:

1. **Sagittal plane:** This vertical plane runs lengthwise from front to back and divides the body, or any of its parts, into right and left portions. The right and left sides do not have to be equal. If the sagittal plane passes through the middle of the body, thus dividing it into equal right and left halves, it

■ **Figure 2-3**   The anatomical position: standing erect, gazing straight ahead, arms down at sides, palms facing forward, fingers extended, legs together, and toes pointing forward. *(Patrick Watson/Pearson Education, Inc.)*

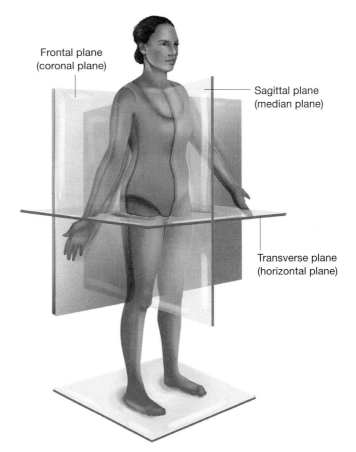

Frontal plane (coronal plane)

Sagittal plane (median plane)

Transverse plane (horizontal plane)

■ **Figure 2-4**   The planes of the body. The sagittal plane is vertical from front to back, the frontal plane is vertical from left to right, and the transverse plane is horizontal.

What's In A Name?

Look for these word parts:
medi/o = middle
trans- = across
-al = pertaining to
-an = pertaining to

is called a **midsagittal** or **median plane**. A cut along the sagittal plane yields a **sagittal section** view of the inside of the body.

2. **Frontal plane:** The frontal, or **coronal plane**, divides the body into front and back portions; a vertical, lengthwise plane is running from side to side. A cut along the frontal plane yields a **frontal** or **coronal section** view of the inside of the body.

3. **Transverse plane:** The transverse, or **horizontal plane**, is a crosswise plane that runs parallel to the ground. This imaginary cut would divide the body, or its parts, into upper and lower portions. A cut along the transverse plane yields a **transverse section** view of the inside of the body.

The terms **cross-section** and **longitudinal section** are frequently used to describe internal views of structures. A lengthwise slice along the long axis of a structure produces a longitudinal section. A slice perpendicular to the long axis of a structure produces a cross-section view.

PRACTICE AS YOU GO

C. Body Plane Matching

Match each body plane to its definition.

1. _____ frontal plane

2. _____ sagittal plane

3. _____ transverse plane

a. divides the body into right and left

b. divides the body into upper and lower

c. divides the body into anterior and posterior

Med Term Tip

As you learn medical terminology, it is important to remember to no longer use common phrases and terms. Many people often use the term *stomach* (an organ) when they actually mean *abdomen* (a body region).

Body Regions

The body is divided into large regions that can easily be identified externally. It is vital to familiarize yourself with both the anatomical name of each region as well as its common name. See Table 2-2 ▪ for a description of each region and Figure 2-5 ▪ to locate each region on the body.

▪ **TABLE 2-2   Terms Describing Body Regions**

Region	Word Parts	Description
abdominal region (ab-DOM-ih-nal)	**abdomin/o** = abdomen **-al** = pertaining to	Abdomen; on anterior side of trunk
brachial region (BRAY-kee-al)	**brachi/o** = arm **-al** = pertaining to	Upper extremities (UE) or arms
cephalic region (seh-FAL-ik)	**cephal/o** = head **-ic** = pertaining to	Head
cervical region (SER-vih-kal)	**cervic/o** = neck **-al** = pertaining to	Neck; connects head to trunk
crural region (KREW-ral)	**crur/o** = leg **-al** = pertaining to	Lower extremities (LE) or legs
dorsum (DOOR-sum)	**dors/o** = back of body	Back; on posterior side of trunk
gluteal region (GLOO-tee-al)	**glute/o** = buttock **-al** = pertaining to	Buttocks; on posterior side of trunk
pelvic region (PEL-vik)	**pelv/o** = pelvis **-ic** = pertaining to	Pelvis; on anterior side of trunk
pubic region (PYOO-bik)	**pub/o** = genital region **-ic** = pertaining to	Region containing external genitals; on anterior side of trunk

■ **TABLE 2-2**   Terms Describing Body Regions (continued)

Region	Word Parts	Description
thoracic region (tho-RASS-ik)	**thorac/o** = chest **-ic** = pertaining to	Chest; on anterior side of trunk; also called *thorax*
trunk		Contains all body regions other than head, neck, and extremities; also called *torso*
vertebral region (VER-teh-bral)	**vertebr/o** = vertebra **-al** = pertaining to	Overlies spinal column or vertebrae; on posterior side of trunk

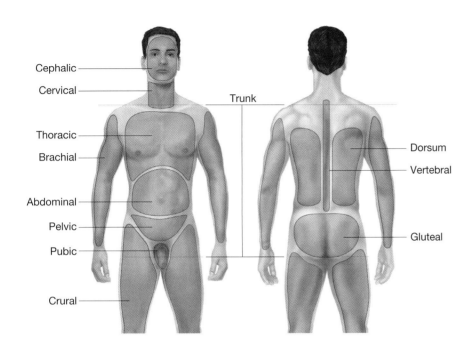

■ **Figure 2-5**   Anterior and posterior views of the body illustrating the location of various body regions.

PRACTICE AS YOU GO

D. Body Region Practice

For each term below, write the corresponding body region.

1. head _____

2. genitals _____

3. leg _____

4. buttocks _____

5. neck _____

6. arm _____

7. back _____

8. chest _____

Body Cavities

abdominal cavity	pericardial cavity (pair-ih-KAR-dee-al)
abdominopelvic cavity (ab-dom-ih-noh-PEL-vik)	peritoneum (pair-ih-toh-NEE-um)
	pleura (PLOO-rah)
cranial cavity (KRAY-nee-al)	pleural cavity (PLOO-ral)
diaphragm (DYE-ah-fram)	spinal cavity
mediastinum (mee-dee-as-TYE-num)	thoracic cavity
parietal layer (pah-RYE-eh-tal)	viscera (VISS-er-ah)
parietal peritoneum	visceral layer (VISS-er-al)
parietal pleura	visceral peritoneum
pelvic cavity	visceral pleura

What's In A Name?

Look for these word parts:
abdomin/o = abdomen
crani/o = skull
pelv/o = pelvis
pariet/o = cavity wall
pleur/o = pleura
spin/o = spine
thorac/o = chest
viscer/o = internal organ
peri- = around
-al = pertaining to
-ic = pertaining to

Med Term Tip

The kidneys are the only major abdominopelvic organ located outside the sac formed by the peritoneum. Because they are found behind this sac, their position is referred to as *retroperitoneal* (**retro-** = behind; **peritone/o** = peritoneum; **-al** = pertaining to).

The body is not a solid structure; it has many open spaces or cavities. These cavities are part of the normal body structure and are illustrated in Figure 2-6 ■. Four major cavities divide the body—two dorsal cavities and two ventral cavities.

The dorsal cavities include the **cranial cavity**, containing the brain, and the **spinal cavity**, containing the spinal cord.

The ventral cavities include the **thoracic cavity** and the **abdominopelvic cavity**. The thoracic cavity contains the two lungs and a central region between them called the **mediastinum**. The heart, aorta, esophagus, trachea, and thymus gland are some of the structures located in the mediastinum. There is an actual physical wall between the thoracic cavity and the abdominopelvic cavity called the **diaphragm**. The diaphragm is a muscle used for breathing. The abdominopelvic cavity is generally subdivided into a superior **abdominal cavity** and an inferior **pelvic cavity**. The organs of the digestive, excretory, and reproductive systems are located in these cavities. The organs within the ventral cavities are referred to as a group as the internal organs or **viscera**. Table 2-3 ■ describes the body cavities and their major organs.

All of the ventral cavities are lined by, and the viscera are encased in, a two-layer membrane called the **pleura** in the thoracic cavity and the **peritoneum** in the abdominopelvic cavity. The outer layer that lines the cavities is called the **parietal layer** (i.e., **parietal pleura** and **parietal peritoneum**), and the inner layer that encases the viscera is called the **visceral layer** (i.e., **visceral pleura** and **visceral peritoneum**).

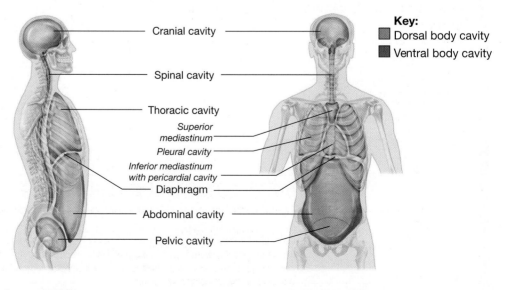

Key:
- Dorsal body cavity
- Ventral body cavity

Cranial cavity
Spinal cavity
Thoracic cavity
Superior mediastinum
Pleural cavity
Inferior mediastinum with pericardial cavity
Diaphragm
Abdominal cavity
Pelvic cavity

Lateral view **Anterior view**

■ **Figure 2-6** The dorsal (red) and ventral (purple) body cavities.

■ **TABLE 2-3** Body Cavities and Their Major Organs

Cavity	Major Organs
Dorsal cavities	
Cranial cavity	Brain
Spinal cavity	Spinal cord
Ventral cavities	
Thoracic cavity	Pleural cavity: lungs
	Pericardial cavity: heart
	Mediastinum: heart, esophagus, trachea, thymus gland, aorta
Abdominopelvic cavities	
Abdominal cavity	Stomach, spleen, liver, gallbladder, pancreas, and portions of the small intestine and colon
Pelvic cavity	Urinary bladder, ureters, urethra, and portions of the small intestine and colon
	Female: uterus, ovaries, fallopian tubes, vagina
	Male: prostate gland, seminal vesicles, portion of vas deferens

Within the thoracic cavity, the pleura is subdivided, forming the **pleural cavity**, containing the lungs, and the **pericardial cavity**, containing the heart. The larger abdominopelvic cavity is usually subdivided into regions in order to precisely refer to different areas. Two different methods of subdividing this cavity are used: the anatomical divisions and the clinical divisions. Choose a method partly on personal preference and partly on which system best describes the patient's condition. See Table 2-4 ■ for a description of these methods for dividing the abdominopelvic cavity.

■ **TABLE 2-4** Methods of Subdividing the Abdominopelvic Cavity

Anatomical Divisions of the Abdomen

- Right hypochondriac (high-poh-KON-dree-ak): Right lateral region of upper row beneath the lower ribs
- Epigastric (ep-ih-GAS-trik): Middle area of upper row above the stomach
- Left hypochondriac: Left lateral region of the upper row beneath the lower ribs
- Right lumbar: Right lateral region of the middle row at the waist
- Umbilical (um-BIL-ih-kal): Central area over the navel
- Left lumbar: Left lateral region of the middle row at the waist
- Right inguinal (ING-gwih-nal): Right lateral region of the lower row at the groin
- Hypogastric (high-poh-GAS-trik): Middle region of the lower row beneath the navel
- Left inguinal: Left lateral region of the lower row at the groin

What's In A Name?

Look for these word parts:
chondr/o = cartilage
gastr/o = stomach
inguin/o = groin
lumb/o = loin (low back)
epi- = above
hypo- = below
-al = pertaining to
-ar = pertaining to
-iac = pertaining to
-ic = pertaining to

Right hypochondriac region | Epigastric region | Left hypochondriac region

Right lumbar region | Umbilical region | Left lumbar region

Right inguinal region | Hypogastric region | Left inguinal region

Med Term Tip

To visualize the nine anatomical divisions, imagine a tic-tac-toe diagram over this region.

Med Term Tip

The term *hypochondriac*, literally meaning *below the cartilage* (of the ribs), has come to refer to a person who believes he or she is sick when there is no obvious cause for illness. These patients commonly complain of aches and pains in the hypochondriac region.

■ **TABLE 2-4**   Methods of Subdividing the Abdominopelvic Cavity (continued)

Clinical Divisions of the Abdomen

- Right upper quadrant (RUQ): Contains majority of liver, gallbladder, small portion of pancreas, right kidney, small intestine, and colon
- Right lower quadrant (RLQ): Contains small intestine and colon, right ovary and fallopian tube, appendix, and right ureter
- Left upper quadrant (LUQ): Contains small portion of liver, spleen, stomach, majority of pancreas, left kidney, small intestine, and colon
- Left lower quadrant (LLQ): Contains small intestine and colon, left ovary and fallopian tube, and left ureter
- Midline organs: uterus, bladder, prostate gland

Liver (majority)
Right kidney
Colon
Pancreas (small portion)
Gallbladder
Small intestine

RIGHT UPPER QUADRANT (RUQ)

Liver (small portion)
Spleen
Left kidney
Stomach
Colon
Pancreas (majority)
Small intestine

LEFT UPPER QUADRANT (LUQ)

RIGHT LOWER QUADRANT (RLQ)

LEFT LOWER QUADRANT (LLQ)

Colon
Small intestine
Right ureter
Appendix
Right ovary (female)
Right fallopian tube (female)

Colon
Small intestine
Left ureter
Left ovary (female)
Left fallopian tube (female)

MIDLINE AREA
Bladder - Uterus (female) - Prostate (male)

PRACTICE AS YOU GO

E. Complete the Statement

1. In the _____ position, the body is standing erect with arms at sides and palms facing forward.

2. The _____ quadrant of the abdomen contains the appendix.

3. The dorsal cavities are the _____ cavity and the _____ cavity.

4. There are _____ anatomical divisions in the abdominal cavity.

5. The _____ region of the abdominal cavity is located in the right lower lateral region near the groin.

6. Within the thoracic cavity, the lungs are found in the _____ cavity and the heart is found in the _____ cavity.

Directional Terms

Directional terms describe the positions of structures relative to other structures or locations in the body. Table 2-5 ■ presents commonly used terms for describing the position of the body or its parts. They are listed in pairs that have opposite meanings; for example, superior versus inferior, anterior versus posterior, medial versus lateral, proximal versus distal, superficial versus deep, and supine versus prone. Directional terms are illustrated in Figure 2-7 ■.

■ **Figure 2-7**   Anterior and lateral views of the body illustrating directional terms.

(Michal Heron/Pearson Education, Inc.)

■ **TABLE 2-5**   Terms for Describing Body Position

Term	Word Parts	Description
superior (soo-PEE-ree-or) or cephalic (seh-FAL-ik)	**super/o** = above **-ior** = pertaining to **cephal/o** = head **-ic** = pertaining to	More toward head, or above another structure Example: Adrenal glands are superior to the kidneys
inferior (in-FEE-ree-or) or caudal (KAWD-al)	**infer/o** = below **-ior** = pertaining to **caud/o** = tail **-al** = pertaining to	More toward feet or tail or below another structure Example: Intestines are inferior to the heart
anterior (an-TEE-ree-or) or ventral (VEN-tral)	**anter/o** = front **-ior** = pertaining to **ventr/o** = belly **-al** = pertaining to	More toward front or belly side of body Example: Navel is located on anterior surface of body
posterior (poss-TEE-ree-or) or dorsal (DOR-sal)	**poster/o** = back **-ior** = pertaining to **dors/o** = back **-al** = pertaining to	More toward back or spinal cord side of body Example: Posterior wall of right kidney was excised

■ **TABLE 2-5**   Terms for Describing Body Position (continued)

Term	Word Parts	Description
medial (MEE-dee-al)	**medi/o** = middle **-al** = pertaining to	Refers to middle or near middle of body or structure Example: Heart is medially located in chest cavity
lateral (LAT-er-al)	**later/o** = side **-al** = pertaining to	Refers to the side Example: Ovaries are located lateral to uterus
proximal (PROK-sim-al)	**proxim/o** = near to **-al** = pertaining to	Located nearer to point of attachment to body Example: In anatomical position, elbow is proximal to hand
distal (DIS-tal)	**dist/o** = away from **-al** = pertaining to	Located farther away from point of attachment to body Example: Hand is distal to elbow
apex (AY-peks)		Tip or summit of an organ Example: We hear the heartbeat by listening over apex of heart
base		Bottom or lower part of organ Example: On X-ray, a fracture was noted at base of skull
superficial		More toward surface of body Example: Cut was superficial
deep		Further away from surface of body Example: Incision into abdominal organ is a deep incision
supine (soo-PINE)		Body is lying horizontally and facing upward Example: Patient is in supine position for abdominal surgery
prone (PROHN)		Body is lying horizontally and facing downward Example: Patient is placed in prone position for spinal surgery

■ **Figure 2-8A**   The supine position. *(Richard Logan/Pearson Education, Inc.)*

■ **Figure 2-8B**   The prone position. *(Richard Logan/Pearson Education, Inc.)*

PRACTICE AS YOU GO

F. Directional Opposites

For each directional term provided, write the term for the "opposite" direction.

1. superior _____

2. prone _____

3. medial _____

4. dorsal _____

5. superficial _____

6. base   _____

7. proximal   _____

8. anterior   _____

9. caudal   _____

Routes and Methods of Drug Administration

aerosol (AIR-oh-sol)

buccal (BUK-al)

eardrops

eyedrops

inhalation (in-hah-LAY-shun)

intracavitary (in-trah-KAV-ih-tair-ee)

intradermal (in-trah-DER-mal)

intramuscular (in-trah-MUS-kyoo-lar)

intrathecal (in-trah-THEE-kal)

intravenous (in-trah-VEE-nus)

oral (OR-al)

parenteral (par-EN-ter-al)

rectal (REK-tal)

subcutaneous (sub-kyoo-TAY-nee-us)

sublingual (sub-LING-gwal)

suppositories (suh-POZ-ih-tor-ees)

topical (TOP-ih-kal)

transdermal (tranz-DER-mal)

vaginal (VAJ-in-al)

The method by which a drug is introduced into the body is referred to as the *route of administration.* To be effective, drugs must be administered by a particular route. In some cases, there may be a variety of routes by which a drug can be given. For instance, the female hormone estrogen can be given orally in pill form or by a patch applied to the skin. The most common routes of administration are described in Table 2-6 ■.

■ **TABLE 2-6**   Common Routes of Drug Administration

Method	Word Parts	Description
oral	or/o = mouth -al = pertaining to	Includes all drugs given by mouth; advantages: ease of administration and slow rate of absorption via the stomach and intestinal wall; disadvantages: slowness of absorption and destruction of some chemical compounds by gastric juices; additionally, some medications, such as aspirin, can have corrosive action on stomach lining
sublingual (sl)	sub- = under lingu/o = tongue -al = pertaining to	Includes drugs held under the tongue and not swallowed; medication is absorbed by blood vessels on underside of the tongue as saliva dissolves it; rate of absorption is quicker than oral route; nitroglycerin to treat angina pectoris (chest pain) is administered by this route

■ **Figure 2-9** Sublingual medication administration. A male patient with a nitroglycerin tablet placed under his tongue. *(Michal Heron/ Pearson Education, Inc.)*

■ **TABLE 2-6**   Common Routes of Drug Administration (continued)

Method	Word Parts	Description
inhalation	**in-** = inward **hal/o** = to breathe	Includes drugs inhaled directly into nose and mouth; **aerosol** (aer/o = air) sprays are administered by this route

■ **Figure 2-10**   Inhalation medication administration. This young girl is using a metered-dose inhaler. *(Michal Heron/Pearson Education, Inc.)*

Method	Word Parts	Description
parenteral	**para-** = beside **enter/o** = intestine **-al** = pertaining to	An invasive method of administering drugs as it requires skin to be punctured by a needle; needle with syringe attached is introduced either under the skin or into a muscle, vein, or body cavity
intracavitary	**intra-** = within **-ary** = pertaining to	Injection into body cavity such as peritoneal cavity or chest cavity; one type of parenteral route of administration
intradermal (ID)	**intra-** = within **derm/o** = skin **-al** = pertaining to	Very shallow injection just under top layer of the skin; commonly used in skin testing for allergies and tuberculosis testing; one type of parenteral route of administration

Intramuscular   Subcutaneous   Intravenous   Intradermal

Epidermis
Dermis
Subcutaneous layer
Muscle

Intramuscular   Subcutaneous   Intravenous   Intradermal

■ **Figure 2-11**   Parenteral medication administration. The angle of needle insertion for four different types of parenteral injections.

Method	Word Parts	Description
intramuscular (IM)	**intra-** = within **muscul/o** = muscle **-ar** = pertaining to	Injection directly into muscle of buttocks, thigh, or upper arm; used when there is a large amount of medication or it is irritating (see again Figure 2-11 ■); one type of parenteral route of administration

■ **TABLE 2-6**   Common Routes of Drug Administration (continued)

Method	Word Parts	Description
intrathecal	**intra-** = within **thec/o** = sheath (meninges) **-al** = pertaining to	Injection into meningeal space surrounding the brain and spinal cord; one type of parenteral route of administration
intravenous (IV)	**intra-** = within **ven/o** = vein **-ous** = pertaining to	Injection into veins; route may be set up to deliver medication very quickly or to deliver continuous drip of medication (see again Figure 2-11); one type of parenteral route of administration
subcutaneous (Subc, Subq)	**sub-** = under **cutane/o** = skin **-ous** = pertaining to	Injection into subcutaneous layer of skin, usually outer part of upper arm, or abdomen (see again Figure 2-11); for example, insulin injection; one type of parenteral route of administration
transdermal	**trans-** = across **derm/o** = skin **-al** = pertaining to	Includes medications that coat underside of a patch, which is applied to skin where it is then absorbed; examples include birth control patches, nicotine patches, and sea sickness patches
rectal	**rect/o** = rectum **-al** = pertaining to	Includes medications introduced directly into rectal cavity in the form of **suppositories** (suppos, supp) or solution; drugs may have to be administered by this route if patient is unable to take them by mouth due to nausea, vomiting, or surgery
topical (top)	**topic/o** = a specific area **-al** = pertaining to	Includes medications applied directly to skin or mucous membranes; distributed in ointment, cream, or lotion form and used to treat skin infections and eruptions
vaginal	**vagin/o** = vagina **-al** = pertaining to	Includes tablets and suppositories that may be inserted vaginally to treat vaginal yeast infections and other irritations
eyedrops		Includes drops used during eye examinations to dilate pupil of eye for better examination of interior of eye; also placed into eye to control eye pressure in glaucoma and treat infections
eardrops		Includes drops placed directly into ear canal for purpose of relieving pain or treating infection
buccal	**bucc/o** = cheek **-al** = pertaining to	Includes drugs placed under lip or between cheek and gum

PRACTICE AS YOU GO

G. Matching Routes of Drug Administration

1. _____ given by mouth
2. _____ injected into muscle
3. _____ breathed into nose or mouth
4. _____ injected into vein
5. _____ applied directly to skin
6. _____ placed under tongue

a. inhalation
b. intravenous
c. topical
d. oral
e. sublingual
f. intramuscular

Abbreviations

AP	anteroposterior	**LUQ**	left upper quadrant
CV	cardiovascular	**MS**	musculoskeletal
ENT	ear, nose, and throat	**OB**	obstetrics
GI	gastrointestinal	**PA**	posteroanterior
GYN	gynecology	**RLQ**	right lower quadrant
ID	intradermal	**RUQ**	right upper quadrant
IM	intramuscular	**sl**	sublingual
IV	intravenous	**Subc, Subq**	subcutaneous
lat	lateral	**suppos, supp**	suppository
LE	lower extremity	**top**	apply topically
LLQ	left lower quadrant	**UE**	upper extremity

Chapter Review

Practice Exercises

A. Prefix Practice

Circle the prefixes in the following terms and define in the space provided.

1. epigastric _____

2. pericardium _____

3. hypochondriac _____

4. retroperitoneal _____

B. Match Organs and Systems

Match each organ to its body system.

1. _____ heart
2. _____ kidneys
3. _____ joints
4. _____ prostate gland
5. _____ hair
6. _____ thyroid gland
7. _____ uterus
8. _____ stomach
9. _____ lungs
10. _____ spleen
11. _____ brain
12. _____ eye
13. _____ muscles
14. _____ ear
15. _____ blood

a. integumentary system
b. digestive system
c. endocrine system
d. female reproductive system
e. nervous system
f. musculoskeletal system
g. male reproductive system
h. respiratory system
i. urinary system
j. cardiovascular system
k. hematic system
l. lymphatic system
m. special senses

C. What's the Abbreviation?

1. musculoskeletal _____

2. lateral _____

3. right upper quadrant _____

4. cardiovascular _____

5. gastrointestinal _____

6. anteroposterior _____

7. obstetrics _____

8. left lower quadrant _____

D. Fill in the blank with the missing corresponding noun or adjective.

Noun	Adjective
1. chest	_____
2. _____	cephalic
3. _____	cervical
4. arm	_____
5. buttocks	_____
6. _____	crural
7. _____	spinal
8. back	_____
9. abdomen	_____
10. _____	cranial

E. Writing Directional Terms

For each term defined below, write the correct combining form that goes with the suffix given, and then write the complete term.

Definition	Combining Form	Term
1. pertaining to near to	_____-al	_____
2. pertaining to above	_____-ior	_____
3. pertaining to the middle	_____-al	_____
4. pertaining to the belly	_____-al	_____
5. pertaining to the tail	_____-al	_____
6. pertaining to front	_____-ior	_____
7. pertaining to the side	_____-al	_____
8. pertaining to back	_____-al	_____
9. pertaining to below	_____-ior	_____
10. pertaining to back	_____-ior	_____

F. Terminology Matching

Match each organ to its body cavity.

1. _____ gallbladder
2. _____ appendix
3. _____ urinary bladder
4. _____ small intestine
5. _____ right kidney
6. _____ left ovary
7. _____ stomach
8. _____ colon
9. _____ right ureter
10. _____ pancreas (majority)

a. right upper quadrant

b. left upper quadrant

c. right lower quadrant

d. left lower quadrant

e. all quadrants

f. midline structure

G. Drug Administration Practice

Name the route of drug administration for the following descriptions.

1. under the tongue _____

2. into the anus or rectum _____

3. applied to the skin _____

4. injected under the first layer of skin _____

5. injected into a muscle _____

6. injected into a vein _____

7. by mouth _____

H. Spelling Practice

Some of the terms below are misspelled. Identify the incorrect terms and spell them correctly in the blank provided.

1. parenteral _____

2. hypokondriac _____

3. integumentery _____

4. cytology _____

5. peritoneum _____

6. inguinal _____

7. intravenus _____

8. saggital _____

9. otorhinolaryngology _____

10. epitheleum _____

I. Fill in the Blank

cardiology	otorhinolaryngology	urology	gynecology
ophthalmology	gastroenterology	dermatology	orthopedics

1. John is a musician who plays an electric bass guitar and is experiencing difficulty in hearing soft voices. He would consult a physician in _____.

2. Ruth is a stock trader with the Chicago Board of Trade. She has had a pounding and racing heartbeat. She would consult a physician specializing in _____.

3. Mary Ann is experiencing excessive bleeding from the uterus. She would consult a _____ doctor.

4. José has fractured his wrist in a fall. A physician in _____ would see him for an examination.

5. A physician who performs eye exams specializes in the field of _____.

6. When her daughter had repeated bladder infections, Mrs. Cortez sought the opinion of a specialist in

    _____.

7. Martha could not get rid of a persistent skin rash with over-the-counter creams. She decided to make an appointment with a specialist in _____.

8. After reviewing his X-ray, the specialist in _____ informed Mr. Sparks that he had a stomach ulcer.

Labeling Exercises

Image A

Write the labels for this figure on the numbered lines provided.

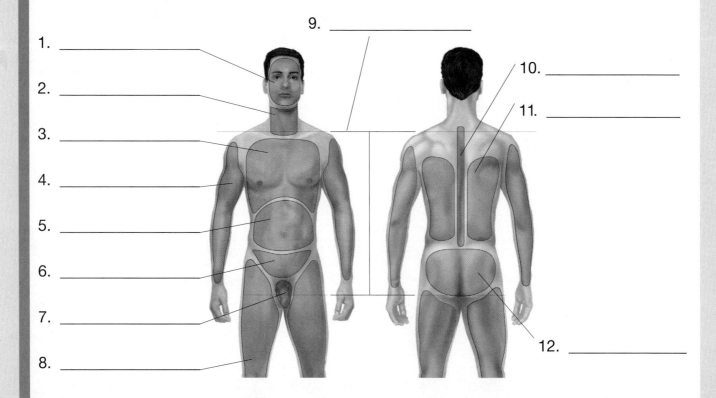

1. _____
2. _____
3. _____
4. _____
5. _____
6. _____
7. _____
8. _____
9. _____
10. _____
11. _____
12. _____

Image B

Write the labels for this figure on the numbered lines provided.

1. _____

2. _____

3. _____

MyLab Medical Terminology™

MyLab Medical Terminology is a premium online homework management system that includes a host of features to help you study. Registered users will find:

- A multitude of activities and assignments built within the MyLab platform

- Powerful tools that track and analyze your results—allowing you to create a personalized learning experience

- Videos and audio pronunciations to help enrich your progress

- Streaming lesson presentations (Guided Lectures) and self-paced learning modules

- A space where you and your instructors can check your progress and manage your assignments

Chapter 3

Integumentary System

Learning Objectives

Upon completion of this chapter, you will be able to

1. Identify and define the combining forms, prefixes, and suffixes introduced in this chapter.
2. Correctly spell and pronounce medical terms and major anatomical structures relating to the integumentary system.
3. List and describe the four purposes of the skin.
4. Describe the layers of the skin and the subcutaneous layer and their functions.
5. List and describe the accessory organs of the skin.
6. Identify and define integumentary system anatomical terms.
7. Identify and define selected integumentary system pathology terms.
8. Identify and define selected integumentary system diagnostic procedures.
9. Identify and define selected integumentary system therapeutic procedures.
10. Identify and define selected medications relating to the integumentary system.
11. Define selected abbreviations associated with the integumentary system.

(Pearson Education, Inc.)

AT A GLANCE

Function

The skin provides a protective two-way barrier between our internal environment and the outside world. It also plays an important role in temperature regulation, houses sensory receptors to detect the environment around us, and secretes important fluids.

Organs

The primary structures that comprise the integumentary system:

skin	**sebaceous glands**
hair	**sweat glands**
nails	

Word Parts

Presented here are the most common word parts (with their meanings) used to build integumentary system terms. For a more comprehensive list, refer to the Terminology section of this chapter.

Combining Forms

albin/o	white	**myc/o**	fungus
cauter/o	to burn	**necr/o**	death
cry/o	cold	**onych/o**	nail
cutane/o	skin	**pedicul/o**	lice
derm/o	skin	**phot/o**	light
dermat/o	skin	**py/o**	pus
diaphor/o	profuse sweating	**rhytid/o**	wrinkle
electr/o	electricity	**sarc/o**	flesh
erythr/o	red	**scler/o**	hard
hidr/o	sweat	**seb/o**	oil
ichthy/o	scaly, dry	**system/o**	system
kerat/o	hard, horny	**trich/o**	hair
leuk/o	white	**ungu/o**	nail
lip/o	fat	**vesic/o**	sac, bladder
melan/o	black	**xer/o**	dry

Suffixes

-derma	skin condition

Prefixes

allo-	other, different from usual
xeno-	foreign

hair, p. 60

Provides some protection; associated with sensory receptors

skin, p. 58

Protective barrier, houses sensory receptors, secretes sweat and sebum, temperature regulation

nail, p. 61

Covers and protects tips of digits

Anatomy and Physiology of the Integumentary System

cutaneous membrane (kyoo-TAY-nee-us)	pathogens (PATH-oh-jenz)
hair	sebaceous glands (sih-BAY-shus)
integument (in-TEG-yoo-ment)	sensory receptors
integumentary system	skin
(in-teg-yoo-MEN-tah-ree)	sweat glands
nails	

The **skin** and its accessory organs—**sweat glands**, **sebaceous glands**, **hair**, and **nails**—are known as the **integumentary system**, with **integument** and **cutaneous membrane** being alternate terms for skin. In fact, the skin is the largest organ of the body and can weigh more than 20 pounds in an adult. The skin serves many purposes for the body: protecting, housing nerve receptors, secreting fluids, and regulating temperature.

The primary function of the skin is protection. It forms a two-way barrier capable of keeping **pathogens** (disease-causing organisms) and harmful chemicals from entering the body. It also stops critical fluids from escaping the body and prevents injury to the internal organs lying underneath the skin.

Sensory receptors that detect temperature, pain, touch, and pressure are located in the skin. The messages for these sensations are conveyed to the spinal cord and brain from the nerve endings in the dermis layer of the skin.

Fluids are produced in two types of skin glands: sweat and sebaceous. Sweat glands assist the body in maintaining its internal temperature by creating a cooling effect as sweat evaporates. The sebaceous glands, or oil glands, produce an oily substance that lubricates the skin's surface.

The structure of skin aids in the regulation of body temperature through a variety of means. As noted previously, the evaporation of sweat cools the body. The body also lowers its internal temperature by dilating superficial blood vessels in the skin. This brings more blood to the surface of the skin, which allows the release of heat. If the body needs to conserve heat, it constricts superficial blood vessels, keeping warm blood away from the surface of the body. Finally, the continuous layer of fat that makes up the subcutaneous layer of the skin acts as insulation.

The Skin

dermis (DER-mis)	hypodermis (high-poh-DER-mis)
epidermis (ep-ih-DER-mis)	subcutaneous layer (sub-kyoo-TAY-nee-us)

The skin is composed of two layers, the superficial **epidermis** and the deeper **dermis**. Underlying the dermis is another layer called the **hypodermis**, or **subcutaneous layer** (see Figure 3-1 ■). The hypodermis is not truly one of the layers of the skin, but because it assists in the functions of the skin, it is studied along with the skin.

Epidermis

basal layer (BAY-sal)	melanocytes (mel-AN-oh-sights)
keratin (KAIR-ah-tin)	stratified squamous epithelium (STRAT-ih-fyde /
melanin (MEL-ah-nin)	SKWAY-mus / ep-ih-THEE-lee-um)

■ **Figure 3-1**   Skin structure, including the layers of the skin, the subcutaneous layer, and the accessory organs: sweat gland, sebaceous gland, and hair.

The epidermis is composed of **stratified squamous epithelium** (see Figure 3-2 ■). This type of epithelial tissue consists of flat, scale-like cells arranged in overlapping layers or strata. The epidermis does not have a blood supply or any connective tissue, so it is dependent for nourishment on the deeper layers of skin.

■ **Figure 3-2**   Photomicrograph showing the two layers of the skin and the subcutaneous layer. *(Jubal Harshaw/ Shutterstock)*

The deepest layer within the epidermis is called the **basal layer**. Cells in this layer continually grow and multiply. New cells that are forming push the old cells toward the outer layer of the epidermis. During this process, the cells shrink, die, and become filled with a hard protein called **keratin**. These dead, overlapping, keratinized cells allow the skin to act as an effective barrier to infection and also make it waterproof.

The basal layer also contains special cells called **melanocytes**, which produce the black pigment **melanin**. Not only is this pigment responsible for the color of the skin, but it also protects against damage from the ultraviolet (UV) rays of the sun. This damage may be in the form of leather-like skin and wrinkles, which are not hazardous, or it may be one of several forms of skin cancer. Dark-skinned people have more melanin and are generally less likely to get wrinkles or skin cancer.

Dermis

collagen fibers (KOL-ah-jen)   **corium** (KOH-ree-um)

The dermis, also referred to as the **corium**, is the deeper layer of skin, located between the epidermis and the subcutaneous layer (see Figure 3-2). Its name means "true skin." Unlike the thinner epidermis, the dermis is living tissue with an excellent blood supply. The dermis itself is composed of connective tissue and **collagen fibers**. Collagen fibers are made from a strong, fibrous protein present in connective tissue, forming a flexible "glue" that gives connective tissue its strength. The dermis houses hair follicles, sweat glands, sebaceous glands, blood vessels, lymph vessels, sensory receptors, nerve fibers, and muscle fibers.

Subcutaneous Layer

lipocytes (LIP-oh-sights)

The subcutaneous layer (or hypodermis) is a continuous layer of fat that separates the dermis from deeper tissues (see Figure 3-2). Composed of fat cells called **lipocytes**, its functions include protecting deeper tissues of the body from trauma, acting as insulation from heat and cold, and serving as a source of energy in a starvation situation.

Accessory Organs

The accessory organs of the skin are the anatomical structures located within the dermis, including the hair, nails, sebaceous glands, and sweat glands.

Hair

arrector pili (ah-REK-tor / pie-lie)   **hair root**
hair follicle (FALL-ih-kl)   **hair shaft**

The fibers that make up hair are composed of the protein keratin, the same hard protein material that fills the cells of the epidermis. The process of hair formation is much like the process of growth in the epidermal layer of the skin. The deeper cells in the **hair root** force older keratinized cells to move upward, forming the **hair shaft**. The hair shaft grows toward the skin surface within the **hair follicle**. Melanin gives hair its color. Sebaceous glands release oil directly into the hair follicle. Each hair has a small slip of smooth muscle attached to it called the **arrector pili** muscle (see Figure 3-3 ■). When this muscle contracts, the hair shaft stands up, resulting in "goose bumps."

■ **Figure 3-3** Structure of a hair and its associated sebaceous gland.

- Epidermis
- Dermis
- Subcutaneous layer

Sebaceous glands
Arrector pili
Shaft of hair
Hair follicle
Hair root
Papilla
Muscle fibers

Nails

cuticle (KYOO-tih-kl)
free edge
lunula (LOO-nyoo-lah)

nail bed
nail body
nail root

Nails are a flat plate of keratin called the **nail body** that covers the top ends of fingers and toes. The nail body is connected to the tissue underneath by the **nail bed**. Nails grow longer from the **nail root**, which is found at the base of the nail and is covered and protected by the soft tissue **cuticle**. The **free edge** is the exposed edge that is trimmed when nails become too long. The light-colored half-moon area at the base of the nail is the **lunula** (see Figure 3-4 ■).

Med Term Tip

Because of its rich blood supply and light color, the nail bed is an excellent place to check patients for low oxygen levels in their blood. Deoxygenated blood is a very dark purple-red and gives skin a bluish tinge called *cyanosis*.

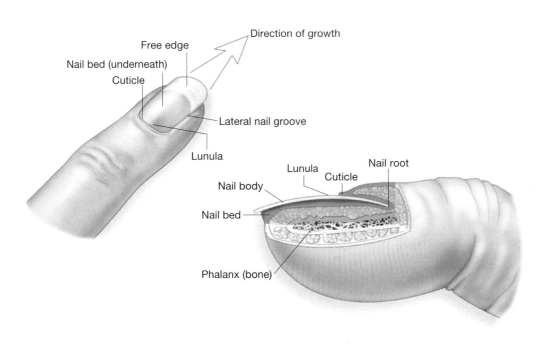

■ **Figure 3-4** External and internal structures of nails.

Sebaceous Glands

sebum

Sebaceous glands, found in the dermis, secrete the oil **sebum**, which lubricates the hair and skin, thereby helping to prevent drying and cracking. These glands secrete sebum directly into hair follicles, rather than a duct (see Figure 3-1). Secretion from the sebaceous glands increases during adolescence, playing a role in the development of acne. Sebum secretion begins to diminish as age increases. A loss of sebum in old age, along with sun exposure, can account for wrinkles and dry skin.

Sweat Glands

apocrine glands (AP-oh-krin)	**sweat duct**
perspiration	**sweat pore**
sudoriferous glands (soo-doh-RIF-er-us)	

What's In A Name?
Look for these word parts:
crin/o = to secrete
-ous = pertaining to

Word Watch
Be careful when using **hydr/o** meaning *water* and **hidr/o** meaning *sweat*.

About 2 million sweat glands, also called **sudoriferous glands**, are found throughout the body. These highly coiled glands are located in the dermis. Sweat travels to the surface of the skin through a **sweat duct**. The surface opening of a sweat duct is called a **sweat pore** (see Figure 3-1).

Sweat glands function to cool the body as sweat evaporates. Sweat or **perspiration** contains a small amount of waste products but is normally colorless and odorless. However, there are sweat glands called **apocrine glands** in the pubic and underarm areas that secrete a thicker sweat, which can produce an odor when it comes into contact with bacteria on the skin. This is what is recognized as body odor.

PRACTICE AS YOU GO

A. Complete the Statement

1. The two layers of skin are the superficial _____ and deeper _____.

2. The _____ separates the dermis from underlying tissue.

3. The _____ layer is the only living layer of the epidermis.

4. The hypodermis is composed primarily of _____.

5. Sensory receptors are located in the _____ layer of skin.

6. Nails and hair are composed of a hard protein called _____.

7. _____ is the pigment that gives skin its color.

8. Another name for the dermis is _____.

9. The nail body is connected to underlying tissue by the _____.

10. _____ glands release their product directly into hair follicles whereas _____ glands release their product into a duct.

Terminology

Word Parts Used to Build Integumentary System Terms

The following lists contain the combining forms, suffixes, and prefixes used to build terms in the remaining sections of this chapter.

Combining Forms

albin/o	white	diaphor/o	profuse sweating	onych/o	nail
angi/o (see Chapter 5)	vessel	electr/o	electricity	pedicul/o	lice
		erythr/o	red	phot/o	light
bas/o	base	esthesi/o (see Chapter 12)	feeling	py/o	pus
bi/o	life			rhytid/o	wrinkle
carcin/o	cancer	hem/o (see Chapter 6)	blood	sarc/o	flesh
cauter/o	to burn			scler/o	hard
chem/o	chemical	hidr/o	sweat	seb/o	oil
cis/o	to cut	ichthy/o	scaly, dry	septic/o (see Chapter 6)	infection
cortic/o (see Chapter 4)	outer layer	kerat/o	hard, horny	system/o	system
		leuk/o	white	trich/o	hair
cry/o	cold	lip/o	fat	ungu/o	nail
cutane/o	skin	melan/o	black	vesic/o	sac
cyt/o	cell	myc/o	fungus	xer/o	dry
derm/o	skin	necr/o	death		
dermat/o	skin				

Suffixes

-al	pertaining to	-ic	pertaining to	-ous	pertaining to
-derma	skin condition	-ism	state of	-phagia (see Chapter 8)	eat, swallow
-ectomy	surgical removal	-itis	inflammation		
		-logy	study of	-plasty	surgical repair
-emia (see Chapter 6)	blood condition	-malacia	abnormal softening	-rrhea	discharge
				-tic	pertaining to
-ia	state, condition	-oma	mass, tumor	-tome	instrument to cut
		-opsy	view of		
-iasis	abnormal condition	-osis	abnormal condition	-ule	small

Prefixes

allo-	other	epi-	above	intra-	within
an-	without	ex-	outward	para-	beside
anti-	against	hyper-	excessive	sub-	under
auto-	self	hypo-	below	xeno-	foreign
de-	without				

Adjective Forms of Anatomical Terms

Term	Word Parts	Definition
cutaneous (kyoo-TAY-nee-us)	cutane/o = skin -ous = pertaining to	Pertaining to skin
dermal (DER-mal)	derm/o = skin -al = pertaining to	Pertaining to skin
dermic (DER-mik)	derm/o = skin -ic = pertaining to	Pertaining to skin
epidermal (ep-ih-DER-mal)	epi- = above derm/o = skin -al = pertaining to	Pertaining to above [upon] skin
hypodermic (high-poh-DER-mik)	hypo- = below derm/o = skin -ic = pertaining to	Pertaining to below skin
intradermal (ID) (in-trah-DER-mal)	intra- = within derm/o = skin -al = pertaining to	Pertaining to within skin
subcutaneous (Subc, Subq) (sub-kyoo-TAY-nee-us)	sub- = under cutane/o = skin -ous = pertaining to	Pertaining to under skin
ungual (UNG-gwal)	ungu/o = nail -al = pertaining to	Pertaining to nails

PRACTICE AS YOU GO

B. Give the adjective form for each anatomical structure.

1. A nail _____

2. The skin _____ or _____

3. Above the skin _____

4. Below the skin _____ or _____

5. Within the skin _____

Pathology

Term	Word Parts	Definition
Medical Specialties		
dermatology (Derm, derm) (der-mah-TAH-oh-jee)	dermat/o = skin -logy = study of	Branch of medicine involving diagnosis and treatment of conditions and diseases of the integumentary system; physician is a *dermatologist*
plastic surgery		Surgical specialty involved in repair, reconstruction, or improvement of body structures such as damaged, missing, or misshapen skin; physician is a *plastic surgeon*
Signs and Symptoms		
abrasion (ah-BRAY-zhun)		A scraping-away of skin surface by friction
anhidrosis (an-high-DROH-sis)	an- = without hidr/o = sweat -osis = abnormal condition	Abnormal condition of no sweat
bulla (BUL-luh)	*Bulla* is the Latin term for bubble	Large blister; larger than a vesicle
comedo (KOM-ee-doh)		Collection of hardened sebum in hair follicle; also called a *blackhead*
contusion		Injury caused by a blow to the body; causes swelling, pain, and bruising; skin is not broken
cyst (SIST)		Fluid-filled sac under the skin

■ Figure 3-5 Cyst.

Term	Word Parts	Definition
depigmentation (dee-pig-men-TAY-shun)	de- = without	Loss of normal skin color or pigment
diaphoresis (dye-ah-foh-REE-sis)	diaphor/o = profuse sweating	Profuse sweating
ecchymosis (ek-ih-MOH-sis)	-osis = abnormal condition	Skin discoloration caused by blood collecting under the skin following blunt trauma to the skin; a bruise

■ Figure 3-6 Male lying supine with large ecchymosis on lateral rib cage and shoulder. *(Michal Heron/Pearson Education, Inc.)*

Pathology (continued)

Term	Word Parts	Definition
erythema (air-ih-THEE-mah)	erythr/o = red hem/o = blood	Redness or flushing of skin
erythroderma (eh-rith-roh-DER-mah)	erythr/o = red -derma = skin condition	Condition of having reddened or flushed skin
eschar (ES-kar)		Thick layer of dead tissue and tissue fluid that develops over deep burn area
fissure (FISH-er)		Crack-like lesion or groove on skin

■ **Figure 3-7** Fissure.

Term	Word Parts	Definition
hirsutism (HER-soo-tizm)	-ism = state of	Excessive hair growth over body
hyperemia (high-per-EE-mee-ah)	hyper- = excessive -emia = blood condition	Redness of skin due to increased blood flow
hyperhidrosis (high-per-high-DROH-sis)	hyper- = excessive hidr/o = sweat -osis = abnormal condition	Abnormal condition of excessive sweat
hyperpigmentation (high-per-pig-men-TAY-shun)	hyper- = excessive	Abnormal amount of pigmentation in skin
lesion (LEE-zhun)		General term for wound, injury, or abnormality
leukoderma (loo-koh-DER-mah)	leuk/o = white -derma = skin condition	Having skin that appears white because normal skin pigment is absent; may be all of the skin or just in some areas
lipoma (lih-POH-mah)	lip/o = fat -oma = mass	Fatty mass
macule (MAK-yool)	-ule = small	Flat, discolored area flush with skin surface; example would be freckle or birthmark

■ **Figure 3-8** Macule.

Pathology (continued)

Term	Word Parts	Definition
necrosis (neh-KROH-sis)	necr/o = death -osis = abnormal condition	Abnormal condition of death
nevus (NEE-vus)		Pigmented skin blemish, birthmark, or mole; usually benign but may become cancerous
nodule (NOD-jool)	-ule = small	Firm, solid mass of cells in skin larger than 0.5 cm in diameter

■ **Figure 3-9**   Nodule.

Term	Word Parts	Definition
onychomalacia (on-ih-koh-mah-LAY-shee-ah)	onych/o = nail -malacia = abnormal softening	Softening of the nails
pallor (PAL-or)		Abnormal paleness of skin
papule (PAP-yool)	-ule = small	Small, solid, circular raised spot on surface of skin less than 0.5 cm in diameter

■ **Figure 3-10**   Papule.

Term	Word Parts	Definition
petechiae (peh-TEE-kee-ee)		Pinpoint purple or red spots from minute hemorrhages under skin; singular is *petechia* (peh-TEE-kee-ah)

■ **Figure 3-11**   Petechiae, pinpoint skin hemorrhages.
(CLS Digital Arts/Shutterstock)

Pathology (continued)

Term	Word Parts	Definition
photosensitivity (foh-toh-sen-sih-TIH-vih-tee)	phot/o = light	Condition in which skin reacts abnormally when exposed to light, such as ultraviolet (UV) rays of the sun
pruritus (proo-RIGH-tus)		Severe itching
purpura (PER-pew-rah)	*Purpura* is the Latin term for purple	Hemorrhages into skin due to fragile blood vessels that appear dark brown/purplish; commonly seen in older adults

■ **Figure 3-12** Purpura, hemorrhaging into the skin due to fragile blood vessels. *(Scimat/Science Source)*

Term	Word Parts	Definition
purulent (PYOOR-yoo-lent)		Containing pus or infection that is producing pus; pus consists of dead bacteria, white blood cells, and tissue debris
pustule (PUS-tyool)	-ule = small	Raised spot on skin containing pus

■ **Figure 3-13** Pustule.

Term	Word Parts	Definition
pyoderma (pye-oh-DER-mah)	py/o = pus -derma = skin condition	Presence of pus on or in layers of skin; sign of bacterial infection
scleroderma (sklair-ah-DER-mah)	scler/o = hard -derma = skin condition	Condition in which skin has lost its elasticity and become hardened
seborrhea (seb-or-EE-ah)	seb/o = oil -rrhea = discharge	Oily discharge
suppurative (SUP-pyoor-ah-tiv)		Containing or producing pus

Pathology (continued)

Term	Word Parts	Definition
ulcer (UL-ser)		Open sore or lesion in skin or mucous membrane

■ **Figure 3-14**   Ulcer.

Term	Word Parts	Definition
urticaria (er-tih-KAIR-ee-ah)	-ia = state, condition	Also called *hives*; skin eruption of pale reddish wheals with severe itching; usually associated with food allergy, stress, or drug reactions
vesicle (VES-ih-kl)	vesic/o = sac	Blister; small, fluid-filled raised spot on skin

■ **Figure 3-15**   Vesicle.

Term	Word Parts	Definition
wheal (HWEEL)		Small, round, swollen area on skin; typically seen in allergic skin reactions such as *hives* and usually accompanied by urticaria

■ **Figure 3-16**   Wheal.

Term	Word Parts	Definition
xeroderma (zeer-oh-DER-mah)	xer/o = dry -derma = skin condition	Condition in which skin is abnormally dry
Skin		
abscess (AB-sess)		Collection of pus in skin
acne (AK-nee)		Inflammatory disease of sebaceous glands and hair follicles resulting in papules and pustules

Pathology (continued)

Term	Word Parts	Definition
acne rosacea (AK-nee / roh-ZAY-shee-ah)		Chronic form of acne seen in adults involving redness, tiny pimples, and broken blood vessels, primarily on nose and cheeks
acne vulgaris (AK-nee / vul-GAIR-is)		Common form of acne seen in teenagers; characterized by comedos, papules, and pustules
albinism (AL-bih-nizm)	albin/o = white -ism = state of	Genetic condition in which body is unable to make melanin; characterized by white hair and skin and red pupils due to lack of pigment; person with albinism is called an *albino*
basal cell carcinoma (BCC) (BAY-sal / sell / kar-sih-NOH-mah)	bas/o = base -al = pertaining to carcin/o = cancer -oma = tumor	Cancerous tumor of basal cell layer of epidermis; frequent type of skin cancer that rarely metastasizes or spreads; these cancers can arise on sun-exposed skin

■ **Figure 3-17**   Basal cell carcinoma. A frequent type of skin cancer that rarely metastasizes. *(Centers for Disease Control and Prevention)*

burn		Damage to skin that can result from exposure to open fire, electricity, ultraviolet (UV) light from the sun, or caustic chemicals; seriousness depends on amount of body surface involved and depth of burn as determined by amount of damage to each layer; skin and burns are categorized as first-degree (superficial), second-degree (partial thickness), or third-degree (full thickness); see Figure 3-18 ■ for a description of damage associated with each degree of burn; extent of burn is estimated using Rule of Nines (see Figure 3-19 ■)

Pathology (continued)

Term	Word Parts	Definition

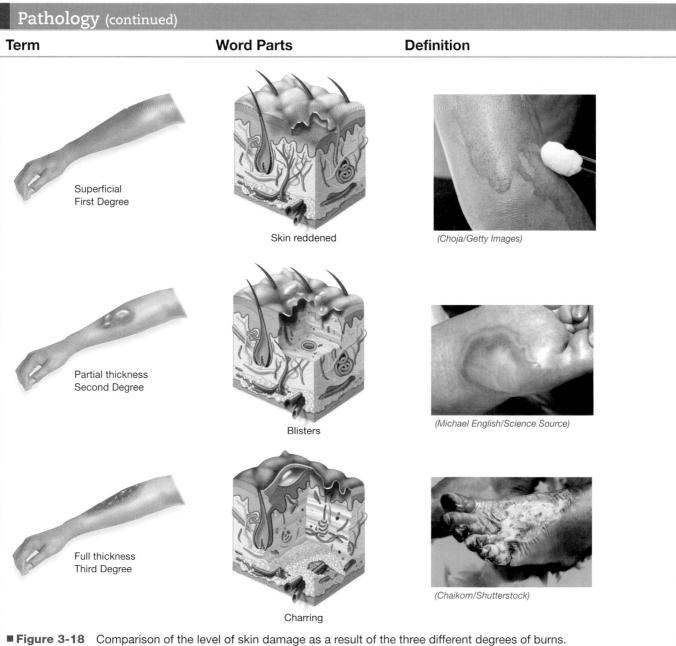

Superficial
First Degree — Skin reddened — *(Choja/Getty Images)*

Partial thickness
Second Degree — Blisters — *(Michael English/Science Source)*

Full thickness
Third Degree — Charring — *(Chaikom/Shutterstock)*

■ **Figure 3-18**   Comparison of the level of skin damage as a result of the three different degrees of burns.

Pathology (continued)

Term	Word Parts	Definition

■**Figure 3-19** Rule of Nines. A method for determining percentage of body burned. Each colored section represents a percentage of the body surface. All sections added together will equal 100%.

Term	Word Parts	Definition
cellulitis (sell-yoo-LYE-tis)	-itis = inflammation	Diffuse, acute infection and inflammation of connective tissue found in skin
cicatrix (SIK-ah-triks)		A scar
decubitus ulcer (decub) (dee-KYOO-bih-tus)	Comes from the Latin word *decumbo*, meaning *lying down*	Open sore caused by pressure over bony prominences cutting off blood flow to overlying skin; can appear in bedridden patients who lie in one position too long and can be difficult to heal; also called *bedsore* or *pressure sore*
dermatitis (der-mah-TYE-tis)	dermat/o = skin -itis = inflammation	Inflammation of skin
dermatosis (der-mah-TOH-sis)	dermat/o = skin -osis = abnormal condition	General term indicating presence of abnormal skin condition
dry gangrene (GANG-green)		Late stages of gangrene characterized by affected area becoming dried, blackened, and shriveled; referred to as *mummified*
eczema (EK-zeh-mah)		Superficial dermatitis of unknown cause accompanied by redness, vesicles, itching, and crusting
gangrene (GANG-green)		Tissue necrosis usually due to deficient blood supply
ichthyosis (ik-thee-OH-sis)	ichthy/o = scaly, dry -osis = abnormal condition	Condition in which skin becomes dry, scaly, and keratinized

Pathology (continued)

Term	Word Parts	Definition
impetigo (im-peh-TYE-goh)		Highly infectious bacterial infection of skin with pustules that rupture and become crusted over

■ **Figure 3-20** Impetigo, a highly contagious bacterial infection. *(Biophoto Associates/Science Source/Getty Images)*

Term	Word Parts	Definition
Kaposi's sarcoma (KAP-oh-seez / sar-KOH-mah)	sarc/o = flesh -oma = tumor	Form of skin cancer frequently seen in acquired immunodeficiency syndrome (AIDS) patients; consists of brownish-purple papules that spread from skin and metastasize to internal organs
keloid (KEE-loyd)		Formation of raised and thickened hypertrophic scar after injury or surgery

■ **Figure 3-21** Keloid.

Term	Word Parts	Definition
keratosis (kair-ah-TOH-sis)	kerat/o = hard, horny -osis = abnormal condition	Term for any skin condition involving overgrowth and thickening of epidermis layer
laceration (lass-er-AY-shun)		Torn or jagged wound; incorrectly used to describe a cut
malignant melanoma (MM) (mah-LIG-nant / mel-ah-NOH-mah)	melan/o = black -oma = tumor	Dangerous form of skin cancer caused by uncontrolled growth of melanocytes; may quickly metastasize or spread to internal organs

■ **Figure 3-22** Malignant melanoma. This photograph demonstrates the highly characteristic color of this tumor. *(National Cancer Institute)*

Pathology (continued)

Term	Word Parts	Definition
pediculosis (peh-dik-yoo-LOH-sis)	pedicul/o = lice -osis = abnormal condition	Infestation with lice; eggs laid by lice are called *nits* and cling tightly to hair
psoriasis (soh-RYE-ah-sis)	-iasis = abnormal condition	Chronic inflammatory condition consisting of papules forming "silvery scale" patches with circular borders

■ **Figure 3-23** This photograph demonstrates the "silvery scale" circular patches that are characteristic of psoriasis. *(Baworn47/Shutterstock)*

Term	Word Parts	Definition
rubella (roo-BELL-ah)		Contagious viral skin infection; commonly called *German measles*
scabies (SKAY-bees)		Contagious skin disease caused by egg-laying mite that burrows through skin and causes redness and intense itching; often seen in children
sebaceous cyst (sih-BAY-shus / SIST)	seb/o = oil	Sac under skin filled with sebum or oil from sebaceous gland; can grow to large size and may need to be excised
squamous cell carcinoma (SCC) (SKWAY-mus / sell / kar-sih-NOH-mah)	carcin/o = cancer -oma = tumor	Cancer of epidermis layer of skin that may invade deeper tissue and metastasize; often begins as sore that does not heal

■ **Figure 3-24** Squamous cell carcinoma. *(National Cancer Institute)*

Term	Word Parts	Definition
strawberry hemangioma (hee-man-jee-OH-mah)	hem/o = blood angi/o = vessel -oma = mass	Congenital collection of dilated blood vessels causing red birthmark that fades a few months after birth

■ **Figure 3-25** Strawberry hemangioma, a birthmark caused by a collection of blood vessels in the skin. *(Gordana Sermek/ Shutterstock)*

Pathology (continued)

Term	Word Parts	Definition
systemic lupus erythematosus (SLE) (sis-TEM-ik / LOO-pus / air-ih-them-ah-TOH-sus)	system/o = system -ic = pertaining to erythr/o = red	Chronic disease of connective tissue that injures skin, joints, kidneys, nervous system, and mucous membranes; autoimmune condition meaning that body's own immune system attacks normal tissue of body; may produce characteristic red, scaly butterfly rash across cheeks and nose
tinea (TIN-ee-ah)		Fungal skin disease resulting in itching, scaling lesions
tinea capitis (TIN-ee-ah / KAP-ih-tis)	*Capitis* is the Latin term for the head	Fungal infection of scalp; commonly called *ringworm*
tinea pedis (TIN-ee-ah / PEE-dis)	*Pedis* is the Latin term for the foot	Fungal infection of foot; commonly called *athlete's foot*
varicella (vair-ih-SELL-ah)		Contagious viral skin infection; commonly called *chickenpox*

■ **Figure 3-26** Varicella or chickenpox, a viral skin infection. In this photograph, the rash is beginning to form scabs. *(Beneda Miroslav/Shutterstock)*

Term	Word Parts	Definition
verruca (ver-ROO-kah)		Commonly called *warts*; benign growth caused by virus; has rough surface removed by chemicals and/or laser therapy
vitiligo (vit-ill-EYE-goh)		Disappearance of pigment from skin in patches, causing milk-white appearance; also called *leukoderma*
wet gangrene (GANG-green)		Area of gangrene that becomes secondarily infected by pus-producing bacteria
Hair		
alopecia (al-oh-PEE-shee-ah)		Absence or loss of hair, especially of head; commonly called *baldness*
carbuncle (KAR-bung-kl)		Furuncle involving several hair follicles
furuncle (FYOO-rung-kl)		Bacterial infection of hair follicle; characterized by redness, pain, and swelling; also called a *boil*
trichomycosis (trik-oh-my-KOH-sis)	trich/o = hair myc/o = fungus -osis = abnormal condition	Abnormal condition of hair fungus

Pathology (continued)

Term	Word Parts	Definition
Nails		
onychia (oh-NIK-ee-ah)	onych/o = nail -ia = state, condition	Infected nail bed
onychomycosis (on-ih-koh-my-KOH-sis)	onych/o = nail myc/o = fungus -osis = abnormal condition	Abnormal condition of nail fungus
onychophagia (on-ih-koh-FAY-jee-ah)	onych/o = nail -phagia = eat, swallow	Nail eating (nail biting)
paronychia (pair-oh-NIK-ee-ah)	para- = beside onych/o = nail -ia = state, condition	Infection of skin fold around a nail

■ **Figure 3-27**   Paronychia.
(Zlikovec/Shutterstock)

PRACTICE AS YOU GO

C. Match each pathology term with its definition.

1. _____ eczema
2. _____ nevus
3. _____ lipoma
4. _____ urticaria
5. _____ bedsore
6. _____ acne rosacea
7. _____ acne vulgaris
8. _____ hirsutism
9. _____ alopecia
10. _____ gangrene
11. _____ scleroderma
12. _____ albinism

a. decubitus ulcer
b. lack of skin pigment
c. acne commonly seen in adults
d. hardened skin
e. redness, vesicles, itching, crusts
f. birthmark
g. excessive hair growth
h. caused by deficient blood supply
i. fatty tumor
j. hives
k. baldness
l. acne of adolescence

Diagnostic Procedures

Term	Word Parts	Definition
Clinical Laboratory Tests		
culture and sensitivity (C&S)		Laboratory test that grows a colony of bacteria removed from infected area in order to identify specific infecting bacteria and then determine its sensitivity to a variety of antibiotics
Biopsy Procedures		
biopsy (BX, bx) (BYE-op-see)	bi/o = life -opsy = view of	Piece of tissue removed by syringe and needle, knife, punch, or brush to examine under a microscope; used to aid in diagnosis
	Word Watch Be careful when using bi- meaning *two* and bi/o meaning *life*.	
excisional biopsy (ek-SIZH-ih-nal)	ex- = outward cis/o = to cut -al = pertaining to	Entire suspicious area of tissue removed for examination
exfoliative cytology (ex-FOH-lee-ah-tiv / sigh-TALL-oh-jee)	ex- = outward cyt/o = cell -logy = study of	Scraping cells from tissue and then examining them under a microscope
frozen section (FS)		Thin piece of tissue cut from frozen specimen for rapid examination under a microscope
fungal scrapings	-al = pertaining to	Scrapings, taken with curette or scraper, of tissue from lesions are placed on growth medium and examined under a microscope to identify fungal growth
punch biopsy		Small cylinder of tissue is removed by an instrument that pierces through tissue like a hole punch
shave biopsy		Using scalpel or razor to remove epidermis or dermis tissue elevated above surface of skin

Therapeutic Procedures

Term	Word Parts	Definition
Skin Grafting		
allograft (AL-oh-graft)	allo- = other	Skin graft from one person to another; donor is usually a cadaver; also called *homograft* (homo- = same)
autograft (AW-toh-graft)	auto- = self	Skin graft from person's own body

■ **Figure 3-28** A freshly applied autograft. Note that the donor skin has been perforated so that it can be stretched to cover a larger burned area. *(Grandriver/Getty Images)*

Therapeutic Procedures (continued)

Term	Word Parts	Definition
dermatome (DER-mah-tohm)	derm/o = skin -tome = instrument to cut	Instrument for cutting skin or thin transplants of skin
dermatoplasty (DER-mah-toh-plas-tee)	dermat/o = skin -plasty = surgical repair	Skin grafting; transplantation of skin
skin graft (SG)		Transfer of skin from normal area to cover another site; used to treat burn victims and after some surgical procedures; also called *dermatoplasty*
xenograft (ZEN-oh-graft)	xeno- = foreign	Skin graft from animal of another species (usually a pig) to a human; also called *heterograft* (hetero- = different)
Surgical Procedures		
cauterization (kaw-ter-ih-ZAY-shun)	cauter/o = to burn	Destruction of tissue by using caustic chemicals, electric currents, or by heating or freezing
cryosurgery (kry-oh-SER-jer-ee)	cry/o = cold	Use of extreme cold to freeze and destroy tissue
curettage (kyoo-reh-TAZH)		Removal of superficial skin lesions with curette (surgical instrument shaped like a spoon) or scraper
debridement (dih-BREED-mint)		Removal of foreign material and dead or damaged tissue from a wound
electrocautery (ee-lek-troh-KAW-teh-ree)	electr/o = electricity	To destroy tissue with electric current
incision and drainage (I&D)	cis/o = to cut	Making an incision to create an opening for drainage of material such as pus
onychectomy (on-ih-KEK-toh-mee)	onych/o = nail -ectomy = surgical removal	Removal of a nail
Plastic Surgery Procedures		
chemabrasion (kee-mah-BRAY-zhun)	chem/o = chemical	Abrasion using chemicals; also called *chemical peel*
dermabrasion (DERM-ah-bray-zhun)	derm/o = skin	Abrasion or rubbing using wire brushes or sandpaper; performed to remove acne scars, tattoos, and scar tissue
laser therapy		Removal of skin lesions and birthmarks using laser beam that emits intense heat and power at close range; laser converts frequencies of light into one small, powerful beam
liposuction (LIP-oh-suk-shun)	lip/o = fat	Removal of fat beneath skin by means of suction
rhytidectomy (rit-ih-DEK-toh-mee)	rhytid/o = wrinkle -ectomy = surgical removal	Surgical removal of excess skin to eliminate wrinkles; commonly referred to as a *face-lift*

PRACTICE AS YOU GO

D. Procedure Matching

Match each procedure term with its definition.

1. _____ debridement   **a.** surgical removal of wrinkled skin

2. _____ cauterization   **b.** instrument to cut thin slices of skin

3. _____ chemabrasion   **c.** removing a piece of tissue for examination

4. _____ dermatoplasty   **d.** use of extreme cold to destroy tissue

5. _____ biopsy   **e.** skin grafting

6. _____ rhytidectomy   **f.** removal of lesions with scraper

7. _____ curettage   **g.** removal of skin with brushes

8. _____ dermabrasion   **h.** removal of damaged skin

9. _____ dermatome   **i.** destruction of tissue with electric current

10. _____ cryosurgery   **j.** chemical peel

Pharmacology

Vocabulary

Term	Word Parts	Definition
broad spectrum		Ability of drug to be effective against wide range of microorganisms
placebo		Inactive, harmless substance used to satisfy patient's desire for medication; also used in research when given to control group of persons in a study in which another group receives a drug; effect of placebo versus drug is then observed
unit dose		Drug dosage system that provides prepackaged, prelabeled, individual medications that are ready for immediate use by patient

Drugs

Classification	Word Parts	Action	Examples
anesthetic (an-es-THET-ik)	an- = without esthesi/o = feeling -tic = pertaining to	Deadens pain when applied to skin	lidocaine, Xylocaine; procaine, Novocain
antibiotic (an-tye-bye-AW-tik)	anti- = against bi/o = life -tic = pertaining to	Kills bacteria causing skin infections	bacitracin/neomycin/polymixinB, Neosporin ointment
antifungal (an-tye-FUNG-al)	anti- = against -al = pertaining to	Kills fungi infecting skin	miconazole, Monistat; clotrimazole, Lotrimin
antiparasitic (an-tye-pair-ah-SIT-ik)	anti- = against -ic = pertaining to	Kills mites or lice	lindane, Kwell; permethrin, Nix
antipruritic (an-tye-proo-RIH-tik)	anti- = against -ic = pertaining to	Reduces severe itching	diphenhydramine, Benadryl; camphor/pramoxine/zinc, Caladryl
antiseptic (an-tih-SEP-tik)	anti- = against septic/o = infection -tic = pertaining to	Kills bacteria in skin cuts and wounds or at surgical site	isopropyl alcohol; hydrogen peroxide
corticosteroid cream (kor-tih-koh-STAIR-oyd)	cortic/o = outer layer	Cream containing a hormone produced by adrenal cortex that has very strong anti-inflammatory properties	hydrocortisone, Cortaid; triamcinolone, Kenalog

Abbreviations

#	number		ii	two
BCC	basal cell carcinoma		iii	three
bid	two times a day		MM	malignant melanoma
BX, bx	biopsy		oint	ointment
C&S	culture and sensitivity		qid	four times a day
decub	decubitus ulcer		SCC	squamous cell carcinoma
Derm, derm	dermatology		SG	skin graft
FS	frozen section		SLE	systemic lupus erythematosus
I&D	incision and drainage		STSG	split-thickness skin graft
i	one		Subc, Subq	subcutaneous
ID	intradermal		tid	three times a day
			UV	ultraviolet

Word Watch

Be careful when using the abbreviation *ID* meaning *intradermal* and *I&D* meaning *incision and drainage*.

x	times

PRACTICE AS YOU GO

E. Give the abbreviation for each term.

1. frozen section _____

2. incision and drainage _____

3. intradermal _____

4. subcutaneous _____

5. ultraviolet _____

6. biopsy _____

7. culture and sensitivity _____

8. basal cell carcinoma _____

9. decubitus ulcer _____

10. dermatology _____

Chapter Review

Real-World Applications

Medical Record Analysis

This Dermatology Consultation Report contains 11 medical terms. Underline each term and write it in the list below the report. Then explain each term as you would for a nonmedical person.

Dermatology Consultation Report

Reason for Consultation:	Possible recurrence of basal cell carcinoma, left cheek
History of Present Illness:	Patient is a 74-year-old male first seen by his regular physician five years ago for persistent facial lesions. Biopsies revealed basal cell carcinoma in two lesions, one on the nasal tip and the other on the left cheek. These were successfully excised. The patient noted that the left cheek lesion returned approximately one year ago. Patient reports pruritus and states the lesion is growing larger.
Results of Physical Exam:	Examination revealed a 10 × 14 mm lesion on left cheek 20 mm anterior to the ear. The lesion displays marked erythema and poorly defined borders. The area immediately around the lesion shows depigmentation with vesicles.
Assessment:	Recurrence of basal cell carcinoma
Recommendations:	Due to the lesion's size, shape, and recurrence, deep excision of the carcinoma through the epidermis and dermis layers followed by dermatoplasty is recommended.

	Term	**Explanation**
1.	_____	_____
2.	_____	_____
3.	_____	_____
4.	_____	_____
5.	_____	_____
6.	_____	_____
7.	_____	_____
8.	_____	_____
9.	_____	_____
10.	_____	_____
11.	_____	_____

Chart Note Transcription

The chart note below contains 10 phrases that can be reworded with a medical term presented in this chapter. Each phrase is identified with an underline. Determine the medical term and write your answers in the spaces provided.

Pearson General Hospital Consultation Report

| Task | Edit | View | Time Scale | Options | Help | Download | Archive | Date: 17 May 2017 |

Current Complaint:	A 64-year-old female with an <u>open sore</u> **1** on her right leg is seen by the <u>specialist in treating diseases of the skin.</u> **2**
Past History:	Patient states she first noticed an area of pain, <u>severe itching,</u> **3** and <u>redness of the skin</u> **4** just below her right knee about six weeks ago. One week later, <u>raised spots containing pus</u> **5** appeared. Patient states the raised spots containing pus ruptured and the open sore appeared.
Signs and Symptoms:	Patient has a deep open sore 5 × 3 cm. It is 4 cm distal to the knee on the lateral aspect of the right leg. It appears to extend into the <u>deeper skin layer,</u> **6** and the edges show signs of <u>tissue death.</u> **7** The open sore has a small amount of drainage but there is no odor. A <u>sample of the drainage that was grown in the lab to identify the microorganism and determine the best antibiotic</u> **8** of the drainage revealed *Staphylococcus* bacteria in the open sore.
Diagnosis:	<u>Inflammation of connective tissue in the skin</u> **9**
Treatment:	<u>Removal of damaged tissue</u> **10** of the open sore followed by application of an antibiotic cream. Patient was instructed to return to the skin disease specialist's office in two weeks, or sooner if the open sore does not heal or if it begins draining pus.

1. _____

2. _____

3. _____

4. _____

5. _____

6. _____

7. _____

8. _____

9. _____

10. _____

Case Study

Below is a case study presentation of a patient with a condition discussed in this chapter. Read the case study and answer the questions below. Some questions will ask for information not included within this chapter. Use your text, a medical dictionary, or any other reference material you choose to answer these questions.

A 40-year-old female is seen in the dermatologist's office, upon the recommendation of her internist, for a workup for suspected SLE. Her presenting symptoms include erythema rash across her cheeks and nose, photosensitivity resulting in raised rash in sun-exposed areas, patches of alopecia, and pain and stiffness in her joints. The dermatologist examines the patient and orders exfoliative cytology and fungal scrapings to rule out other sources of the rash. Her internist had already placed the patient on oral anti-inflammatory medication for joint pain. The dermatologist orders corticosteroid cream for the rash. The patient is advised to use a sunscreen and make a follow-up appointment for results of the biopsy.

(Monkey Business Images/Shutterstock)

Questions

1. What pathological condition does the internist think this patient might have? Look this condition up in a reference source, and include a short description of it. SLE is an autoimmune disease. Use a reference source to look up the name of another autoimmune disease.

_____

_____

2. List and define each of the patient's presenting symptoms in your own words.

_____

_____

3. What diagnostic tests did the dermatologist perform? Describe them in your own words. Why were they important in helping the dermatologist make a diagnosis?

_____

_____

4. Each physician initiated a treatment. Describe them in your own words.

_____

_____

5. What do you think the term *workup* means?

_____

_____

Practice Exercises

A. Complete the Term

For each definition given below, fill in the blank with the word part that completes the term.

Definition	Term
1. use of cold to destroy tissue	_____surgery
2. abnormal softening of the nail	_____malacia
3. skin graft from one person to another	_____graft
4. abnormal condition of death	_____osis
5. profuse sweating	_____esis
6. skin graft from another species to a human	_____graft
7. abnormal condition of not sweating	an_____osis
8. oily discharge	_____rrhea
9. abnormal condition of lice	_____osis
10. using suction to remove fat from under skin	_____suction
11. study of the skin	_____logy
12. abnormal condition of hair fungus	_____mycosis
13. scaly skin	_____osis
14. surgical removal of wrinkles	_____ectomy
15. dry skin condition	_____derma

B. Describe the Type of Burn

1. first-degree _____

2. second-degree _____

3. third-degree _____

C. Define the Term

1. macule _____

2. papule _____

3. cyst _____

4. fissure _____

5. pustule _____

6. wheal _____

7. vesicle _____

8. ulcer _____

9. nodule _____

10. laceration _____

D. Word Building Practice

The combining form **dermat/o** refers to the skin. Use it to write a term that means:

1. inflammation of the skin _____

2. any abnormal skin condition _____

3. an instrument for cutting the skin _____

4. specialist in skin _____

5. surgical repair of the skin _____

6. study of the skin _____

The combining form **melan/o** means *black*. Use it to write a term that means:

7. black tumor _____

8. black cell _____

The suffix **-derma** means *skin*. Use it to write a term that means:

9. hardened skin _____

10. white skin _____

11. red skin _____

The combining form **onych/o** refers to the nail. Use it to write a term that means:

12. abnormal softening of the nails _____

13. infection around the nail _____

14. nail eating (biting) _____

15. removal of the nail _____

E. Using Abbreviations

Fill in each blank with the appropriate abbreviation.

1. Mrs. Brown developed a(n) _____ from laying supine too long.

2. _____ is an autoimmune disease attacking connective tissue.

3. The _____ test identified a bacterial infection.

4. The black mole tumor turned out be _____.

5. A(n) _____ was necessary to cover the burn.

6. A(n) _____ was performed to drain the pus from the abscess.

7. _____ often begins as a sore that does not heal, while a _____ tumor forms in the basal layer of the epidermis.

8. _____ treats conditions of the integumentary system.

F. Fill in the Blank

impetigo	tinea	keloid	exfoliative cytology	xeroderma
petechiae	frozen section	paronychia	scabies	Kaposi's sarcoma

1. The winter climates can cause dry skin. The medical term for this is _____.

2. Kim has experienced small, pinpoint, purplish spots caused by bleeding under the skin. This is called _____.

3. Janet has a fungal skin disease. This is called _____.

4. A contagious skin disease caused by a mite is _____.

5. An infection around the entire nail is called _____.

6. A form of skin cancer affecting AIDS patients is called _____.

7. Latrivia has a bacterial skin infection that results in pustules crusting and rupturing. It is called _____.

8. James's burn scar became a hypertrophic _____.

9. For a(n) _____ test, cells scraped off the skin are examined under a microscope.

10. During surgery, a(n) _____ was ordered for a rapid exam of tissue cut from a tumor.

G. Pharmacology Challenge

Fill in the classification for each drug description, then match the brand name.

Drug Description	Classification	Brand Name
1. _____ kills fungi	_____	a. Kwell
2. _____ reduces severe itching	_____	b. Cortaid
3. _____ kills mites and lice	_____	c. Benadryl
	_____	d. Neosporin
4. _____ powerful anti-inflammatory	_____	e. Monistat
5. _____ deadens pain	_____	f. Xylocaine
6. _____ kills bacteria		

H. Spelling Practice

Some of the following terms are misspelled. Identify the incorrect terms and spell them correctly in the blank provided.

1. anesthetic _____

2. chemobrasion _____

3. rytidectomy _____

4. urticaria _____

5. hyperhydrosis _____

6. peronychia _____

7. varicella _____

8. sebaceous _____

9. decubitis _____

10. purulent _____

I. Complete the Statement

1. The accessory organs of the skin include the _____, _____, _____, and _____.

2. The deepest (living) layer of the epidermis is the _____.

3. _____ is the pigment responsible for skin color.

4. The dermis is composed of connective tissue and _____ fibers.

5. The subcutaneous layer is a continuous layer of _____ that separates the skin from deeper tissues.

6. Hair and nails are composed of the hard protein _____.

7. _____ is responsible for lubricating the hair and skin.

8. Most of the sweat glands in the body are _____ glands.

MyLab Medical Terminology™

MyLab Medical Terminology is a premium online homework management system that includes a host of features to help you study. Registered users will find:

- A multitude of activities and assignments built within the MyLab platform

- Powerful tools that track and analyze your results—allowing you to create a personalized learning experience

- Videos and audio pronunciations to help enrich your progress

- Streaming lesson presentations (Guided Lectures) and self-paced learning modules

- A space where you and your instructors can check your progress and manage your assignments

Labeling Exercises

Image A

Write the labels for this figure on the numbered lines provided.

Image B

Write the labels for this figure on the numbered lines provided.

4. _____

5. _____

6. _____

7. _____

8. _____

9. _____

1. _____

2. _____

3. _____

Image C

Write the labels for this figure on the numbered lines provided.

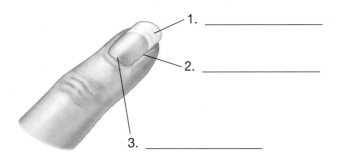

1. _____

2. _____

3. _____

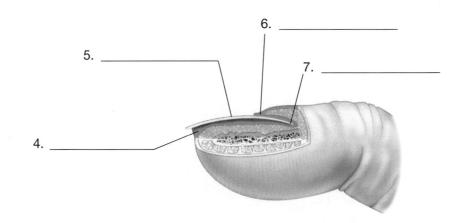

5. _____

6. _____

7. _____

4. _____

Chapter 4

Musculoskeletal System

Learning Objectives

Upon completion of this chapter, you will be able to

1. Identify and define the combining forms, suffixes, and prefixes introduced in this chapter.
2. Correctly spell and pronounce medical terms and major anatomical structures relating to the musculoskeletal system.
3. Locate and describe the major organs of the musculoskeletal system and their functions.
4. Correctly place bones in either the axial or the appendicular skeleton.
5. List and describe the components of a long bone.
6. Identify bony projections and depressions.
7. Identify the parts of a synovial joint.
8. Describe the characteristics of the three types of muscle tissue.
9. Use movement terminology correctly.
10. Identify and define musculoskeletal system anatomical terms.
11. Identify and define selected musculoskeletal system pathology terms.
12. Identify and define selected musculoskeletal system diagnostic procedures.
13. Identify and define selected musculoskeletal system therapeutic procedures.
14. Identify and define selected medications relating to the musculoskeletal system.
15. Define selected abbreviations associated with the musculoskeletal system.

(Pearson Education, Inc.)

AT A GLANCE

Function

The skeletal system consists of 206 bones that make up the internal framework of the body, called the skeleton. The skeleton supports the body, protects internal organs, serves as a point of attachment for skeletal muscles for body movement, produces blood cells, and stores minerals.

Organs

The primary structures that comprise the skeletal system:

bones   **joints**

Word Parts

Presented here are the most common word parts (with their meanings) used to build skeletal system terms. For a more comprehensive list, refer to the Terminology section of this chapter.

Combining Forms

ankyl/o	stiff joint	**metatars/o**	metatarsus
arthr/o	joint	**myel/o**	bone marrow, spinal cord
articul/o	joint	**orth/o**	straight
burs/o	sac	**oste/o**	bone
carp/o	carpus	**patell/o**	patella
cervic/o	neck	**pector/o**	chest
chondr/o	cartilage	**ped/o**	child; foot
clavicul/o	clavicle	**pelv/o**	pelvis
coccyg/o	coccyx	**phalang/o**	phalanges
cortic/o	outer layer	**pod/o**	foot
cost/o	rib	**prosthet/o**	addition
crani/o	skull	**pub/o**	pubis
femor/o	femur	**radi/o**	radius; ray (X-ray)
fibul/o	fibula	**sacr/o**	sacrum
humer/o	humerus	**scapul/o**	scapula
ili/o	ilium	**scoli/o**	crooked
ischi/o	ischium	**spin/o**	spine
kyph/o	hump	**spondyl/o**	vertebrae
lamin/o	lamina (part of vertebra)	**stern/o**	sternum
lord/o	bent backward	**synovi/o**	synovial membrane
lumb/o	loin (low back between ribs and pelvis)	**synov/o**	synovial membrane
		tars/o	tarsus
mandibul/o	mandible	**thorac/o**	chest
maxill/o	maxilla	**tibi/o**	tibia
medull/o	inner region	**uln/o**	ulna
metacarp/o	metacarpus	**vertebr/o**	vertebra

Suffixes

-blast	immature
-clasia	to surgically break
-desis	to fuse
-listhesis	slipping
-logic	pertaining to study of
-porosis	porous

Prefixes

dis-	apart
non-	not

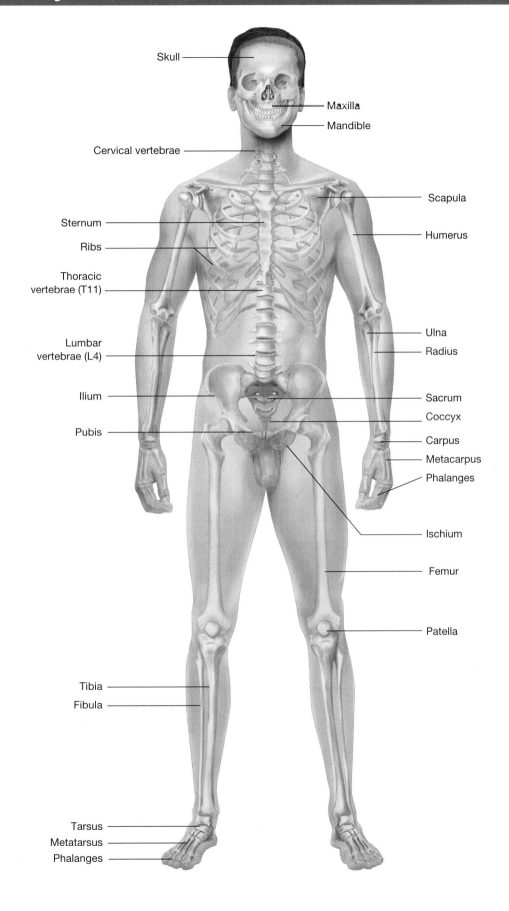

Skull

Maxilla

Mandible

Cervical vertebrae

Scapula

Sternum

Humerus

Ribs

Thoracic
vertebrae (T11)

Lumbar
vertebrae (L4)

Ulna

Radius

Ilium

Sacrum

Coccyx

Pubis

Carpus

Metacarpus

Phalanges

Ischium

Femur

Patella

Tibia

Fibula

Tarsus

Metatarsus

Phalanges

Anatomy and Physiology of the Skeletal System

bone marrow   ligaments (LIG-ah-ments)

bones   skeleton

joints

Each bone in the human body is a unique organ that carries its own blood supply, nerves, and lymphatic vessels. When these **bones** are connected to each other, it forms the framework of the body called a **skeleton.** The skeleton protects vital organs and stores minerals. **Bone marrow** is the site of blood cell production. A **joint** is the place where two bones meet and are held together by **ligaments.** This gives flexibility to the skeleton. The skeleton, joints, and muscles work together to produce movement.

Bones

cartilage (KAR-tih-lij)   osteoblasts (OSS-tee-oh-blasts)

osseous tissue (OSS-ee-us)   osteocytes (OSS-tee-oh-sights)

ossification (oss-ih-fih-KAY-shun)

Bones, also called **osseous tissue**, are one of the hardest materials in the body. Bones are formed from a gradual process beginning before birth called **ossification.** The first model of the skeleton, made of **cartilage**, is formed in the fetus. **Osteoblasts**, immature bone cells, gradually replace the cartilage with bone. In a fully adult bone, the osteoblasts have matured into **osteocytes** that work to maintain the bone. The formation of strong bones is greatly dependent on an adequate supply of minerals such as calcium (Ca) and phosphorus (P).

Bone Structure

articular cartilage (ar-TIK-yoo-lar)   long bones

cancellous bone (KAN-sel-us)   medullary cavity (MED-yoo-lair-ee)

compact bone   periosteum (pair-ee-OSS-tee-um)

cortical bone (KOR-tih-kal)   red bone marrow

diaphysis (dye-AF-ih-sis)   short bones

epiphysis (eh-PIF-ih-sis)   spongy bone

flat bones   yellow bone marrow

irregular bones

Several different types of bones are found throughout the body and fall into four categories based on their shape: **long bones**, **short bones**, **flat bones**, and **irregular bones** (see Figure 4-1 ■). Long bones are longer than they are wide; examples are the femur and humerus. Short bones are roughly as long as they are wide; examples are the carpals and tarsals. Flat bones are usually plate-shaped bones such as the sternum, scapulae, and pelvis. Irregular bones received their name because the shapes of the bones are very irregular; for example, the vertebrae are irregular bones.

The majority of bones in the human body are long bones. These bones have similar structure with a central shaft or **diaphysis** that widens at each end, which is called an **epiphysis**. Each epiphysis is covered by a layer of **articular cartilage** that acts as a cushion and prevents the bones in a joint from rubbing directly on each other. The remaining surface of each bone is covered with a thin connective tissue membrane called the **periosteum**, which contains numerous blood vessels,

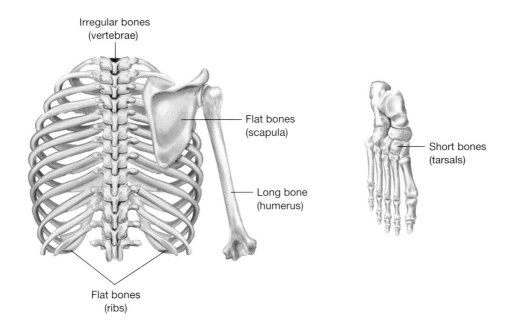

Irregular bones (vertebrae)

Flat bones (scapula)

Long bone (humerus)

Short bones (tarsals)

Flat bones (ribs)

nerves, and lymphatic vessels. The dense and hard exterior surface bone is called **cortical** or **compact bone**. **Cancellous** or **spongy bone** is found inside the bone. As its name indicates, spongy bone has spaces in it, giving it a spongelike appearance. These spaces contain **red bone marrow**, which manufactures most of the blood cells and is found in some parts of all bones.

The center of the diaphysis contains an open canal called the **medullary cavity**. Early in life, this cavity also contains red bone marrow, but as a person ages, the red bone marrow of the medullary cavity gradually converts to **yellow bone marrow**, which consists primarily of fat cells. Figure 4-2 ■ contains an illustration of the structure of long bones.

> **Med Term Tip**
>
> The term *diaphysis* comes from the Greek term meaning *to grow between*.

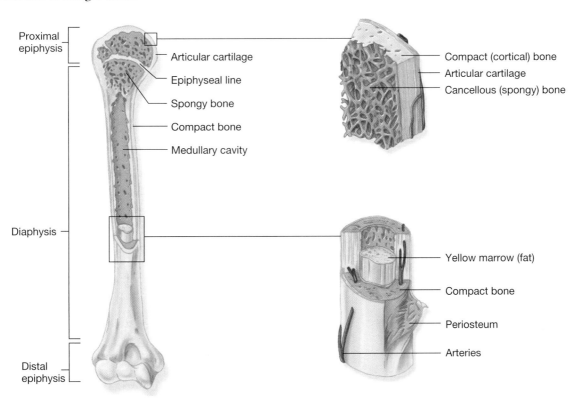

Proximal epiphysis

Articular cartilage
Epiphyseal line
Spongy bone
Compact bone
Medullary cavity

Compact (cortical) bone
Articular cartilage
Cancellous (spongy) bone

Diaphysis

Yellow marrow (fat)

Compact bone

Periosteum

Arteries

Distal epiphysis

■ **Figure 4-2** Components of a long bone. The entire long bone is on the left side, accompanied by a blow-up of the proximal epiphysis and a section of the diaphysis.

Bone Projections and Depressions

condyle (KON-dile)　　　　　　　　neck

epicondyle (ep-ih-KON-dile)　　　　process

fissure (FISH-er)　　　　　　　　　sinus (SIGH-nus)

foramen (for-AY-men)　　　　　　　trochanter (troh-KAN-ter)

fossa (FOSS-ah)　　　　　　　　　tubercle (TOO-ber-kl)

head　　　　　　　　　　　　　　tuberosity (too-ber-OSS-ih-tee)

Med Term Tip

The elbow, commonly referred to as the *funny bone*, is actually a projection of the ulna called the *olecranon process*.

Bones have many projections and depressions; some are rounded and smooth in order to articulate with another bone in a joint. Others are rough to provide muscles with attachment points. The general term for any bony projection is a **process**. Then there are specific terms to describe the different shapes and locations of various processes. These terms are commonly used on operative reports and in physicians' records for clear identification of areas on the individual bones. Some of the common bony processes include the following:

1. The **head** is a large, smooth, ball-shaped end on a long bone. It may be separated from the body or shaft of the bone by a narrow area called the **neck**.
2. A **condyle** refers to a smooth, rounded portion at the end of a bone.
3. The **epicondyle** is a projection located above or on a condyle.
4. The **trochanter** refers to a large rough process for the attachment of a muscle.
5. A **tubercle** is a small, rough process that provides the attachment for tendons and muscles.
6. The **tuberosity** is a large, rough process that provides the attachment for tendons and muscles.

   See Figure 4-3 ■ for an illustration of the processes found on the femur.

   Additionally, bones have hollow regions or depressions, the most common of which are the:

7. **Sinus**: a hollow cavity within a bone.
8. **Foramen**: a smooth, round opening for nerves and blood vessels.
9. **Fossa**: a shallow cavity or depression on the surface of a bone.
10. **Fissure**: a slit-type opening.

What's In A Name?

Look for this word part:

epi- = above

PRACTICE AS YOU GO

A. Complete the Statement

1. Bone is also called _____ tissue.
2. A(n) _____ is the place where two bones meet and are held together by _____.
3. The central shaft of a long bone is the _____ and one of the wide ends is a(n) _____.
4. Three bony processes are _____, _____, and _____.
5. Two bony depressions are _____ and _____.

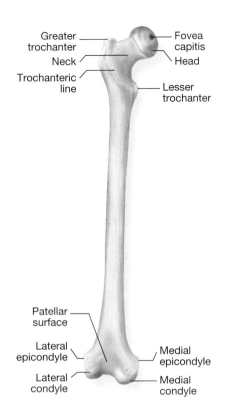

Greater trochanter

Neck

Trochanteric line

Fovea capitis

Head

Lesser trochanter

Patellar surface

Lateral epicondyle

Lateral condyle

Medial epicondyle

Medial condyle

■ **Figure 4-3** Bony processes found on the femur.

Skeleton

appendicular skeleton (ap-en-DIK-yoo-lar)   **axial skeleton** (AK-see-al)

The human skeleton has two divisions: the **axial skeleton** and the **appendicular skeleton**. Figures 4-4 ■ and 4-8 illustrate these two skeletons.

Axial Skeleton

cervical vertebrae

coccyx (KOK-siks)

cranium (KRAY-nee-um)

ethmoid bone (ETH-moyd)

facial bones

frontal bone

hyoid bone (HIGH-oyd)

intervertebral disk (in-ter-VER-teh-bral)

lacrimal bone (LAK-rim-al)

lumbar vertebrae

mandible (MAN-dih-bl)

maxilla (mak-SIL-ah)

nasal bone

occipital bone (ok-SIP-ih-tal)

palatine bone (PAL-ah-tyne)

parietal bone (pah-RYE-eh-tal)

rib cage

sacrum (SAY-krum)

sphenoid bone (SFEE-noyd)

sternum (STER-num)

temporal bone (TEM-por-al)

thoracic vertebrae

vertebral column (VER-teh-bral)

vomer bone (VOH-mer)

zygomatic bone (zye-goh-MAT-ik)

The axial skeleton includes the bones of the head, neck, spine, chest, and trunk of the body (see Figure 4-4). These bones form the central axis for the whole body and protect many of the internal organs such as the brain, lungs, and heart.

The head or skull is divided into two parts consisting of the **cranium** and **facial bones**. These bones surround and protect the brain, eyes, ears, nasal cavity, and oral cavity from injury. The muscles for chewing and moving the head are attached to the cranial bones. The cranium encases the brain and consists

■ **Figure 4-4** Bones of the axial skeleton. Number of bones in each section of the axial skeleton is indicated in parentheses.

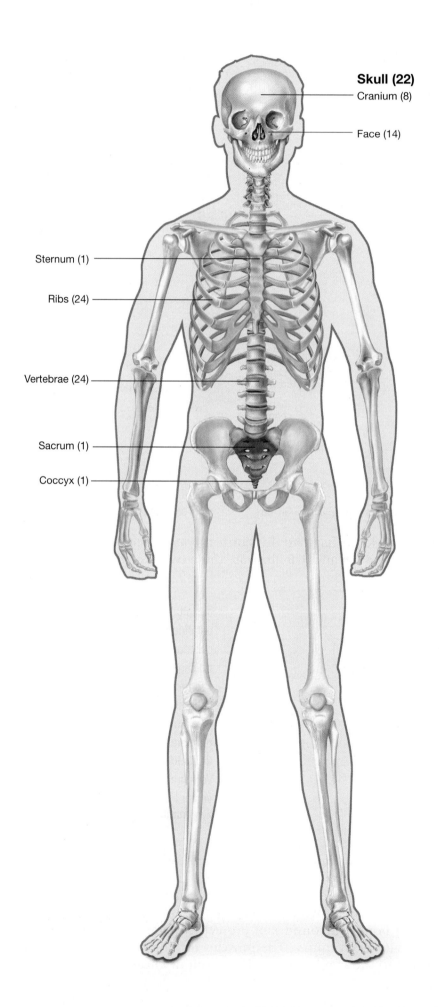

of the **frontal, parietal, temporal, ethmoid, sphenoid,** and **occipital bones.** The facial bones surround the mouth, nose, and eyes, and include the **mandible, maxilla, zygomatic, vomer, palatine, nasal,** and **lacrimal bones.** The cranial and facial bones are illustrated in Figure 4-5 ■ and described in Table 4-1 ■.

The **hyoid bone** is a single U-shaped bone suspended in the neck between the mandible and larynx. It is a point of attachment for swallowing and speech muscles.

The trunk of the body consists of the **vertebral column, sternum,** and **rib cage.** The vertebral or spinal column is divided into five sections: **cervical vertebrae, thoracic vertebrae, lumbar vertebrae, sacrum,** and **coccyx** (see Figure 4-6 ■ and Table 4-2 ■). Located between each pair of vertebrae, from the cervical through the lumbar regions, is an **intervertebral disk.** Each disk is composed of fibrocartilage to provide a cushion between the vertebrae. The rib cage has 12 pairs of ribs attached at the back to the vertebral column. Ten of the pairs are also attached to the sternum in the front (see Figure 4-7 ■). The lowest two pairs are called *floating ribs* and

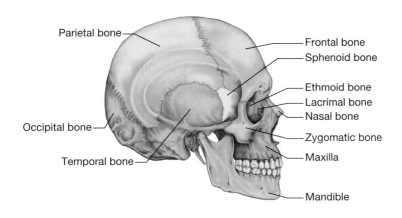

■ **Figure 4-5** Bones of the skull. Note: the palatine and vomer bones are not visible in sagittal view. *(Stihii/Shutterstock)*

■ **TABLE 4-1** Bones of the Skull

Name	Number	Description
Cranial Bones		
Frontal bone	1	Forehead
Parietal bones	2	Upper sides of cranium and roof of skull
Occipital bone	1	Back and base of skull
Temporal bones	2	Sides and base of cranium
Sphenoid bone	1	Bat-shaped bone that forms part of base of skull and floor and sides of eye orbit
Ethmoid bone	1	Forms part of eye orbit, nose, and floor of cranium
Facial Bones		
Lacrimal bones	2	Inner corner of each eye
Nasal bones	2	Form part of nasal septum and support bridge of nose
Maxilla	1	Upper jaw
Mandible	1	Lower jawbone; only movable bone of the skull
Zygomatic bones	2	Cheekbones
Vomer bone	1	Base of nasal septum
Palatine bone	1	Hard palate (PAL-et) roof of oral cavity and floor of nasal cavity

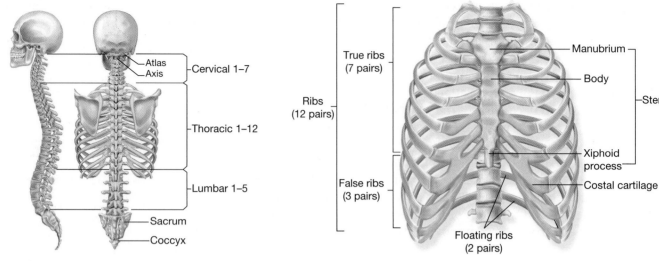

■ **Figure 4-6**   Divisions of the vertebral column.   ■ **Figure 4-7**   The structure of the rib cage.

■ **TABLE 4-2**   Bones of the Vertebral/Spinal Column

Name	Number	Description
Cervical vertebrae	7	Vertebrae in the neck region
Thoracic vertebrae	12	Vertebrae in the chest region with ribs attached
Lumbar vertebrae	5	Vertebrae in the small of the back, about waist level
Sacrum	1	Five vertebrae that become fused into one triangular-shaped flat bone at the base of the vertebral column
Coccyx	1	Three to five very small vertebrae attached to the sacrum; often become fused

are attached only to the vertebral column. The rib cage serves to provide support for organs, such as the heart and lungs.

Appendicular Skeleton

carpus (KAR-pus)

clavicle (KLAV-ih-kl)

femur (FEE-mer)

fibula (FIB-yoo-lah)

humerus (HYOO-mer-us)

ilium (IL-ee-um)

innominate bone (ih-NOM-ih-nit)

ischium (ISS-kee-um)

lower extremities

metacarpus (met-ah-KAR-pus)

metatarsus (met-ah-TAR-sus)

os coxae (OSS / KOK-see)

patella (pah-TEL-ah)

pectoral girdle (PEK-toh-ral)

pelvic girdle (PEL-vik)

phalanges (fah-LAN-jeez)

pubis (PYOO-bis)

radius (RAY-dee-us)

scapula (SKAP-yoo-lah)

tarsus (TAR-sus)

tibia (TIB-ee-ah)

ulna (UL-nah)

upper extremities

The appendicular skeleton consists of the **pectoral girdle**, **upper extremities (UE)**, **pelvic girdle**, and **lower extremities (LE)** (see Figure 4-8 ■). These are the bones for the appendages or limbs and, along with the muscles attached to them, are responsible for body movement.

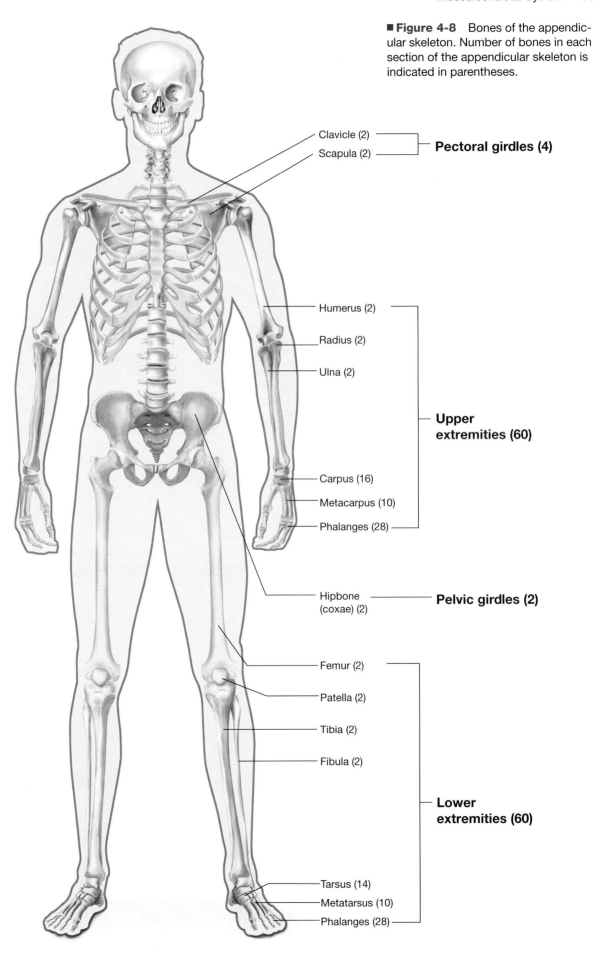

■ **Figure 4-8** Bones of the appendicular skeleton. Number of bones in each section of the appendicular skeleton is indicated in parentheses.

Clavicle (2)
Scapula (2)
Pectoral girdles (4)

Humerus (2)

Radius (2)

Ulna (2)

Upper extremities (60)

Carpus (16)

Metacarpus (10)

Phalanges (28)

Hipbone (coxae) (2)
Pelvic girdles (2)

Femur (2)

Patella (2)

Tibia (2)

Fibula (2)

Lower extremities (60)

Tarsus (14)

Metatarsus (10)

Phalanges (28)

The pectoral girdle consists of the **clavicle** and **scapula** bones. It functions to attach the upper extremity, or arm, to the axial skeleton by articulating with the sternum anteriorly and the vertebral column posteriorly. The bones of the upper extremity include the **humerus, ulna, radius, carpus, metacarpus,** and **phalanges**. These bones are illustrated in Figure 4-9 ■ and described in Table 4-3 ■.

■ **Figure 4-9** Anatomical and common names for the pectoral girdle and upper extremity.

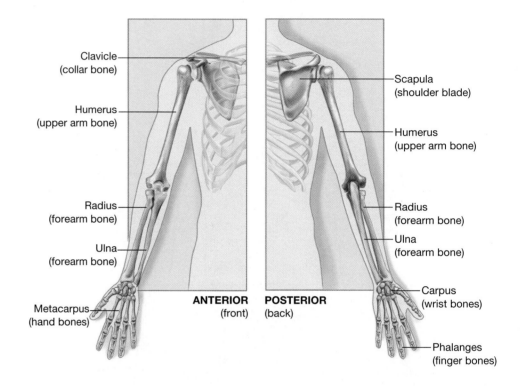

■ **TABLE 4-3**   Bones of the Pectoral Girdle and Upper Extremity

Name	Number	Description
Pectoral Girdle		
Clavicle	2	Collar bone
Scapula	2	Shoulder blade
Upper Extremity		
Humerus	2	Upper arm bone
Radius	2	Forearm bone on thumb side of lower arm
Ulna	2	Forearm bone on little finger side of lower arm
Carpus (carpal bones)	16	Bones of wrist
Metacarpus (metacarpal bones)	10	Bones in palm of hand
Phalanges	28	Finger bones; three in each finger and two in each thumb

The pelvic girdle is called the **os coxae** or the **innominate bone** or hipbone and contains the **ilium, ischium,** and **pubis**. It articulates with the sacrum posteriorly to attach the lower extremity, or leg, to the axial skeleton. The lower extremity bones include the **femur, patella, tibia, fibula, tarsus, metatarsus,** and phalanges. These bones are illustrated in Figure 4-10 ■ and described in Table 4-4 ■.

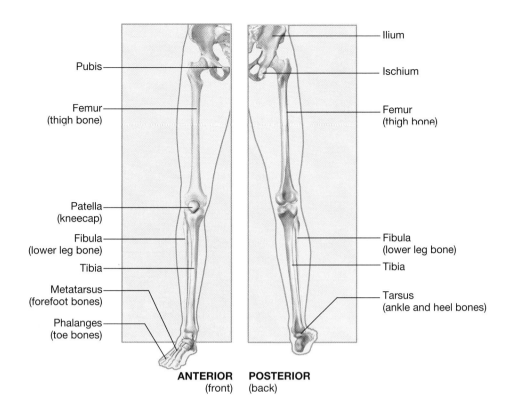

Pubis

Femur
(thigh bone)

Patella
(kneecap)

Fibula
(lower leg bone)

Tibia

Metatarsus
(forefoot bones)

Phalanges
(toe bones)

Ilium

Ischium

Femur
(thigh bone)

Fibula
(lower leg bone)

Tibia

Tarsus
(ankle and heel bones)

ANTERIOR   **POSTERIOR**
(front)   (back)

■ **Figure 4-10** Anatomical and common names for the pelvic girdle and lower extremity.

■ **TABLE 4-4**   **Bones of the Pelvic Girdle and Lower Extremity**

Name	Number	Description
Pelvic Girdle/Os Coxae		
Ilium	2	Part of the hipbone
Ischium	2	Part of the hipbone
Pubis	2	Part of the hipbone
Lower Extremity		
Femur	2	Upper leg bone; thigh bone
Patella	2	Kneecap
Tibia	2	Shin bone; thicker lower leg bone
Fibula	2	Thinner long bone in lateral side of lower leg
Tarsus (tarsal bones)	14	Ankle and heel bones
Metatarsus (metatarsal bones)	10	Forefoot bones
Phalanges	28	Toe bones; three in each toe and two in each great toe

Joints

articulation (ar-tik-yoo-LAY-shun)
bursa (BER-sah)
cartilaginous joints (kar-tih-LAJ-ih-nus)
fibrous joints (FYE-bruss)
joint capsule

range of motion
synovial fluid
synovial joint (sin-OH-vee-al)
synovial membrane

What's In A Name?

Look for these word parts:
articul/o = joint
fibr/o = fibers
synovi/o = synovial membrane
-al = pertaining to
-ous = pertaining to

Joints are formed when two or more bones meet. This is also referred to as an **articulation**. There are three types of joints determined by the amount of movement allowed between the bones: **synovial joints**, **cartilaginous joints**, and **fibrous joints** (see Figure 4-11 ■).

Skull

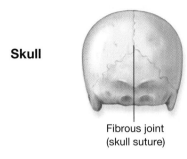

Fibrous joint
(skull suture)

Pelvis

Cartilaginous joint

Hand

Synovial joint

■ **Figure 4-11** Examples of three types of joints found in the body.

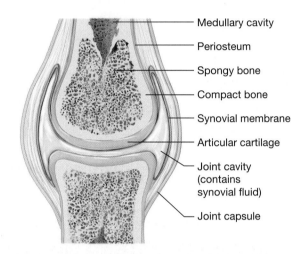

Medullary cavity

Periosteum

Spongy bone

Compact bone

Synovial membrane

Articular cartilage

Joint cavity (contains synovial fluid)

Joint capsule

■ **Figure 4-12** Structure of a generalized synovial joint.

Most joints are freely moving synovial joints (see Figure 4-12 ■), which are enclosed by an elastic **joint capsule**. The joint capsule is lined with **synovial membrane**, which secretes **synovial fluid** to lubricate the joint. As noted earlier, the ends of bones in a synovial joint are covered by a layer of articular cartilage. Cartilage is very tough, but still flexible. It withstands high levels of stress to act as a shock absorber for the joint and prevents bone from rubbing against bone. Cartilage is found in several other areas of the body, such as the nasal septum, external ear, eustachian tube, larynx, trachea, bronchi, and intervertebral disks. One example of a synovial joint is the ball-and-socket joint found at the shoulder or hip. The ball rotating in the socket allows for a wide range of motion. Bands of strong connective tissue called ligaments bind bones together at the joint. The maximum amount of movement allowed at a joint is referred to as its **range of motion** (ROM). Range of motion is measured in degrees of a circle.

Some synovial joints contain a saclike structure called a **bursa**, which is composed of connective tissue and lined with synovial membrane. Most commonly found between bones and ligaments or tendons, bursas function to reduce friction. Some common bursa locations are the elbow, knee, and shoulder joints.

Not all joints are freely moving. Fibrous joints allow almost no movement since the ends of the bones are joined by thick fibrous tissue, which may even fuse into solid bone. The sutures of the skull are an example of a fibrous joint. Cartilaginous joints allow for slight movement but hold bones firmly in place by a solid piece of cartilage. An example of this type of joint is the pubic symphysis, the point at which the left and right pubic bones meet in the front of the lower abdomen.

Med Term Tip

Bursitis is an inflammation of the bursa located between bony prominences such as at the shoulder. *Housemaid's knee*, a term thought to have originated from the damage to the knees that occurred when maids knelt to scrub floors, is a form of bursitis and carries the medical name *prepatellar bursitis*.

PRACTICE AS YOU GO

B. Give the Anatomical Name

1. kneecap _____

2. ankle bones _____

3. collar bone _____

4. thigh bone _____

5. toe bones _____

6. wrist bones _____

7. shin bone _____

8. shoulder blade _____

9. finger bones _____

Terminology

Word Parts Used to Build Skeletal System Terms

The following lists contain the combining forms, suffixes, and prefixes used to build terms in the remaining sections of this chapter.

Combining Forms

ankyl/o	stiff joint	kyph/o	hump	prosthet/o	addition
arthr/o	joint	lamin/o	lamina	pub/o	pubis
burs/o	bursa	lord/o	bent backward	radi/o	radius, ray (X-ray)
carp/o	carpus	lumb/o	loin	sacr/o	sacrum
cervic/o	neck	mandibul/o	mandible	sarc/o	flesh
chondr/o	cartilage	maxill/o	maxilla	scapul/o	scapula
clavicul/o	clavicle	medull/o	inner region	scoli/o	crooked
coccyg/o	coccyx	metacarp/o	metacarpus	spin/o	spine
cortic/o	outer layer	metatars/o	metatarsus	spondyl/o	vertebra
cost/o	rib	myel/o	bone marrow, spinal cord	stern/o	sternum
crani/o	skull			synov/o	synovial membrane
cutane/o	skin	orth/o	straight		
erythr/o	red	oste/o	bone	system/o	system
femor/o	femur	patell/o	patella	tars/o	tarsus
fibul/o	fibula	path/o	disease	thorac/o	chest
humer/o	humerus	ped/o	child; foot	tibi/o	tibia
ili/o	ilium	phalang/o	phalanges	uln/o	ulna
ischi/o	ischium	pod/o	foot	vertebr/o	vertebra

Suffixes

-ac	pertaining to	-iatry	medical treatment	-ous	pertaining to
-al	pertaining to	-ic	pertaining to	-pathy	disease
-algia	pain	-itis	inflammation	-plasty	surgical repair
-ar	pertaining to	-listhesis	slipping	-porosis	porous
-ary	pertaining to	-logic	pertaining to study of	-scope	instrument for viewing
-centesis	puncture to withdraw fluid	-logy	study of	-scopic	pertaining to visually examining
-clasia	surgically break	-malacia	abnormal softening		
-desis	to fuse	-metry	process of measuring	-scopy	process of visually examining
-eal	pertaining to			-stenosis	narrowing
-ectomy	surgical removal	-oma	tumor	-tic	pertaining to
-genic	producing	-ory	pertaining to	-tome	instrument to cut
-gram	record	-osis	abnormal condition		
-graph	to record	-otomy	cutting into		
-graphy	process of recording				

Prefixes

anti-	against	inter-	between	per-	through
bi-	two	intra-	within	pre-	before
dis-	apart	non-	not	sub-	under
ex-	outward				

Adjective Forms of Anatomical Terms

Term	Word Parts	Definition
carpal (KAR-pal)	carp/o = carpus -al = pertaining to	Pertaining to carpus
cervical (SER-vih-kal)	cervic/o = neck -al = pertaining to	Pertaining to neck
clavicular (klah-VIK-yoo-lar)	clavicul/o = clavicle -ar = pertaining to	Pertaining to clavicle
coccygeal (kok-SIH-jee-al)	coccyg/o = coccyx -eal = pertaining to	Pertaining to coccyx
cortical (KOR-tih-kal)	cortic/o = outer layer -al = pertaining to	Pertaining to outer layer
costal (KOS-tal)	cost/o = rib -al = pertaining to	Pertaining to rib
cranial (KRAY-nee-al)	crani/o = skull -al = pertaining to	Pertaining to skull
femoral (FEM-or-al)	femor/o = femur -al = pertaining to	Pertaining to femur

Adjective Forms of Anatomical Terms (continued)

Term	Word Parts	Definition
fibular (FIB-yoo-lar)	fibul/o = fibula -ar = pertaining to	Pertaining to fibula
humeral (HYOO-mer-al)	humer/o = humerus -al = pertaining to	Pertaining to humerus
iliac (IL-ee-ak)	ili/o = ilium -ac = pertaining to	Pertaining to ilium
intervertebral (in-ter-VER-teh-bral)	inter- = between vertebr/o = vertebra -al = pertaining to	Pertaining to between vertebrae
intracranial (in-trah-KRAY-nee-al)	intra- = within crani/o = skull -al = pertaining to	Pertaining to within skull
ischial (ISS-kee-al)	ischi/o = ischium -al = pertaining to	Pertaining to ischium
lumbar (LUM-bar)	lumb/o = low back -ar = pertaining to	Pertaining to low back
mandibular (man-DIB-yoo-lar)	mandibul/o = mandible -ar = pertaining to	Pertaining to mandible
maxillary (MAK-sih-lair-ee)	maxill/o = maxilla -ary = pertaining to	Pertaining to maxilla
medullary (MED-yoo-lair-ee)	medull/o = inner region -ary = pertaining to	Pertaining to inner region
metacarpal (met-ah-KAR-pal)	metacarp/o = metacarpus -al = pertaining to	Pertaining to metacarpus
metatarsal (met-ah-TAR-sal)	metatars/o = metatarsus -al = pertaining to	Pertaining to metatarsus
patellar (pah-TEL-ar)	patell/o = patella -ar = pertaining to	Pertaining to patella
phalangeal (fah-LAN-jee-al)	phalang/o = phalanges -eal = pertaining to	Pertaining to phalanges
pubic (PYOO-bik)	pub/o = pubis -ic = pertaining to	Pertaining to pubis
radial (RAY-dee-al)	radi/o = radius -al = pertaining to	Pertaining to radius
sacral (SAY-kral)	sacr/o = sacrum -al = pertaining to	Pertaining to sacrum
scapular (SKAP-yoo-lar)	scapul/o = scapula -ar = pertaining to	Pertaining to scapula
spinal (SPY-nal)	spin/o = spine -al = pertaining to	Pertaining to spine
sternal (STER-nal)	stern/o = sternum -al = pertaining to	Pertaining to sternum
tarsal (TAR-sal)	tars/o = tarsus -al = pertaining to	Pertaining to tarsus

Adjective Forms of Anatomical Terms (continued)

Term	Word Parts	Definition
thoracic (tho-RASS-ik)	thorac/o = thorax -ic = pertaining to	Pertaining to thorax
tibial (TIB-ee-al)	tibi/o = tibia -al = pertaining to	Pertaining to tibia
ulnar (UL-nar)	uln/o = ulna -ar = pertaining to	Pertaining to ulna
vertebral (VER-teh-bral)	vertebr/o = vertebra -al = pertaining to	Pertaining to a vertebra

PRACTICE AS YOU GO

C. Adjective Form Practice

Give the adjective form for the following bones.

1. femur _____
2. sternum _____
3. clavicle _____
4. coccyx _____
5. maxilla _____
6. tibia _____
7. patella _____
8. phalanges _____
9. humerus _____
10. pubis _____

Pathology

Term	Word Parts	Definition
Medical Specialties		
chiropractic (kye-roh-PRAK-tik)	-tic = pertaining to	Healthcare profession concerned with diagnosis and treatment of malalignment conditions of spine and musculoskeletal system with intention of affecting nervous system and improving health; healthcare professional is a *chiropractor*

Pathology (continued)

Term	Word Parts	Definition
orthopedics (Orth, ortho) (or-thoh-PEE-diks)	orth/o = straight ped/o = child, foot -ic = pertaining to	Branch of medicine specializing in diagnosis and treatment of conditions of musculoskeletal system; also called *orthopedic surgery*; physician is an *orthopedist* or *orthopedic surgeon*; name derived from straightening (orth/o) deformities in children (ped/o)
orthotics (or-THOT-iks)	orth/o = straight -tic = pertaining to	Healthcare profession specializing in making orthopedic appliances such as braces and splints; person skilled in making and adjusting these appliances is an *orthotist*; *orthotic* is the appliance
podiatry (poh-DYE-ah-tree)	pod/o = foot -iatry = medical treatment	Healthcare profession specializing in diagnosis and treatment of disorders of feet and lower legs; healthcare professional is a *podiatrist*
prosthetics (pross-THET-iks)	prosthet/o = addition -ic = pertaining to	Healthcare profession specializing in making artificial body parts; person skilled in making and adjusting prostheses is a *prosthetist*; *prosthesis* is a manufactured substitute for any missing body part, such as an artificial leg
rheumatology (roo-mah-TALL-oh-jee)	-logy = study of	Branch of medicine (subspecialty of internal medicine) specializing in diagnosis and treatment of musculoskeletal and autoimmune conditions affecting joints, muscles, and bones; physician is a *rheumatologist*
Signs and Symptoms		
arthralgia (ar-THRAL-jee-ah)	arthr/o = joint -algia = pain	Joint pain
bursitis (ber-SIGH-tis)	burs/o = bursa -itis = inflammation	Inflammation of a bursa
callus (KAL-us)		Mass of bone tissue that forms at fracture site during its healing
chondromalacia (kon-droh-mah-LAY-shee-ah)	chondr/o = cartilage -malacia = abnormal softening	Softening of cartilage
crepitation (krep-ih-TAY-shun)		Noise produced by bones or cartilage rubbing together in conditions such as arthritis; also called *crepitus*
ostealgia (oss-tee-AL-jee-ah)	oste/o = bone -algia = pain	Bone pain
synovitis (sin-oh-VIGH-tis)	synov/o = synovial membrane -itis = inflammation	Inflammation of synovial membrane

Pathology (continued)

Term	Word Parts	Definition
Fractures		

closed fracture		Fracture in which there is no open skin wound; also called a *simple fracture*

■ **Figure 4-13**   A) Closed (or simple) fracture and B) open (or compound) fracture.

Colles' fracture (KAW-leez)		Common type of wrist fracture

■ **Figure 4-14**   Colles' fracture.
(Akawath/Shutterstock)

comminuted fracture (kom-ih-NYOOT-ed)		Fracture in which bone is shattered, splintered, or crushed into many small pieces or fragments
compound fracture		Fracture in which bone has broken through skin; also called an *open fracture* (see Figure 4-13B)

Pathology (continued)

Term	Word Parts	Definition
compression fracture		Fracture involving loss of height of a vertebral body; may be result of trauma, but in older people, especially women, may be caused by conditions like osteoporosis
fracture (FX, Fx)		Broken bone

■ **Figure 4-15** Figure illustrating the fracture lines seen in different types of fractures. (*Alila Medical Media/Shutterstock*)

Transverse   Oblique   Spiral   Greenstick   Comminuted

Term	Word Parts	Definition
greenstick fracture		Fracture in which there is an incomplete break; one side of bone is broken and other side is bent; fracture type commonly found in children due to their softer and more pliable bone structure
impacted fracture		Fracture in which bone fragments are pushed into each other
oblique fracture (oh-BLEEK)		Fracture at an angle to bone

■ **Figure 4-16** X-ray showing oblique fracture of the humerus. (*Puwadol Jaturawutthichai/Shutterstock*)

Term	Word Parts	Definition
pathologic fracture (path-oh-LOJ-ik)	path/o = disease -logic = pertaining to study of	Fracture caused by diseased or weakened bone
spiral fracture	-al = pertaining to	Fracture in which fracture line spirals around shaft of bone; can be caused by twisting injury and is often slower to heal than other types of fractures
stress fracture		Slight fracture caused by repetitive, low-impact forces, like running, rather than single, forceful impact

Pathology (continued)

Term	Word Parts	Definition
transverse fracture		Complete fracture that is straight across bone at right angles to long axis of bone

■ **Figure 4-17** X-ray showing transverse fracture of radius and ulna. *(Puwadol Jaturawutthichai/Shutterstock)*

Bones

Term	Word Parts	Definition
chondroma (kon-DROH-mah)	chondr/o = cartilage -oma = tumor	Tumor, usually benign, that forms in cartilage
Ewing's sarcoma (YOO-ingz / sar-KOH-mah)	sarc/o = flesh -oma = tumor	Malignant growth found in shaft of long bones that spreads through periosteum; removal is treatment of choice because tumor will metastasize or spread to other organs
exostosis (eks-oss-TOH-sis)	ex- = outward oste/o = bone -osis = abnormal condition	Bony, outward projection from surface of a bone; also called *bone spur*
myeloma (my-eh-LOH-mah)	myel/o = bone marrow -oma = tumor	Tumor that forms in bone marrow tissue
osteochondroma (oss-tee-oh-kon-DROH-mah)	oste/o = bone chondr/o = cartilage -oma = tumor	Tumor, usually benign, that consists of both bone and cartilage tissue
osteogenic sarcoma (oss-tee-oh-JEN-ik / sar-KOH-mah)	oste/o = bone -genic = producing sarc/o = flesh -oma = tumor	Most common type of bone cancer; usually begins in osteocytes found at ends of long bones; also called *osteosarcoma*
osteoma (OSS-tee-oh-mah)	oste/o = bone -oma = tumor	Tumor found in bone tissue
osteomalacia (oss-tee-oh-mah-LAY-shee-ah)	oste/o = bone -malacia = abnormal softening	Softening of bones caused by deficiency of calcium; thought to be caused by insufficient sunlight and vitamin D in children

Pathology (continued)

Term	Word Parts	Definition
osteomyelitis (oss-tee-oh-my-eh-LYE-tis)	oste/o = bone myel/o = bone marrow -itis = inflammation	Inflammation of bone and bone marrow
osteopathy (oss-tee-OP-ah-thee)	oste/o = bone -pathy = disease	General term for bone disease
osteoporosis (oss-tee-oh-poh-ROH-sis)	oste/o = bone -porosis = porous	Decrease in bone mass producing a thinning and weakening of bone with resulting fractures; bone becomes more porous, especially in spine and pelvis
Paget's disease (PAH-jets)		Fairly common metabolic disease of bone from unknown causes; usually attacks middle-aged and older adults and is characterized by bone destruction and deformity; named for Sir James Paget, a British surgeon
rickets (RIK-ets)		Deficiency in calcium and vitamin D found in early childhood that results in bone deformities, especially bowed legs

Spinal Column

Term	Word Parts	Definition
ankylosing spondylitis (ang-kih-LOH-sing / spon-dih-LYE-tis)	ankyl/o = stiff joint spondyl/o = vertebra -itis = inflammation	Inflammatory spinal condition resembling rheumatoid arthritis and results in gradual stiffening and fusion of vertebrae; more common in men than in women
herniated nucleus pulposus (HNP) (HER-nee-ay-ted / NOO-klee-us / pul-POH-sus)		Herniation or protrusion of intervertebral disk; also called *herniated disk* or *ruptured disk*; may require surgery
kyphosis (kye-FOH-sis)	kyph/o = hump -osis = abnormal condition	Abnormal increase in outward curvature of thoracic spine; also known as *hunchback* or *humpback*; see Figure 4-19 ■ for illustration of abnormal spine curvatures

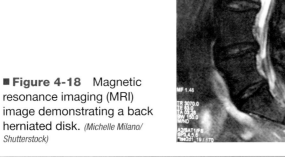

■ **Figure 4-18** Magnetic resonance imaging (MRI) image demonstrating a back herniated disk. *(Michelle Milano/ Shutterstock)*

Pathology (continued)

Term	Word Parts	Definition

■ **Figure 4-19** Abnormal spinal curvatures: kyphosis, lordosis, and scoliosis.

Kyphosis (excessive posterior thoracic curvature - hunchback)

Lordosis (excessive anterior lumbar curvature - swayback)

Scoliosis (lateral curvature)

Term	Word Parts	Definition
lordosis (lor-DOH-sis)	lord/o = bent backward -osis = abnormal condition	Abnormal increase in forward curvature of lumbar spine; also known as *swayback*
scoliosis (skoh-lee-OH-sis)	scoli/o = crooked -osis = abnormal condition	Abnormal lateral curvature of spine; see again Figure 4-19 for illustration of abnormal spine curvatures
spina bifida (SPY-nah / BIF-ih-dah)	spin/o = spine bi- = two	Congenital anomaly occurring when vertebra fails to fully form around spinal cord; see also Figure 12-12C
spinal stenosis (steh-NOH-sis)	spin/o = spine -al = pertaining to	Narrowing of spinal canal causing pressure on cord and nerves

> **Word Watch**
>
> Watch how the term *stenosis* is used in this condition. It most often appears as the suffix **-stenosis**. However, in this case, it is used as a freestanding word.

Term	Word Parts	Definition
spondylolisthesis (spon-dih-loh-liss-THEE-sis)	spondyl/o = vertebra -listhesis = slipping	Forward sliding of lumbar vertebra over vertebra below it
spondylosis (spon-dih-LOH-sis)	spondyl/o = vertebra -osis = abnormal condition	Specifically refers to ankylosing of spine, but commonly used in reference to any degenerative condition of vertebral column

Pathology (continued)

Term	Word Parts	Definition
whiplash		Cervical muscle and ligament sprain or strain as a result of sudden movement forward and backward of head and neck; can occur as a result of rear-end auto collision
Joints		
bunion (BUN-yun)		Inflammation of bursa of first metatarsophalangeal joint (base of big toe)
dislocation	dis- = apart	Occurs when bones in a joint are displaced from normal alignment and ends of bones are no longer in contact
gout (GOWT)		Type of arthritis presenting as pain and swelling usually in first metatarsophalangeal joint; caused by high uric acid blood level resulting in uric acid crystals being deposited in soft tissue; more common in men
osteoarthritis (OA) (oss-tee-oh-ar-THRY-tis)	oste/o = bone arthr/o = joint -itis = inflammation	Arthritis resulting in degeneration of bones and joints, especially those bearing weight; results in bone rubbing against bone; also called *degenerative joint disease (DJD)*
prepatellar bursitis (pree-pah-TELL-ar / ber-SIGH-tis)	pre- = before patell/o = patella -ar = pertaining to burs/o = bursa -itis = inflammation	Pain and swelling in bursa located between patella and skin; seen often in persons who kneel frequently; commonly called *housemaid's knee*
rheumatoid arthritis (RA) (ROO-mah-toyd / ar-THRY-tis)	arthr/o = joint -itis = inflammation	Chronic form of arthritis with inflammation of joints, swelling, stiffness, pain, and changes in cartilage that can result in crippling deformities; considered to be autoimmune disease

■ **Figure 4-20**   Patient with typical rheumatoid arthritis contractures. *(Michal Heron/Pearson Education, Inc.)*

Pathology (continued)

Term	Word Parts	Definition
sprain		Damage to ligaments surrounding a joint due to overstretching, but no dislocation of joint or fracture of bone
subluxation (sub-luks-AY-shun)	sub- = under	Incomplete dislocation; joint alignment is disrupted, but ends of bones remain in contact
systemic lupus erythematosus (SLE) (sis-TEM-ik / LOO-pus / air-ih-them-ah-TOH-sus)	system/o = system -ic = pertaining to erythr/o = red	Chronic inflammatory autoimmune disease of connective tissue affecting many systems that may include joint pain and arthritis; may be mistaken for rheumatoid arthritis
talipes (TAL-ih-peez)		Congenital deformity causing misalignment of ankle joint and foot; also referred to as *clubfoot*

PRACTICE AS YOU GO

D. Pathology Matching

Match each term to its definition.

_____ **1.** chondromalacia

_____ **2.** exostosis

_____ **3.** rheumatoid arthritis

_____ **4.** subluxation

_____ **5.** bunion

_____ **6.** spina bifida

_____ **7.** kyphosis

_____ **8.** osteoporosis

_____ **9.** orthotics

_____ **10.** comminuted

a. abnormal outward curvature of thoracic spine

b. an incomplete dislocation

c. thinning and weakening of the bone

d. bone spur

e. softening of cartilage

f. braces and splints

g. inflammation at base of big toe

h. shattered fracture

i. a congenital anomaly

j. considered to be an autoimmune disease

Diagnostic Procedures

Term	Word Part	Definition
Diagnostic Imaging		
arthrogram (AR-throh-gram)	arthr/o = joint -gram = record	X-ray record of a joint, usually taken after joint has been injected by contrast medium
arthrography (ar-THROG-rah-fee)	arthr/o = joint -graphy = process of recording	Process of X-raying a joint, usually after injection of contrast medium into joint space

Diagnostic Procedures (continued)

Term	Word Part	Definition
bone scan	■ **Figure 4-21** Photograph illustrating the appearance of a bone scan. The darker regions are produced by bone areas that take up more of the radioactive dye. *(Susan Law Cain/Shutterstock)*	Nuclear medicine procedure in which patient is given radioactive dye and then scanning equipment is used to visualize bones; especially useful in identifying stress fractures, observing progress of treatment for osteomyelitis, and locating cancer metastases to bone
dual-energy X-ray absorptiometry (DXA, DEXA) (ab-sorp-shee-AHM-eh-tree)	-metry = process of measuring	Measurement of bone density using low-dose X-ray for purpose of detecting osteoporosis
myelogram (MY-eh-loh-gram)	myel/o = spinal cord -gram = record	X-ray record of spinal column after injection of opaque dye
myelography (my-eh-LOG-rah-fee)	myel/o = spinal cord -graphy = process of recording	Study of spinal column after injecting opaque contrast material; particularly useful in identifying herniated nucleus pulposus pinching a spinal nerve

Med Term Tip

The combining form **myel/o** means *marrow* and is used for both the spinal cord and bone marrow. To the ancient Greek philosophers and physicians, the spinal cord appeared to be much like the marrow found in the medullary cavity of a long bone.

Term	Word Part	Definition
radiograph (RAY-dee-oh-graf)	radi/o = ray -graph = record	Image produced by X-rays striking photographic film; commonly referred to as an *X-ray*
radiography (ray-dee-OG-rah-fee)	radi/o = ray -graphy = process of recording	Diagnostic imaging procedure using X-rays to study internal structure of body; especially useful for visualizing bones and joints

Endoscopic Procedures

Term	Word Part	Definition
arthroscope (AR-throh-skohp)	arthr/o = joint -scope = instrument for viewing	Instrument used to view inside a joint

Diagnostic Procedures (continued)

Term	Word Part	Definition
arthroscopy (ar-THROS-koh-pee)	arthr/o = joint -scopy = process of visually examining	Examination of interior of a joint by entering joint with *arthroscope*; arthroscope contains small television camera that allows physician to view interior of joint on monitor during procedure; some joint conditions can be repaired during arthroscopy

Therapeutic Procedures

Term	Word Part	Definition
Medical Treatments		
arthrocentesis (ar-throh-sen-TEE-sis)	arthr/o = joint -centesis = puncture to withdraw fluid	Involves insertion of a needle into joint cavity in order to remove or aspirate fluid; may be done to remove excess fluid from a joint or to obtain fluid for examination
orthotic (or-THOT-ik)	orth/o = straight -tic = pertaining to	Orthopedic appliance, such as brace or splint, used to prevent or correct deformities
prosthesis (pross-THEE-sis)	prosthet/o = addition	Artificial device used as a substitute for body part that is either congenitally missing or absent as a result of accident or disease; example would be an artificial leg
Surgical Procedures		
amputation (am-pyoo-TAY-shun)		Partial or complete removal of a limb for a variety of reasons, including tumors, gangrene, intractable pain, crushing injury, or uncontrollable infection
arthroclasia (ar-throh-KLAY-zee-ah)	arthr/o = joint -clasia = surgically break	To forcibly break loose a fused joint while patient is under anesthetic; fusion usually caused by buildup of scar tissue or adhesions
arthrodesis (ar-throh-DEE-sis)	arthr/o = joint -desis = to fuse	Procedure to stabilize a joint by fusing bones together
arthroscopic surgery (ar-throh-SKOP-ik)	arthr/o = joint -scopic = pertaining to visually examining	Performing a surgical procedure while using arthroscope to view internal structure, such as a joint
arthrotomy (ar-THROT-oh-mee)	arthr/o = joint -otomy = cutting into	Surgical procedure that cuts into a joint capsule
bone graft		Piece of bone taken from patient used to take the place of removed bone or bony defect at another site
bunionectomy (bun-yun-EK-toh-mee)	-ectomy = surgical removal	Removal of bursa at joint of great toe
bursectomy (ber-SEK-toh-mee)	burs/o = bursa -ectomy = surgical removal	Surgical removal of a bursa
chondrectomy (kon-DREK-toh-mee)	chondr/o = cartilage -ectomy = surgical removal	Surgical removal of cartilage
chondroplasty (KON-droh-plas-tee)	chondr/o = cartilage -plasty = surgical repair	Surgical repair of cartilage
craniotomy (kray-nee-OT-oh-mee)	crani/o = skull -otomy = cutting into	Surgical procedure that cuts into skull

Therapeutic Procedures (continued)

Term	Word Part	Definition
laminectomy (lam-ih-NEK-toh-mee)	lamin/o = lamina -ectomy = surgical removal	Removal of vertebral posterior arch to correct severe back problems and pain caused by compression of spinal nerve
osteoclasia (oss-tee-oh-KLAY-zee-ah)	oste/o = bone -clasia = surgically break	Surgical procedure involving intentional breaking of bone to correct a deformity
osteotome (OSS-tee-oh-tohm)	oste/o = bone -tome = instrument to cut	Instrument used to cut bone
osteotomy (oss-tee-OT-ah-mee)	oste/o = bone -otomy = cutting into	Surgical procedure that cuts into a bone
percutaneous diskectomy (per-kyoo-TAY-nee-us / dis-KEK-toh-mee)	per- = through cutane/o = skin -ous = pertaining to -ectomy = surgical removal	Thin catheter tube is inserted into intervertebral disk through skin and herniated or ruptured disk material is sucked out or a laser is used to vaporize it
spinal fusion	spin/o = spine -al = pertaining to	Surgical immobilization of adjacent vertebrae; may be done for several reasons, including correction for herniated disk
synovectomy (sin-oh-VEK-toh-mee)	synov/o = synovial membrane -ectomy = surgical removal	Surgical removal of synovial membrane
total hip arthroplasty (THA) (AR-throh-plas-tee)	arthr/o = joint -plasty = surgical repair	Surgical reconstruction of hip by implanting prosthetic or artificial hip joint; also called *total hip replacement (THR)*

■ **Figure 4-22** Prosthetic hip joint. *(Alex Mit/Shutterstock)*

Term	Word Part	Definition
total knee arthroplasty (TKA) (AR-throh-plas-tee)	arthr/o = joint -plasty = surgical repair	Surgical reconstruction of knee joint by implanting prosthetic knee joint; also called *total knee replacement (TKR)*

Fracture Care

Term	Word Part	Definition
cast		Application of solid material to immobilize extremity or portion of body as a result of fracture, dislocation, or severe injury; may be made of plaster of Paris or fiberglass
fixation		Procedure to stabilize fractured bone while it heals; *external fixation* includes casts, splints, and pins inserted through skin; *internal fixation* includes pins, plates, rods, screws, and wires that are applied during *open reduction*

Therapeutic Procedures (continued)

Term	Word Part	Definition
reduction		Correcting fracture by realigning bone fragments; *closed reduction* is doing manipulation without entering body; *open reduction* is process of making surgical incision at site of fracture to do reduction; necessary when bony fragments need to be removed or *internal fixation*, such as plates or pins, is required
traction		Applying a pulling force on fractured or dislocated limb or vertebral column in order to restore normal alignment

PRACTICE AS YOU GO

E. Procedure Matching

Match each term to its definition.

_____ **1.** reduction

_____ **2.** osteoclasia

_____ **3.** bone scan

_____ **4.** radiograph

_____ **5.** prosthesis

_____ **6.** arthrodesis

a. an X-ray

b. fusing bones to stabilize a joint

c. intentional breaking of a bone

d. replacement body part

e. realigning bone fragments

f. nuclear medicine procedure

Pharmacology

Classification	Word Parts	Action	Examples
bone reabsorption inhibitors		Conditions that result in weak and fragile bones, such as osteoporosis and Paget's disease, are improved by medications that inhibit reabsorption of bones	alendronate, Fosamax; ibandronate, Boniva
calcium supplements and vitamin D therapy		Maintaining high blood levels of calcium in association with vitamin D helps maintain bone density; used to treat osteomalacia, osteoporosis, and rickets	calcium carbonate, Oystercal, Tums; calcium citrate, Cal-Citrate, Citracal
corticosteroids	**cortic/o** = outer layer	Natural or synthetic adrenal cortex hormone; has very strong anti-inflammatory properties; particularly useful in treating rheumatoid arthritis	prednisone; methylprednisolone, Medrol; dexamethasone, Decadron
nonsteroidal anti-inflammatory drugs (NSAIDs)	**non-** = not **-al** = pertaining to **anti-** = against **-ory** = pertaining to	Large group of drugs (other than corticosteroids) that provide mild pain relief and anti-inflammatory benefits for conditions such as arthritis	ibuprofen, Advil, Motrin; naproxen, Aleve, Naprosyn; aspirin, Bayer's, Bufferin

Abbreviations

AE	above elbow	**NSAID**	nonsteroidal anti-inflammatory drug
AK	above knee	**OA**	osteoarthritis
BDT	bone density testing	**ORIF**	open reduction–internal fixation
BE	below elbow	**Orth, ortho**	orthopedics
BK	below knee	**P**	phosphorus
C1, C2, etc.	first cervical vertebra, second cervical vertebra, etc.	**RA**	rheumatoid arthritis
Ca	calcium	**RLE**	right lower extremity
DJD	degenerative joint disease	**ROM**	range of motion
DXA, DEXA	dual-energy X-ray absorptiometry	**RUE**	right upper extremity
FX, Fx	fracture	**SLE**	systemic lupus erythematosus
HNP	herniated nucleus pulposus	**T1, T2, etc.**	first thoracic vertebra, second thoracic vertebra, etc.
JRA	juvenile rheumatoid arthritis	**THA**	total hip arthroplasty
L1, L2, etc.	first lumbar vertebra, second lumbar vertebra, etc.	**THR**	total hip replacement
LE	lower extremity	**TKA**	total knee arthroplasty
LLE	left lower extremity	**TKR**	total knee replacement
LUE	left upper extremity	**UE**	upper extremity

PRACTICE AS YOU GO

F. What's the Abbreviation?

1. total knee replacement _____

2. herniated nucleus pulposus _____

3. upper extremity _____

4. fifth lumbar vertebra _____

5. above the knee _____

6. fracture _____

7. nonsteroidal anti-inflammatory drug _____

SECTION II: MUSCULAR SYSTEM

AT A GLANCE

Function

Muscles are bundles, sheets, or rings of tissue that produce movement by contracting and pulling on the structures to which they are attached.

Organs

The primary structure that comprises the muscular system:

muscles

Word Parts

Presented here are the most common word parts (with their meanings) used to build muscular system terms. For a more comprehensive list, refer to the Terminology section of this chapter.

Combining Forms

duct/o	to bring	**myos/o**	muscle
extens/o	to stretch out	**phon/o**	sound
fasci/o	fibrous band	**physic/o**	body
fibr/o	fibers	**plant/o**	sole of foot
flex/o	to bend	**rotat/o**	to revolve
habilitat/o	ability	**ten/o**	tendon
hydr/o	water	**tend/o**	tendon
kinesi/o	movement	**tendin/o**	tendon
muscul/o	muscle	**therm/o**	heat
my/o	muscle	**vers/o**	to turn

Suffixes

-asthenia	weakness
-ion	action
-kinesia	movement
-phoresis	carrying
-tonia	tone
-trophic	pertaining to development

Prefixes

ab-	away from
ad-	toward
circum-	around
e-	outward

Frontalis

Orbicularis oris

Sternocleidomastoid

Trapezius

Deltoid

Pectoralis

Biceps brachii

Rectus abdominis

Brachioradialis

External oblique

Sartorius

Rectus femoris

Vastus medialis

Tibialis anterior

Gastrocnemius

Anatomy and Physiology of the Muscular System

muscle fibers   muscles

Muscles are bundles of parallel **muscle fibers**. As these fibers contract (shorten in length) they produce movement of or within the body. The movement may take the form of bringing two bones closer together, pushing food through the digestive system, or pumping blood through blood vessels. In addition to producing movement, muscles also hold the body erect and generate heat.

Types of Muscles

cardiac muscle   smooth muscle

involuntary muscles   voluntary muscles

skeletal muscle

The three types of muscle tissue are **skeletal muscle**, **smooth muscle**, and **cardiac muscle** (see Figure 4-23 ■). Muscle tissue may be either voluntary or involuntary. **Voluntary muscles** are those muscles for which a person consciously chooses to contract and for how long and how hard to contract them. The skeletal muscles of the arm and leg are examples of this type of muscle. **Involuntary muscles** are the muscles under the control of the subconscious regions of the brain. The smooth muscles found in internal organs and cardiac muscles are examples of involuntary muscle tissue.

Skeletal muscle

Cardiac muscle

Smooth muscle

■ **Figure 4-23** The three types of muscles: skeletal, smooth, and cardiac.

Skeletal Muscle

fascia (FASH-ee-ah)
motor neurons
myoneural junction (my-oh-NOO-ral)

neuromuscular junction
(noo-roh-MUS-kyoo-lar)
striated muscles (STRY-ay-ted)

tendon (TEN-dun)

A skeletal muscle is directly or indirectly attached to a bone and produces voluntary movement of the skeleton. It is also referred to as a **striated muscle** because of its striped appearance under a microscope (see Figure 4-24 ■). Each muscle is wrapped in layers of fibrous connective tissue called **fascia**. The fascia tapers at each end of a skeletal muscle to form a very strong **tendon**. The tendon then inserts into the periosteum covering a bone to anchor the muscle to the bone. Skeletal muscles are stimulated by **motor neurons** of the nervous system. The point at which the motor nerve contacts a muscle fiber is called the **myoneural junction** or the **neuromuscular junction**.

> **Med Term Tip**
>
> The human body has more than 400 skeletal muscles, which account for almost 50% of the body's weight.

Smooth Muscle

visceral muscle (VISS-er-ral)

Smooth muscle tissue is found in association with internal organs. For this reason, it is also referred to as **visceral muscle**. The name *smooth muscle* refers to the muscle's microscopic appearance; it lacks the striations of skeletal muscle (see again Figure 4-24). Smooth muscle is found in the walls of hollow organs, such as the stomach; tube-shaped organs, such as the respiratory airways; and blood vessels. It is responsible for the involuntary muscle action associated with movement of the internal organs, such as churning food, constricting a blood vessel, and uterine contractions.

> **What's In A Name?**
>
> Look for these word parts:
> **cardi/o** = heart
> **muscul/o** = muscle
> **my/o** = muscle
> **neur/o** = nerve
> **viscer/o** = internal organ
> **-al** = pertaining to
> **-ar** = pertaining to

Cardiac Muscle

myocardium (my-oh-KAR-dee-um)

Cardiac muscle, or **myocardium**, makes up the wall of the heart (see again Figure 4-24). With each involuntary contraction, the heart squeezes to pump blood out of its chambers and through the blood vessels. This muscle is more thoroughly described in Chapter 5, Cardiovascular System.

	Visceral (smooth)	**Skeletal** (striated)	**Cardiac** (striated)
Contracts	Slowly	Rapidly	Rapidly
Found	Viscera, blood vessels	Trunk, extremities, head and neck	Heart
Control	Involuntary	Voluntary	Involuntary

■ **Figure 4-24**
Characteristics of the three types of muscles.

PRACTICE AS YOU GO

G. Complete the Statement

1. Another name for visceral muscle is _____ muscle.

2. Nerves contact skeletal muscle fibers at the _____ junction.

3. The three types of muscle are _____, _____, and _____.

Naming Skeletal Muscles

biceps (BYE-seps)

extensor carpi

external oblique

flexor carpi

gluteus maximus (GLOO-tee-us / MAKS-ih-mus)

rectus abdominis (REK-tus / ab-DOM-ih-nis)

sternocleidomastoid (ster-noh-kly-doh-MAS-toyd)

The name of a muscle often reflects its location, origin and insertion, size, action, fiber direction, or number of attachment points, as illustrated by the following examples:

- **Location:** the term **rectus abdominis** means *straight* (rectus) abdominal muscle.
- **Origin and insertion:** the **sternocleidomastoid** is named for its two origins (**stern/o** for sternum and **cleid/o** for clavicle) and single insertion (mastoid process).
- **Size:** when gluteus, meaning rump area, is combined with maximus, meaning large, we have the term **gluteus maximus**.
- **Action:** the **flexor carpi** and **extensor carpi** muscles are named as such because they produce flexion and extension at the wrist.
- **Fiber direction:** the **external oblique** muscle is an abdominal muscle whose fibers run at an oblique angle.
- **Number of attachment points:** the prefix **bi-**, meaning two, can form the medical term **biceps**, which refers to the muscle in the upper arm that has two heads or connecting points.

What's In A Name?
Look for these word parts:
cleid/o = clavicle
extens/o = to stretch out
flex/o = to bend
stern/o = sternum
-al = pertaining to
bi- = two
ex- = outward

Skeletal Muscle Actions

action

antagonistic pairs

insertion

origin

Skeletal muscles are attached to two different bones and overlap a joint. When a muscle contracts, the two bones move, but not usually equally. The less movable of the two bones is considered to be the starting point of the muscle and is called the **origin**. The more movable bone is considered to be where the muscle ends and is called the **insertion** (see Figure 4-25 ■). The type of movement a muscle produces is called its **action**. Muscles are often arranged around joints in **antagonistic pairs**, meaning that they produce opposite actions. For example, one muscle will bend a joint while its antagonist is responsible for straightening the joint. Some common terminology for muscle actions are described in Table 4-5 ■.

■ **Figure 4-25**   Origin and insertion of a muscle

Origins

Biceps brachii

Insertion

Action-Flexion

■ **TABLE 4-5**   Muscle Actions Grouped by Antagonistic Pairs

Action	Word Parts	Description
abduction (ab-DUK-shun)	**ab-** = away from **duct/o** = to bring **-ion** = action	Movement away from midline of the body (see Figure 4-26 ■)
adduction (ah-DUK-shun)	**ad-** = toward **duct/o** = to bring **-ion** = action	Movement toward midline of the body (see again Figure 4-26)
flexion (FLEK-shun)	**flex/o** = to bend **-ion** = action	Act of bending or being bent (see Figure 4-27 ■)

180°

abduction to 180°

adduction to 50°

0°

180°   160°

Flexion to 160°

0° Extension

■ **Figure 4-26**   Abduction and adduction of the shoulder joint. *(Patrick Watson/Pearson Education, Inc.)*

■ **Figure 4-27**   Flexion and extension of the elbow joint. *(Patrick Watson/Pearson Education, Inc.)*

■ **TABLE 4-5**   Muscle Actions Grouped by Antagonistic Pairs (continued)

Action	Word Parts	Description
extension (eks-TEN-shun)	**extens/o** = to stretch out **-ion** = action	Movement that brings limb into or toward a straight condition (see again Figure 4-27)
dorsiflexion (dor-sih-FLEK-shun)	**dors/o** = back of body **flex/o** = to bend **-ion** = action	Backward bending, as of hand or foot (see Figure 4-28A ■)
plantar flexion (PLAN-tar / FLEK-shun)	**plant/o** = sole of foot **-ar** = pertaining to **flex/o** = to bend **-ion** = action	Bending sole of foot; pointing toes downward (see Figure 4-28B ■)

A   B

■ **Figure 4-28**   Dorsiflexion (A) and plantar flexion (B) of the ankle joint.   *(Alan Poulsons Photography/Shutterstock)*

eversion (ee-VER-zhun)	**e-** = outward **vers/o** = to turn **-ion** = action	Turning outward (see Figure 4-29 ■)
inversion (in-VER-zhun)	**in-** = inward **vers/o** = to turn **-ion** = action	Turning inward (see again Figure 4-29)
pronation (proh-NAY-shun)		To turn downward or backward as with the hand or foot (see Figure 4-30 ■)
supination (soo-pih-NAY-shun)		Turning the palm or foot upward (see again Figure 4-30)
elevation		To raise a body part, as in shrugging the shoulders
depression		A downward movement, as in dropping the shoulders

The circular actions described below are an exception to the antagonistic pair arrangement.

circumduction (ser-kum-DUK-shun)	**circum-** = around **duct/o** = to bring **-ion** = action	Movement in a circular direction from a central point as if drawing a large, imaginary circle in the air
opposition	**Med Term Tip** Primates are the only animals with opposable thumbs.	Moving thumb away from palm; the ability to move the thumb into contact with the other fingers
rotation	**rotat/o** = to revolve **-ion** = action	Moving around a central axis

■ TABLE 4-5   Muscle Actions Grouped by Antagonistic Pairs (continued)

■ Figure 4-29   Eversion and inversion of the foot.
(Patrick Watson/Pearson Education, Inc.)

■ Figure 4-30   Pronation and supination of the forearm.
(Patrick Watson/Pearson Education, Inc.)

PRACTICE AS YOU GO

H. Terminology Matching

Match each term to its definition.

1. _____ abduction		**a.**	backward bending of the foot
2. _____ rotation		**b.**	bending the foot to point toes toward the ground
3. _____ plantar flexion		**c.**	straightening motion
4. _____ extension		**d.**	motion around a central axis
5. _____ dorsiflexion		**e.**	motion away from the body
6. _____ flexion		**f.**	moving the thumb away from the palm
7. _____ adduction		**g.**	motion toward the body
8. _____ opposition		**h.**	bending motion

Terminology
Word Parts Used to Build Muscular System Terms

The following lists contain the combining forms, suffixes, and prefixes used to build terms in the remaining sections of this chapter.

Combining Forms

bi/o = life	**hydr/o** = water	**phon/o** = sound
carp/o = carpus	**kinesi/o** = movement	**physic/o** = body
cry/o = cold	**later/o** = side	**ten/o** = tendon
electr/o = electricity	**muscul/o** = muscle	**tend/o** = tendon
fasci/o = fibrous band	**my/o** = muscle	**tendin/o** = tendon
fibr/o = fibers	**myos/o** = muscle	**therm/o** = heat
habilitat/o = ability	**necr/o** = death	

Suffixes

-al = pertaining to	**-ic** = pertaining to	**-phoresis** = carrying
-algia = pain	**-itis** = inflammation	**-plasty** = surgical repair
-ar = pertaining to	**-kinesia** = movement	**-rrhaphy** = suture
-asthenia = weakness	**-logy** = study of	**-rrhexis** = rupture
-desis = to fuse	**-opsy** = view of	**-therapy** = treatment
-dynia = pain	**-otomy** = cutting into	**-tonia** = tone
-gram = record	**-ous** = pertaining to	**-trophic** = pertaining to development
-graphy = process of recording	**-pathy** = disease	**-trophy** = development

Prefixes

a- = without	**hyper-** = excessive	**re-** = again
brady- = slow	**hypo-** = insufficient	**ultra-** = beyond
dys- = abnormal; difficult	**poly-** = many	
epi- = above	**pseudo-** = false	

Adjective Forms of Anatomical Terms

Term	Word Parts	Definition
fascial (FASH-ee-al)	fasci/o = fibrous band -al = pertaining to	Pertaining to fascia
muscular (MUS-kyoo-lar)	muscul/o = muscle -ar = pertaining to	Pertaining to muscles
musculoskeletal (mus-kyoo-loh-SKEL-eh-tal)	muscul/o = muscle -al = pertaining to	Pertaining to muscles and skeleton
tendinous (TEN-dih-nus)	tendin/o = tendon -ous = pertaining to	Pertaining to tendons

Pathology

Term	Word Parts	Definition
Medical Specialties		
kinesiology (kih-nee-see-ALL-oh-jee)	kinesi/o = movement -logy = study of	Science that studies movement, how it is produced, and muscles involved
occupational therapy (OT)	-al = pertaining to	Assists persons to regain, develop, and improve skills important for independent functioning (activities of daily living); specialist is *occupational therapist*
physical medicine	physic/o = body -al = pertaining to	Branch of medicine focused on restoring function; primarily cares for patients with musculoskeletal and nervous system disorders; physician is *physiatrist*
physical therapy (PT)	physic/o = body -al = pertaining to	Evaluation and treatment of disorders and rehabilitation of people using physical methods such as heat, cold, massage, and exercise; specialist is *physical therapist*
Signs and Symptoms		
adhesion		Scar tissue forming in fascia surrounding muscle, making it difficult to stretch muscle
atonia	a- = without -tonia = tone	Lack of muscle tone
atrophy (AT-rah-fee)	a- = without -trophy = development	Poor muscle development as a result of muscle disease, nervous system disease, or lack of use; commonly referred to as *muscle wasting*
bradykinesia (brad-ee-kih-NEE-zee-ah)	brady- = slow -kinesia = movement	Having slow movements
contracture (kon-TRAK-chur)		Abnormal shortening of muscle fibers, tendons, or fascia, making it difficult to stretch muscle
dyskinesia (dis-kih-NEE-zee-ah)	dys- = difficult, abnormal -kinesia = movement	Having difficult or abnormal movement
dystonia	dys- = abnormal -tonia = tone	Having abnormal muscle tone
hyperkinesia (high-per-kih-NEE-zee-ah)	hyper- = excessive -kinesia = movement	Having excessive amount of movement
hypertonia	hyper- = excessive -tonia = tone	Having excessive muscle tone
hypertrophy (high-PER-troh-fee)	hyper- = excessive -trophy = development	Increase in muscle bulk as a result of use, as with lifting weights
hypokinesia (high-poh-kih-NEE-zee-ah)	hypo- = insufficient -kinesia = movement	Having insufficient amount of movement
hypotonia	hypo- = insufficient -tonia = tone	Having insufficient muscle tone
intermittent claudication (klaw-dih-KAY-shun)		Attacks of severe pain and lameness caused by ischemia of muscles, typically calf muscles; brought on by walking even very short distances

Pathology (continued)

Term	Word Parts	Definition
myalgia (my-AL-jee-ah)	my/o = muscle -algia = pain	Muscle pain
myasthenia (my-as-THEE-nee-ah)	my/o = muscle -asthenia = weakness	Muscle weakness
myotonia	my/o = muscle -tonia = tone	Muscle tone
spasm		Sudden, involuntary, strong muscle contraction
tenodynia (ten-oh-DIN-ee-ah)	ten/o = tendon -dynia = pain	Tendon pain
Muscles		
fibromyalgia (figh-broh-my-AL-jee-ah)	fibr/o = fibers my/o = muscle -algia = pain	Condition with widespread aching and pain in muscles and soft tissue
lateral epicondylitis (ep-ih-kon-dih-LYE-tis)	later/o = side -al = pertaining to epi- = above -itis = inflammation	Inflammation of muscle attachment to lateral epicondyle of elbow; often caused by strongly gripping; commonly called *tennis elbow*
muscular dystrophy (MD) (MUS-kyoo-lar / DIS-troh-fee)	muscul/o = muscle -ar = pertaining to dys- = abnormal -trophy = development	Inherited disease causing progressive muscle degeneration, weakness, and atrophy
myopathy (my-OP-ah-thee)	my/o = muscle -pathy = disease	General term for muscle disease
myorrhexis (my-oh-REK-sis)	my/o = muscle -rrhexis = rupture	Tearing a muscle
necrotizing fasciitis (NF) (NEK-ruh-tye-zing / fash-ee-EYE-tis)	necr/o = death fasci/o = fibrous band -itis = inflammation	Infection, usually bacterial, that results in death of body's soft tissue (skin, fat, and fascia); commonly called *flesh-eating disease*
polymyositis (pol-ee-my-oh-SIGH-tis)	poly- = many myos/o = muscle -itis = inflammation	Simultaneous inflammation of two or more muscles
pseudohypertrophic muscular dystrophy (soo-doh-high-per-TROH-fik)	pseudo- = false hyper- = excessive -trophic = pertaining to development muscul/o = muscle -ar = pertaining to dys- = abnormal -trophy = development	Type of inherited muscular dystrophy in which muscle tissue is gradually replaced by fatty tissue, giving appearance of a healthy and strong muscle; also called *Duchenne's muscular dystrophy*
torticollis (tor-tih-KALL-iss)		Severe neck spasms pulling head to one side; commonly called *wryneck* or a *crick in the neck*
Tendons, Muscles, and/or Ligaments		
carpal tunnel syndrome (CTS)	carp/o = carpus -al = pertaining to	Repetitive motion disorder with pain caused by compression of finger flexor tendons and median nerve as they pass through carpal tunnel of wrist

Pathology (continued)

Term	Word Parts	Definition
ganglion cyst (GANG-lee-on)		Cyst that forms on tendon sheath, usually on hand, wrist, or ankle
repetitive motion disorder		Group of chronic disorders involving tendon, muscle, joint, and nerve damage, resulting from tissue being subjected to pressure, vibration, or repetitive movements for prolonged periods
rotator cuff injury		Rotator cuff consists of joint capsule of shoulder joint reinforced by tendons from several shoulder muscles; high degree of flexibility at shoulder joint puts rotator cuff at risk for strain and tearing
strain		Damage to muscle, tendons, or ligaments due to overuse or overstretching
tendinitis (ten-dih-NIGH-tis)	tendin/o = tendon -itis = inflammation	Inflammation of a tendon

PRACTICE AS YOU GO

I. Terminology Matching

Match each term to its definition.

_____ **1.** adhesion

_____ **2.** lateral epicondylitis

_____ **3.** carpal tunnel syndrome

_____ **4.** myasthenia

_____ **5.** spasm

_____ **6.** muscular dystrophy

_____ **7.** dyskinesia

_____ **8.** intermittent claudication

a. repetitive motion disorder

b. typically occurs in the calf muscles

c. inherited condition

d. scar tissue

e. sudden, involuntary muscle contraction

f. difficult or abnormal movement

g. *tennis elbow*

h. muscle weakness

Diagnostic Procedures

Term	Word Parts	Definition
Clinical Laboratory Test		
creatine kinase (CK) (KREE-ah-teen / KYE-nase)		Muscle enzyme found in skeletal muscle and cardiac muscle; blood levels become elevated in disorders such as heart attack, muscular dystrophy, and other skeletal muscle pathologies; also known as *creatine phosphokinase (CPK)*

Diagnostic Procedures (continued)

Term	Word Parts	Definition
Additional Diagnostic Procedures		
deep tendon reflexes (DTR)		Muscle contraction in response to a stretch caused by striking muscle tendon with a reflex hammer; test used to determine if muscles are responding properly
electromyogram (EMG) (ee-lek-troh-MY-oh-gram)	electr/o = electricity my/o = muscle -gram = record	Hardcopy record produced by electromyography
electromyography (EMG) (ee-lek-troh-my-OG-rah-fee)	electr/o = electricity my/o = muscle -graphy = process of recording	Study and record of strength and quality of muscle contractions as a result of electrical stimulation
muscle biopsy (BYE-op-see)	bi/o = life -opsy = view of	Removal of muscle tissue for pathological examination

Therapeutic Procedures

Term	Word Parts	Definition
Rehabilitation Procedures		
activities of daily living (ADLs)		Activities usually performed during a normal day, such as eating, dressing, and washing
cryotherapy (kry-oh-THAIR-ah-pee)	cry/o = cold -therapy = treatment	Use of cold in a treatment
gait training		Assisting patient to learn to walk again or how to use assistive device (such as crutches or walker) to walk
hydrotherapy (high-droh-THAIR-ah-pee)	hydr/o = water -therapy = treatment	Application of warm water as a treatment; can be done in baths, swimming pools, and whirlpools
massage		Kneading or applying pressure by hands to part of body to promote muscle relaxation and reduce tension
mobilization		Treatments such as exercise, massage, and physical manipulation to restore movement to joints and soft tissue
passive range of motion (PROM)		Putting a joint through available range of motion without assistance from patient
phonophoresis (foh-noh-foh-REE-sis)	phon/o = sound -phoresis = carrying	Use of ultrasound waves to introduce medication across skin and into subcutaneous tissues
rehabilitation	re- = again habilitat/o = ability	Process of treatment and exercise that can help person with disability attain maximum function and well-being

■ **Figure 4-31** An occupational therapist assisting a patient with learning independence in activities of daily living *(Lisa S./Shutterstock)*

Therapeutic Procedures (continued)

Term	Word Parts	Definition
therapeutic exercise (thair-ah-PYOO-tik)	-ic = pertaining to	Exercise planned and carried out to achieve specific physical benefit, such as improved range of motion, muscle strengthening, or cardiovascular function
thermotherapy (ther-moh-THAIR-ah-pee)	therm/o = heat -therapy = treatment	Applying heat—often in form of moist, hot packs—to body for therapeutic purposes
ultrasound (US)	ultra- = beyond	Use of high-frequency sound waves to create heat in soft tissues under skin; particularly useful for treating injuries to muscles, tendons, and ligaments, as well as muscle spasms

■ Figure 4-32 Ultrasound treatment to thoracic (neck and upper back) region. *(Microgen/Shutterstock)*

Med Term Tip

Ultrasound waves serve two very different purposes, one of which is for diagnostic imaging. The echoes of these high-frequency waves bouncing off internal structures are captured by a computer and used to generate an image. The other purpose is for the therapeutic treatment of muscle pain and spasms. The same high-frequency sound waves cause the molecules they strike to vibrate, thereby generating heat deep in the muscle tissue.

Surgical Procedures

Term	Word Parts	Definition
carpal tunnel release	carp/o = carpus -al = pertaining to	Surgical cutting of ligament in wrist to relieve nerve pressure caused by carpal tunnel syndrome, which can result from repetitive motion such as typing
fasciotomy (fash-ee-OT-oh-mee)	fasci/o = fibrous band -otomy = cutting into	Surgical procedure that cuts into fascia
myoplasty (MY-oh-plas-tee)	my/o = muscle -plasty = surgical repair	Surgical procedure to repair a muscle
myorrhaphy (my-OR-ah-fee)	my/o = muscle -rrhaphy = suture	To suture a muscle
tendoplasty (TEN-doh-plas-tee)	tend/o = tendon -plasty = surgical repair	Surgical procedure to repair a tendon
tendotomy (ten-DOT-oh-mee)	tend/o = tendon -otomy = cutting into	Surgical procedure that cuts into a tendon
tenodesis (ten-oh-DEE-sis)	ten/o = tendon -desis = fuse	Surgical procedure to stabilize a joint by anchoring down tendons of muscles that move joint
tenoplasty (TEN-oh-plas-tee)	ten/o = tendon -plasty = surgical repair	Surgical procedure to repair a tendon
tenorrhaphy (teh-NOR-ah-fee)	ten/o = tendon -rrhaphy = suture	To suture a tendon

Pharmacology

Classification	Word Parts	Action	Examples
skeletal muscle relaxants	-al = pertaining to	Medication to relax skeletal muscles in order to reduce muscle spasms; also called *antispasmodics*	cyclobenzaprine, Flexeril; carisoprodol, Soma

Abbreviations

ADLs	activities of daily living	**MD**	muscular dystrophy
CK	creatine kinase	**NF**	necrotizing fasciitis
CPK	creatine phosphokinase	**OT**	occupational therapy
CTS	carpal tunnel syndrome	**PROM**	passive range of motion
DTR	deep tendon reflex	**PT**	physical therapy
EMG	electromyogram	**US**	ultrasound
IM	intramuscular		

PRACTICE AS YOU GO

J. What's the Abbreviation?

1. intramuscular _____

2. deep tendon reflex _____

3. muscular dystrophy _____

4. electromyogram _____

5. carpal tunnel syndrome _____

Chapter Review

Real-World Applications

Medical Record Analysis

This Discharge Summary contains 10 medical terms. Underline each term and write it in the list below the report. Then explain each term as you would to a nonmedical person.

Discharge Summary

Admitting Diagnosis:	Osteoarthritis bilateral knees
Final Diagnosis:	Osteoarthritis bilateral knees with right TKA
History of Present Illness:	Patient is a 68-year-old male. He reports experiencing occasional knee pain and swelling since he injured his knees playing football in high school. These symptoms became worse while he was in his 50s and working on a concrete surface. The right knee has always been more painful than the left. He saw his orthopedic surgeon six months ago because of constant knee pain and swelling severe enough to interfere with sleep and all activities. He required a cane to walk. Radiographs indicated severe bilateral osteoarthritis. He is admitted to the hospital at this time for TKR right knee.
Summary of Hospital Course:	Patient tolerated the surgical procedure well. He began intensive physical therapy for lower-extremity therapeutic exercise and gait training with a walker. He received occupational therapy instruction in ADLs, especially dressing and personal care. He was able to transfer himself out of bed by the third post-op day and was able to ambulate 150 ft with a walker and dress himself on the fifth post-op day.
Discharge Plans:	Patient was discharged home with his wife one week post-op. He will continue rehabilitation as an outpatient. Return to office for post-op checkup in one week.

Term **Explanation**

1.
2.
3.
4.
5.
6.
7.
8.
9.
10.

Chart Note Transcription

The chart note below contains 11 phrases that can be reworded with a medical term presented in this chapter. Each phrase is identified with an underline. Determine the medical term and write your answers in the space provided.

Pearson General Hospital Consultation Report

Task	Edit	View	Time Scale	Options	Help	Download	Archive	Date: 17 May 2017

Current Complaint:	An 82-year-old female was transported to the Emergency Room via ambulance with severe left hip pain following a fall on the ice.
Past History:	Patient suffered a <u>broken wrist bone</u> **1** two years earlier that required <u>immobilization by solid material</u>. **2** Following this <u>broken bone,</u> **3** her <u>physician who specializes in treatment of bone conditions</u> **4** diagnosed her with moderate <u>porous bones</u> **5** on the basis of a <u>low-dose X-ray for bone density</u>. **6**
Signs and Symptoms:	Patient reported severe left hip pain, rating it as 8 on a scale of 1 to 10. She held her hip <u>in a bent position</u> **7** and could not tolerate <u>movement toward a straight position</u>. **8** X-rays of the left hip and leg were taken.
Diagnosis:	<u>Shattered broken bone</u> **9** in the neck of the left <u>thigh bone</u>. **10**
Treatment:	<u>Implantation of an artificial hip joint</u> **11** on the left.

1. _____

2. _____

3. _____

4. _____

5. _____

6. _____

7. _____

8. _____

9. _____

10. _____

11. _____

Case Study

Below is a case study presentation of a patient with a condition discussed in this chapter. Read the case study and answer the questions below. Some questions will ask for information not included within this chapter. Use your text, a medical dictionary, or any other reference material you choose to answer these questions.

Mary Pearl, age 60, has come into the physician's office complaining of swelling, stiffness, and arthralgia, especially in her elbows, wrists, and hands. A bone scan revealed acute inflammation in multiple joints with damaged articular cartilage, and an erythrocyte sedimentation rate blood test indicated a significant level of acute inflammation in the body. A diagnosis of acute episode of rheumatoid arthritis was made. The physician ordered nonsteroidal anti-inflammatory medication and physical therapy. The therapist initiated a treatment program of hydrotherapy and therapeutic exercises.

(Monkey Business Images/ Shutterstock)

Questions

1. What pathological condition does this patient have? Look this condition up in a reference source and include a short description of it.

2. What type of long-term damage may occur in a patient with rheumatoid arthritis?

3. Describe the other major type of arthritis mentioned in this textbook.

4. What two diagnostic procedures did the physician order? Describe them in your own words. What were the results? (One of these procedures is described in Chapter 6 of this text.)

5. What treatments were ordered? Explain what the physical therapy procedures involve.

6. This patient is experiencing an acute episode. Explain what this phrase means and contrast it with chronic.

Practice Exercises

A. Word Building Practice

The combining form **oste/o** refers to *bone*. Use it to write a term that means:

1. bone cell   _____

2. immature bone cell   _____

3. porous bone   _____

4. disease of the bone   _____

5. cutting into a bone   _____

6. instrument to cut bone   _____

7. inflammation of the bone and bone marrow   _____

8. abnormal softening of bone   _____

9. bone and cartilage tumor   _____

The combining form **my/o** refers to *muscle*. Use it to write a term that means:

10. muscle disease   _____

11. surgical repair of muscle   _____

12. suture of muscle   _____

13. record of muscle electricity _____

14. muscle weakness   _____

The combining form **ten/o** refers to *tendons*. Use it to write a term that means:

15. tendon pain   _____

16. tendon suture _____

The combining form **arthr/o** refers to the *joints*. Use it to write a term that means:

17. to fuse a joint   _____

18. surgical repair of a joint   _____

19. cutting into a joint   _____

20. inflammation of a joint   _____

21. puncture to withdraw fluid from a joint   _____

22. pain in the joints   _____

The combining form **chondr/o** refers to *cartilage*. Use it to write a term that means:

23. surgical removal of cartilage   _____

24. cartilage tumor   _____

25. abnormal softening of cartilage _____

B. Spinal Column Practice

Name the five regions of the spinal column and indicate the number of bones in each area.

Name	**Number of Bones**
1. _____	_____
2. _____	_____
3. _____	_____
4. _____	_____
5. _____	_____

C. Complete the Term

For each definition given below, fill in the blank with the word part that completes the term.

Definition	**Term**
1. porous bone	osteo_____
2. a ruptured muscle	_____rrhexis
3. crooked (lateral curvature of) spine	_____osis
4. abnormal muscle tone	dys_____
5. the study of movement	_____logy
6. abnormal forward curvature of lumbar spine	_____osis
7. forward slipping of a vertebra	spondylo_____
8. withdrawing fluid from a joint	_____centesis
9. movement away from body	_____duction
10. bone and joint inflammation	_____arthritis
11. to surgically break a bone	osteo_____
12. abnormal softening of cartilage	_____malacia
13. pertaining to muscles	_____ar
14. muscle weakness	my_____
15. inflammation of a tendon	_____itis
16. inflammation of a bursa	_____itis
17. bone marrow tumor	_____oma
18. to fuse a joint	arthro_____

D. Fill in the Blank

carpal tunnel syndrome	rickets	spondylolisthesis	systemic lupus
scoliosis	osteogenic sarcoma	lateral epicondylitis	erythematosus
herniated nucleus pulposus	osteoporosis	pseudohypertrophic muscular dystrophy	

1. Mrs. Lewis, age 84, broke her hip. Her physician will be running tests for what potential ailment? _____

2. Jamie, age six months, is being given orange juice and vitamin supplements to avoid what condition? _____

3. George has severe elbow pain after playing tennis four days in a row. He may have _____.

4. Marshall's doctor told him that he had a ruptured disk. The medical term for this is _____.

5. Mr. Jefferson's physician has discovered a tumor at the end of his femur. He has been admitted to the hospital for a biopsy to rule out what type of bone cancer? _____

6. The school nurse has asked Janelle to bend over so that she may examine her back to see if she is developing a lateral curve. What is the nurse looking for? _____

7. Gerald has experienced a gradual loss of muscle strength over the past five years even though his muscles look large and healthy. The doctors believe he has an inherited muscle disease. What is that disease? _____

8. Roberta has suddenly developed arthritis in her hands and knees. Rheumatoid arthritis had been ruled out, but what other autoimmune disease might Roberta have? _____

9. Mark's X-ray demonstrated forward sliding of a lumbar vertebra; the radiologist diagnosed _____.

10. The orthopedist determined that Marcia's repetitive wrist movements at work caused her to develop _____.

E. Know Your Bones

For each bone listed below, give its division of the skeleton (axial or appendicular), the total number in the body, and its common name.

	Division	**Number**	**Common Name**
1. maxilla	_____	_____	_____
2. carpus	_____	_____	_____
3. scapula	_____	_____	_____
4. patella	_____	_____	_____
5. sternum	_____	_____	_____
6. femur	_____	_____	_____
7. metatarsus	_____	_____	_____
8. tibia	_____	_____	_____
9. clavicle	_____	_____	_____
10. zygomatic bone	_____	_____	_____

F. Using Abbreviations

Fill in the blank with the appropriate abbreviation.

1. The pain in her wrist and hand was determined to be _____.

2. The _____ showed clear evidence of osteoporosis.

3. _____ is an inherited disease with progressive muscle degeneration.

4. Mrs. Mendez underwent a(n) _____ after breaking her hip.

5. He had a(n) _____ to study the strength and quality of muscle contractions.

6. _____ is an arthritis resulting from an autoimmune condition.

7. The young boy fell from the tree and has a greenstick _____.

8. The physician recommended a(n) _____ like ibuprofen for her mild pain.

G. Define the Term

1. chondroplasty _____

2. bradykinesia _____

3. osteoporosis _____

4. lordosis _____

5. atrophy _____

6. myeloma _____

7. prosthesis _____

8. craniotomy _____

9. arthrocentesis _____

10. bursitis _____

H. Pharmacology Challenge

Fill in the classification for each drug description, then match the brand name.

Drug Description	Classification	Brand Name
1. _____ Treats mild pain and is an anti-inflammatory	_____	a. Flexeril
2. _____ Hormone with anti-inflammatory properties	_____	b. Aleve
3. _____ Reduces muscle spasms	_____	c. Fosamax
4. _____ Treats conditions of weakened bones	_____	d. Oystercal
5. _____ Maintains blood calcium levels	_____	e. Medrol

I. Identify the rehabilitation procedure described by each phrase.

1. kneading or applying pressure by hands _____

2. treatment to restore movement _____

3. using water for treatment purposes _____

4. high-frequency sound waves to create heat _____

5. use of heat for treatment purposes _____

6. medication introduced by ultrasound waves _____

7. use of cold for treatment purposes _____

8. learning to walk again _____

J. Fracture Type Matching

1. _____ comminuted

2. _____ greenstick

3. _____ compound

4. _____ simple

5. _____ impacted

6. _____ transverse

7. _____ oblique

8. _____ spiral

a. fracture line is at an angle

b. fracture line curves around the bone

c. bone is splintered or crushed

d. bone is pressed into itself

e. fracture line is straight across bone

f. skin has been broken

g. no open wound

h. bone only partially broken

K. Spelling Practice

Some of the following terms are misspelled. Identify the incorrect terms and spell them correctly in the blank provided.

1. tendinous   _____

2. psudohypertrophic   _____

3. polymyocitis   _____

4. electromyography   _____

5. ankylosing   _____

6. osteocondroma   _____

7. spondilosis   _____

8. laminectomy   _____

9. corticosteroid   _____

10. exosstosis   _____

MyLab Medical Terminology™

MyLab Medical Terminology is a premium online homework management system that includes a host of features to help you study. Registered users will find:

- A multitude of activities and assignments built within the MyLab platform

- Powerful tools that track and analyze your results—allowing you to create a personalized learning experience

- Videos and audio pronunciations to help enrich your progress

- Streaming lesson presentations (Guided Lectures) and self-paced learning modules

- A space where you and your instructors can check your progress and manage your assignments

Labeling Exercises

Image A

Write the labels for this figure on the numbered lines provided.

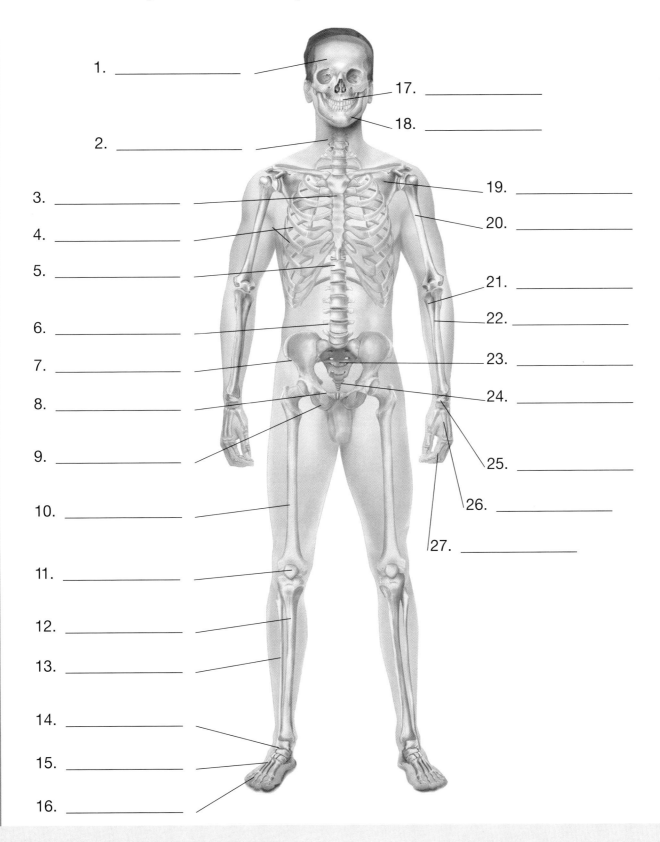

1. _____

2. _____

3. _____

4. _____

5. _____

6. _____

7. _____

8. _____

9. _____

10. _____

11. _____

12. _____

13. _____

14. _____

15. _____

16. _____

17. _____

18. _____

19. _____

20. _____

21. _____

22. _____

23. _____

24. _____

25. _____

26. _____

27. _____

Image B

Write the labels for this figure on the numbered lines provided.

1. _____

2. _____

3. _____

4. _____

5. _____

6. _____

7. _____

8. _____

Image C

Write the labels for this figure on the numbered lines provided.

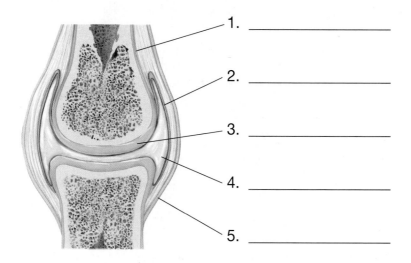

1. _____

2. _____

3. _____

4. _____

5. _____

Chapter 5

Cardiovascular System

Learning Objectives

Upon completion of this chapter, you will be able to

1. Identify and define the combining forms, suffixes, and prefixes introduced in this chapter.
2. Correctly spell and pronounce medical terms and major anatomical structures relating to the cardiovascular system.
3. Describe the major organs of the cardiovascular system and their functions.
4. Describe the anatomy of the heart.
5. Describe the flow of blood through the heart.
6. Explain how the electrical conduction system controls the heartbeat.
7. List and describe the characteristics of the three types of blood vessels.
8. Define *pulse* and *blood pressure*.
9. Identify and define cardiovascular system anatomical terms.
10. Identify and define selected cardiovascular system pathology terms.
11. Identify and define selected cardiovascular system diagnostic procedures.
12. Identify and define selected cardiovascular system therapeutic procedures.
13. Identify and define selected medications relating to the cardiovascular system.
14. Define selected abbreviations associated with the cardiovascular system.

(Pearson Education, Inc.)

AT A GLANCE

Function

The cardiovascular system consists of the pump and vessels that distribute blood to all areas of the body. This system allows for the delivery of needed substances to the cells of the body as well as for the removal of wastes.

Organs

The primary structures that comprise the cardiovascular system:

blood vessels   **heart**

- **arteries**
- **capillaries**
- **veins**

Word Parts

Presented here are the most common word parts (with their meanings) used to build cardiovascular system terms. For a more comprehensive list, refer to the Terminology section of this chapter.

Combining Forms

angi/o	vessel	**sept/o**	wall
aort/o	aorta	**son/o**	sound
arteri/o	artery	**sphygm/o**	pulse
arteriol/o	arteriole	**steth/o**	chest
ather/o	fatty substance	**thromb/o**	clot
atri/o	atrium	**valv/o**	valve
cardi/o	heart	**valvul/o**	valve
coron/o	heart	**varic/o**	dilated vein
embol/o	plug	**vascul/o**	blood vessel
fibrin/o	fibers	**vas/o**	vessel
isch/o	to hold back	**ven/o**	vein
myocardi/o	heart muscle	**ventricul/o**	ventricle
phleb/o	vein	**venul/o**	venule

Suffixes

-cardia	heart condition	**-spasm**	involuntary muscle contraction
-manometer	instrument to measure pressure	**-tension**	pressure
-ole	small	**-tonic**	pertaining to tone
-pressor	to press down	**-ule**	small

Prefixes

di-	two

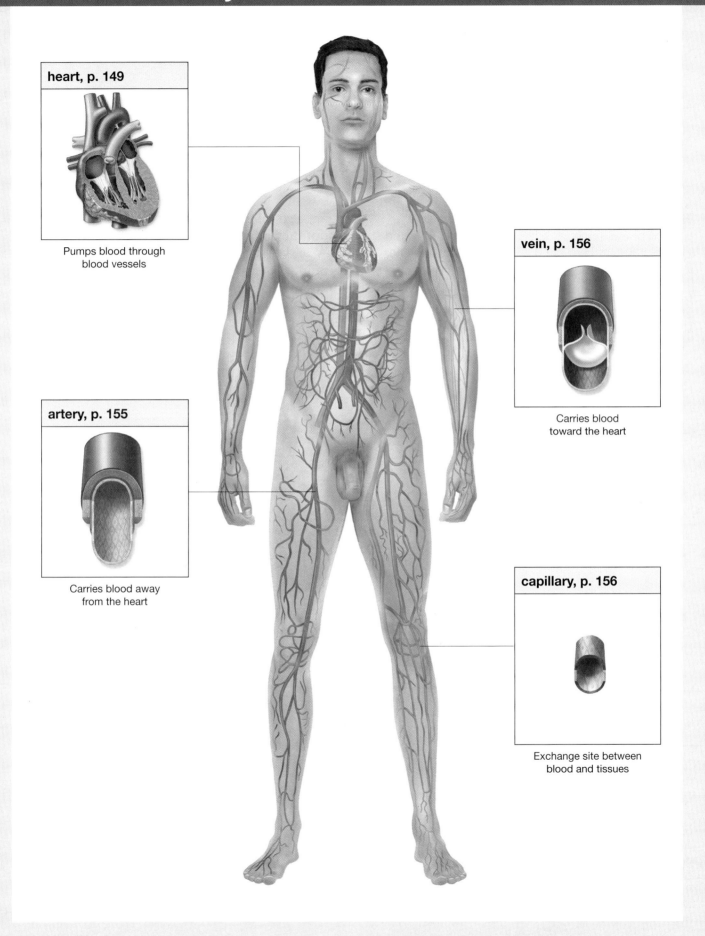

heart, p. 149

Pumps blood through blood vessels

artery, p. 155

Carries blood away from the heart

vein, p. 156

Carries blood toward the heart

capillary, p. 156

Exchange site between blood and tissues

Anatomy and Physiology of the Cardiovascular System

arteries

blood vessels

capillaries

carbon dioxide

circulatory system

deoxygenated (dee-OK-sih-jen-ay-ted)

heart

oxygen

oxygenated (OK-sih-jen-ay-ted)

pulmonary circulation (PULL-mon-air-ee / ser-kyoo-LAY-shun)

systemic circulation (sis-TEM-ik / ser-kyoo-LAY-shun)

veins

The cardiovascular (CV) system, also called the **circulatory system**, maintains the distribution of blood throughout the body and is composed of the **heart** and the **blood vessels**—**arteries**, **capillaries**, and **veins**.

The circulatory system is composed of two parts: the **pulmonary circulation** and the **systemic circulation**. The pulmonary circulation, between the heart and lungs, transports **deoxygenated** blood to the lungs to get oxygen, and then back to the heart. The systemic circulation carries **oxygenated** blood away from the heart to the tissues and cells, and then back to the heart (see Figure 5-1 ■). In this way, all the body's cells receive blood and oxygen.

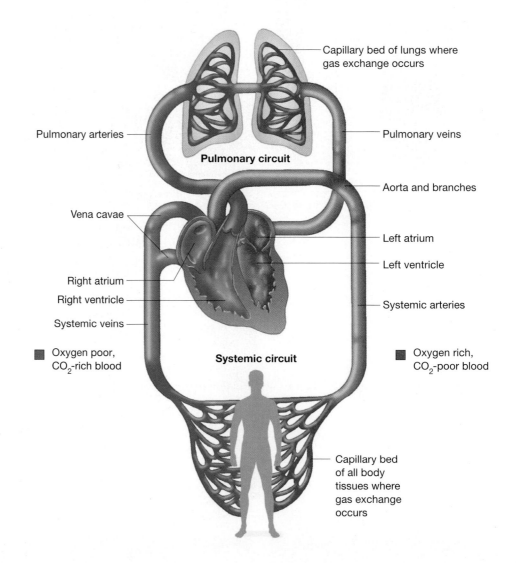

■ Figure 5-1 A schematic of the circulatory system illustrating the pulmonary circulation picking up oxygen from the lungs and the systemic circulation delivering oxygen to the body.

In addition to distributing **oxygen** and other nutrients, such as glucose and amino acids, the cardiovascular system also collects the waste products from the body's cells. **Carbon dioxide** and other waste products produced by metabolic reaction are transported by the cardiovascular system to the lungs, liver, and kidneys, where they are eliminated from the body.

Heart

apex (AY-peks) **cardiac muscle** (KAR-dee-ak)

The heart, a muscular pump made up of **cardiac muscle** fibers, could be considered a muscle rather than an organ. It has four chambers, or cavities, and beats an average of 60–100 beats per minute (bpm) or about 100,000 times in one day. Each time the cardiac muscle contracts, blood is ejected from the heart and pushed throughout the body within the blood vessels.

The heart is located in the mediastinum in the center of the chest cavity; however, it is not exactly centered; more of the heart is on the left side of the mediastinum than the right (see Figure 5-2 ■). At about the size of a fist and shaped like an upside-down pear, the heart lies directly behind the sternum. The tip of the heart at the lower edge is called the **apex**.

> **Med Term Tip**
>
> Your heart is approximately the size of your clenched fist and pumps 4,000 gallons of blood each day. It will beat at least three billion times during your lifetime.

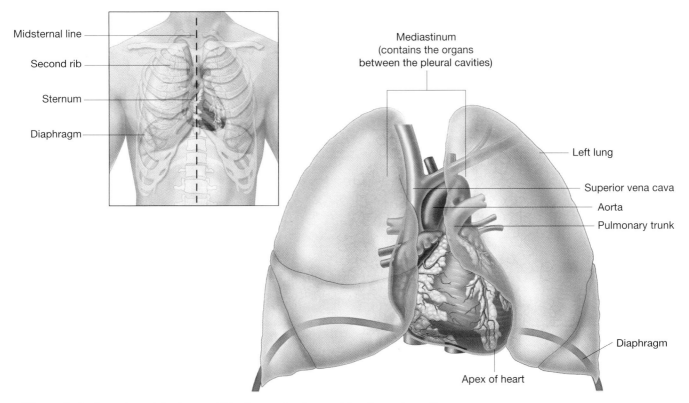

Midstern line
Second rib
Sternum
Diaphragm

Mediastinum (contains the organs between the pleural cavities)

Left lung
Superior vena cava
Aorta
Pulmonary trunk
Diaphragm
Apex of heart

■ **Figure 5-2** Location of the heart within the mediastinum of the thoracic cavity.

Med Term Tip

The layers of the heart become important when studying the disease conditions affecting the heart. For instance, when the prefix **endo-** is added to *carditis*, forming *endocarditis*, we know that the inflammation is within the "inner layer of the heart." In discussing the muscular action of the heart, the combining form **my/o**, meaning *muscle*, is added to *cardium* to form the word *myocardium*. The diagnosis *myocardial infarction* (MI), or heart attack, means that the patient has an infarct or "dead tissue in the muscle of the heart." The prefix **peri-**, meaning *around*, when added to the word *cardium* refers to the sac surrounding the heart. Therefore, *pericarditis* is an "inflammation of the outer sac of the heart."

Heart Layers

endocardium (en-doh-KAR-dee-um)
epicardium (ep-ih-KAR-dee-um)
myocardium (my-oh-KAR-dee-um)
parietal pericardium (pah-RYE-eh-tal / pair-ih-KAR-dee-um)

pericardium (pair-ih-KAR-dee-um)
visceral pericardium (VISS-er-al / pair-ih-KAR-dee-um)

The wall of the heart is quite thick and is composed of three layers (see Figure 5-3 ■):

1. The **endocardium** is the inner layer of the heart lining the heart chambers. It is a very smooth, thin layer that serves to reduce friction as the blood passes through the heart chambers.
2. The **myocardium** is the thick, muscular middle layer of the heart. Contraction of this muscle layer develops the pressure required to pump blood through the blood vessels.
3. The **epicardium** is the outer layer of the heart. The heart is enclosed within a double-layered pleural sac, called the **pericardium**. The epicardium is the **visceral pericardium**, or inner layer of the sac. The outer layer of the sac is the **parietal pericardium**. Fluid between the two layers of the sac reduces friction as the heart beats.

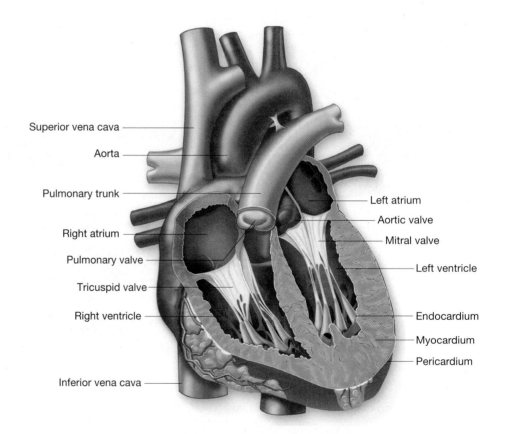

Superior vena cava
Aorta
Pulmonary trunk
Right atrium
Pulmonary valve
Tricuspid valve
Right ventricle
Inferior vena cava

Left atrium
Aortic valve
Mitral valve
Left ventricle
Endocardium
Myocardium
Pericardium

■ **Figure 5-3** Internal view of the heart illustrating the heart chambers, heart layers, and major blood vessels associated with the heart.

Heart Chambers

atria (AY-tree-ah)

interatrial septum (in-ter-AY-tree-al /
    SEP-tum)

interventricular septum
    (in-ter-ven-TRIK-yoo-lar / SEP-tum)

ventricles (VEN-trih-kulz)

The heart is divided into four chambers or cavities (see again Figure 5-3). There are two **atria**, or upper chambers, and two **ventricles**, or lower chambers. These chambers are divided into right and left sides by walls called the **interatrial septum** and the **interventricular septum**. The atria are the receiving chambers of the heart. Blood returning to the heart via veins first collects in the atria. The ventricles are the pumping chambers. They have a much thicker myocardium and their contraction ejects blood out of the heart and into the great arteries.

> **Med Term Tip**
>
> The term *ventricle* comes from the Latin term *venter*, which means *little belly*. Although it originally referred to the abdomen and then the stomach, it came to stand for any hollow region inside an organ.

Heart Valves

aortic valve (ay-OR-tik)

atrioventricular valve
    (ay-tree-oh-ven-TRIK-yoo-lar)

bicuspid valve (bye-KUSS-pid)

cusps

mitral valve (MY-tral)

pulmonary valve (PULL-mon-air-ee)

semilunar valve (sem-ee-LOO-nar)

tricuspid valve (trye-KUSS-pid)

Four valves act as restraining gates to control the direction of blood flow. They are situated at the entrances and exits to the ventricles (see Figure 5-4 ■). Properly functioning valves allow blood to flow only in a forward direction by blocking it from returning to the previous chamber.

Anterior

Pulmonary valve
(right semilunar valve)

Aortic valve
(left semilunar valve)

Mitral valve
(left atrioventricular valve)

Tricuspid valve
(right atrioventricular valve)

Posterior

■ **Figure 5-4** Superior view of heart valves illustrating position, size, and shape of each valve.

The four valves are:

1. **Tricuspid valve:** an **atrioventricular valve** (AV), meaning that it controls the opening between the right atrium and the right ventricle. Once the blood enters the right ventricle, it cannot go back up into the atrium again. The prefix **tri-**, meaning three, indicates that this valve has three leaflets or **cusps.**
2. **Pulmonary valve:** a **semilunar valve**, with the prefix **semi-** meaning *half* and the term **lunar** meaning *moon,* indicate that this valve looks like a half moon. Located between the right ventricle and the pulmonary artery, this valve prevents blood that has been ejected into the pulmonary artery from returning to the right ventricle as it relaxes.
3. **Mitral valve:** also called the **bicuspid valve**, indicating that it has two cusps. Blood flows through this atrioventricular valve to the left ventricle and cannot go back up into the left atrium.
4. **Aortic valve:** a semilunar valve located between the left ventricle and the aorta. Blood leaves the left ventricle through this valve and cannot return to the left ventricle.

Blood Flow Through the Heart

aorta (ay-OR-tah)
diastole (dye-ASS-toh-lee)
inferior vena cava (VEE-nah / KAY-vah)
pulmonary artery (PULL-mon-air-ee)
pulmonary veins
superior vena cava
systole (SIS-toh-lee)

The flow of blood through the heart is very orderly (see Figure 5-5 ■). It progresses through the heart to the lungs, where it receives oxygen; then goes back to the heart; and then out to the body tissues and parts. The normal process of blood flow is:

1. Deoxygenated blood from all the tissues in the body enters a relaxed right atrium via two large veins called the **superior vena cava** and **inferior vena cava.**
2. The right atrium contracts and blood flows through the tricuspid valve into the relaxed right ventricle.
3. The right ventricle then contracts and blood is pumped through the pulmonary valve into the **pulmonary artery**, which carries it to the lungs for oxygenation.
4. The left atrium receives blood returning to the heart after being oxygenated by the lungs. This blood enters the relaxed left atrium from the four **pulmonary veins.**
5. The left atrium contracts and blood flows through the mitral valve into the relaxed left ventricle.
6. When the left ventricle contracts, the blood is pumped through the aortic valve and into the **aorta**, the largest artery in the body. The aorta carries blood to all parts of the body.

It can be seen that the heart chambers alternate between relaxing, in order to fill, and contracting to push blood forward. The period of time a chamber is relaxed is **diastole**. The contraction phase is **systole**.

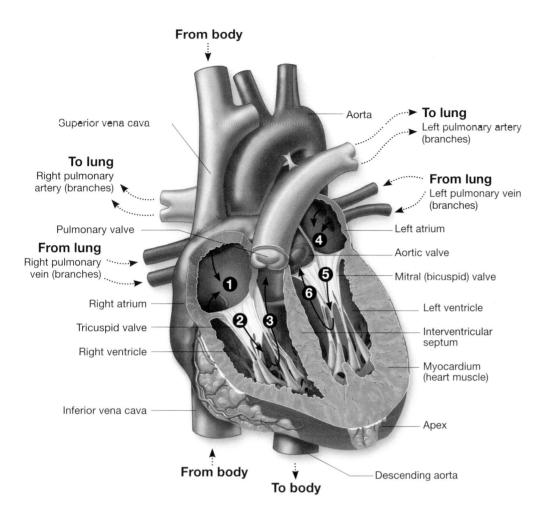

From body

Superior vena cava

To lung
Right pulmonary
artery (branches)

Pulmonary valve

From lung
Right pulmonary
vein (branches)

Right atrium

Tricuspid valve

Right ventricle

Inferior vena cava

From body

Aorta

To lung
Left pulmonary artery
(branches)

From lung
Left pulmonary vein
(branches)

Left atrium

Aortic valve

Mitral (bicuspid) valve

Left ventricle

Interventricular
septum

Myocardium
(heart muscle)

Apex

Descending aorta

To body

■ Figure 5-5 The path of blood flow through the chambers of the left and right side of the heart, including the veins delivering blood to the heart and arteries receiving blood ejected from the heart.

Conduction System of the Heart

atrioventricular bundle
atrioventricular node
autonomic nervous system (aw-toh-NOM-ik / NER-vus / SIS-tem)
bundle branches

bundle of His
pacemaker
Purkinje fibers (per-KIN-jee)
sinoatrial node (sigh-noh-AY-tree-al)

The heart rate is regulated by the **autonomic nervous system**; therefore, there is no voluntary control over the beating of the heart. Special tissue within the heart is responsible for conducting an electrical impulse stimulating the different chambers to contract in the correct order.

The path that the impulses travel is as follows (see Figure 5-6 ■):

1. The **sinoatrial (SA, S-A) node**, or **pacemaker**, is where the electrical impulses begin. From the sinoatrial node, a wave of electricity travels through the atria, causing them to contract, or go into systole.
2. The **atrioventricular node** is stimulated.
3. This node transfers the stimulation wave to the **atrioventricular bundle** (formerly called **bundle of His**).
4. The electrical signal next travels down the **bundle branches** within the interventricular septum.
5. The **Purkinje fibers** out in the ventricular myocardium are stimulated, resulting in ventricular systole.

What's In A Name?
Look for these word parts:
atri/o = atrium
-al = pertaining to
-ic = pertaining to
auto- = self

Med Term Tip
The atrioventricular bundle was originally named the *bundle of His* in recognition of the Swiss cardiologist who first discovered these fibers. Current medical terminology usage has moved away from eponyms and toward anatomically descriptive terms for naming structures.

■ **Figure 5-6** The conduction system of the heart; traces the path of the electrical impulse that stimulates the heart chambers to contract in the correct sequence.

Superior vena cava

Aorta

Left atrium

1. Sinoatrial node (pacemaker)

Internodal pathway

2. Atrioventricular node

3. Atrioventricular bundle (bundle of His)

4. Bundle branches

5. Purkinje fibers

Purkinje fibers

Interventricular septum

Med Term Tip

The electrocardiogram, referred to as an EKG or ECG, is a measurement of the electrical activity of the heart (see Figure 5-7 ■). This can give the physician information about the health of the heart, especially the myocardium.

■ **Figure 5-7** An electrocardiogram (EKG or ECG) wave record of the electrical signal as it moves through the conduction system of the heart. This signal stimulates the chambers of the heart to contract and relax in the proper sequence.

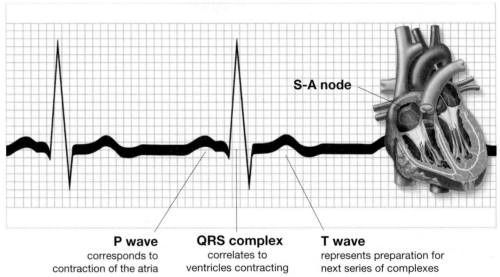

S-A node

P wave
corresponds to contraction of the atria

QRS complex
correlates to ventricles contracting

T wave
represents preparation for next series of complexes

PRACTICE AS YOU GO

A. Complete the Statement

1. The study of the heart is called _____.

2. The three layers of the heart are _____, _____, and _____.

3. The impulse for the heartbeat (the pacemaker) originates in the _____.

4. Arteries carry blood _____ the heart.

5. The four heart valves are _____, _____, _____, and _____.

6. The _____ are the receiving chambers of the heart and the _____ are the pumping chambers.

7. The _____ circulation carries blood to and from the lungs.

8. The pointed tip of the heart is called the _____.

9. The _____ divides the heart into left and right halves.

10. _____ is the contraction phase of the heartbeat and _____ is the relaxation phase.

Blood Vessels

lumen (LOO-men)

There are three types of blood vessels: arteries, capillaries, and veins (see Figure 5-8 ■). These are the pipes that circulate blood throughout the body. The **lumen** is the channel within these vessels through which blood flows.

Arteries

arterioles (ar-TEER-ee-ohlz)   **coronary arteries** (KOR-ah-nair-ee / AR-ter-eez)

The arteries are the large, thick-walled vessels that carry the blood away from the heart. The walls of arteries contain a thick layer of smooth muscle that can contract or relax to change the size of the arterial lumen. The pulmonary artery carries deoxygenated blood from the right ventricle to the lungs. The largest

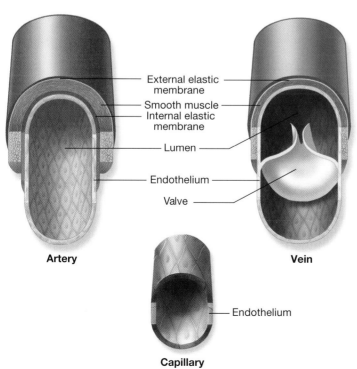

Artery

External elastic membrane
Smooth muscle
Internal elastic membrane
Lumen
Endothelium
Valve

Vein

Endothelium

Capillary

■ **Figure 5-8** Comparative structure of arteries, capillaries, and veins.

■ **Figure 5-9** The coronary arteries.

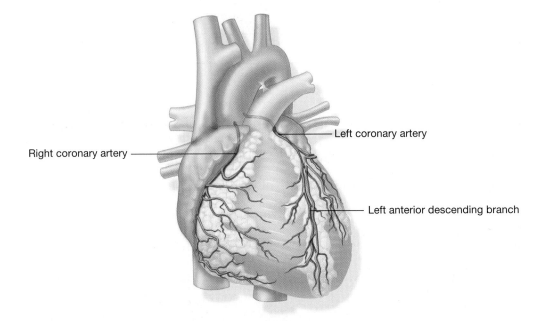

■ **Figure 5-9** The coronary arteries.

Right coronary artery

Left coronary artery

Left anterior descending branch

Med Term Tip

The term *coronary*, from the Latin word for crown, describes how the great vessels encircle the heart as they emerge from the top of the heart.

artery, the aorta, begins from the left ventricle of the heart and carries oxygenated blood to all the body systems. The **coronary arteries** then branch from the aorta and provide blood to the myocardium (see Figure 5-9 ■). As they travel through the body, the arteries branch into progressively smaller-sized arteries. The smallest of the arteries, called **arterioles**, deliver blood to the capillaries. Figure 5-10 ■ illustrates the major systemic arteries.

Capillaries

capillary bed

Capillaries are a network of tiny blood vessels referred to as a **capillary bed**. Arterial blood flows into a capillary bed, and venous blood flows back out. Capillaries are very thin walled, allowing for the diffusion of the oxygen and nutrients from the blood into the body tissues (see Figure 5-8). Likewise, carbon dioxide and waste products are able to diffuse out of the body tissues and into the bloodstream to be carried away. Since the capillaries are so small in diameter, the blood will not flow as quickly through them as it does through the arteries and veins. This means that the blood has time for an exchange of nutrients, oxygen, and waste material to take place. As blood exits a capillary bed, it returns to the heart through a vein.

Veins

venules (VEN-yools)

The veins carry blood back to the heart (see Figure 5-8). Blood leaving capillaries first enters small **venules**, which then merge into larger veins. Veins have much thinner walls than arteries, causing them to collapse easily. The veins also have valves that allow the blood to move only toward the heart. These valves prevent blood from backflowing, ensuring that blood always flows toward the heart. The two large veins that enter the heart are the superior vena cava, which carries blood from the upper body, and the inferior vena cava, which carries blood from the lower body. Blood pressure in the veins is much lower than in the arteries. Muscular action against the veins and skeletal muscle contractions help in the movement of blood. Figure 5-11 ■ illustrates the major systemic veins.

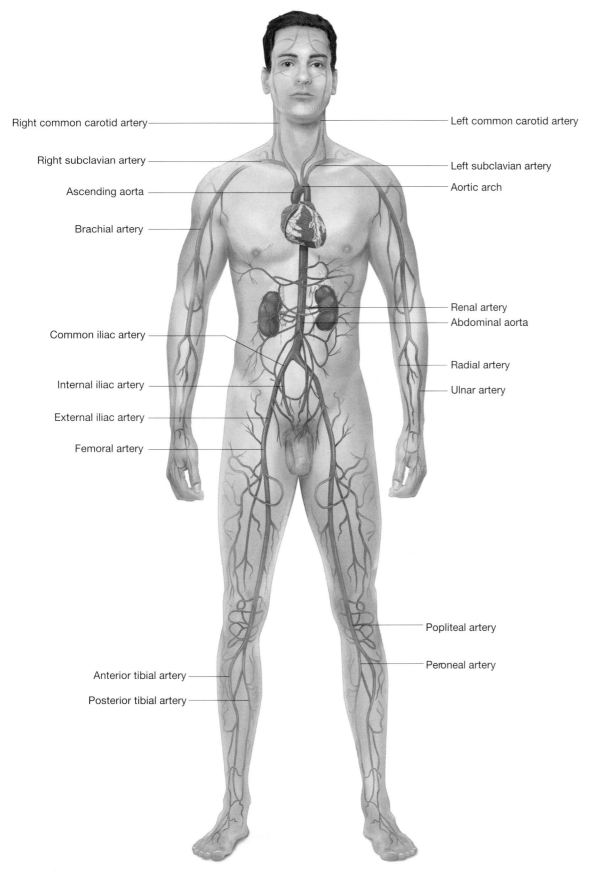

Right common carotid artery

Right subclavian artery

Ascending aorta

Brachial artery

Common iliac artery

Internal iliac artery

External iliac artery

Femoral artery

Anterior tibial artery

Posterior tibial artery

Left common carotid artery

Left subclavian artery

Aortic arch

Renal artery

Abdominal aorta

Radial artery

Ulnar artery

Popliteal artery

Peroneal artery

■ **Figure 5-10**   The major arteries of the body.

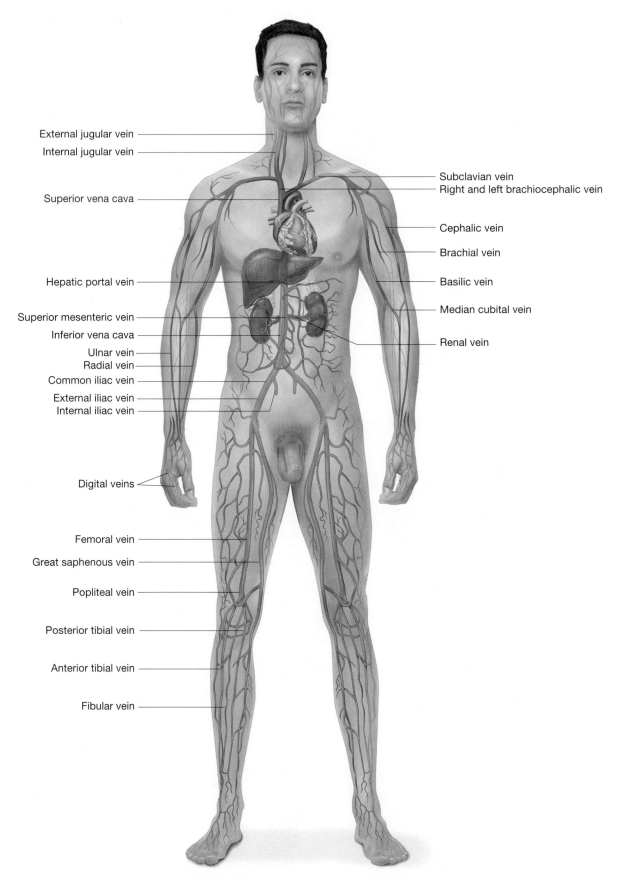

External jugular vein

Internal jugular vein

Superior vena cava

Hepatic portal vein

Superior mesenteric vein

Inferior vena cava

Ulnar vein

Radial vein

Common iliac vein

External iliac vein

Internal iliac vein

Digital veins

Femoral vein

Great saphenous vein

Popliteal vein

Posterior tibial vein

Anterior tibial vein

Fibular vein

Subclavian vein

Right and left brachiocephalic vein

Cephalic vein

Brachial vein

Basilic vein

Median cubital vein

Renal vein

■ **Figure 5-11**   The major veins of the body.

Pulse and Blood Pressure

blood pressure   pulse

diastolic pressure (dye-ah-STOL-ik)   systolic pressure (sis-TOL-ik)

Blood pressure (BP) is a measurement of the force exerted by blood against the wall of a blood vessel. During ventricular systole, blood is under a lot of pressure from the ventricular contraction, giving the highest blood pressure reading—the **systolic pressure**. The **pulse**(P) felt at the wrist or throat is the surge of blood caused by the heart contraction. This is why pulse rate is normally equal to heart rate. During ventricular diastole, blood is not being pushed by the heart at all and the blood pressure reading drops to its lowest point—the **diastolic pressure**. Therefore, to see the full range of what is occurring with blood pressure, both numbers are required. Blood pressure is also affected by several other characteristics of the blood and the blood vessels. These include the elasticity of the arteries, the diameter of the blood vessels, the viscosity of the blood, the volume of blood flowing through the vessels, and the amount of resistance to blood flow.

Med Term Tip

The instrument used to measure blood pressure is called a *sphygmomanometer*. The combining form **sphygm/o** means *pulse* and the suffix **-manometer** means *instrument to measure pressure*. A blood pressure reading is reported as two numbers, for example, 120/80. The 120 is the systolic pressure and the 80 is the diastolic pressure. There is no one "normal" blood pressure number. The normal blood pressure for an adult is a systolic pressure less than 120 and diastolic pressure less than 80.

PRACTICE AS YOU GO

B. Complete the Statement

1. The three types of blood vessels are _____, _____, and _____.

2. _____ carry blood toward the heart.

3. _____ carry blood away from the heart.

4. Diffusion of oxygen and nutrients from blood into body tissues occurs in the _____.

5. The highest blood pressure is the _____ pressure and the lowest blood pressure is the _____ pressure.

Terminology

Word Parts Used to Build Cardiovascular System Terms

The following lists contain the combining forms, suffixes, and prefixes used to build terms in the remaining sections of this chapter.

Combining Forms

angi/o	vessel	**cardi/o**	heart	**fibrin/o**	fibers
aort/o	aorta	**coron/o**	heart	**hem/o** (see Chapter 6)	blood
arteri/o	artery	**corpor/o**	body		
arteriol/o	arteriole	**cutane/o**	skin	**isch/o**	to hold back
ather/o	fatty substance	**duct/o**	to bring	**lip/o**	fat
atri/o	atrium	**electr/o**	electricity	**my/o**	muscle
bi/o	life	**embol/o**	plug	**myocardi/o**	heart muscle

Combining Forms (continued)

orth/o	straight	**sept/o**	a wall	**varic/o**	dilated vein
pector/o	chest	**son/o**	sound	**vas/o**	vessel
peripher/o (see Chapter 12)	away from center	**sphygm/o**	pulse	**vascul/o**	blood vessel
		steth/o	chest	**ven/o**	vein
phleb/o	vein	**thromb/o**	clot	**ventricul/o**	ventricle
pulmon/o	lung	**valv/o**	valve	**venul/o**	venule
scler/o	hard	**valvul/o**	valve		

Suffixes

-ac	pertaining to	**-logy**	study of	**-rrhexis**	rupture
-al	pertaining to	**-lytic**	destruction	**-sclerosis**	hardening
-ar	pertaining to	**-manometer**	instrument to measure pressure	**-scope**	instrument for viewing
-ary	pertaining to				
-cardia	heart condition	**-megaly**	enlarged	**-spasm**	involuntary muscle contraction
-eal	pertaining to	**-ole**	small		
		-oma	mass	**-stenosis**	narrowing
-ectomy	surgical removal	**-ose**	pertaining to	**-tension**	pressure
-gram	record	**-ous**	pertaining to	**-therapy**	treatment
-graphy	process of recording			**-tic**	pertaining to
-ia	condition	**-pathy**	disease	**-tonic**	pertaining to tone
-ic	pertaining to	**-plasty**	surgical repair	**-ule**	small
-itis	inflammation	**-pressor**	to press down		

Prefixes

a-	without	**hypo-**	insufficient	**re-**	again
anti-	against	**inter-**	between	**tachy-**	fast
brady-	slow	**intra-**	within	**tetra-**	four
de-	without	**per-**	through	**trans-**	across
endo-	inner	**peri-**	around	**ultra-**	beyond
extra-	outside of	**poly-**	many		
hyper-	excessive	**pre-**	before		

Adjective Forms of Anatomical Terms

Term	Word Parts	Definition
aortic (ay-OR-tik)	aort/o = aorta -ic = pertaining to	Pertaining to aorta
arterial (ar-TEE-ree-al)	arteri/o = artery -al = pertaining to	Pertaining to artery

Adjective Forms of Anatomical Terms (continued)

Term	Word Parts	Definition
arteriolar (ar-teer-ee-OH-lar)	arteriol/o = arteriole -ar = pertaining to	Pertaining to arteriole
atrial (AY-tree-al)	atri/o = atrium -al = pertaining to	Pertaining to atrium
atrioventricular (AV, A-V) (ay-tree-oh-ven-TRIK-yoo-lar)	atri/o = atrium ventricul/o = ventricle -ar = pertaining to	Pertaining to atrium and ventricle
cardiac (KAR-dee-ak)	cardi/o = heart -ac = pertaining to	Pertaining to heart
coronary (KOR-ah-nair-ee)	coron/o = heart -ary = pertaining to	Pertaining to heart
corporeal (kor-POH-ree-al)	corpor/o = body -eal = pertaining to	Pertaining to body
interatrial (in-ter-AY-tree-al)	inter- = between atri/o = atrium -al = pertaining to	Pertaining to between the atria
interventricular (in-ter-ven-TRIK-yoo-lar)	inter- = between ventricul/o = ventricle -ar = pertaining to	Pertaining to between the ventricles
myocardial (my-oh-KAR-dee-al)	myocardi/o = heart muscle -al = pertaining to	Pertaining to heart muscle
valvular (VAL-vyoo-lar)	valvul/o = valve -ar = pertaining to	Pertaining to a valve
vascular (VAS-kyoo-lar)	vascul/o = blood vessel -ar = pertaining to	Pertaining to a blood vessel
venous (VEE-nus)	ven/o = vein -ous = pertaining to	Pertaining to a vein
ventricular (ven-TRIK-yoo-lar)	ventricul/o = ventricle -ar = pertaining to	Pertaining to a ventricle
venular (VEN-yoo-lar)	venul/o = venule -ar = pertaining to	Pertaining to venule

PRACTICE AS YOU GO

C. Give the adjective form for each anatomical structure/location.

1. The heart _____

2. Between the ventricles _____

3. An artery _____

4. A small vein _____

5. The heart muscle _____

6. An atrium _____

Pathology

Term	Word Parts	Definition
Medical Specialties		
cardiology (kar-dee-ALL-oh-jee)	cardi/o = heart -logy = study of	Branch of medicine involving diagnosis and treatment of conditions and diseases of cardio-vascular system; physician is a *cardiologist*
cardiovascular technologist/technician	cardi/o = heart vascul/o = blood vessel -ar = pertaining to	Healthcare professional trained to perform variety of diagnostic and therapeutic procedures including electrocardiography, echocardiography, and exercise stress tests
Signs and Symptoms		
angiitis (an-jee-EYE-tis)	angi/o = vessel -itis = inflammation	Inflammation of a vessel
angiospasm (AN-jee-oh-spazm)	angi/o = vessel -spasm = involuntary muscle contraction	Involuntary muscle contraction of smooth muscle in wall of a vessel; narrows vessel
angiostenosis (an-jee-oh-steh-NOH-sis)	angi/o = vessel -stenosis = narrowing	Narrowing of a vessel
embolus (EM-boh-lus)	embol/o = plug	Obstruction of blood vessel by blood clot that has broken off from thrombus somewhere else in body and traveled to point of obstruction; if it occurs in coronary artery, may result in myocardial infarction

Artery
Embolus

■ **Figure 5-12**   Illustration of an embolus floating in an artery. The embolus will become lodged in a blood vessel that is smaller than it is, resulting in occlusion of that artery.

Term	Word Parts	Definition
infarct (IN-farkt)		Area of tissue within organ or part that undergoes necrosis (death) following loss of its blood supply
ischemia (iss-KEE-mee-ah)	isch/o = to hold back hem/o = blood -ia = condition	Localized and temporary deficiency of blood supply due to obstruction to circulation
murmur (MUR-mur)		A sound, in addition to normal heart sounds, arising from blood flowing through heart; extra sound may or may not indicate a heart abnormality
orthostatic hypotension (or-thoh-STAT-ik)	orth/o = straight hypo- = insufficient -tension = pressure	Sudden drop in blood pressure a person experiences when standing straight up suddenly
palpitations (pal-pih-TAY-shunz)		Pounding, racing heartbeats
plaque (PLAK)		Yellow, fatty deposit of lipids in artery that is hallmark of atherosclerosis; also called an *atheroma*

Pathology (continued)

Term	Word Parts	Definition
regurgitation (ree-ger-jih-TAY-shun)	re- = again	To flow backward; in cardiovascular system this refers to backflow of blood through a valve
thrombus (THROM-bus)	thromb/o = clot	Blood clot forming within blood vessel; may partially or completely occlude blood vessel

■ **Figure 5-13** Development of an atherosclerotic plaque that progressively narrows the lumen of an artery.

Heart

Term	Word Parts	Definition
angina pectoris (an-JYE-nah / PEK-tor-is)	pector/o = chest	Condition in which there is severe pain with sensation of constriction around heart; caused by deficiency of oxygen to heart muscle; commonly called *chest pain* (CP)
cardiac arrest	cardi/o = heart -ac = pertaining to	Complete stopping of heart activity
cardiac tamponade (KAR-dee-ak / tam-poh-NADE)	cardi/o = heart -ac = pertaining to	Pressure on heart as a result of fluid buildup around heart inside pericardial sac; heart becomes unable to pump blood effectively
cardiomegaly (kar-dee-oh-MEG-ah-lee)	cardi/o = heart -megaly = enlarged	Enlarged heart
cardiomyopathy (kar-dee-oh-my-OP-ah-thee)	cardi/o = heart my/o = muscle -pathy = disease	General term for disease of myocardium; can be caused by alcohol abuse, parasites, viral infection, and congestive heart failure; one of most common reasons a patient may require heart transplant
congenital septal defect (CSD)	sept/o = a wall -al = pertaining to	Hole, present at birth, in septum between two heart chambers; results in mixture of oxygenated and deoxygenated blood; can be an *atrial septal defect* (ASD) and a *ventricular septal defect* (VSD)
congestive heart failure (CHF) (kon-JESS-tiv)		Pathological condition of heart in which there is reduced outflow of blood from left side of heart because left ventricle myocardium has become too weak to efficiently pump blood; results in weakness, breathlessness, and edema

Pathology (continued)

Term	Word Parts	Definition
coronary artery disease (CAD) (KOR-ah-nair-ee)	coron/o = heart -ary = pertaining to	Insufficient blood supply to heart muscle due to obstruction of one or more coronary arteries; may be caused by atherosclerosis and may cause angina pectoris and myocardial infarction

Med Term Tip

All types of cardiovascular disease have been the number one killer of Americans since the 19th century. This disease kills more people annually than cancer.

Plaque

■ **Figure 5-14** Formation of an atherosclerotic plaque within a coronary artery; may lead to coronary artery disease, angina pectoris, and myocardial infarction.

Term	Word Parts	Definition
endocarditis (en-doh-kar-DYE-tis)	endo- = inner cardi/o = heart -itis = inflammation	Inflammation of lining membranes of heart; may be due to bacteria or to abnormal immunological response; in bacterial endocarditis, mass of bacteria that forms is referred to as *vegetation*
heart valve prolapse (PROH-laps)		Condition in which cusps or flaps of heart valve are too loose and fail to shut tightly, allowing blood to flow backward through valve when heart chamber contracts; most commonly occurs in mitral valve, but may affect any of heart valves; also called *heart valve incompetence* or *heart valve insufficiency*
heart valve stenosis (steh-NOH-sis)	-stenosis = narrowing	Condition in which cusps or flaps of heart valve are too stiff and are unable to open fully (making it difficult for blood to flow through) or shut tightly (allowing blood to flow backward); condition may affect any of heart valves
myocardial infarction (MI) (my-oh-KAR-dee-al / in-FARK-shun)	myocardi/o = heart muscle -al = pertaining to	Condition caused by partial or complete occlusion or closing of one or more of coronary arteries; symptoms include squeezing pain or heavy pressure in middle of chest (angina pectoris); delay in treatment could result in death; also referred to as a *heart attack*; see Figure 5-15 ■

Pathology (continued)

Term	Word Parts	Definition

■ **Figure 5-15** External and cross-sectional view of an infarct caused by a myocardial infarction.

Term	Word Parts	Definition
myocarditis (my-oh-kar-DYE-tis)	myocardi/o = heart muscle -itis = inflammation	Inflammation of muscle layer of heart wall
pericarditis (pair-ih-kar-DYE-tis)	peri- = around cardi/o = heart -itis = inflammation	Inflammation of pericardial sac around heart
tetralogy of Fallot (teh-TRALL-oh-jee / fal-LOH)	tetra- = four -logy = study of	Combination of four congenital anomalies: pulmonary stenosis, interventricular septal defect, improper placement of aorta, and hypertrophy of right ventricle; needs immediate surgery to correct
valvulitis (val-vyoo-LYE-tis)	valvul/o = valve -itis = inflammation	Inflammation of a heart valve
Arrhythmias		
arrhythmia (ah-RITH-mee-ah)	a- = without -ia = condition	Irregularity in heartbeat or action; comes in many different forms; may be too fast, too slow, or irregular pattern; some are not serious, while others are life-threatening
bundle branch block (BBB)		Occurs when electrical impulse is blocked from traveling down bundle of His or bundle branches; results in ventricles beating at different rate than atria; also called a *heart block*
bradycardia (brad-ee-KAR-dee-ah)	brady- = slow -cardia = heart condition	Condition of having a slow heart rate, typically less than 60 beats/minute; highly trained aerobic persons may normally have a slow heart rate

Pathology (continued)

Term	Word Parts	Definition
fibrillation (fib) (fih-brill-AY-shun)		Extremely serious arrhythmia characterized by abnormal quivering or contraction of heart fibers; when this occurs in ventricles, cardiac arrest and death can occur; emergency equipment to defibrillate, or convert heart to normal beat, is necessary
flutter		Arrhythmia in which atria beat too rapidly, but in regular pattern
premature atrial contraction (PAC) (AY-tree-al)	pre- = before atri/o = atrium -al = pertaining to	Arrhythmia in which atria contract earlier than they should
premature ventricular contraction (PVC) (ven-TRIK-yoo-lar)	pre- = before ventricul/o = ventricle -ar = pertaining to	Arrhythmia in which ventricles contract earlier than they should
tachycardia (tak-ee-KAR-dee-ah)	tachy- = fast -cardia = heart condition	Condition of having a fast heart rate, typically more than 100 beats/minute while at rest

Blood Vessels

Term	Word Parts	Definition
aneurysm (AN-yoo-rizm)		Weakness in wall of artery resulting in localized widening of artery; although aneurysm may develop in any artery, common sites include aorta in abdomen and cerebral arteries in brain

Right kidney

Abdominal aorta

Aneurysm

Inferior vena cava

■ **Figure 5-16** Illustration of a large aneurysm in the abdominal aorta that has ruptured.

Term	Word Parts	Definition
arteriorrhexis (ar-tee-ree-oh-REK-sis)	arteri/o = artery -rrhexis = rupture	Ruptured artery; may occur if aneurysm ruptures arterial wall
arteriosclerosis (AS) (ar-tee-ree-oh-skleh-ROH-sis)	arteri/o = artery -sclerosis = hardening	Thickening, hardening, and loss of elasticity of walls of arteries; most often due to atherosclerosis
atheroma (ath-er-OH-mah)	ather/o = fatty substance -oma = mass	Deposit of fatty substance in wall of artery that bulges into and narrows lumen of artery; characteristic of atherosclerosis; also called a *plaque*

Pathology (continued)

Term	Word Parts	Definition
atherosclerosis (ath-er-oh-skleh-ROH-sis)	ather/o = fatty substance -sclerosis = hardening	Most common form of arteriosclerosis; caused by formation of yellowish plaques of cholesterol on inner walls of arteries (see again Figures 5-13 and 5-14)
coarctation of the aorta (CoA) (koh-ark-TAY-shun)		Severe congenital narrowing of aorta
deep vein thrombosis (DVT) (throm-BOH-sis)	thromb/o = clot	Formation of blood clot in a vein deep in the body, most commonly the legs; embolus breaking off from this thrombosis would travel to lungs and block blood flow through lungs
hemorrhoid (HEM-oh-royd)	hem/o = blood	Varicose veins in anal region
hypertension (HTN) (high-per-TEN-shun)	hyper- = excessive -tension = pressure	Blood pressure (BP) above normal range; *essential* or *primary hypertension* occurs directly from cardiovascular disease; *secondary hypertension* refers to high blood pressure resulting from another disease such as kidney disease
hypotension (high-poh-TEN-shun)	hypo- = insufficient -tension = pressure	Decrease in blood pressure (BP); can occur in shock, infection, cancer, anemia, or as death approaches
patent ductus arteriosus (PDA) (PAY-tent / DUK-tus / ar-tee-ree-OH-sis)	duct/o = to bring arteri/o = artery	Congenital heart anomaly in which fetal connection between pulmonary artery and aorta fails to close at birth; condition may be treated with medication and resolve with time; however, in some cases, surgery is required
peripheral vascular disease (PVD)	peripher/o = away from center -al = pertaining to vascul/o = blood vessel -ar = pertaining to	Any abnormal condition affecting blood vessels outside heart; symptoms may include pain, pallor, numbness, and loss of circulation and pulse
phlebitis (fleh-BYE-tis)	phleb/o = vein -itis = inflammation	Inflammation of a vein
polyarteritis (pol-ee-ar-ter-EYE-tis)	poly- = many arteri/o = artery -itis = inflammation	Inflammation of several arteries
Raynaud's phenomenon (ray-NOZ)		Periodic ischemic attacks affecting extremities of body, especially fingers, toes, ears, and nose; affected extremities become cyanotic and very painful; attacks are brought on by arterial constriction due to extreme cold or emotional stress
thrombophlebitis (throm-boh-fleh-BYE-tis)	thromb/o = clot phleb/o = vein -itis = inflammation	Inflammation of vein resulting in formation of blood clots within vein
varicose veins (VAIR-ih-kohs)	varic/o = dilated vein -ose = pertaining to	Swollen and distended veins, usually in legs

PRACTICE AS YOU GO

D. Terminology Matching

Match each term to its definition.

1. _____ arrhythmia
2. _____ thrombus
3. _____ bradycardia
4. _____ murmur
5. _____ phlebitis
6. _____ hypotension
7. _____ varicose veins
8. _____ tetralogy of Fallot
9. _____ valve prolapse
10. _____ plaque

a. swollen, distended veins
b. inflammation of vein
c. serious congenital anomaly
d. slow heart rate
e. cusps are too loose
f. irregular heartbeat
g. an extra heart sound
h. clot in blood vessel
i. low blood pressure
j. fatty deposit in artery

Diagnostic Procedures

Term	Word Parts	Definition
Medical Procedures		
auscultation (oss-kul-TAY-shun)		Process of listening to sounds within body by using a stethoscope
sphygmomanometer (sfig-moh-mah-NOM-eh-ter)	sphygm/o = pulse -manometer = instrument to measure pressure	Instrument for measuring blood pressure (BP); also referred to as *blood pressure cuff*

■ **Figure 5-17** Using a sphygmoma-nometer to measure blood pressure.
(Michal Heron/Pearson Education, Inc.)

Term	Word Parts	Definition
stethoscope (STETH-oh-skohp)	steth/o = chest -scope = instrument for viewing	Instrument for listening to body sounds (auscultation), such as chest, heart, or intestines

Diagnostic Procedures (continued)

Term	Word Parts	Definition
Clinical Laboratory Tests		
cardiac biomarkers (KAR-dee-ak)	cardi/o = heart -ac = pertaining to bi/o = life	Blood test to determine level of proteins specific to heart muscle in blood; increase in these proteins may indicate heart muscle damage such as myocardial infarction; proteins include creatine kinase (CK) and troponin
serum lipoprotein level (SEER-um / lip-oh-PROH-teen)	lip/o = fat	Blood test to measure amount of cholesterol and triglycerides in blood; indicator of atherosclerosis risk
Diagnostic Imaging		
angiogram (AN-jee-oh-gram)	angi/o = vessel -gram = record	X-ray record of vessel taken during angiography
angiography (an-jee-OG-rah-fee)	angi/o = vessel -graphy = process of recording	X-rays taken after injection of opaque material into blood vessel; can be performed on aorta as aortic angiography, on heart as angiocardiography, and on brain as cerebral angiography
cardiac scan	cardi/o = heart -ac = pertaining to	Patient is given radioactive thallium intravenously and then scanning equipment is used to visualize heart; especially useful in determining myocardial damage
Doppler ultrasonography (DOP-ler / ul-trah-son-OG-rah-fee)	ultra- = beyond son/o = sound -graphy = process of recording	Measurement of sound-wave echoes as they bounce off tissues and organs to produce an image; procedure is used to measure velocity of blood moving through blood vessels to look for blood clots or deep vein thromboses
echocardiography (ECHO) (ek-oh-kar-dee-OG-rah-fee)	cardi/o = artery -graphy = process of recording	Noninvasive diagnostic procedure using ultrasound to visualize internal cardiac structures; cardiac valve activity can be evaluated using this method
Cardiac Function Tests		
cardiac catheterization (CC, cath) (KAR-dee-ak / kath-eh-ter-ih-ZAY-shun)	cardi/o = heart -ac = pertaining to	Passage of thin-tube catheter through blood vessel leading to heart; done to detect abnormalities, to collect cardiac blood samples, and to determine blood pressure within heart
catheter (KATH-eh-ter)		Flexible tube inserted into body for purpose of moving fluids into or out of body; in the cardiovascular system, a catheter is used to place dye into blood vessels so they may be visualized on X-rays
electrocardiogram (ECG, EKG) (ee-lek-troh-KAR-dee-oh-gram)	electr/o = electricity cardi/o = heart -gram = record	Hardcopy record produced by electrocardiography
electrocardiography (ee-lek-troh-kar-dee-OG-rah-fee)	electr/o = electricity cardi/o = heart -graphy = process of recording	Process of recording electrical activity of heart; useful in diagnosis of abnormal cardiac rhythm and heart muscle (myocardium) damage

Diagnostic Procedures (continued)

Term	Word Parts	Definition
Holter monitor		Portable ECG monitor worn by patient for a period of a few hours to a few days to assess heart and pulse activity as person goes through activities of daily living; used to assess patient who experiences chest pain and unusual heart activity during exercise and normal activities
stress testing		Method for evaluating cardiovascular fitness; patient is placed on treadmill or bicycle and then subjected to steadily increasing levels of work; EKG and oxygen levels are taken while patient exercises; test is stopped if abnormalities occur on EKG; also called *exercise test* or *treadmill test*

■ **Figure 5-18**   Man undergoing a stress test on a treadmill while physician monitors his condition. *(Serafino Mozzo/Shutterstock)*

Therapeutic Procedures

Term	Word Parts	Definition
Medical Procedures		
cardiopulmonary resuscitation (CPR) (kar-dee-oh-PULL-mon-air-ee / ree-suss-ih-TAY-shun)	cardi/o = heart pulmon/o = lung -ary = pertaining to	Procedure to restore cardiac output and oxygenated air to lungs for person in cardiac arrest; combination of chest compressions (to push blood out of heart) and artificial respiration (to blow air into lungs) is performed by one or two CPR-trained rescuers
defibrillation (dee-fib-rih-LAY-shun)	de- = without	Procedure that converts serious irregular heartbeats, such as fibrillation, by giving electric shocks to heart using instrument called defibrillator; also called *cardioversion*; automated external defibrillators (AEDs) are portable devices that automatically detect life-threatening arrhythmias and deliver appropriate electrical shock; designed to be used by nonmedical personnel and found in public places such as shopping malls and schools

■ **Figure 5-19**   An emergency medical technician positions defibrillator paddles on the chest of a supine male patient. *(Floyd Jackson/Pearson Education, Inc.)*

Therapeutic Procedures (continued)

Term	Word Parts	Definition
extracorporeal circulation (ECC) (eks-trah-kor-POR-ee-al)	extra- = outside of corpor/o = body -eal = pertaining to	During open-heart surgery, routing of blood to heart-lung machine so it can be oxygenated and pumped to rest of body
implantable cardioverter-defibrillator (ICD) (KAR-dee-oh-ver-ter / dee-FIB-rih-lay-ter)	cardi/o = heart de- = without	Device implanted in heart that delivers electrical shock to restore normal heart rhythm; particularly useful for persons who experience ventricular fibrillation
pacemaker implantation		Electrical device that substitutes for natural pacemaker of heart; controls beating of heart by series of rhythmic electrical impulses; external pacemaker has electrodes on outside of body; internal pacemaker has electrodes surgically implanted within chest wall

■ **Figure 5-20** X-ray showing a pacemaker implanted in the left side of the chest and the electrode wires running to the heart muscle. *(Chaikom/Shutterstock)*

Term	Word Parts	Definition
sclerotherapy (SKLAIR-oh-thair-ah-pee)	scler/o = hard -therapy = treatment	Medical treatment for varicose veins; injection of solution (usually salt solution) directly into varicose vein; irritates lining of vessel, causing it to collapse and stick together
thrombolytic therapy (throm-boh-LIT-ik / THAIR-ah-pee)	thromb/o = clot -lytic = destruction	Process in which drugs, such as streptokinase (SK) or tissue plasminogen activator (tPA), are injected into a blood vessel to dissolve clots and restore blood flow
Surgical Procedures		
aneurysmectomy (an-yoo-riz-MEK-toh-mee)	-ectomy = surgical removal	Surgical removal of sac of an aneurysm
arterial anastomosis (ar-TEE-ree-al / ah-nas-toh-MOH-sis)	arteri/o = artery -al = pertaining to	Surgical joining together of two arteries; performed if artery is severed or if damaged section of artery is removed
atherectomy (ath-er-EK-toh-mee)	ather/o = fatty substance -ectomy = surgical removal	Surgical procedure to remove deposit of fatty substance, atheroma, from artery
coronary artery bypass graft (CABG) (KOR-ah-nair-ee)	coron/o = heart -ary = pertaining to	Open-heart surgery in which blood vessel from another location in body (often a leg vein) is grafted to route blood around blocked coronary artery
embolectomy (em-boh-LEK-toh-mee)	embol/o = plug -ectomy = surgical removal	Removal of embolus or clot from blood vessel
endarterectomy (end-ar-teh-REK-toh-mee)	endo- = inner arteri/o = artery -ectomy = surgical removal	Removal of diseased or damaged inner lining of artery; usually performed to remove atherosclerotic plaques
heart transplantation		Replacement of diseased or malfunctioning heart with donor's heart

Therapeutic Procedures (continued)

Term	Word Parts	Definition
intracoronary artery stent (in-trah-KOR-ah-nair-ee / AR-ter-ee)	intra- = within coron/o = heart -ary = pertaining to	Placement of stent within coronary artery to treat coronary ischemia due to atherosclerosis

■ **Figure 5-21** The process of placing a stent in a blood vessel. A) A catheter is used to place a collapsed stent next to an atherosclerotic plaque; B) stent is expanded; C) catheter is removed, leaving the expanded stent behind.

A   B   C

| **ligation and stripping** (lye-GAY-shun) | | Surgical treatment for varicose veins; damaged vein is tied off (ligation) and removed (stripping) |
| **percutaneous transluminal coronary angioplasty** (PTCA) (per-kyoo-TAY-nee-us / trans-LOO-mih-nal / KOR-ah-nair-ee / AN-jee-oh-plas-tee) | per- = through cutane/o = skin -ous = pertaining to trans- = across -al = pertaining to angi/o = vessel -plasty = surgical repair | Method for treating localized coronary artery narrowing; balloon catheter is inserted through skin into coronary artery and inflated to dilate narrow blood vessel |

■ **Figure 5-22** Balloon angioplasty: A) deflated balloon catheter is approaching an atherosclerotic plaque; B) plaque is compressed by inflated balloon; C) plaque remains compressed after balloon catheter is removed.

A   B   C

stent		Stainless steel tube placed within blood vessel or duct to widen lumen (see again Figure 5-21 ■)
valve replacement		Removal of diseased heart valve and replacement with artificial valve
valvoplasty (VAL-voh-plas-tee)	valv/o = valve -plasty = surgical repair	Surgical procedure to repair a heart valve

Pharmacology

Classification	Word Parts	Action	Examples
ACE inhibitor drugs		Produce vasodilation and decrease blood pressure	benazepril, Lotensin; catopril, Capoten
antiarrhythmic (an-tye-ah-RHYTH-mik)	anti- = against a- = without -ic = pertaining to	Reduces or prevents cardiac arrhythmias	flecainide, Tambocor; ibutilide, Corvert
anticoagulant (an-tye-koh-AG-yoo-lant)	anti- = against	Prevents blood clot formation	heparin; warfarin, Coumadin
antilipidemic (an-tye-lip-ih-DEEM-ik)	anti- = against lip/o = fat -ic = pertaining to	Reduces amount of cholesterol and lipids in bloodstream; treats hyperlipidemia	atorvastatin, Lipitor; simvastatin, Zocor
antiplatelet agents	anti- = against	Inhibit ability of platelets to clump together as part of blood clot	clopidogrel, Plavix; aspirin; ticlopidine, Ticlid
beta-blocker drugs		Treat hypertension and angina pectoris by lowering heart rate	metoprolol, Lopressor; propranolol, Inderal
calcium channel blocker drugs		Treat hypertension, angina pectoris, and congestive heart failure by causing heart to beat less forcefully and less often	diltiazem, Cardizem; nifedipine, Procardia
cardiotonic (kar-dee-oh-TAHN-ik)	cardi/o = heart -tonic = pertaining to tone	Increases force of cardiac muscle contraction; treats congestive heart failure	digoxin, Lanoxin
diuretic (dye-yoo-RET-ik)	-tic = pertaining to	Increases urine production by kidneys, which works to reduce plasma and therefore blood volume, resulting in lower blood pressure	furosemide, Lasix
fibrinolytic (fye-brin-oh-LIT-ik)	fibrin/o = fibers -lytic = destruction	Dissolves existing blood clots	tissue plasminogen activator (tPA); alteplase, Activase
vasodilator (vay-zoh-DYE-lay-ter)	vas/o = vessel	Relaxes smooth muscle in walls of arteries, thereby increasing diameter of blood vessel; used for two main purposes: increasing circulation to ischemic area and reducing blood pressure	nitroglycerin, Nitro-Dur; hydralazine, Apresoline
vasopressor (vay-zoh-PRESS-or)	vas/o = vessel -pressor = to press down	Contracts smooth muscle in walls of blood vessels; raises blood pressure	dopamine, Myocard-DX; vasopressin, Vasostrict

PRACTICE AS YOU GO

E. Procedure Matching

Match each procedure to its definition.

1. _____ cardiac biomarkers   a. visualizes heart after patient is given radioactive thallium

2. _____ Doppler ultrasound   b. uses ultrasound to visualize heart beating

3. _____ Holter monitor   c. blood test that indicates heart muscle damage

4. _____ cardiac scan   d. uses treadmill to evaluate cardiac fitness

5. _____ stress testing   e. removes varicose veins

6. _____ echocardiography   f. clot-dissolving drugs

7. _____ extracorporeal circulation g. measures velocity of blood moving through blood vessels

8. _____ ligation and stripping   h. balloon angioplasty

9. _____ thrombolytic therapy   i. use of a heart-lung machine

10. _____ PTCA   j. portable EKG monitor

Abbreviations

AED	automated external defibrillator	CoA	coarctation of the aorta
AF	atrial fibrillation	CP	chest pain
AMI	acute myocardial infarction	CPR	cardiopulmonary resuscitation
AS	arteriosclerosis	CSD	congenital septal defect
ASD	atrial septal defect	CV	cardiovascular
ASHD	arteriosclerotic heart disease	DVT	deep vein thrombosis
AV, A-V	atrioventricular	ECC	extracorporeal circulation
BBB	bundle branch block (L for left; R for right)	ECG, EKG	electrocardiogram
BP	blood pressure	ECHO	echocardiography
bpm	beats per minute	fib	fibrillation
CABG	coronary artery bypass graft	HTN	hypertension
CAD	coronary artery disease	ICD	implantable cardioverter-defibrillator
cath	catheterization	ICU	intensive care unit
CC	cardiac catheterization, chief complaint	IV	intravenous
CCU	coronary care unit	LVH	left-ventricular hypertrophy
CHF	congestive heart failure	MI	myocardial infarction, mitral insufficiency
CK	creatine kinase	mm Hg	millimeters of mercury

Abbreviations (continued)

MR	mitral regurgitation		**S1**	first heart sound
MS	mitral stenosis		**S2**	second heart sound

> **Word Watch**
> Be careful using the abbreviation *MS*, which can mean either *mitral stenosis* or *multiple sclerosis*.

MVP	mitral valve prolapse		**SA, S-A**	sinoatrial
P	pulse		**SK**	streptokinase
PAC	premature atrial contraction		**tPA**	tissue plasminogen activator
PDA	patent ductus arteriosus		**V fib**	ventricular fibrillation
PTCA	percutaneous transluminal coronary angioplasty		**VSD**	ventricular septal defect
PVC	premature ventricular contraction		**VT**	ventricular tachycardia
PVD	peripheral vascular disease			

PRACTICE AS YOU GO

F. What's the Abbreviation?

1. mitral valve prolapse _____
2. ventricular septal defect _____
3. percutaneous transluminal coronary angioplasty _____
4. ventricular fibrillation _____
5. deep vein thrombosis _____
6. arteriosclerotic heart disease _____
7. coarctation of the aorta _____
8. tissue plasminogen activator _____
9. cardiovascular _____
10. extracorporeal circulation _____

Chapter Review

Real-World Applications

Medical Record Analysis

This Discharge Summary contains 13 medical terms. Underline each term and write it in the list below the report. Then explain each term as you would to a nonmedical person.

Date: 6/1/2017
Patient: Juanita Johnson
Patient complaint: Severe pain in the right ankle with any movement of lower limb.

Discharge Summary

Admitting Diagnosis:	Difficulty breathing, hypertension, tachycardia
Final Diagnosis:	CHF secondary to mitral valve prolapse
History of Present Illness:	Patient was brought to the Emergency Room by her family because of difficulty breathing and palpitations. Patient reports having experienced these symptoms for the past six months, but this episode is more severe than any previous. Upon admission in the ER, heart rate was 120 beats per minute and blood pressure was 180/110. The results of an EKG and cardiac biomarkers were normal. She was admitted for a complete workup for tachycardia and hypertension.
Summary of Hospital Course:	Patient underwent a full battery of diagnostic tests. A prolapsed mitral valve was observed by echocardiography. A stress test had to be stopped early due to onset of severe difficulty in breathing. Angiocardiography failed to demonstrate significant CAD. Blood pressure and tachycardia were controlled with medications. At discharge, HR was 88 beats per minute and blood pressure was 165/98.
Discharge Plans:	There was no evidence of a myocardial infarction or significant CAD. Patient was placed on a low-salt and low-cholesterol diet. She received instructions on beginning a carefully graded exercise program. She is to continue her medications. If symptoms are not controlled by these measures, a mitral valvoplasty will be considered.

Term   **Explanation**

1.
2.
3.
4.
5.
6.
7.
8.
9.
10.
11.
12.
13.

Chart Note Transcription

The chart note below contains 11 phrases that can be reworded with a medical term presented in this chapter. Each phrase is identified with an underline. Determine the medical term and write your answers in the space provided.

Pearson General Hospital Coronary Care Unit

Task   Edit   View   Time Scale   Options   Help Download   Archive   Date: 17 May 2017

Current Complaint:	A 56-year-old male was admitted to the Cardiac Care Unit from the Emergency Room with left arm pain, severe <u>pain around the heart</u>, **1** <u>an abnormally slow heartbeat</u>, **2** and nausea and vomiting.
Past History:	Patient reports no heart problems prior to this episode. He has taken medication for <u>high blood pressure</u> **3** for the past five years. His family history is significant for a father and brother who both died in their 50s from <u>death of heart muscle</u>. **4**
Signs and Symptoms:	Patient reports severe pain around the heart that radiates into his left jaw and arm. A <u>record of the heart's electrical activity</u> **5** and a <u>blood test to determine the amount of heart damage</u> **6** were abnormal.
Diagnosis:	An acute <u>death of heart muscle</u> **4** resulting from <u>insufficient blood flow to heart muscle due to obstruction of coronary artery</u>. **7**
Treatment:	First, provide supportive care during the acute phase. Second, evaluate heart damage by <u>passing a thin tube through a blood vessel into the heart to detect abnormalities</u> **8** and <u>evaluate heart fitness by having patient exercise on a treadmill</u>. **9** Finally, perform surgical intervention by either <u>inflating a balloon catheter to dilate a narrow vessel</u> **10** or by <u>open heart surgery to create a shunt around a blocked vessel</u>. **11**

1. _____

2. _____

3. _____

4. _____

5. _____

6. _____

7. _____

8. _____

9. _____

10. _____

11. _____

Case Study

Below is a case study presentation of a patient with a condition discussed in this chapter. Read the case study and answer the questions below. Some questions will ask for information not included within this chapter. Use your text, a medical dictionary, or any other reference material you choose to answer these questions.

(Christopher Coates/Shutterstock)

Mr. Thomas is a 62-year-old man who has been diagnosed with an acute myocardial infarction with the following symptoms and history. His chief complaint is a persistent, crushing chest pain that radiates to his left arm, jaw, neck, and shoulder blade. He describes the pain, which he has had for the past 12 hours, as a "squeezing" sensation around his heart. He has also suffered nausea, dyspnea, and diaphoresis. He has a low-grade temperature and his blood pressure is within a normal range at 130/82. He states that he smokes two packs of cigarettes a day, is overweight by 50 pounds, and has a family history of hypertension and coronary artery disease. He leads a relatively sedentary lifestyle.

Questions

1. What is the common name for Mr. Thomas's acute condition? Look this condition up in a reference source and include a short description of it.

   _____

   _____

2. What do you think the phrase "chief complaint" means?

   _____

   _____

3. What is the medical term for this patient's chief complaint? Define this term.

   _____

   _____

4. List and define each of the patient's additional symptoms in your own words. (These terms appear in other chapters of this book or use a medical dictionary.)

   _____

   _____

5. Using your text as a resource, name and describe three diagnostic tests that may be performed to determine the extent of the patient's heart damage.

   _____

   _____

6. What risk factors for developing heart disease does Mr. Thomas have? What changes should he make?

   _____

   _____

Practice Exercises

A. Word Building Practice

The combining form **cardi/o** refers to the *heart.* Use it to write a term that means:

1. pertaining to the heart _____
2. disease of the heart muscle _____
3. enlargement of the heart _____
4. fast heart condition _____
5. slow heart condition _____
6. record of heart electricity _____

The combining form **angi/o** refers to the *vessel.* Use it to write a term that means:

7. vessel narrowing _____
8. vessel inflammation _____
9. involuntary muscle contraction of a vessel _____

The combining form **arteri/o** refers to the *artery.* Use it to write a term that means:

10. pertaining to an artery _____
11. hardening of an artery _____
12. small artery _____

Add the appropriate prefix to **carditis** to form the term that matches each definition:

13. inflammation of the inner lining of the heart _____
14. inflammation of the outer layer of the heart _____
15. inflammation of the muscle of the heart _____

B. Anatomical Adjectives

Fill in the blank with the missing noun or adjective.

Noun	Adjective
1. aorta	_____
2. atrium	_____
3. _____	cardiac
4. vein	_____
5. _____	arteriolar
6. _____	ventricular
7. valve	_____
8. heart muscle	_____
9. venule	_____
10. _____	coronary
11. _____	vascular
12. _____	arterial

C. Complete the Term

For each definition given below, fill in the blank with the word part that completes the term.

Definition	Term
1. record of a vessel	_____gram
2. fast heart condition	tachy _____
3. heart muscle disease	_____myopathy
4. inflammation of inner lining of heart	_____carditis
5. hardening of an artery	_____sclerosis
6. excessive pressure	hyper _____
7. fatty substance mass	_____oma
8. vein inflammation	_____itis
9. clot destruction	_____lytic
10. surgical removal of a plug	_____ectomy
11. pertaining to within the heart	_____coronary
12. surgical repair of a valve	_____plasty

D. Complete the Statement

1. The _____ circulation carries blood between the heart and lungs, while the _____ circulation carries blood between the heart and the cells and tissues of the body.

2. The _____ is composed of cardiac muscle.

3. The right and left sides of the heart are divided by the _____.

4. The atrioventricular valves are the _____ and _____. The semilunar valves are the _____ and _____.

5. The _____ is the pacemaker of the heart.

6. The _____ arteries carry blood to the heart muscle.

7. _____ is the force exerted by blood against the wall of a blood vessel.

8. A network of tiny blood vessels is referred to as a(n) _____.

E. Using Abbreviations

Fill in each blank with the appropriate abbreviation.

1. A(n) _____ is an arrhythmia, also called a heart block.

2. In a(n) _____, there is partial or complete occlusion of a coronary artery.

3. A(n) _____ occurs when there is an early contraction of an atrium.

4. A(n) _____ is used to diagnose cardiac arrhythmias.

5. A(n) _____ uses ultrasound to visualize cardiac structures.

6. The coronary artery was dilated during a(n) _____ procedure.

7. During open-heart surgery, _____ is used to oxygenate and circulate blood.

8. Doppler ultrasonography was used to look for a(n) _____.

9. In _____, the myocardium is too weak to efficiently pump blood.

10. _____ means that at birth there is a hole in the septum between two heart chambers.

F. Define the Term

1. catheter _____

2. infarct _____

3. thrombus _____

4. palpitation _____

5. regurgitation _____

6. aneurysm _____

7. cardiac arrest _____

8. fibrillation _____

9. myocardial infarction _____

10. hemorrhoid _____

G. Fill in the Blank

angiography	murmur	varicose veins	echocardiogram
pacemaker	CHF	defibrillation	angina pectoris
Holter monitor	hypertension	MI	CCU

1. Tiffany was born with a congenital condition resulting in an abnormal heart sound called a(n) _____.

2. Joseph suffered an arrhythmia resulting in cardiac arrest. The emergency team used an instrument to give electric shocks to the heart to create a normal heart rhythm. This procedure is called _____.

3. Marguerite has been placed on a low-sodium diet and medication to bring her blood pressure down to a normal range. She suffers from _____.

4. Tony has had an artificial device called a(n) _____ inserted to control the beating of his heart by producing rhythmic electrical impulses.

5. Derrick's physician determined that he had _____ after examining his legs and finding swollen, tortuous veins.

6. Laura has persistent chest pains that require medication. The term for the pain is _____.

7. La Tonya will be admitted to what hospital unit after surgery to correct her heart condition? _____

8. Stephen is going to have a coronary artery bypass graft to correct the blockage in his coronary arteries. He recently suffered a heart attack as a result of this occlusion. His attack is called a(n) _____.

9. Stephen's physician scheduled a(n) _____, an X-ray to determine the extent of his blood vessel damage.

10. Maria is scheduled to have a diagnostic procedure that uses ultrasound to produce an image of the heart valves. She is going to have a(n) _____.

11. Eric must wear a device for 24 hours that will keep track of his heart activity as he performs his normal daily routine. This device is called a(n) _____.

12. Lydia is 82 years old and is suffering from a heart condition that causes weakness, edema, and breathlessness. Her heart failure is the cause of her lung congestion. This condition is called _____.

H. Pharmacology Challenge

Fill in the classification for each drug description, then match the brand name.

Drug Description	Classification	Brand Name
1. _____ prevents arrhythmia	_____	a. tPA
2. _____ reduces cholesterol	_____	b. Coumadin
3. _____ increases force of heart contraction	_____	c. Cardizem
4. _____ increases urine production	_____	d. Nitro-Dur
5. _____ prevents blood clots	_____	e. Tambocor
6. _____ dissolves blood clots	_____	f. Lanoxin
7. _____ relaxes smooth muscle in artery wall	_____	g. Lipitor
8. _____ causes heart to beat less forcefully	_____	h. Lasix

I. Spelling Practice

Some of the following terms are misspelled. Identify the incorrect terms and spell them correctly in the blank provided.

1. cardiomiopathy _____

2. tackycardia _____

3. ischemia _____

4. auscultation _____

5. arteriosclerosis _____

6. aneurysm _____

7. catheterization _____

8. infraction _____

9. arhythmia _____

10. angitis _____

MyLab Medical Terminology™

MyLab Medical Terminology is a premium online homework management system that includes a host of features to help you study. Registered users will find:

• A multitude of activities and assignments built within the MyLab platform

• Powerful tools that track and analyze your results—allowing you to create a personalized learning experience

• Videos and audio pronunciations to help enrich your progress

• Streaming lesson presentations (Guided Lectures) and self-paced learning modules

• A space where you and your instructors can check your progress and manage your assignments

Labeling Exercises

Image A

Write the labels for this figure on the numbered lines provided.

1. _____

2. _____

3. _____

4. _____

5. _____

6. _____

7. _____

8. _____

9. _____

10. _____

11. _____

12. _____

Image B

Write the labels for this figure on the numbered lines provided.

1. _____

2. _____

3. _____

4. _____

5. _____

6. _____

7. _____

8. _____

9. _____

10. _____

11. _____

12. _____

13. _____

14. _____

15. _____

16. _____

17. _____

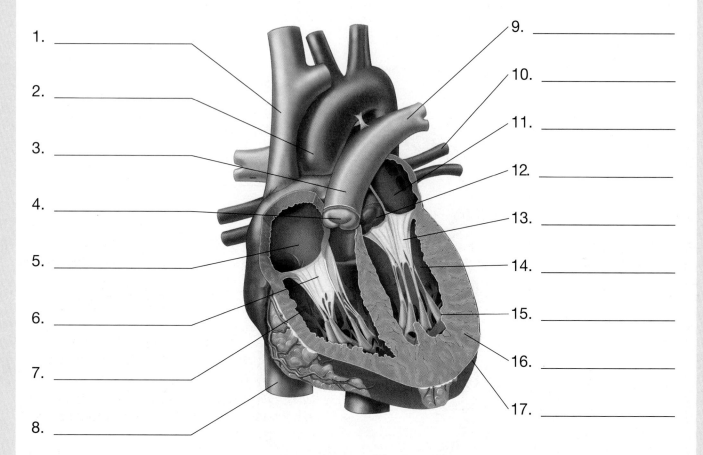

Chapter 6

Blood and the Lymphatic and Immune Systems

Learning Objectives

Upon completion of this chapter, you will be able to

1. Identify and define the combining forms and suffixes introduced in this chapter.
2. Gain the ability to pronounce medical terms and major anatomical structures.
3. List the major components, structures, and organs of the blood and lymphatic and immune systems and their functions.
4. Describe the blood typing systems.
5. Discuss immunity, the immune response, and standard precautions.
6. Identify and define blood and lymphatic and immune system anatomical terms.
7. Identify and define selected blood and lymphatic and immune system pathology terms.
8. Identify and define selected blood and lymphatic and immune system diagnostic procedures.
9. Identify and define selected blood and lymphatic and immune system therapeutic procedures.
10. Identify and define selected medications associated with blood and the lymphatic and immune systems.
11. Define selected abbreviations associated with blood and the lymphatic and immune systems.

(Pearson Education, Inc.)

SECTION I: BLOOD

AT A GLANCE

Function

Blood transports gases, nutrients, and wastes to all areas of the body either attached to red blood cells or dissolved in the plasma. White blood cells fight infection and disease, and platelets initiate the blood-clotting process.

Organs

The primary components that comprise blood:

formed elements   **plasma**

- **erythrocytes**
- **leukocytes**
- **platelets**

Word Parts

Presented here are the most common word parts (with their meanings) used to build blood terms. For a more comprehensive list, refer to the Terminology section of this chapter.

Combining Forms

agglutin/o	clumping	**hemat/o**	blood
bas/o	base	**morph/o**	shape
chrom/o	color	**myel/o**	bone marrow, spinal cord
coagul/o	clotting	**neutr/o**	neutral
eosin/o	rosy red	**phag/o**	eat, swallow
fus/o	pouring	**sanguin/o**	blood
granul/o	granules	**septic/o**	infection
hem/o	blood		

Suffixes

-apheresis	removal, carry away	**-phil**	attracted to
-crit	separation of	**-philia**	condition of being attracted to
-cytic	pertaining to cells	**-philic**	pertaining to being attracted to
-cytosis	more than the normal number of cells	**-plastic**	pertaining to formation
		-plastin	formation
-emia	blood condition	**-poiesis**	formation
-globin	protein	**-rrhagic**	pertaining to abnormal flow
-oid	resembling	**-stasis**	standing still
-penia	abnormal decrease, too few		

Blood Illustrated

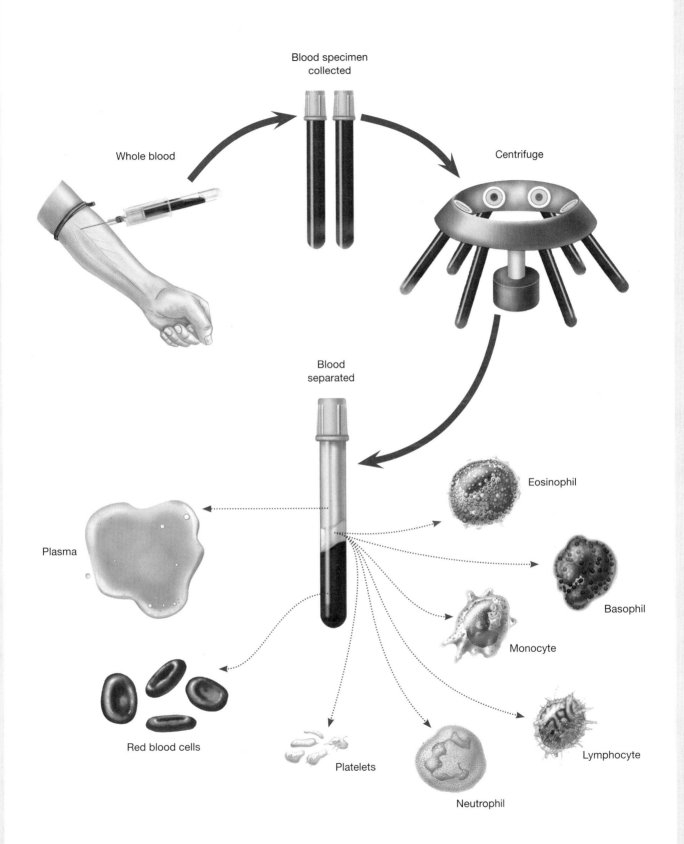

Blood specimen
collected

Whole blood

Centrifuge

Blood
separated

Plasma

Eosinophil

Basophil

Monocyte

Red blood cells

Platelets

Lymphocyte

Neutrophil

Anatomy and Physiology of Blood

erythrocytes (eh-RITH-roh-sights)

formed elements

hematopoiesis (hee-mah-toh-poy-EE-sis)

leukocytes (LOO-koh-sights)

plasma (PLAZ-mah)

platelets (PLAYT-lets)

red blood cells

white blood cells

The average adult has about five liters of blood that circulates throughout the body within the blood vessels of the cardiovascular system. Blood is a mixture of cells floating in watery **plasma**. As a group, these cells are referred to as **formed elements**, but there are three different kinds: **erythrocytes** (or **red blood cells**), **leukocytes** (or **white blood cells**), and **platelets**. Blood cells are produced in the red bone marrow by a process called **hematopoiesis**. Plasma and erythrocytes are responsible for transporting substances, leukocytes protect the body from invading microorganisms, and platelets play a role in controlling bleeding.

Plasma

albumin (al-BYOO-min)

amino acids (ah-MEE-noh)

calcium (KAL-see-um)

creatinine (kree-AT-in-in)

fats

fibrinogen (fye-BRIN-oh-jen)

gamma globulin (GAM-ah / GLOB-yoo-lin)

globulins (GLOB-yoo-lins)

glucose (GLOO-kohs)

plasma proteins

potassium (poh-TASS-ee-um)

sodium

urea (yoo-REE-ah)

Liquid plasma composes about 55% of whole blood in the average adult and is 90–92% water. The remaining 8–10% portion of plasma is dissolved substances, especially **plasma proteins** such as **albumin**, **globulins**, and **fibrinogen**. Albumin helps transport fatty substances that cannot dissolve in the watery plasma. There are three main types of globulins; the most commonly known one, **gamma globulin**, acts as an antibody. Fibrinogen is a blood-clotting protein. In addition to the plasma proteins, smaller amounts of other important substances are also dissolved in the plasma for transport: **calcium**, **potassium**, **sodium**, **glucose**, **amino acids**, **fats**, and waste products such as **urea** and **creatinine**.

Erythrocytes

bilirubin (bil-ih-ROO-bin)

enucleated (ee-NOO-klee-ay-ted)

hemoglobin (hee-moh-GLOH-bin)

Erythrocytes, or red blood cells (RBCs), are biconcave disks that are **enucleated**, meaning they no longer contain a nucleus (see Figure 6-1 ■). Red blood cells appear red in color because they contain **hemoglobin**, an iron-containing pigment. Hemoglobin is the part of the red blood cell that picks up oxygen from the lungs and delivers it to the tissues of the body.

There are about 5 million erythrocytes per cubic millimeter of blood. The total number in an average-sized adult is 35 trillion, with males having more red blood cells than females. Erythrocytes have an average lifespan of 120 days, and then the spleen removes the worn-out and damaged ones from circulation. Much of the red blood cell, such as the iron, can be reused, but one portion, **bilirubin**, is a waste product disposed of by the liver.

Erythrocytes

Red blood cells

■ **Figure 6-1** The biconcave disk shape of erythrocytes (red blood cells).

Leukocytes

Basophil

Eosinophil

Monocyte

Neutrophil

Lymphocyte

■ **Figure 6-2** The five different types of leukocytes (white blood cells).

Leukocytes

agranulocytes (ah-GRAN-yoo-loh-sights)
granulocytes (GRAN-yoo-loh-sights)
pathogens (PATH-oh-jenz)

Leukocytes, also referred to as white blood cells (WBCs), provide protection against the invasion of **pathogens** such as bacteria, viruses, and other foreign material. In general, white blood cells have a spherical shape with a large nucleus, and there are about 8,000 per cubic millimeter of blood (see Figure 6-2 ■). There are five different types of white blood cells, each with its own strategy for protecting the body. The five can be subdivided into two categories: **granulocytes** (with granules in the cytoplasm) and **agranulocytes** (without granules in the cytoplasm). The name and function of each type is presented in Table 6-1 ■.

Platelets

agglutinate (ah-GLOO-tih-nayt)
fibrin (FYE-brin)
hemostasis (hee-moh-STAY-sis)
prothrombin (proh-THROM-bin)
thrombin (THROM-bin)
thrombocyte (THROM-boh-sight)
thromboplastin (throm-boh-PLAS-tin)

Platelet, the modern term for **thrombocyte**, refers to the smallest of all the formed blood elements. Platelets are not whole cells, but rather are formed when the

> **Med Term Tip**
> Your body makes about 2 million erythrocytes every second. Of course, it must then destroy 2 million every second to maintain a relatively constant 30 trillion red blood cells.

> **What's In A Name?**
> Look for these word parts:
> **bas/o** = base
> **eosin/o** = rosy red
> **granul/o** = granules
> **lymph/o** = lymph
> **neutr/o** = neutral
> **path/o** = disease
> **-cyte** = cell
> **-gen** = that which produces
> **-phil** = attracted to
> **a-** = without
> **mono-** = one

> **Med Term Tip**
> A *phagocyte* is a cell that has the ability to ingest (**phag/o** = eat; **-cyte** = cell) and digest bacteria and other foreign particles. This process, *phagocytosis*, is critical for the control of bacteria within the body.

■ **TABLE 6–1** Leukocyte Classification

Leukocyte	Function
Granulocytes	
Basophils (basos) (BAY-soh-fillz)	Release histamine and heparin to damaged tissues
Eosinophils (eosins, eos) (ee-oh-SIN-oh-fillz)	Destroy parasites and increase during allergic reactions
Neutrophils (NOO-troh-fillz)	Engulf foreign and damaged cells (phagocytosis); most numerous of the leukocytes
Agranulocytes	
Monocytes (monos) (MON-oh-sights)	Engulf foreign and damaged cells (phagocytosis)
Lymphocytes (lymphs) (LIM-foh-sights)	Play several different roles in immune response

■ **Figure 6-3** Platelet structure.

cytoplasm of a large precursor cell shatters into small platelike fragments (see Figure 6-3 ■). There are between 200,000 and 300,000 per cubic millimeter in the body.

Platelets play a critical part in the blood-clotting process or **hemostasis**. They **agglutinate** or clump together into small clusters when a blood vessel is cut or damaged. Platelets also release a substance called **thromboplastin**, which, in the presence of calcium, reacts with **prothrombin** (a clotting protein in the blood) to form **thrombin**. Then thrombin, in turn, works to convert fibrinogen to **fibrin**, which eventually becomes the meshlike blood clot.

Blood Typing

ABO system   Rh factor
blood typing

Each person's blood is different due to the presence of antigens or markers on the surface of erythrocytes. Before a person receives a blood transfusion, it is important to do **blood typing**. This laboratory test determines if the donated blood is compatible with the recipient's blood. There are many different subgroups of blood markers, but the two most important ones are the **ABO system** and **Rh factor**.

ABO System

type A   type 0
type AB   universal donor
type B   universal recipient

In the ABO blood system, there are two possible red blood cell markers, A and B. A marker is one method by which cells identify themselves. A person with an A marker is said to have **type A** blood. Type A blood produces anti-B antibodies that will attack type B blood. The presence of a B marker indicates **type B** blood and anti-A antibodies (that will attack type A blood). If both markers are present, the blood is **type AB** and does not contain any antibodies. Therefore, type AB blood will not attack any other blood type. The absence of either an A or a B marker results in **type 0** blood, which contains both anti-A and anti-B antibodies. Type O blood will attack all other blood types (A, B, and AB). For further information on antibodies, refer to the lymphatic section later in this chapter.

Because type O blood does not have either the A or B marker, its red blood cells will not be attacked by the antibodies in type A, type B, or type AB blood. For this reason, a person with type O blood is referred to as a **universal donor**. In extreme cases, type O blood may be given to a person with any of the other blood types. Similarly, type AB blood is the **universal recipient**. A person with type AB blood has no antibodies against the other blood types and, therefore, in extreme cases, can receive any type of blood.

Rh Factor

Rh-negative   Rh-positive

Rh factor is not as difficult to understand as the ABO system. A person with the Rh factor on his or her red blood cells is said to be **Rh-positive** (Rh+). Since this person has the factor, he or she will not make anti-Rh antibodies. A person without the Rh factor is **Rh-negative** (Rh−) and will produce anti-Rh antibodies. Therefore, an Rh+ person may receive both an Rh+ and an Rh− transfusion, but an Rh− person can receive only Rh− blood.

PRACTICE AS YOU GO

A. Complete the Statement

1. The process whereby cells ingest and destroy bacteria within the body is _____.

2. The formed elements of blood are the _____, _____, and _____.

3. The fluid portion of blood is called _____.

4. The medical term for blood clotting is _____.

5. The two most important subgroups of blood markers are the _____ and _____.

Terminology

Word Parts Used to Build Blood Terms

The following lists contain the combining forms, suffixes, and prefixes used to build terms in the remaining sections of this chapter.

Combining Forms

bas/o	base	fus/o	pouring	myel/o	bone marrow
chrom/o	color	hem/o	blood	neutr/o	neutral
coagul/o	clotting	hemat/o	blood	phleb/o	vein
cyt/o	cell	leuk/o	white	sanguin/o	blood
eosin/o	rosy red	lip/o	fat	septic/o	infection
erythr/o	red	lymph/o	lymph	thromb/o	clot
fibrin/o	fibers	morph/o	shape		

Suffixes

-apheresis	removal, carry away	-ic	pertaining to	-philia	condition of being attracted to
-crit	separation of	-ion	action	-philic	pertaining to being attracted to
-cyte	cell	-logy	study of		
-cytic	pertaining to cells	-lytic	destruction	-plastic	pertaining to formation
-cytosis	more than the normal number of cells	-oid	resembling		
		-oma	mass	-rrhage	abnormal flow
-emia	blood condition	-otomy	cutting into	-rrhagic	pertaining to abnormal flow
-globin	protein	-ous	pertaining to		
-ia	condition	-penia	too few	-tic	pertaining to

Prefixes

a-	without	dys-	abnormal	pan-	all
an-	without	homo-	same	poly-	many
anti-	against	hyper-	excessive	trans-	across
auto-	self	hypo-	insufficient		
contra-	against	mono-	one		

Adjective Forms of Anatomical Terms

Term	Word Parts	Definition
basophilic (bay-soh-FILL-ik)	bas/o = base -philic = pertaining to being attracted to	Pertaining to [a leukocyte] that attracts a basic pH stain
eosinophilic (ee-oh-sin-oh-FILL-ik)	eosin/o = rosy red -philic = pertaining to being attracted to	Pertaining to [a leukocyte] that attracts a rosy red stain
erythrocytic (eh-rith-roh-SIT-ik)	erythr/o = red -cytic = pertaining to cells	Pertaining to a red blood cell
fibrinous (FYE-brin-us)	fibrin/o = fibers -ous = pertaining to	Pertaining to fibers
hematic (hee-MAT-ik)	hemat/o = blood -ic = pertaining to	Pertaining to blood
leukocytic (loo-koh-SIT-ik)	leuk/o = white -cytic = pertaining to cells	Pertaining to a white blood cell
lymphocytic (lim-foh-SIT-ik)	lymph/o = lymph -cytic = pertaining to cells	Pertaining to a [white] cell formed in lymphatic tissue
monocytic (mon-oh-SIT-ik)	mono- = one -cytic = pertaining to cells	Pertaining to a [white] cell with a single, large nucleus
neutrophilic (noo-troh-FILL-ik)	neutr/o = neutral -philic = pertaining to being attracted to	Pertaining to [a leukocyte] that attracts a neutral pH stain
sanguineous (sang-GWIN-ee-us)	sanguin/o = blood -ous = pertaining to	Pertaining to blood

> **Word Watch**
> The term *sanguineous* has an unusual spelling; an *e* is added between the word root, **sanguin**, and the suffix, **-ous**.

Term	Word Parts	Definition
thrombocytic (throm-boh-SIT-ik)	thromb/o = clot -cytic = pertaining to cells	Pertaining to a clotting cell; a platelet
thrombotic (throm-BOT-ik)	thromb/o = clot -tic = pertaining to	Pertaining to a clot

PRACTICE AS YOU GO

B. Give the adjective form for each anatomical structure.

1. Blood   _____ or _____

2. White cell   _____

3. Clotting cell   _____

4. Fibers   _____

5. Red cell   _____

Pathology

Term	Word Parts	Definition
Medical Specialties		
hematology (hee-mah-TALL-oh-jee)	hemat/o = blood -logy = study of	Branch of medicine specializing in treatment of diseases and conditions of blood; physician is a *hematologist*
Signs and Symptoms		
coagulate (koh-AG-yoo-late)	coagul/o = clotting	To convert from a liquid to a gel or solid, as in blood coagulation
dyscrasia (dis-KRAY-zee-ah)	dys- = abnormal -ia = condition	General term indicating presence of a disease affecting blood
hematoma (hee-mah-TOH-mah)	hemat/o = blood -oma = mass	Collection of blood under skin as result of blood escaping into tissue from damaged blood vessels; commonly referred to as a *bruise*
	Word Watch The term *hematoma* is confusing. Its simple translation is *blood mass.* However, it is used to refer to blood that has leaked out of a blood vessel and has pooled in the tissues causing swelling.	
hemorrhage (HEM-eh-rij)	hem/o = blood -rrhage = abnormal flow	Blood flowing out of blood vessel (i.e., bleeding)
thrombus (THROM-bus)	thromb/o = clot	Hard collection of fibrin, blood cells, and tissue debris that is end result of hemostasis or blood-clotting process; thrombus is helpful to body by stopping bleeding, as in skin laceration; however, it is hurtful to body if it occurs within a blood vessel, as in myocardial infarction; commonly referred to as a *blood clot*

■ **Figure 6-4** Electronmicrograph showing a thrombus composed of fibrin, red blood cells, and tissue debris. *(Juan Gaertner/Shutterstock)*

Term	Word Parts	Definition
Blood		
hemophilia (hee-moh-FILL-ee-ah)	hem/o = blood -philia = condition of being attracted to	Hereditary blood disease in which blood-clotting time is prolonged due to lack of one vital clotting factor; transmitted by sex-linked trait from females to males, appearing almost exclusively in males
hyperlipidemia (high-per-lip-ih-DEE-mee-ah)	hyper- = excessive lip/o = fat -emia = blood condition	Condition of having too high a level of lipids such as cholesterol in bloodstream; risk factor for developing atherosclerosis and coronary artery disease
pancytopenia (pan-sigh-toh-PEE-nee-ah)	pan- = all cyt/o = cell -penia = too few	Having too few of all cells
septicemia (sep-tih-SEE-mee-ah)	septic/o = infection -emia = blood condition	Having bacteria or their toxins in bloodstream; *sepsis* is term that means *putrefaction* or *infection;* commonly referred to as *blood poisoning*

Pathology (continued)

Term	Word Parts	Definition
Erythrocytes		
anemia (ah-NEE-mee-ah)	an- = without -emia = blood condition	Large group of conditions characterized by reduction in number of red blood cells or amount of hemoglobin in blood; results in less oxygen reaching tissues
aplastic anemia (ay-PLAS-tik / ah-NEE-mee-ah)	a- = without -plastic = pertaining to formation an- = without -emia = blood condition	Severe form of anemia that develops as a consequence of loss of functioning red bone marrow; results in decrease in number of all formed elements; treatment may eventually require bone marrow transplant
erythrocytosis (eh-rith-roh-sigh-TOH-sis)	erythr/o = red -cytosis = more than normal number of cells	Condition of having too many red blood cells
erythropenia (eh-rith-roh-PEE-nee-ah)	erythr/o = red -penia = too few	Condition of having too few red blood cells
hemolytic anemia (hee-moh-LIT-ik / ah-NEE-mee-ah)	hem/o = blood -lytic = destruction an- = without -emia = blood condition	Anemia that develops as result of destruction of erythrocytes
hemolytic reaction (hee-moh-LIT-ik)	hem/o = blood -lytic = destruction	Destruction of patient's erythrocytes that occurs when receiving a transfusion of incompatible blood type; also called *transfusion reaction*
hypochromic anemia (high-poh-KROHM-ik / ah-NEE-mee-ah)	hypo- = insufficient chrom/o = color -ic = pertaining to an- = without -emia = blood condition	Anemia resulting from having insufficient hemoglobin in erythrocytes; named because hemoglobin molecule is responsible for dark red color of erythrocytes
iron-deficiency anemia	an- = without -emia = blood condition	Anemia resulting from not having sufficient iron to manufacture hemoglobin
pernicious anemia (PA) (per-NISH-us / ah-NEE-mee-ah)	an- = without -emia = blood condition	Anemia associated with insufficient absorption of vitamin B_{12} by digestive system; vitamin B_{12} is necessary for erythrocyte production
polycythemia vera (pol-ee-sigh-THEE-mee-ah / VAIR-ah)	poly- = many cyt/o = cell hem/o = blood -ia = condition	Production of too many red blood cells by bone marrow; blood becomes too thick to easily flow through blood vessels
sickle cell anemia	an- = without -emia = blood condition	Genetic disorder in which erythrocytes take on abnormal curved or "sickle" shape; cells are fragile and are easily damaged, leading to hemolytic anemia

Normal red blood cells   **Sickled cells**

■ **Figure 6-5** Comparison of normal-shaped erythrocytes and the abnormal sickle shape noted in patients with sickle cell anemia.

Pathology (continued)

Term	Word Parts	Definition
thalassemia (thal-ah-SEE-mee-ah)	-emia = blood condition	Genetic disorder in which body is unable to make functioning hemoglobin, resulting in anemia
Leukocytes		
leukemia (loo-KEE-mee-ah)	leuk/o = white -emia = blood condition	Cancer located in red bone marrow tissue responsible for producing white blood cells; results in large number of abnormal and immature leukocytes circulating in bloodstream
leukocytosis (loo-koh-sigh-TOH-sis)	leuk/o = white -cytosis = more than normal number of cells	Condition of having too many white blood cells
leukopenia (loo-koh-PEE-nee-ah)	leuk/o = white -penia = too few	Condition of having too few white blood cells
lymphocytic leukemia (lim-foh-SIT-ik / loo-KEE-mee-ah)	lymph/o = lymph -cytic = pertaining to cells leuk/o = white -emia = blood condition	Type of leukemia in which abnormal white blood cells are lymphocytes; may be acute (rapid onset and progression) or chronic (slow onset and progression)
myeloid leukemia (MY-eh-loyd / loo-KEE-mee-ah)	myel/o = bone marrow -oid = resembling leuk/o = white -emia = blood condition	Type of leukemia in which abnormal leukocytes are granulocytes (usually neutrophils); may be acute (rapid onset and progression) or chronic (slow onset and progression)
Platelets		
thrombocytopenia (throm-boh-sigh-toh-PEE-nee-ah)	thromb/o = clot cyt/o = cell -penia = too few	Condition of having too few platelets
thrombocytosis (throm-boh-sigh-TOH-sis)	thromb/o = clot -cytosis = more than normal number of cells	Condition of having too many platelets

PRACTICE AS YOU GO

C. Terminology Matching

Match each term to its definition.

1. _____ thalassemia
2. _____ dyscrasia
3. _____ hematoma
4. _____ anemia
5. _____ hemophilia

a. disease in which blood does not clot

b. condition with reduced number of RBCs

c. mass of blood

d. type of anemia

e. general term for blood disorders

Diagnostic Procedures

Term	Word Parts	Definition
Clinical Laboratory Tests		
blood analyzer		Automated machine that analyzes different characteristics of blood specimen, such as complete blood count, erythrocyte sedimentation rate, and blood-clotting tests
blood culture and sensitivity (C&S)		Sample of blood is incubated in laboratory to check for bacterial growth; if bacteria are present, they are identified and tested to determine to which antibiotics they are sensitive
complete blood count (CBC)		Combination of blood tests including red blood cell count (RBC), white blood cell count (WBC), hemoglobin (Hgb), hematocrit (Hct), white blood cell differential, and platelet count
erythrocyte sedimentation rate (ESR, sed rate) (eh-RITH-roh-sight / sed-ih-men-TAY-shun)	erythr/o = red -cyte = cell	Blood test to determine rate at which mature red blood cells settle out of blood after addition of anticoagulant; indicates presence of inflammatory disease
hematocrit (HCT, Hct, crit) (hee-MAT-oh-krit)	hemat/o = blood -crit = separation of	Blood test to measure volume of red blood cells (erythrocytes) within total volume of blood
hemoglobin (Hgb, Hb) (hee-moh-GLOH-bin)	hem/o = blood -globin = protein	Blood test to measure amount of hemoglobin present in given volume of blood
platelet count (PLAYT-let)		Determines number of platelets in given volume of blood
prothrombin time (pro-time, PT) (proh-THROM-bin)	thromb/o = clot	Indicates blood's coagulation abilities by measuring how long it takes for a clot to form after prothrombin has been activated
red blood cell count (RBC)		Determines number of erythrocytes in volume of blood; decrease in red blood cells may indicate anemia; increase may indicate polycythemia
red blood cell morphology	morph/o = shape -logy = study of	Determines diseases such as sickle cell anemia through examination of specimen of blood for abnormalities in shape (morphology) of erythrocytes
white blood cell count (WBC)		Measures number of leukocytes in volume of blood; increase may indicate presence of infection or disease such as leukemia; decrease in white blood cells may be caused by radiation therapy or chemotherapy
white blood cell differential (diff) (diff-er-EN-shal)		Determines number of each variety of leukocytes in volume of blood
Medical Procedures		
bone marrow aspiration (as-pih-RAY-shun)		Removed by aspiration with a needle, a sample of bone marrow is examined for diseases such as leukemia or aplastic anemia
phlebotomy (fleh-BOT-oh-mee)	phleb/o = vein -otomy = cutting into	Incision into vein in order to remove blood for diagnostic test; also called *venipuncture*

■ **Figure 6-6** Phlebotomist using a needle to withdraw blood. *(Michal Heron/Pearson Education, Inc.)*

Therapeutic Procedures

Term	Word Parts	Definition
Medical Procedures		
autologous transfusion (aw-TALL-oh-gus / trans-FYOO-zhun)	auto- = self	Procedure for collecting and storing patient's own blood several weeks prior to actual need; can then be used to replace blood lost during surgical procedure
blood transfusion (trans-FYOO-zhun)	trans- = across fus/o = pouring -ion = action	Artificial transfer of blood into bloodstream **Med Term Tip** Before a patient receives a blood transfusion, the laboratory performs a **type and cross-match**. This test first double-checks the blood type of both the donor's and recipient's blood. Then a cross-match is performed. This process mixes together small samples of both bloods and observes the mixture for adverse reactions.
bone marrow transplant (BMT)		Patient receives red bone marrow from donor after patient's own bone marrow has been destroyed by radiation or chemotherapy
homologous transfusion (hoh-MALL-oh-gus / trans-FYOO-zhun)	homo- = same	Replacement of blood by transfusion of blood received from another person
packed red cells		Transfusion in which most of plasma, leukocytes, and platelets have been removed, leaving only erythrocytes
plasmapheresis (plaz-mah-fah-REE-sis)	-apheresis = removal, carry away	Method of removing plasma from body without depleting formed elements; whole blood is removed and cells and plasma are separated; cells are returned to patient along with donor plasma transfusion
whole blood		Transfusion of a mixture of both plasma and formed elements

Pharmacology

Vocabulary

Term	Word Parts	Definition
additive		Sum of action of two (or more) drugs given; in this case, total strength of medications is equal to sum of strength of each individual drug
contraindication (kon-trah-in-dih-KAY-shun)	contra- = against	Condition in which particular drug should not be used
drug interaction		Occurs when effect of one drug is altered because it was taken at the same time as another drug
potentiation (poh-ten-shee-AY-shun)		Giving patient a second drug to boost (potentiate) effect of another drug; total strength of drugs is greater than sum of strength of individual drugs

Drugs

Classification	Word Parts	Action	Examples
anticoagulant (an-tye-koh-AG-yoo-lant)	anti- = against coagul/o = clotting	Prevents blood clot formation; commonly referred to as *blood thinner*	heparin, HepLock; warfarin, Coumadin

Pharmacology (continued)

Classification	Word Parts	Action	Examples
antihemorrhagic (an-tye-hem-eh-RAJ-ik)	anti- = against hem/o = blood -rrhagic = pertaining to abnormal flow	Prevents or stops hemorrhaging; *hemostatic agent*	aminocaproic acid, Amicar; vitamin K
antiplatelet agents (an-tee-PLAYT-let)	anti- = against	Interferes with action of platelets; prolongs bleeding time; used to prevent heart attacks and strokes	clopidogrel, Plavix; ticlopidine, Ticlid
fibrinolytic (fye-brin-oh-LIT-ik)	fibrin/o = fibers -lytic = destruction	Able to dissolve existing blood clots	alteplase, Activase; tissue plasminogen activator; Tenecteplase
hematinic (hee-mah-TIN-ik)	hemat/o = blood -ic = pertaining to	Increases number of erythrocytes or amount of hemoglobin in blood	epoetin alfa, Procrit; darbepoetin alfa, Aranesp

PRACTICE AS YOU GO

D. Procedure Matching

Match each procedure term with its definition.

1. _____ phlebotomy
2. _____ ESR
3. _____ plasmapheresis
4. _____ whole blood
5. _____ culture and sensitivity

a. method of removing plasma from the body
b. mixture of plasma and formed elements
c. removal of blood from a vein
d. test for bacterial growth
e. test that indicates presence of inflammatory disease

Abbreviations

ā	before	CBC	complete blood count
ac	before meals	CLL	chronic lymphocytic leukemia
ALL	acute lymphocytic leukemia	CML	chronic myeloid leukemia
AML	acute myeloid leukemia	diff	differential
ante	before	eosins, eos	eosinophils
basos	basophils	ESR, sed rate	erythrocyte sedimentation rate
BMT	bone marrow transplant	et	and
c̄	with	HCT, Hct, crit	hematocrit

Abbreviations (continued)

Hgb, Hb	hemoglobin	**PMN, polys**	polymorphonuclear neutrophil
lymphs	lymphocytes	**PT, pro-time**	prothrombin time
monos	monocytes	**RBC**	red blood cell
noc	night	**Rh+**	Rh-positive
$\bar{p}$	after	**Rh−**	Rh-negative
PA	pernicious anemia	$\bar{s}$	without
pc	after meals	**segs**	segmented neutrophils
PCV	packed cell volume	**WBC**	white blood cell

PRACTICE AS YOU GO

E. What's the Abbreviation?

1. acute lymphocytic leukemia _____

2. bone marrow transplant _____

3. eosinophils _____

4. hematocrit _____

5. pernicious anemia _____

6. complete blood count _____

7. differential _____

8. white blood cell _____

9. night _____

10. after meals _____

AT A GLANCE

Function

The lymphatic system consists of a network of lymph vessels that pick up excess tissue fluid, cleanse it, and return it to the circulatory system. It also picks up fats that have been absorbed by the digestive system. The immune system fights disease and infections.

Organs

The primary structures that comprise the lymphatic and immune systems:

lymph nodes	**spleen**
lymphatic vessels	**thymus gland**
	tonsils

Word Parts

Presented here are the most common word parts (with their meanings) used to build lymphatic and immune system terms. For a more comprehensive list, refer to the Terminology section of this chapter.

Combining Forms

adenoid/o	adenoids	**lymphangi/o**	lymph vessel
axill/o	axilla (underarm)	**nucle/o**	nucleus
immun/o	protection	**splen/o**	spleen
inguin/o	groin region	**thym/o**	thymus gland
lymph/o	lymph	**tonsill/o**	tonsils
lymphaden/o	lymph node		

Suffixes

-edema	swelling	**-phage**	to eat
-globulin	protein	**-toxic**	pertaining to poison

The Lymphatic and Immune Systems Illustrated

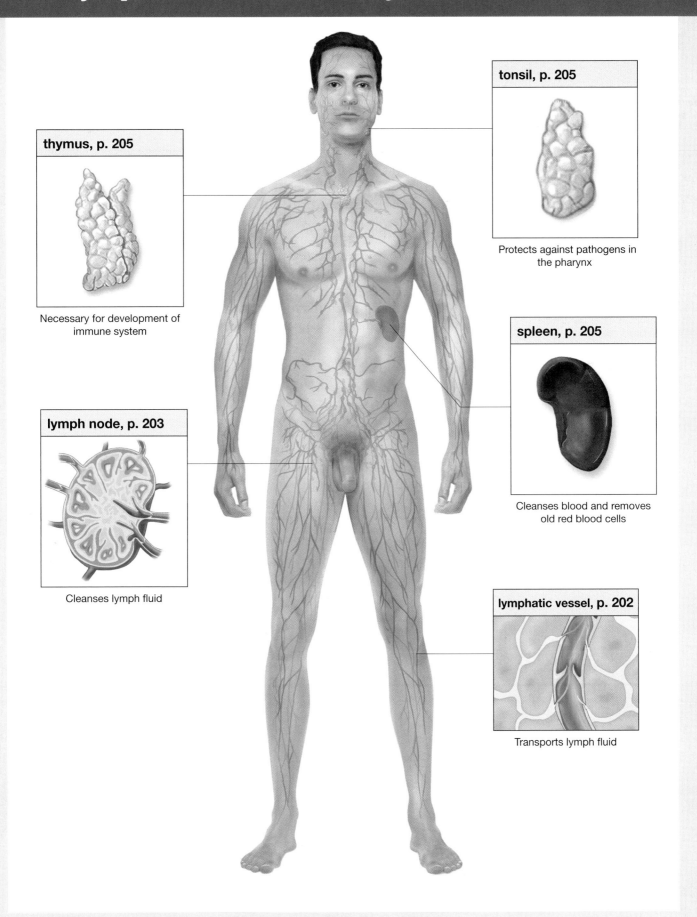

thymus, p. 205

Necessary for development of immune system

tonsil, p. 205

Protects against pathogens in the pharynx

spleen, p. 205

Cleanses blood and removes old red blood cells

lymph node, p. 203

Cleanses lymph fluid

lymphatic vessel, p. 202

Transports lymph fluid

Anatomy and Physiology
of the Lymphatic and Immune Systems

Med Term Tip

The term *lymph* comes from the Latin word *lympha* meaning *clear spring water*. Although a very pale, clear yellow, lymph appears crystal clear when compared to the other body fluid, blood.

Med Term Tip

The term *lacteal* describes the appearance of lymph fluid inside the lacteal vessels. After absorbing fats from a meal, the suspended fat molecules turn the lymph fluid a milky white.

lacteals (LAK-tee-als)   spleen
lymph (LIMF)   thymus gland (THIGH-mus)
lymph nodes   tonsils (TAHN-sulls)
lymphatic vessels (lim-FAT-ik)

The lymphatic system consists of a network of **lymphatic vessels**, **lymph nodes**, the **spleen**, the **thymus gland**, and the **tonsils**. These organs perform several quite diverse functions for the body. First, they collect excess tissue fluid through-out the body and return it to the circulatory system. The fluid, once inside a lymphatic vessel, is referred to as **lymph**. Lymph vessels located around the small intestines, called **lacteals**, are able to pick up absorbed fats for transport. Additionally, the lymphatic system works with the immune system to form the groups of cells, tissues, organs, and molecules that serve as the body's primary defense against the invasion of pathogens. These systems work together, defend-ing the body against foreign invaders and substances, as well as removing the body's own cells that have become diseased.

Lymphatic Vessels

lymphatic capillaries (KAP-ih-lair-eez)   thoracic duct
lymphatic ducts   valves
right lymphatic duct

The lymphatic vessels form an extensive network of ducts throughout the entire body. However, unlike the circulatory system, these vessels are not in a closed loop. Instead, they serve as one-way pipes conducting lymph from the tissues toward the thoracic cavity (see Figure 6-7 ■). These vessels begin as very small **lymphatic capillaries** in the tissues. Excessive tissue fluid enters these capillaries to begin the trip back to the circulatory system. The capillaries merge into larger

■ **Figure 6-7** Lymphatic vessels (green) pick up excess tissue fluid, purify it in lymph nodes, and return it to the circulatory system.

■ **Figure 6-8**   A) Lymphatic vessel with valves within tissue cells; B) Photomicrograph of lymphatic vessel with valve clearly visible. *(Michael Abbey/Science Source.)*

lymphatic vessels. This is a very low-pressure system, so these vessels have **valves** along their length to ensure that lymph can only move forward toward the thoracic cavity (see Figure 6-8 ■). These vessels finally drain into one of two large **lymphatic ducts**, the **right lymphatic duct** or the **thoracic duct**. The smaller right lymphatic duct drains the right arm and the right side of the head, neck, and chest. This duct empties lymph into the right subclavian vein. The larger thoracic duct drains lymph from the rest of the body and empties into the left subclavian vein (see Figure 6-9 ■).

Lymph Nodes

lymph glands

Lymph nodes are small organs composed of lymphatic tissue located along the route of the lymphatic vessels. These nodes, also referred to as **lymph glands**, house lymphocytes and antibodies and therefore work to remove pathogens and cell debris as lymph passes through them on its way back to the thoracic cavity (see Figure 6-10 ■). Lymph nodes also serve to trap and destroy cells from cancerous tumors. Although found throughout the body, lymph nodes are particularly concentrated in several regions. For example, lymph nodes concentrated in the neck region drain lymph from the head. See again Figure 6-9 and Table 6-2 ■ for a description of some of the most important sites for lymph nodes.

> **What's In A Name?**
>
> Look for these word parts:
> **thorac/o** = chest
> **-ic** = pertaining to

> **Med Term Tip**
>
> The term *capillary* is also used to describe the minute blood vessels within the circulatory system. This is one of several general medical terms, such as valves, cilia, and hair, that are used across several systems.

> **Med Term Tip**
>
> In surgical procedures to remove a malignancy from an organ, such as a breast, the adjacent lymph nodes are also tested for cancer. If cancerous cells are found in the tested lymph nodes, the disease is said to have spread or *metastasized*. Tumor cells may then spread to other parts of the body by means of the lymphatic system.

■ **TABLE 6-2**   Sites for Lymph Nodes

Name	Location	Function
axillary (AK-sih-lair-ee)	armpits	Drain arms and shoulder region; cancer cells from breasts may be present
cervical (SER-vih-kal)	neck	Drain head and neck; may be enlarged during upper respiratory infections
inguinal (ING-gwih-nal)	groin	Drain legs and lower pelvis
mediastinal (mee-dee-as-TYE-nal)	chest	Drain chest cavity

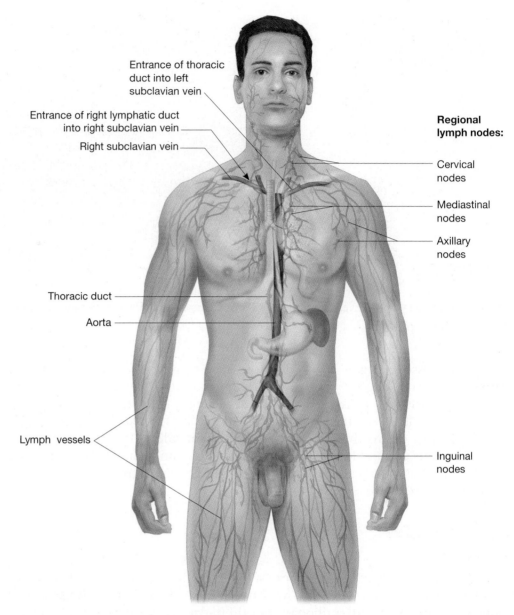

Entrance of thoracic
duct into left
subclavian vein

Entrance of right lymphatic duct
into right subclavian vein

Right subclavian vein

**Regional
lymph nodes:**

Cervical
nodes

Mediastinal
nodes

Axillary
nodes

Thoracic duct

Aorta

Lymph vessels

Inguinal
nodes

■ **Figure 6-9** Location of lymph vessels, lymphatic ducts, and areas of lymph node
concentrations.

Location of lymphocytes
and antibodies

Lymphatic vessel
(with valves)
entering lymph node

Lymphatic vessel
leaving lymph node

■ **Figure 6-10** Structure of a lymph node.

Tonsils

adenoids (AD-eh-noydz)

lingual tonsils (LING-gwal)

palatine tonsils (PAL-ah-tyne)

pharyngeal tonsils (fair-IN-jee-al)

pharynx (FAIR-inks)

The tonsils are collections of lymphatic tissue located on each side of the throat or **pharynx** (see Figure 6-11 ■). There are three sets of tonsils: **palatine tonsils**, **pharyngeal tonsils** (commonly referred to as the **adenoids**), and **lingual tonsils**. All tonsils contain a large number of leukocytes and act as filters to protect the body from the invasion of pathogens through the digestive or respiratory systems. Tonsils are not vital organs and can safely be removed if they become a continuous site of infection.

Spleen

blood sinuses

macrophages (MAK-roh-fay-jez)

The spleen, located in the upper left quadrant of the abdomen, consists of lymphatic tissue that is highly infiltrated with blood vessels (see Figure 6-12 ■). These vessels spread out into slow-moving **blood sinuses**. The spleen filters out and destroys old red blood cells, recycles the iron, and also stores some of the blood supply for the body. Phagocytic **macrophages** line the blood sinuses in the spleen to engulf and remove pathogens. Because the blood is moving through the organ slowly, the macrophages have time to carefully identify pathogens and worn-out red blood cells. The spleen is also not a vital organ and can be removed due to injury or disease. However, without the spleen, a person's susceptibility to a bloodstream infection may be increased.

Thymus Gland

T cells

T lymphocytes

thymosin (THIGH-moh-sin)

The thymus gland, located in the upper portion of the mediastinum, is essential for the proper development of the immune system (see Figure 6-13 ■). It assists the body with the immune function and the development of antibodies. This organ's hormone, **thymosin**, changes lymphocytes to **T lymphocytes** (simply called **T cells**), which play an important role in the immune response. The thymus is active in the unborn child and throughout childhood until adolescence, when it begins to shrink in size.

Immunity

acquired immunity

active acquired immunity

bacteria (bak-TEE-ree-ah)

cancerous tumors

fungi (FUN-jeye)

immune response

immunity (im-YOO-nih-tee)

immunizations (im-yoo-nih-ZAY-shuns)

natural immunity

passive acquired immunity

protozoans (proh-toh-ZOH-anz)

toxins

vaccinations (vak-sih-NAY-shuns)

viruses

Immunity is the body's ability to defend itself against pathogens, such as **bacteria**, **viruses**, **fungi**, **protozoans**, **toxins**, and **cancerous tumors**. Immunity comes in two forms: **natural immunity** and **acquired immunity**. Natural immunity, also called *innate immunity*, is not specific to a particular disease and does not require prior exposure to the pathogenic agent. A good example of natural immunity is the

■ **Figure 6-11** The shape of a tonsil.

What's In A Name?
Look for these word parts:
lingu/o = tongue
palat/o = palate
pharyng/o = pharynx
-al = pertaining to
-eal = pertaining to
-ine = pertaining to

What's In A Name?
Look for these word parts:
macro- = large
-phage = to eat

■ **Figure 6-12** The shape of the spleen.

What's In A Name?
Look for these word parts:
lymph/o = lymph
-cyte = cell

■ **Figure 6-13** The shape of the thymus gland.

What's In A Name?
Look for this word part:
-ous = pertaining to

Figure 6-14 Enhanced photomicrograph showing a macrophage (purple) attacking bacillus *Escherichia coli* (green). *(Sebastian Kaulitzki/ Shutterstock)*

macrophage. These leukocytes are present throughout all the tissues of the body, but are concentrated in areas of high exposure to invading bacteria, like the lungs and digestive system. They are very active phagocytic cells, ingesting and digesting any pathogen they encounter (see Figure 6-14 ■).

Acquired immunity is the body's response to a specific pathogen and may be established either passively or actively. **Passive acquired immunity** results when a person receives protective substances produced by another human or animal. This may take the form of maternal antibodies crossing the placenta to a baby or an antitoxin or gamma globulin injection. **Active acquired immunity** develops following direct exposure to the pathogenic agent. The agent stimulates the body's **immune response**, a series of different mechanisms all geared to neutralize the agent. For example, a person typically can catch chickenpox only once because once the body has successfully fought the virus, it will be able to more quickly recognize and kill it in the future. **Immunizations**, or **vaccinations**, are special types of active acquired immunity. Instead of actually being exposed to the infectious agent and having the disease, a person is exposed to a modified or weakened pathogen that is still capable of stimulating the immune response but not actually causing the disease.

Immune Response

antibody (AN-tih-bod-ee)	cellular immunity
antibody-mediated immunity	cytotoxic (sigh-toh-TOK-sik)
antigen–antibody complex	humoral immunity (HYOO-mor-al)
antigens (AN-tih-jens)	immunoglobulin (Ig)
B cells	(im-yoo-noh-GLOB-yoo-lin)
B lymphocytes	natural killer (NK) cells
cell-mediated immunity	pathogenic (path-oh-JEN-ik)

Disease-causing, or **pathogenic**, agents are recognized as being foreign because they display proteins that are different from a person's own natural proteins. Those foreign proteins, called **antigens**, stimulate the immune response. The immune response consists of two distinct and different processes: **humoral immunity** (also called **antibody-mediated immunity**) and **cellular immunity** (also called **cell-mediated immunity**).

Humoral immunity refers to the production of **B lymphocytes**, also called **B cells**, which respond to antigens by producing a protective protein, called an **antibody** (also referred to as an **immunoglobulin**). Antibodies combine with the antigen to form an **antigen–antibody complex**. This complex either targets the foreign

What's In A Name?

Look for these word parts:
cyt/o = cell
immun/o = protection
lymph/o = lymph
path/o = disease
-al = pertaining to
-ar = pertaining to
-cyte = cell
-gen = that which produces
-genic = producing
-globulin = protein
-toxic = pertaining to poison
anti- = against

Med Term Tip

The term *humoral* comes from the Latin word for *liquid*. It is the old-fashioned term to refer to the fluids of the body.

substance for phagocytosis or prevents the infectious agent from damaging healthy cells.

Cellular immunity involves the production of T cells and **natural killer** (NK) **cells**. These defense cells are **cytotoxic**, meaning that they physically attack and destroy pathogenic cells.

Standard Precautions

cross-infection

healthcare-associated infection (HAI)

nosocomial infection (noh-soh-KOH-mee-al)

Occupational Safety and Health
   Administration (OSHA)

reinfection

self-inoculation

Hospitals and other healthcare settings contain a large number of infective pathogens. Patients and healthcare workers are exposed to each other's pathogens and sometimes become infected. An infection acquired in this manner, as a result of hospital exposure, is referred to as a **nosocomial infection** or a **healthcare-associated infection** (HAI). Nosocomial infections can spread in several ways. **Cross-infection** occurs when a person, either a patient or healthcare worker, acquires a pathogen from another patient or healthcare worker. **Reinfection** takes place when a patient becomes infected again with the same pathogen that originally brought him or her to the hospital. **Self-inoculation** occurs when a person becomes infected in a different part of the body by a pathogen from another part of his or her own body—such as intestinal bacteria spreading to the urethra.

With the appearance of the hepatitis B virus (HBV) in the mid-1960s and the human immunodeficiency virus (HIV) in the mid-1980s, the fight against spreading infections took on even greater significance. In 1987 the **Occupational Safety and Health Administration** (OSHA) issued mandatory guidelines to ensure that all employees at risk of exposure to body fluids are provided with personal protective equipment. These guidelines state that all human blood, tissue, and body fluids must be treated as if they were infected with HIV, HBV, or other bloodborne pathogens. These guidelines were expanded in 1992, 1996, and 2011 to encourage the fight against not just bloodborne pathogens, but all nosocomial infections spread by contact with blood, mucous membranes, nonintact skin, and all body fluids (including amniotic fluid, vaginal secretions, pleural fluid, cerebrospinal fluid, peritoneal fluid, pericardial fluid, and semen). These guidelines are commonly referred to as the Standard Precautions:

1. Wash or sanitize hands before putting on and after removing gloves, and before and after working with each patient or patient equipment.
2. Wear gloves when in contact with any body fluid, mucous membrane, or nonintact skin, or if you have chapped hands, a rash, or open sores.
3. Wear a nonpermeable gown or apron during procedures that are likely to expose you to any body fluid, mucous membrane, or nonintact skin.
4. Wear a mask and protective equipment or a face shield when in contact with patients who are coughing frequently, or if body fluid droplets or splashes are likely.
5. Wear a facemask and eyewear that seal close to the face during procedures that cause body tissues to be vaporized.
6. Remove for proper cleaning any shared equipment—such as a thermometer, stethoscope, or blood pressure cuff—that has come into contact with body fluids, mucous membrane, or nonintact skin.

What's In A Name?
Look for these word parts:
-al = pertaining to
re- = again

Med Term Tip
The term *nosocomial* comes from the Greek word *nosokomeion*, meaning hospital.

Med Term Tip
The simple act of thoroughly washing your hands is the most effective method of preventing the spread of infectious diseases.

PRACTICE AS YOU GO

F. Complete the Statement

1. The organs of the lymphatic system other than lymphatic vessels and lymph nodes are the
_____, _____, and _____.

2. The two lymph ducts are the _____ and _____.

3. The primary concentrations of lymph nodes are the _____,
_____, _____, and _____ regions.

4. _____ immunity develops following direct exposure to a pathogen.

5. Humoral immunity is also referred to as _____ immunity.

Terminology

Word Parts Used to Build Lymphatic and Immune System Terms

The following lists contain the combining forms, suffixes, and prefixes used to build terms in the remaining sections of this chapter.

Combining Forms

adenoid/o	adenoids	lymph/o	lymph	pneumon/o (see Chapter 7)	lung
axill/o	axilla, underarm	lymphaden/o	lymph node	rhin/o	nose
conjunctiv/o (see Chapter 13)	conjunctiva	lymphangi/o	lymph vessel	sarc/o	flesh
		myel/o	bone marrow	splen/o	spleen
cortic/o	outer layer	nas/o	nose	thym/o	thymus gland
dermat/o	skin	nucle/o	nucleus	tonsill/o	tonsils
immun/o	protection	path/o	disease		
inguin/o	groin				

Suffixes

-al	pertaining to	-graphy	process of recording	-logy	study of
-ar	pertaining to			-megaly	enlarged
-ary	pertaining to	-ia	condition	-oma	tumor
-atic	pertaining to	-iasis	abnormal condition	-osis	abnormal condition
-ectomy	surgical removal				
-edema	swelling	-ic	pertaining to	-pathy	disease
-gram	record	-itis	inflammation	-therapy	treatment

Prefixes

anti-	against	auto-	self	mono-	one

Adjective Form of Anatomical Terms

Term	Word Parts	Definition
axillary (AK-sih-lair-ee)	axill/o = axilla, underarm -ary = pertaining to	Pertaining to underarm region
inguinal (ING-gwih-nal)	inguin/o = groin -al = pertaining to	Pertaining to groin region
lymphangial (lim-FAN-jee-al)	lymphangi/o = lymph vessel -al = pertaining to	Pertaining to lymph vessels
lymphatic (lim-FAT-ik)	lymph/o = lymph -atic = pertaining to	Pertaining to lymph
splenic (SPLEN-ik)	splen/o = spleen -ic = pertaining to	Pertaining to spleen
thymic (THIGH-mik)	thym/o = thymus gland -ic = pertaining to	Pertaining to thymus gland
tonsillar (TAHN-sih-lar)	tonsill/o = tonsils -ar = pertaining to	Pertaining to tonsils

PRACTICE AS YOU GO

G. Give the adjective form for each anatomical structure.

1. Spleen _____
2. Lymph _____
3. Tonsil _____
4. Thymus gland _____
5. Lymph vessel _____

Pathology

Term	Word Parts	Definition
Medical Specialties		
allergist (AL-er-jist)		Physician who specializes in testing for and treating allergies
immunology (im-yoo-NALL-oh-jee)	immun/o = protection -logy = study of	Branch of medicine concerned with diagnosis and treatment of infectious diseases and other disorders of immune system; physician is an *immunologist*
pathology (pah-THOL-oh-jee)	path/o = disease -logy = study of	Branch of medicine concerned with determining underlying causes and development of diseases; physician is a *pathologist*

Pathology (continued)

Term	Word Parts	Definition
Signs and Symptoms		
hives		Appearance of wheals as part of allergic reaction
inflammation (in-flah-MAY-shun)		Tissues' response to injury from pathogens or physical agents; characterized by redness, pain, swelling, and feeling hot to the touch

■ **Figure 6-15** Inflammation as illustrated by cellulitis of the nose. Note that the area is red and swollen. It is also painful and hot to touch. *(ARENA Creative/Shutterstock)*

Word Watch

The terms *inflammation* and *inflammatory* are spelled with two *m*'s, while *inflame* and *inflamed* each have only one *m*. These may be the most commonly misspelled terms by medical terminology students.

Term	Word Parts	Definition
lymphedema (limf-eh-DEE-mah)	lymph/o = lymph -edema = swelling	Edema appearing in extremities due to obstruction of lymph flow through lymphatic vessels
splenomegaly (spleh-noh-MEG-ah-lee)	splen/o = spleen -megaly = enlarged	Enlarged spleen
urticaria (er-tih-KAIR-ee-ah)		Severe itching associated with hives, usually linked to food allergy, stress, or drug reactions
Allergic Reactions		
allergic asthma (ah-LER-jik / AZ-mah)	-ic = pertaining to	Inflammation and narrowing of airways triggered by inhaling an allergen; symptoms include wheezing, coughing, and shortness of breath
allergic conjunctivitis (ah-LER-jik / kon-junk-tih-VYE-tis)	-ic = pertaining to conjunctiv/o = conjunctiva -itis = inflammation	Inflammation of the conjunctiva (protective membrane over front of eyeball) caused by allergens in the air
allergic rhinitis (ah-LER-jik / rye-NYE-tis)	-ic = pertaining to rhin/o = nose -itis = inflammation	Allergic reaction caused by inhaling an allergen such as pollen, animal dander, or mold; symptoms may include sneezing, runny nose, congestion, post-nasal drip, cough, and itchy, watery eyes; commonly called *hay fever*
allergy (AL-er-jee)		Hypersensitivity to common substance in environment or to medication; substance causing allergic reaction is called *allergen*
anaphylactic shock (an-ah-fih-LAK-tik)		Life-threatening condition resulting from a severe allergic reaction; examples of instances that may trigger this reaction include bee stings, medications, or ingestion of foods; circulatory and respiratory problems occur, including respiratory distress, hypotension, edema, tachycardia, and convulsions; also called *anaphylaxis*

Pathology (continued)

Term	Word Parts	Definition
contact dermatitis (der-mah-TYE-tis)	dermat/o = skin -itis = inflammation	Skin irritation caused by skin coming into direct contact with an allergen; symptoms may include redness, itching, rash, and blisters; common allergens are poison ivy, soaps, fragrances, and jewelry
Lymphatic System		
adenoiditis (ad-eh-noyd-EYE-tis)	adenoid/o = adenoids -itis = inflammation	Inflammation of adenoids
autoimmune disease	auto- = self	Disease resulting from body's immune system attacking its own cells as if they were pathogens; examples include systemic lupus erythematosus, rheumatoid arthritis, and multiple sclerosis
elephantiasis (el-eh-fan-TYE-ah-sis)	-iasis = abnormal condition	Inflammation, obstruction, and destruction of lymph vessels resulting in enlarged tissues due to edema
Hodgkin's disease (HD) (HOJ-kins)		Also called *Hodgkin's lymphoma*; cancer of lymphatic cells found in concentration in lymph nodes; named after Thomas Hodgkin, a British physician, who first described it
lymphadenitis (lim-fad-en-EYE-tis)	lymphaden/o = lymph node -itis = inflammation	Inflammation of lymph nodes; referred to as *swollen glands*
lymphadenopathy (lim-fad-eh-NOP-ah-thee)	lymphaden/o = lymph node -pathy = disease	General term for lymph node diseases
lymphangioma (lim-fan-jee-OH-mah)	lymphangi/o = lymph vessel -oma = tumor	Tumor in a lymphatic vessel
lymphoma (lim-FOH-mah)	lymph/o = lymph -oma = tumor	Tumor in lymphatic tissue
mononucleosis (mono) (mon-oh-noo-klee-OH-sis)	mono- = one nucle/o = nucleus -osis = abnormal condition	Acute infectious disease with large number of abnormal mononuclear lymphocytes; caused by Epstein–Barr virus; abnormal liver function may occur; commonly called *kissing disease* since virus can be spread by saliva

> **Med Term Tip**
>
> *Mononuclear* is a term occasionally used to describe any cell that has a large, single, round nucleus, including lymphocytes and monocytes. This is opposed to having a lobed nucleus like the other white blood cells.

Term	Word Parts	Definition
non-Hodgkin's lymphoma (NHL)	lymph/o = lymph -oma = tumor	Cancer of lymphatic tissues other than Hodgkin's lymphoma

■ **Figure 6-16** Photo of the neck of a patient with non-Hodgkin's lymphoma showing swelling associated with enlarged lymph nodes. *(Dr. P. Marazzi/Science Source)*

Pathology (continued)

Term	Word Parts	Definition
thymoma (thigh-MOH-mah)	thym/o = thymus gland -oma = tumor	Tumor of thymus gland
tonsillitis (tahn-sill-EYE-tis)	tonsill/o = tonsils -itis = inflammation	Inflammation of tonsils
Immune System		
acquired immunodeficiency syndrome (AIDS) (im-yoo-noh-dih-FIH-shen-see / SIN-drohm)	immun/o = protection	Disease involving defect in cell-mediated immunity system; syndrome of opportunistic infections occurring in final stages of infection with human immunodeficiency virus (HIV); virus attacks T4 lymphocytes and destroys them, reducing person's ability to fight infection
AIDS-related complex (ARC)		Early stage of AIDS; there is a positive test for virus, but only mild symptoms of weight loss, fatigue, skin rash, and anorexia
graft versus host disease (GVHD)		Serious complication of bone marrow transplant (graft); immune cells from donor bone marrow attack recipient's (host's) tissues
human immunodeficiency virus (HIV) (im-yoo-noh-dih-FIH-shen-see)	immun/o = protection	Virus that causes AIDS; also known as a *retrovirus*

■ **Figure 6-17** Color enhanced scanning electron micrograph of HIV virus (red) infecting T-helper cells (blue). *(Illustration Forest/Shutterstock)*

Term	Word Parts	Definition
immunocompromised (im-yoo-noh-KOM-proh-myzd)	immun/o = protection	Having immune system that is unable to respond properly to pathogens; also called *immunodeficiency disorder*
Kaposi's sarcoma (KS) (KAP-oh-seez / sar-KOH-mah)	sarc/o = flesh -oma = tumor	Form of skin cancer frequently seen in patients with AIDS; consists of brownish-purple papules that spread from skin and metastasize to internal organs; named for dermatologist Moritz Kaposi
multiple myeloma (my-eh-LOH-mah)	myel/o = bone marrow -oma = tumor	Originates in plasma cells (type of lymphocyte responsible for making antibodies); over time, these malignant cells collect in bone marrow, resulting in a bone marrow tumor; may spread to skeleton
opportunistic infections		Infectious diseases associated with patients who have compromised immune systems and therefore lowered resistance to infections and parasites; may be result of HIV infection

Pathology (continued)

Term	Word Parts	Definition
pneumocystis pneumonia (PCP) (noo-moh-SIS-tis / noo-MOH-nee-ah)	pneumon/o = lung -ia = condition	Pneumonia common in patients with weakened immune systems, such as AIDS patients, caused by *Pneumocystis jiroveci* fungus
sarcoidosis (sar-koyd-OH-sis)	-osis = abnormal condition	Autoimmune disease of unknown cause that forms fibrous lesions commonly appearing in lymph nodes, liver, skin, lungs, spleen, eyes, and small bones of hands and feet
severe combined immunodeficiency syndrome (SCIDS)	immun/o = protection	Disease seen in children born with nonfunctioning immune system; often these children are forced to live in sealed sterile rooms

Nosocomial Infections

Term	Word Parts	Definition
carbapenem-resistant Enterobacteriaceae (CRE) **infection** (kar-bah-PEN-em / ree-ZISS-tent / en-ter-oh-bak-teer-ee-AY-see-ee)		Infection by group of bacteria that have resistance to powerful group of antibiotics called *carbapenems;* almost all infections occur in healthcare settings, especially among patients with ventilators, urinary catheters, intravenous catheters, or on long-term antibiotics
Clostridium difficile (C. diff) **infection** (klaw-STRIH-dee-um / dif-ee-SEEL)		Infection with *C. diff* bacteria causes inflammation of colon; symptoms may include diarrhea, nausea, fever, and abdominal pain; most commonly occurs in persons with conditions requiring extended use of antibiotics; infection spread through contact with contaminated feces
methicillin-resistant *Staphylococcus aureus* (MRSA) **infection** (meth-ih-SIL-in / ree-ZISS-tent / staf-ih-loh-KOK-us / OR-ee-iss)		Infecting bacteria are resistant to many common antibiotics, such as methicillin, oxacillin, penicillin, and amoxicillin; spread through contact with contaminated surface, often improperly washed hands

PRACTICE AS YOU GO

H. Terminology Matching

Match each term to its definition.

1. _____ allergy

2. _____ hives

3. _____ Hodgkin's disease

4. _____ sarcoidosis

5. _____ graft vs. host disease

a. seen in an allergic reaction

b. complication of bone marrow transplant

c. a hypersensitivity reaction

d. a type of cancer

e. autoimmune disease

Diagnostic Procedures

Term	Word Parts	Definition
Clinical Laboratory Tests		
antinuclear antibody (ANA) test (an-tee-NOO-klee-ar / AN-tee-bod-ee)	anti- = against nucle/o = nucleus -ar = pertaining to	Blood test to assist in diagnosis of autoimmune diseases; antinuclear antibodies are produced by persons with autoimmune disease; presence of these antibodies in blood indicates that person's immune system is attacking body's cells
HIV antigen/antibody immunoassay (im-yoo-noh-ASS-ay)	anti- = against immun/o = protection	Blood test for HIV infection; tests for both HIV antigens and antibodies; foreign viral proteins (HIV antigen) can be detected very shortly after exposure, and antibodies produced by body in response to HIV infection can be detected two to eight weeks after exposure; antibody-only test can also be performed using saliva
Diagnostic Imaging		
lymphangiogram (lim-FAN-jee-oh-gram)	lymphangi/o = lymph vessel -gram = record	X-ray record of lymphatic vessels produced by lymphangiography
lymphangiography (lim-fan-jee-OG-rah-fee)	lymphangi/o = lymph vessel -graphy = process of recording	X-ray taken of lymph vessels after injection of dye into foot; lymph flow through chest is traced
magnetic resonance imaging (MRI) (REZ-oh-nens)	-ic = pertaining to	Use of electromagnetic energy to produce image of soft tissues in any plane of body; atoms behave differently when placed in strong magnetic field; when body is exposed to this magnetic field, nuclei of body's atoms emit radio-frequency signals that can be used to create an image

■ **Figure 6-18** Magnetic resonance image (MRI) showing a sagittal view of the brain, oral cavity, nasal cavity, and spinal cord. *(MriMan/Shutterstock)*

Additional Diagnostic Procedures

Term	Word Parts	Definition
Monospot		Blood test for infectious mononucleosis
skin allergy testing		Form of allergy testing in which the body is exposed to allergens through light scratch, injection, patch, or prick on skin

■ **Figure 6-19** A) Skin allergy testing; patient is exposed to allergens through light scratch in the skin. B) Positive allergy test results. Inflammation indicates person is allergic to that substance. *(Anthony Ricci/Shutterstock)* A B

Therapeutic Procedures

Term	Word Parts	Definition
Medical Procedures		
allergy shots		Type of immunotherapy; person receives regular injections of tiny amounts of allergen to which he or she is allergic; injection is too small to cause allergic reaction, but large enough to stimulate immune system; over time, person's sensitivity to allergen reduces

Therapeutic Procedures (continued)

Term	Word Parts	Definition
immunotherapy (IM-yoo-noh-thair-ah-pee)	immun/o = protection -therapy = treatment	Giving patient injection of immunoglobulins or antibodies in order to treat disease; antibodies may be produced by another person or animal, for example, antivenom for snake bites; more recent developments include treatments to boost activity of immune system, especially to treat cancer and AIDS
vaccination (vak-sih-NAY-shun)		Exposure to weakened pathogen that stimulates immune response and antibody production in order to confer protection against full-blown disease; also called *immunization*
Surgical Procedures		
adenoidectomy (ad-eh-noyd-EK-toh-mee)	adenoid/o = adenoids -ectomy = surgical removal	Surgical removal of adenoids
lymphadenectomy (lim-fad-eh-NEK-toh-mee)	lymphaden/o = lymph node -ectomy = surgical removal	Surgical removal of lymph node; usually done to test for malignancy
splenectomy (spleh-NEK-toh-mee)	splen/o = spleen -ectomy = surgical removal	Surgical removal of spleen
thymectomy (thigh-MEK-toh-mee)	thym/o = thymus gland -ectomy = surgical removal	Surgical removal of thymus gland
tonsillectomy (tahn-sih-LEK-toh-mee)	tonsill/o = tonsils -ectomy = surgical removal	Surgical removal of tonsils

Pharmacology

Classification	Word Parts	Action	Examples
antihistamine (an-tih-HIST-ah-meen)	anti- = against	Blocks effects of histamine released by body during allergic reaction	cetirizine, Zyrtec; diphenhydramine, Benadryl
corticosteroids (kor-tih-koh-STAIR-oydz)	cortic/o = outer layer	Natural or synthetic adrenal cortex hormone; has very strong anti-inflammatory properties; particularly useful in treating autoimmune diseases	prednisone; methylprednisolone, Solu-Medrol
immunosuppressants (im-yoo-noh-suh-PRESS-antz)	immun/o = protection	Block certain actions of immune system; required to prevent rejection of transplanted organ	mycophenolate mofetil, CellCept; cyclosporine, Neoral
nasal steroids (NAY-zal)	nas/o = nose -al = pertaining to	Nose spray; reduces inflammation and treats symptoms of nasal rhinitis	fluticasone, Flonase; triamcinolone, Nasacort
protease inhibitor drugs (PROH-tee-ays)		Inhibit protease, enzyme that viruses need to reproduce	indinavir, Crixivan; saquinavir, Fortovase
reverse transcriptase inhibitor drugs (trans-KRIP-tays)		Inhibit reverse transcriptase, enzyme needed by viruses to reproduce	lamivudine, Epivir; zidovudine, Retrovir

PRACTICE AS YOU GO

I. Procedure Matching

Match each procedure term with its definition.

1. _____ ANA test

2. _____ vaccination

3. _____ corticosteroid

4. _____ Monospot

5. _____ lymphangiography

a. test for mononucleosis

b. an X-ray

c. immunization

d. has strong anti-inflammatory properties

e. assists in diagnosis of autoimmune disease

Abbreviations

AIDS	acquired immunodeficiency syndrome	**Ig**	immunoglobulins (IgA, IgD, IgE, IgG, IgM)
ANA	antinuclear antibody	**KS**	Kaposi's sarcoma
ARC	AIDS-related complex	**mono**	mononucleosis
C. diff	*Clostridium difficile*	**MRSA**	methicillin-resistant *Staphylococcus aureus*
CRE	carbapenem-resistant *Enterobacteriaceae*	**NHL**	non-Hodgkin's lymphoma
GVHD	graft versus host disease	**NK**	natural killer cells
HAI	healthcare-associated infection	**PCP**	pneumocystis pneumonia
HD	Hodgkin's disease	**SCIDS**	severe combined immunodeficiency syndrome
HIV	human immunodeficiency virus		

PRACTICE AS YOU GO

J. What's the Abbreviation?

1. acquired immunodeficiency syndrome   _____

2. AIDS-related complex   _____

3. human immunodeficiency virus   _____

4. mononucleosis   _____

5. Kaposi's sarcoma   _____

6. immunoglobulin   _____

7. severe combined immunodeficiency syndrome   _____

8. pneumocystis pneumonia   _____

Chapter Review

Real-World Applications

Medical Record Analysis

This Discharge Summary contains 10 medical terms. Underline each term and write it in the list below the report. Then explain each term as you would to a nonmedical person.

Discharge Summary

Admitting Diagnosis:	Splenomegaly, weight loss, diarrhea, fatigue, chronic cough
Final Diagnosis:	Non-Hodgkin's lymphoma of spleen; splenectomy
History of Present Illness:	Patient is a 36-year-old businessman who was first seen in the office with complaints of feeling generally "run-down," intermittent diarrhea, weight loss, and, more recently, a dry cough. He states he has been aware of these symptoms for approximately six months. Monospot and HIV antigen/antibody immunoassay are both negative. In spite of a 35-pound weight loss, he has abdominal swelling and splenomegaly was detected. He was admitted to the hospital for further evaluation and treatment.
Summary of Hospital Course:	Full-body MRI confirmed splenomegaly and located a 3-cm encapsulated tumor in the spleen. Biopsies taken from the splenic tumor confirmed the diagnosis of non-Hodgkin's lymphoma. The patient underwent splenectomy for removal of the tumor.
Discharge Plans:	Patient was discharged home following recovery from the splenectomy. The abdominal swelling and diarrhea were resolved, but the dry cough persisted. He was referred to a cancer clinic for evaluation for chemotherapy.

Term	Explanation
1. _____	_____
2. _____	_____
3. _____	_____
4. _____	_____
5. _____	_____
6. _____	_____
7. _____	_____
8. _____	_____
9. _____	_____
10. _____	_____

Chart Note Transcription

The chart note below contains 10 phrases that can be reworded with a medical term presented in this chapter. Each phrase is identified with an underline. Determine the medical term and write your answers in the space provided.

Pearson General Hospital Consultation Report

Task	Edit	View	Time Scale	Options	Help	Download	Archive	Date: 17 May 2017

Current Complaint:	Patient is a 22-year-old female referred to the <u>specialist in treating blood disorders</u> **1** by her internist. Her complaints include fatigue, weight loss, and easy bruising.
Past History:	Patient had normal childhood diseases. She is a college student and was feeling well until symptoms gradually appeared starting approximately three months ago.
Signs and Symptoms:	An <u>immunoassay test for HIV exposure</u> **2** was normal. The <u>measure of the blood's coagulation abilities</u> **3** indicated that the blood took too long to form a clot. A <u>blood test to count all the blood cells</u> **4** reported <u>too few red blood cells</u> **5** and <u>too few clotting cells.</u> **6** There were <u>too many white blood cells,</u> **7** but they were immature and abnormal. A <u>sample of bone marrow obtained for microscopic examination</u> **8** found an excessive number of immature white blood cells.
Diagnosis:	<u>Cancer of the white blood cell–forming bone marrow</u> **9**
Treatment:	Aggressive chemotherapy for the <u>cancer of the white blood cell–forming bone marrow</u> **9** and <u>replacement blood from another person</u> **10** to replace the erythrocytes and platelets.

1. _____

2. _____

3. _____

4. _____

5. _____

6. _____

7. _____

8. _____

9. _____

10. _____

Case Study

Below is a case study presentation of a patient with a condition discussed in this chapter. Read the case study and answer the questions below. Some questions will ask for information not included within this chapter. Use your text, a medical dictionary, or any other reference material you choose to answer these questions.

A two-year-old boy is being seen by a hematologist. The child's symptoms include the sudden onset of high fevers, thrombopenia, epistaxis, gingival bleeding, petechiae, and ecchymoses after minor traumas. The physician has ordered a bone marrow aspiration to confirm the clinical diagnosis of acute lymphocytic leukemia (ALL). If the diagnosis is positive, the child will be placed immediately on intensive chemotherapy. The physician has informed the parents that treatment produces remission in 90% of children with ALL, especially those between the ages of two and eight.

(Flashon Studio/Shutterstock)

Questions

1. What pathological condition does the hematologist suspect? Look this condition up in a reference source and include a short description of it.

_____

_____

2. List and define each of the patient's presenting symptoms in your own words.

_____

_____

3. What diagnostic test did the physician perform? Describe it in your own words.

_____

_____

4. Explain the phrase "clinical diagnosis" in your own words.

_____

_____

5. If the suspected diagnosis is correct, explain the treatment that will begin.

_____

_____

6. What do you think the term *remission* means?

_____

_____

Practice Exercises

A. Word Building Practice

The combining form **splen/o** refers to the *spleen*. Use it to write a term that means:

1. enlargement of the spleen _____

2. surgical removal of the spleen _____

3. cutting into the spleen _____

The combining form **lymph/o** refers to the *lymph*. Use it to write a term that means:

4. lymph cells _____

5. tumor of the lymph system _____

The combining form **lymphaden/o** refers to the *lymph nodes*. Use it to write a term that means:

6. disease of a lymph gland _____

7. tumor of a lymph gland _____

8. inflammation of a lymph gland _____

The combining form **immun/o** refers to the *immune system*. Use it to write a term that means:

9. specialist in the study of the immune system _____

10. immune protein _____

11. study of the immune system _____

The combining form **hemat/o** refers to *blood*. Use it to write a term that means:

12. relating to the blood _____

13. blood tumor or mass _____

14. blood formation _____

The combining form **hem/o** refers to *blood*. Use it to write a term that means:

15. blood destruction _____

16. blood protein _____

The suffix **-penia** refers to *too few (cells)*. Use it to write a term that means:

17. too few white (cells) _____

18. too few red (cells) _____

19. too few of all cells _____

The suffix **-cytosis** refers to *more than the normal number of cells*. Use it to write a term that means:

20. more than the normal number of white cells _____

21. more than the normal number of red cells _____

22. more than the normal number of clotting cells _____

The suffix **-cyte** refers to *cells*. Use it to write a term that means:

23. red cell _____

24. white cell _____

25. lymph cell _____

B. Using Abbreviations

Fill in each blank with the appropriate abbreviation.

1. The _____ test showed a low volume of red blood cells.

2. Infection by the _____ virus may result in _____, a severe immune system disease.

3. The results of the _____ indicated the presence of an inflammatory disease.

4. _____ is a potential complication following a bone marrow transplant.

5. A(n) _____ was ordered to determine if there was a bacterial infection in the blood.

6. _____ is a type of pneumonia common in immunocompromised persons.

7. Before surgery, a(n) _____ was performed to check the blood's coagulation ability.

8. Further tests were needed to determine if the acute leukemia was _____ or _____.

9. The formed elements of the blood include _____, _____, and platelets.

10. Vitamin B$_{12}$ injections are used to treat _____.

C. Complete the Term

For each definition given below, fill in the blank with the word part that completes the term.

Definition	Term
1. more than normal number of red cells	erythro _____
2. blood condition with excessive fat	hyperlipid _____
3. too few white (cells)	leuko _____
4. blood protein	hemo _____
5. cutting into a vein	_____ otomy
6. clot destruction	_____ lytic
7. study of shape	_____ logy
8. separation of blood	hemato _____
9. study of disease	_____ logy
10. swelling with lymph	lymph _____
11. lymph vessel tumor	_____ oma
12. protection treatment	_____ therapy
13. surgical removal of tonsils	_____ ectomy
14. bone marrow tumor	_____ oma
15. enlarged spleen	_____ megaly

D. Fill in the Blank

Kaposi's sarcoma	mononucleosis	Hodgkin's disease	aplastic
polycythemia vera	anaphylactic shock	autoimmune diseases	pernicious
pneumocystis	HIV		

1. The condition characterized by the production of too many red blood cells is called _____.

2. The Epstein–Barr virus is thought to be responsible for _____ infectious disease.

3. A life-threatening allergic reaction is _____.

4. The virus responsible for causing AIDS is _____.

5. A cancer that is seen frequently in AIDS patients is _____.

6. An ANA test is used to test for _____.

7. Malignant tumors concentrate in lymph nodes with this disease: _____.

8. A type of pneumonia seen in AIDS patients is _____ pneumonia.

9. _____ anemia is a severe form of anemia caused by nonfunctioning red bone marrow.

10. _____ anemia is the result of a vitamin B_{12} deficiency.

E. Pharmacology Challenge

Fill in the classification for each drug description, then match the brand name.

Drug Description	Classification	Brand Name
1. _____ inhibits enzyme needed for viral reproduction	_____	a. HepLock
2. _____ prevents blood clot formation	_____	b. Activase
3. _____ stops bleeding	_____	c. Solu-Medrol
4. _____ blocks effects of histamine	_____	d. Amicar
5. _____ prevents rejection of a transplanted organ	_____	e. Epivir
6. _____ dissolves existing blood clots	_____	f. CellCept
7. _____ increases number of erythrocytes	_____	g. Procrit
8. _____ strong anti-inflammatory properties	_____	h. Zyrtec
9. _____ interferes with action of platelets	_____	i. Plavix

F. Terminology Matching

Match each term to its definition.

1. _____ culture and sensitivity		a. measure of blood's clotting ability
2. _____ hematocrit		b. counts number of each type of blood cell
3. _____ complete blood count		c. examines cells for abnormal shape
4. _____ erythrocyte sedimentation rate		d. checks blood for bacterial growth and best antibiotic to use
5. _____ prothrombin time		e. determines number of each type of white blood cell
6. _____ white cell differential		f. measures percent of whole blood that is red blood cells
7. _____ red cell morphology		g. an indicator of the presence of an inflammatory condition

G. Define the Term

1. immunotherapy _____
2. Monospot _____
3. opportunistic infection _____
4. urticaria _____
5. inflammation _____
6. homologous transfusion _____
7. pernicious anemia _____
8. leukemia _____
9. hemorrhage _____
10. septicemia _____

H. Anatomical Adjectives

Fill in the blank with the missing noun or adjective.

Noun	Adjective
1. underarm	_____
2. blood	_____
3. _____	lymphangial
4. _____	fibrinous
5. _____	splenic
6. _____	thymic
7. clotting cell	_____
8. white cell	_____
9. red cell	_____
10. _____	tonsillar

I. Spelling Practice

Some of the following terms are misspelled. Identify the incorrect terms and spell them correctly in the blank provided.

1. tonsilitis _____
2. sanguineous _____
3. immunosuppressants _____
4. sarcoidosis _____
5. inflamation _____
6. phlebotomy _____
7. autolgous _____
8. thrombocytosis _____
9. pancytopeenia _____
10. dyscrasea _____

J. Complete the Statement

1. Erythrocytes contain _____, a protein than binds oxygen for transport.

2. The five types of leukocytes are _____, _____, _____,

   _____, and _____.

3. _____ is the modern term for thrombocyte.

4. Type O blood is the universal _____ and Type AB blood is the universal _____.

5. Lymphatic vessels located around the intestines are called _____.

6. _____ are located along lymphatic vessels and work to trap and destroy pathogens.

7. The _____ filters out and destroys old erythrocytes.

8. Natural killer cells are part of _____ immunity.

MyLab Medical Terminology™

MyLab Medical Terminology is a premium online homework management system that includes a host of features to help you study. Registered users will find:

- A multitude of activities and assignments built within the MyLab platform
- Powerful tools that track and analyze your results—allowing you to create a personalized learning experience
- Videos and audio pronunciations to help enrich your progress
- Streaming lesson presentations (Guided Lectures) and self-paced learning modules
- A space where you and your instructors can check your progress and manage your assignments

Labeling Exercises

Image A

Write the labels for this figure on the numbered lines provided.

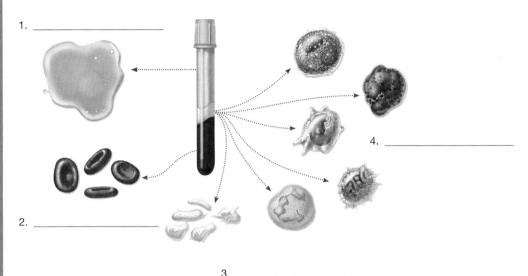

1. _____

2. _____

3. _____

4. _____

Image B

Write the labels for this figure on the numbered lines provided.

1. _____

2. _____

3. _____

4. _____

Image C

Write the labels for this figure on the numbered lines provided.

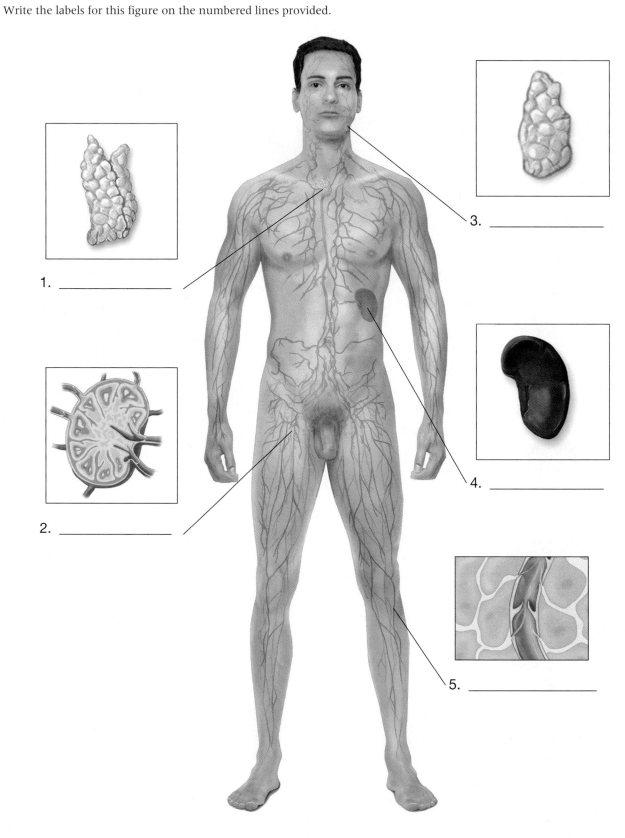

1. _____

2. _____

3. _____

4. _____

5. _____

Chapter 7

Respiratory System

Learning Objectives

Upon completion of this chapter, you will be able to

1. Identify and define the combining forms and suffixes introduced in this chapter.
2. Correctly spell and pronounce medical terms and major anatomical structures relating to the respiratory system.
3. Locate and describe the major organs of the respiratory system and their functions.
4. List and describe the lung volumes and capacities.
5. Describe the process of respiration.
6. Identify and define respiratory system anatomical terms.
7. Identify and define selected respiratory system pathology terms.
8. Identify and define selected respiratory system diagnostic procedures.
9. Identify and define selected respiratory system therapeutic procedures.
10. Identify and define selected medications relating to the respiratory system.
11. Define selected abbreviations associated with the respiratory system.

RESPIRATORY SYSTEM

AT A GLANCE

Function

The organs of the respiratory system are responsible for bringing fresh air into the lungs, exchanging oxygen for carbon dioxide between the air sacs of the lungs and the bloodstream, and exhaling the stale air.

Organs

The primary structures that comprise the respiratory system:

nasal cavity	trachea
pharynx	bronchial tubes
larynx	lungs

Word Parts

Presented here are the most common word parts (with their meanings) used to build respiratory system terms. For a more comprehensive list, refer to the Terminology section of this chapter.

Combining Forms

aer/o	air	muc/o	mucus
alveol/o	alveolus	nas/o	nose
anthrac/o	coal	ox/o, ox/i	oxygen
atel/o	incomplete	pharyng/o	pharynx
bronch/o	bronchus	pleur/o	pleura
bronchi/o	bronchus	pneum/o	lung, air
bronchiol/o	bronchiole	pneumon/o	lung, air
coni/o	dust	pulmon/o	lung
cyan/o	blue	rhin/o	nose
cyst/o	sac	sept/o	wall
diaphragmat/o	diaphragm	sinus/o	sinus
epiglott/o	epiglottis	somn/o	sleep
hal/o	to breathe	spir/o	breathing
laryng/o	larynx	trache/o	trachea
lob/o	lobe	tuss/o	cough

Suffixes

-capnia	carbon dioxide	-pnea	breathing
-osmia	smell	-ptysis	spitting
-phonia	voice	-thorax	chest
-phylaxis	protection		

Respiratory System Illustrated

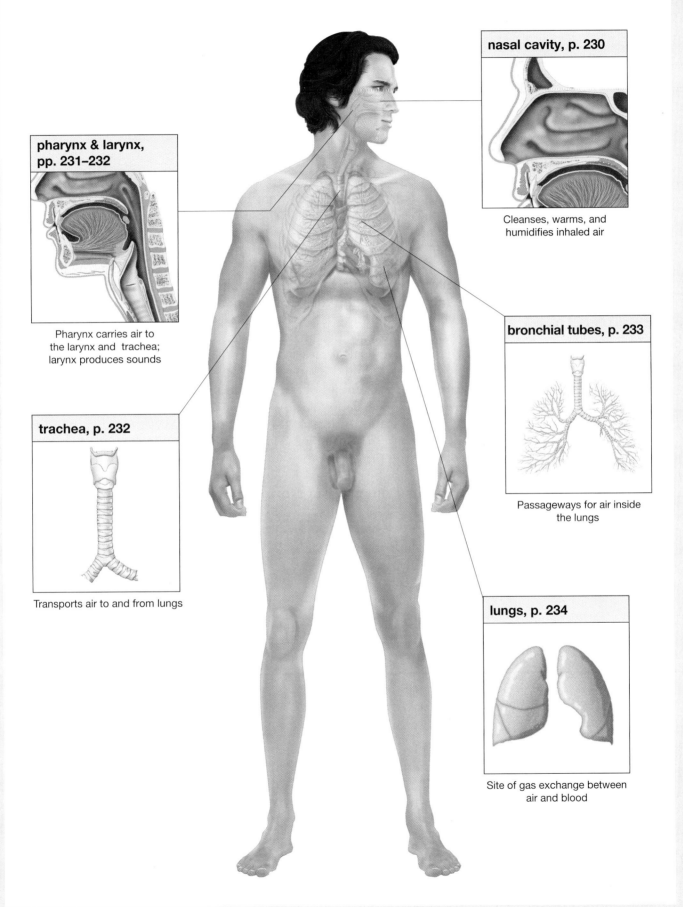

nasal cavity, p. 230

Cleanses, warms, and humidifies inhaled air

pharynx & larynx, pp. 231–232

Pharynx carries air to the larynx and trachea; larynx produces sounds

bronchial tubes, p. 233

Passageways for air inside the lungs

trachea, p. 232

Transports air to and from lungs

lungs, p. 234

Site of gas exchange between air and blood

Anatomy and Physiology of the Respiratory System

bronchial tubes (BRONG-kee-al)	**lungs**
carbon dioxide	**nasal cavity** (NAY-zal)
exhalation (eks-hah-LAY-shun)	**oxygen** (OK-sih-jen)
external respiration	**pharynx** (FAIR-inks)
inhalation (in-hah-LAY-shun)	**trachea** (TRAY-kee-ah)
internal respiration	**ventilation**
larynx (LAIR-inks)	

The organs of the respiratory system include the **nasal cavity, pharynx, larynx, trachea, bronchial tubes**, and **lungs**. These organs function together to perform the mechanical and, for the most part, unconscious mechanism of respiration. The cells of the body require the continuous delivery of oxygen and removal of carbon dioxide. The respiratory system works in conjunction with the cardiovascular system to deliver oxygen to all the cells of the body. The process of respiration must be continuous; interruption for even a few minutes can result in brain damage and/or death.

The process of respiration can be subdivided into three distinct parts: **ventilation, external respiration**, and **internal respiration**. Ventilation is the flow of air between the outside environment and the lungs. **Inhalation** is the flow of air into the lungs, and **exhalation** is the flow of air out of the lungs. Inhalation brings fresh **oxygen** (O_2) into the air sacs, while exhalation removes **carbon dioxide** (CO_2) from the body.

External respiration refers to the exchange of oxygen and carbon dioxide that takes place in the lungs. These gases diffuse in opposite directions between the air sacs of the lungs and the bloodstream. Oxygen enters the bloodstream from the air sacs to be delivered throughout the body. Carbon dioxide leaves the bloodstream and enters the air sacs to be exhaled from the body.

Internal respiration is the process of oxygen and carbon dioxide exchange at the cellular level when oxygen leaves the bloodstream and is delivered to the tissues. Oxygen is needed for the body cells' metabolism, all the physical and chemical changes within the body that are necessary for life. The by-product of metabolism is the formation of a waste product, carbon dioxide. The carbon dioxide enters the bloodstream from the tissues and is transported back to the lungs for disposal.

Nasal Cavity

cilia (SIL-ee-ah)	**nasal septum**
mucus (MYOO-kus)	**palate** (PAL-et)
mucous membrane	**paranasal sinuses** (pair-ah-NAY-zal)
nares (NAIR-eez)	

The process of ventilation begins with the nasal cavity. Air enters through two external openings in the nose called the **nares**. The nasal cavity is divided down the middle by the **nasal septum**, a cartilaginous plate. The **palate** in the roof of the mouth separates the nasal cavity above from the mouth below. The walls of the nasal cavity and the nasal septum are made up of flexible cartilage covered with **mucous membrane** (see Figure 7-1 ■). In fact, much of the respiratory tract is covered with mucous membrane, which secretes a sticky fluid, **mucus**, to help cleanse the air by trapping dust and bacteria. Since this membrane is also wet, it moisturizes inhaled air as it passes by the surface of the cavity. Very small hairs or **cilia** line the opening to the nose (as well as much of the airways)

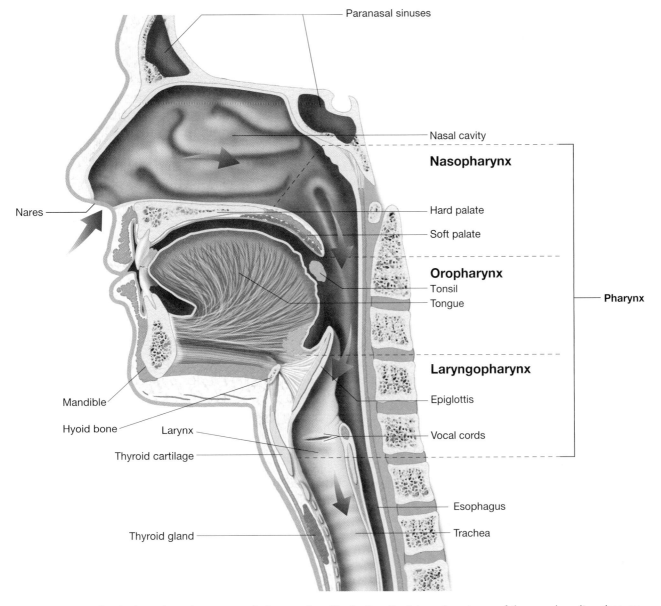

■ **Figure 7-1**   Sagittal section of upper respiratory system illustrating the internal anatomy of the nasal cavity, pharynx, larynx, and trachea.

and filter out large dirt particles before they can enter the lungs. Capillaries in the mucous membranes warm inhaled air as it passes through the airways. Additionally, several **paranasal sinuses**, or air-filled cavities, are located within the facial bones. The sinuses act as an echo chamber during sound production and give resonance to the voice.

> **Word Watch**
> The term *cilia* means *hair*, and there are other body systems that have cilia or cilialike processes. For example, when discussing the eye, *cilia* means *eyelashes*.

Pharynx

adenoids (AD-eh-noydz)
auditory tube
eustachian tube (yoo-STAY-shee-en)
laryngopharynx (lah-ring-goh-FAIR-inks)
lingual tonsils (LING-gwal)

nasopharynx (nay-zoh-FAIR-inks)
oropharynx (or-oh-FAIR-inks)
palatine tonsils (PAL-ah-tyne)
pharyngeal tonsils (fair-IN-jee-al)

> **What's In A Name?**
> Look for these word parts:
> **audit/o** = hearing
> **lingu/o** = tongue
> **-al** = pertaining to
> **-ory** = pertaining to

Air next enters the pharynx, also referred to as the *throat*, which is used by both the respiratory and digestive systems. At the end of the pharynx, air enters the trachea while food and liquids are shunted into the esophagus.

The pharynx is roughly a five-inch-long tube consisting of three parts: the upper **nasopharynx**, middle **oropharynx**, and lower **laryngopharynx** (see again Figure 7-1). Three pairs of tonsils (collections of lymphatic tissue) are located in the pharynx. Tonsils are strategically placed to help keep pathogens from entering the body through either the air breathed or food and liquid swallowed. The nasopharynx, behind the nose, contains the **adenoids** or **pharyngeal tonsils**. The oropharynx, behind the mouth, contains the **palatine tonsils** and the **lingual tonsils**. Tonsils are considered a part of the lymphatic system and are discussed in Chapter 6.

The opening of the **eustachian** or **auditory tube** is also found in the nasopharynx. The other end of this tube is in the middle ear. Each time a person swallows, this tube opens to equalize air pressure between the middle ear and the outside atmosphere.

Larynx

epiglottis (ep-ih-GLOT-iss)	**thyroid cartilage** (THIGH-royd / KAR-tih-lij)
glottis (GLOT-iss)	**vocal cords**

The larynx, or *voice box*, is a muscular structure located between the pharynx and the trachea and contains the **vocal cords** (see again Figure 7-1 and Figure 7-2 ■). The vocal cords are not actually cordlike in structure, but rather they are folds of membranous tissue that produce sound by vibrating as air passes through the **glottis**, the opening between the two vocal cords.

A flap of cartilaginous tissue, the **epiglottis**, sits above the glottis and provides protection against food and liquid being inhaled into the lungs. The epiglottis covers the larynx and trachea during swallowing and shunts food and liquid from the pharynx into the esophagus. The walls of the larynx are composed of several cartilage plates held together with ligaments and muscles. One of these cartilages, the **thyroid cartilage**, forms what is known as the *Adam's apple*. The thyroid cartilage is generally larger in males than in females and helps to produce the deeper male voice.

Trachea

The trachea, also called the *windpipe*, is the passageway for air that extends from the pharynx and larynx down to the main bronchi (see Figure 7-3 ■). Measuring approximately four inches in length, it is composed of smooth muscle and cartilage rings and is lined by mucous membrane and cilia. Therefore, it also assists in cleansing, warming, and moisturizing air as it travels to the lungs.

■ **Figure 7-2** The vocal cords within the larynx, superior view from the pharynx. *(CNRI/Science Source)*

■ **Figure 7-3** Structure of the trachea, which extends from the larynx above to the main bronchi below.

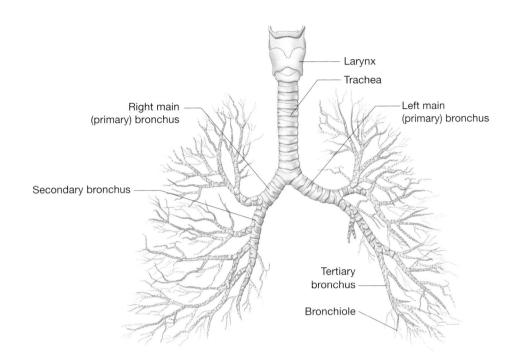

■ **Figure 7-4** The bronchial tree. Note how each main bronchus enters a lung and then branches into smaller and smaller primary bronchi, secondary bronchi, and bronchioles.

Labels in figure:
- Larynx
- Trachea
- Right main (primary) bronchus
- Left main (primary) bronchus
- Secondary bronchus
- Tertiary bronchus
- Bronchiole

Bronchial Tubes

alveoli (al-VEE-oh-lye)
bronchioles (BRONG-kee-ohlz)
bronchus (BRONG-kus)

pulmonary capillaries
respiratory membrane

What's In A Name?

Look for these word parts:
bronchi/o = bronchus
-ole = small

The distal end of the trachea divides to form the left and right main (primary) bronchi. Each **bronchus** enters one of the lungs and branches repeatedly to form secondary and tertiary bronchi. Each branch becomes narrower until the narrowest branches, the **bronchioles**, are formed (see Figure 7-4 ■). Each bronchiole terminates in a small group of air sacs, called **alveoli**. Each lung has approximately 150 million alveoli. The walls of alveoli are elastic, giving them the ability to expand to hold air and then recoil to their original size. A network of **pulmonary capillaries** from the pulmonary blood vessels tightly encases each alveolus (see Figure 7-5 ■). In fact, the walls of the alveoli and capillaries are

Med Term Tip

The respiratory system can be thought of as an upside-down tree and its branches. The trunk of the tree consists of the pharynx, larynx, and trachea. The trachea then divides into two branches, the bronchi. Each bronchus further divides into smaller and smaller branches. In fact, this branching system of tubes is referred to as the *bronchial tree*.

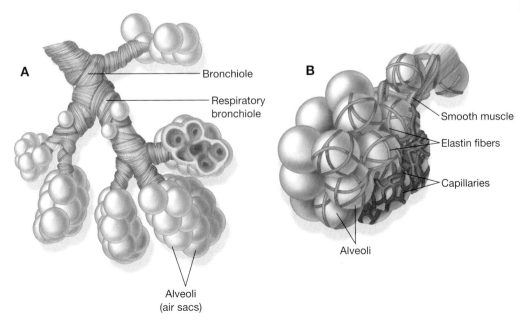

Labels in figure:
- A
- B
- Bronchiole
- Respiratory bronchiole
- Smooth muscle
- Elastin fibers
- Capillaries
- Alveoli
- Alveoli (air sacs)

■ **Figure 7-5** A) Each bronchiole terminates in an alveolar sac, a group of alveoli. B) Alveoli encased by network capillaries, forming the respiratory membrane.

so tightly associated with each other they are referred to as a single unit, the **respiratory membrane**. The exchange of oxygen and carbon dioxide between the air within the alveolus and the blood inside the capillaries takes place across the respiratory membrane.

Lungs

apex	parietal pleura (pah-RYE-eh-tal)
base	pleura (PLOO-rah)
hilum (HYE-lum)	pleural cavity
lobes	serous fluid (SEER-us)
mediastinum (mee-dee-as-TYE-num)	visceral pleura (VISS-er-al)

Each lung is the total collection of the bronchi, bronchioles, and alveoli. They are spongy to the touch because they contain air. The lungs are protected by a double membrane called the **pleura**. The pleura's outer membrane is the **parietal pleura**, which also lines the wall of the chest cavity. The inner membrane, or **visceral pleura**, adheres to the surface of the lungs. The pleural membrane is folded in such a way that it forms a sac around each lung, referred to as the **pleural cavity**. There is normally slippery, watery **serous fluid** between the two layers of the pleura that reduces friction when the two layers rub together as the lungs repeatedly expand and contract.

The lungs contain divisions or **lobes**. There are three lobes in the larger right lung (right upper, right middle, and right lower lobes) and two in the left lung (left upper and left lower lobes). The pointed superior portion of each lung is the **apex**, while the broader lower area is the **base**. Entry of structures like the bronchi, pulmonary blood vessels, and nerves into each lung occurs along its medial border in an area called the **hilum**. The lungs within the thoracic cavity are protected from puncture and damage by the ribs. The area between the right and left lung is called the **mediastinum** and contains the heart, aorta, esophagus, thymus gland, and trachea. See Figure 7-6 ■ for an illustration of the lungs within the chest cavity.

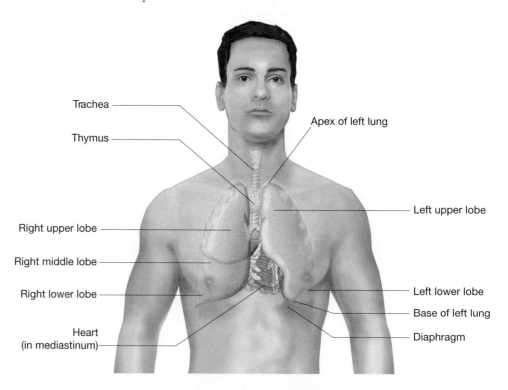

Trachea
Thymus
Apex of left lung
Left upper lobe
Right upper lobe
Right middle lobe
Right lower lobe
Left lower lobe
Base of left lung
Diaphragm
Heart (in mediastinum)

■ **Figure 7-6** Position of the lungs within the thoracic cavity; anterior view illustrating regions of the lungs and their relationship to other thoracic organs.

PRACTICE AS YOU GO

A. Complete the Statement

1. The organs of the respiratory system are _____, _____, _____, _____, _____, and _____.

2. The passageway for food, liquids, and air is the _____.

3. The _____ helps to keep food out of the respiratory tract.

4. The right lung has _____ lobes; the left lung has _____ lobes.

5. The air sacs at the ends of the bronchial tree are called _____.

6. The term for the double membrane around the lungs is _____.

7. The small branches of the bronchi are the _____ and the air sacs are the _____.

Lung Volumes and Capacities

pulmonary function test   **respiratory therapist**

For some types of medical conditions, like emphysema, it is important to measure the volume of air flowing in and out of the lungs to determine lung capacity. Lung volumes are measured by **respiratory therapists** to aid in determining the functioning level of the respiratory system. Collectively, these measurements are called **pulmonary function tests**. Table 7-1 ■ lists and defines the four lung volumes and four lung capacities.

> **What's In A Name?**
> Look for these word parts:
> **spir/o** = breathing
> **-ory** = pertaining to
> **re-** = again

Respiratory Muscles

diaphragm   **intercostal muscles** (in-ter-KOS-tal)

Air moves in and out of the lungs due to the difference between the atmospheric pressure and the pressure within the chest cavity. The **diaphragm**, the muscle separating the abdomen from the thoracic cavity, produces this difference

> **What's In A Name?**
> Look for these word parts:
> **cost/o** = ribs
> **-al** = pertaining to
> **inter-** = between

■ **TABLE 7-1**   Lung Volumes and Capacities

Term	Definition
Tidal volume (TV)	Amount of air that enters lungs in a single inhalation or leaves lungs in a single exhalation of quiet breathing; in an adult this is normally 500 mL*
Inspiratory reserve volume (IRV)	Amount of air that can be forcibly inhaled after normal inspiration; also called *complemental air*, generally measures around 3,000 mL*
Expiratory reserve volume (ERV)	Amount of air that can be forcibly exhaled after normal, quiet exhalation; also called *supplemental air*, approximately 1,000 mL*
Residual volume (RV)	Air remaining in lungs after forced exhalation; about 1,500 mL* in an adult
Inspiratory capacity (IC)	Volume of air inhaled after normal exhale
Functional residual capacity (FRC)	Air that remains in lungs after normal exhalation has taken place
Vital capacity (VC)	Total volume of air that can be exhaled after maximum inhalation; amount will be equal to sum of TV, IRV, and ERV
Total lung capacity (TLC)	Volume of air in lungs after maximal inhalation

*There is a normal range for measurements of volume of air exchanged; numbers given are for average measurement.

■ **Figure 7-7** A) Bell jar apparatus demonstrating how downward movement of the diaphragm results in air flowing into the lungs. B) Action of the intercostal muscles lifts the ribs to assist the diaphragm in enlarging the volume of the thoracic cavity.

Expiration — **Inspiration**

Med Term Tip

Diaphragmatic breathing is taught to singers and public speakers. You can practice this type of breathing by allowing your abdomen to expand during inhalation and contract during exhalation while your shoulders remain motionless.

in pressure. To do this, the diaphragm contracts and moves downward. This increase in thoracic cavity volume causes a decrease in pressure, or negative thoracic pressure, within the chest cavity. Air then flows into the lungs (inhalation) to equalize the pressure. The **intercostal muscles** between the ribs assist in inhalation by raising the rib cage to further enlarge the thoracic cavity. See Figure 7-7 ■ for an illustration of the role of the diaphragm in inhalation. Similarly, when the diaphragm and intercostal muscles relax, the thoracic cavity becomes smaller. This produces an increase in pressure within the cavity, or positive thoracic pressure, and air flows out of the lungs, resulting in exhalation. Therefore, a quiet, unforced exhalation is a passive process since it does not require any muscle contraction. When a forceful inhalation or exhalation is required, additional chest and neck muscles become active to create larger changes in thoracic pressure.

Respiratory Rate

vital signs

Respiratory rate (measured in breaths per minute) is one of the body's **vital signs** (VS), along with heart rate, temperature, and blood pressure. The respiratory rate is normally regulated by the level of CO_2 in the blood. When the CO_2 level is high, breathing is more rapid to expel the excess. Likewise, when CO_2 levels drop, the respiratory rate will also drop.

■ TABLE 7-2   Respiratory Rates for Different Age Groups

Age	Respirations Per Minute
Newborn	30–60
1-year-old	18–30
16-year-old	16–20
Adult	12–20

When the respiratory rate falls outside the range of normal, it may indicate an illness or medical condition. For example, when a patient is running an elevated temperature and has shortness of breath (SOB) due to pneumonia, the respiratory rate may increase dramatically. Or a brain injury or some medications, such as those for pain, can cause a decrease in the respiratory rate. See Table 7-2 ■ for normal respiratory rate ranges for different age groups.

PRACTICE AS YOU GO

B. Lung Volumes and Capacities Matching

1. _____ tidal volume
2. _____ residual volume
3. _____ vital capacity
4. _____ inspiratory reserve volume
5. _____ total lung capacity
6. _____ expiratory reserve volume
7. _____ inspiratory capacity
8. _____ functional residual capacity

a. air that can be exhaled after a maximum inhalation
b. air forcibly exhaled after normal quiet exhalation
c. air that enters lungs in a single inhalation
d. air still in lungs after normal exhalation
e. air inhaled after normal exhale
f. air in lungs after forced exhalation
g. air in lungs after a maximal inhalation
h. air forcibly inhaled after normal inspiration

Terminology

Word Parts Used to Build Respiratory System Terms

The following lists contain the combining forms, suffixes, and prefixes used to build terms in the remaining sections of this chapter.

Combining Forms

aer/o	air	atel/o	incomplete	carcin/o	cancer
alveol/o	alveolus	bi/o	life	cardi/o	heart
angi/o	vessel	bronch/o	bronchus	coni/o	dust
anthrac/o	coal	bronchi/o	bronchus	cortic/o	outer layer
arteri/o	artery	bronchiol/o	bronchiole	cyan/o	blue

Combining Forms (continued)

cyst/o	sac	**myc/o**	fungus	**py/o**	pus
cyt/o	cell	**nas/o**	nose	**rhin/o**	nose
diaphragmat/o	diaphragm	**orth/o**	straight	**sept/o**	wall
embol/o	plug	**ot/o**	ear	**sinus/o**	sinus
epiglott/o	epiglottis	**ox/i**	oxygen	**somn/o**	sleep
fibr/o	fibers	**ox/o**	oxygen	**spir/o**	breathing
hem/o	blood	**pharyng/o**	pharynx	**thorac/o**	chest
hist/o	tissue	**pleur/o**	pleura	**trache/o**	trachea
laryng/o	larynx	**pneum/o**	air	**tuss/o**	cough
lob/o	lobe	**pneumon/o**	lung		
muc/o	mucus	**pulmon/o**	lung		

Suffixes

-al	pertaining to	-ism	state of	-plasm	formation
-algia	pain	-itis	inflammation	-plasty	surgical repair
-ar	pertaining to	-logy	study of	-plegia	paralysis
-ary	pertaining to	-lytic	destruction	-pnea	breathing
-capnia	carbon dioxide	-meter	instrument to measure	-ptysis	spitting
-centesis	puncture to withdraw fluid	-metry	process of measuring	-rrhagia	abnormal flow condition
-dynia	pain	-oma	tumor	-rrhea	discharge
-eal	pertaining to	-ory	pertaining to	-scope	instrument for viewing
-ectasis	dilation	-osis	abnormal condition	-scopy	process of visually examining
-ectomy	surgical removal	-osmia	smell		
-emia	blood condition	-ostomy	surgically create an opening	-spasm	involuntary muscle contraction
-genic	produced by	-otomy	cutting into	-stenosis	narrowing
-gram	record	-ous	pertaining to	-thorax	chest
-graphy	process of recording	-phonia	voice	-tic	pertaining to
-ia	condition	-phylaxis	protection		
-ic	pertaining to				

Prefixes

a-	without	endo-	within	poly-	many
an-	without	eu-	normal	pro-	before
anti-	against	hyper-	excessive	re-	again
brady-	slow	hypo-	insufficient	tachy-	fast
de-	without	pan-	all		
dys-	difficult, abnormal	para-	beside		

Adjective Forms of Anatomical Terms

Term	Word Parts	Definition
alveolar (al-VEE-oh-lar)	alveol/o = alveolus -ar = pertaining to	Pertaining to alveoli
bronchial (BRONG-kee-al)	bronchi/o = bronchus -al = pertaining to	Pertaining to a bronchus
bronchiolar (brong-KEE-oh-lar)	bronchiol/o = bronchiole -ar = pertaining to	Pertaining to a bronchiole
diaphragmatic (dye-ah-frag-MAT-ik)	diaphragmat/o = diaphragm -ic = pertaining to	Pertaining to diaphragm
epiglottic (ep-ih-GLOT-ik)	epiglott/o = epiglottis -ic = pertaining to	Pertaining to epiglottis
laryngeal (lair-IN-jee-al)	laryng/o = larynx -eal = pertaining to	Pertaining to larynx
lobar (LOH-bar)	lob/o = lobe -ar = pertaining to	Pertaining to a lobe (of the lung)
mucous (MYOO-kus)	muc/o = mucus -ous = pertaining to	Pertaining to mucus
nasal (NAY-zal)	nas/o = nose -al = pertaining to	Pertaining to nose or nasal cavity
nasopharyngeal (nay-zoh-fah-RIN-jee-al)	nas/o = nose pharyng/o = pharynx -eal = pertaining to	Pertaining to nose and pharynx
paranasal (pair-ah-NAY-zal)	para- = beside nas/o = nose -al = pertaining to	Pertaining to beside the nose
pharyngeal (fair-IN-jee-al)	pharyng/o = pharynx -eal = pertaining to	Pertaining to pharynx
pleural (PLOO-ral)	pleur/o = pleura -al = pertaining to	Pertaining to pleura
pulmonary (PULL-mon-air-ee)	pulmon/o = lung -ary = pertaining to	Pertaining to lung
septal (SEP-tal)	sept/o = wall -al = pertaining to	Pertaining to wall (i.e., nasal septum)
thoracic (tho-RASS-ik)	thorac/o = chest -ic = pertaining to	Pertaining to chest
tracheal (TRAY-kee-al)	trache/o = trachea -al = pertaining to	Pertaining to trachea

PRACTICE AS YOU GO

C. Give the adjective form for each anatomical structure.

1. The larynx _____
2. The lung _____
3. Beside the nose _____
4. An alveolus _____
5. The nose _____
6. The diaphragm _____

Pathology

Term	Word Parts	Definition
Medical Specialties		
internal medicine		Branch of medicine involving diagnosis and treatment of diseases and conditions of internal organs such as respiratory system; physician is an *internist*
otorhinolaryngology (ENT) (oh-toh-rye-noh-lair-in-GALL-oh-jee)	ot/o = ear rhin/o = nose laryng/o = larynx -logy = study of	Branch of medicine involving diagnosis and treatment of conditions and diseases of ear, nose, and throat region; physician is *otorhinolaryngologist*; this medical specialty may also be referred to as *otolaryngology*
pulmonology (pull-mon-NALL-oh-jee)	pulmon/o = lung -logy = study of	Branch of medicine involved in diagnosis and treatment of diseases and disorders of respiratory system; physician is *pulmonologist*
respiratory therapy	re- = again spir/o = breathing -ory = pertaining to	Allied health specialty that assists patients with respiratory and cardiopulmonary disorders; duties of *respiratory therapist* include conducting pulmonary function tests, monitoring oxygen and carbon dioxide levels in blood, administering breathing treatments, and ventilator management
thoracic surgery (tho-RASS-ik)	thorac/o = chest -ic = pertaining to	Branch of medicine involving diagnosis and treatment of conditions and diseases of respiratory system by surgical means; physician is *thoracic surgeon*
Signs and Symptoms		
anosmia (an-OZ-mee-ah)	an- = without -osmia = smell	Lack of sense of smell

Pathology (continued)

Term	Word Parts	Definition
anoxia (an-OK-see-ah)	an- = without ox/o = oxygen -ia – condition	Condition of receiving almost no oxygen from inhaled air
aphonia (ah-FOH-nee-ah)	a- = without -phonia = voice	Condition of being unable to produce sounds
apnea (AP-nee-ah)	a- = without -pnea = breathing	Not breathing
asphyxia (as-FIK-see-ah)	a- = without -ia = condition	Lack of oxygen that can lead to unconsciousness and death if not corrected immediately; also called *asphyxiation* or *suffocation*; common causes include drowning, foreign body in respiratory tract, poisoning, and electric shock
aspiration (as-pih-RAY-shun)	spir/o = breathing	Refers to withdrawing fluid from body cavity using suction; for example, using long needle and syringe to withdraw fluid from pleural cavity, or using vacuum pump to remove phlegm from patient's airway; additionally, refers to inhaling food, liquid, or foreign object into airways, which may lead to development of pneumonia
bradypnea (brad-ip-NEE-ah)	brady- = slow -pnea = breathing	Breathing too slowly; low respiratory rate
bronchiectasis (brong-kee-EK-tah-sis)	bronchi/o = bronchus -ectasis = dilation	Dilated bronchus
bronchospasm (BRONG-koh-spazm)	bronch/o = bronchus -spasm = involuntary muscle contraction	Involuntary muscle spasm of smooth muscle in the wall of bronchus
Cheyne–Stokes respiration (CHAIN / STOHKS / res-pir-AY-shun)	re- = again spir/o = breathing	Abnormal breathing pattern in which there are long periods (10–60 seconds) of apnea followed by deeper, more rapid breathing; named for John Cheyne, a Scottish physician, and Sir William Stokes, an Irish surgeon
clubbing		Abnormal widening and thickening of ends of fingers and toes associated with chronic oxygen deficiency; seen in patients with chronic respiratory conditions or circulatory problems
crackles		Abnormal crackling or bubbling sound made during inspiration; usually indicates presence of fluid or mucus in small airways; also called *rales*

Pathology (continued)

Term	Word Parts	Definition
cyanosis (sigh-ah-NOH-sis)	cyan/o = blue -osis = abnormal condition	Refers to bluish tint of skin that is receiving insufficient amount of oxygen or circulation

■ **Figure 7-8** A cyanotic infant. Note the bluish tinge to the skin around the lips, chin, and nose. *(St Bartholomew's Hospital, London/Science Source)*

Term	Word Parts	Definition
dysphonia (dis-FOH-nee-ah)	dys- = difficult, abnormal -phonia = voice	Condition of having difficulty producing sounds or producing abnormal sounds
dyspnea (DISP-nee-ah)	dys- = difficult -pnea = breathing	Term describing difficult or labored breathing
epistaxis (ep-ih-STAK-sis)		Nosebleed
eupnea (yoop-NEE-ah)	eu- = normal -pnea = breathing	Normal breathing and respiratory rate
hemoptysis (hee-MOP-tih-sis)	hem/o = blood -ptysis = spitting	To cough up blood or blood-stained sputum
hemothorax (hee-moh-THOH-raks)	hem/o = blood -thorax = chest	Presence of blood in chest cavity
hypercapnia (high-per-KAP-nee-ah)	hyper- = excessive -capnia = carbon dioxide	Condition of having excessive carbon dioxide in body
hyperpnea (high-PERP-nee-ah)	hyper- = excessive -pnea = breathing	Taking deep breaths
hyperventilation (high-per-ven-tih-LAY-shun)	hyper- = excessive	Breathing both too fast (tachypnea) and too deep (hyperpnea)

> **Med Term Tip**
>
> When divers wish to hold their breath longer, they first hyperventilate (breathe faster and deeper) in order to get rid of as much CO_2 as possible. This will hold off the urge to breathe, allowing a diver to stay submerged longer.

Term	Word Parts	Definition
hypocapnia (high-poh-KAP-nee-ah)	hypo- = insufficient -capnia = carbon dioxide	Insufficient level of carbon dioxide in body; very serious problem because it is presence of carbon dioxide that stimulates respiration, not absence of oxygen; therefore, person with low carbon dioxide levels would respond with increased respiratory rate
hypopnea (high-POP-nee-ah)	hypo- = insufficient -pnea = breathing	Taking shallow breaths

Pathology (continued)

Term	Word Parts	Definition
hypoventilation (high-poh-ven-tih-LAY-shun)	hypo- = insufficient	Breathing both too slow (bradypnea) and too shallow (hypopnea)
hypoxemia (high-pok-SEE-mee-ah)	hypo- = insufficient ox/o = oxygen -emia = blood condition	Condition of having insufficient amount of oxygen in bloodstream
hypoxia (high-POK-see-ah)	hypo- = insufficient ox/o = oxygen -ia = condition	Condition of receiving insufficient amount of oxygen from inhaled air
laryngoplegia (lah-ring-goh-PLEE-jee-ah)	laryng/o = larynx -plegia = paralysis	Paralysis of muscles controlling larynx
orthopnea (or-THOP-nee-ah)	orth/o = straight -pnea = breathing	Term describing dyspnea worsened by lying flat; patient feels able to breathe easier while sitting straight up; common occurrence in those with pulmonary disease
pansinusitis (pan-sigh-nus-EYE-tis)	pan- = all sinus/o = sinus -itis = inflammation	Inflammation of all paranasal sinuses
patent (PAY-tent)		Open or unblocked, such as patent airway
phlegm (FLEM)		Thick mucus secreted by membranes lining respiratory tract; when phlegm is coughed through mouth, is called *sputum*; phlegm is examined for color, odor, and consistency and tested for presence of bacteria, viruses, and fungi
pleural rub (PLOO-ral)	pleur/o = pleura -al = pertaining to	Grating sound made when two layers of pleura rub together during respiration; caused when one surface becomes thicker as a result of inflammation or other disease conditions; rub can be felt through fingertips when placed on chest wall or heard through stethoscope
pleurodynia (ploor-oh-DIN-ee-ah)	pleur/o = pleura -dynia = pain	Pleural pain
pyothorax (pye-oh-THOH-raks)	py/o = pus -thorax = chest	Presence of pus in chest cavity; indicates bacterial infection
rhinitis (rye-NYE-tis)	rhin/o = nose -itis = inflammation	Inflammation of nasal cavity
rhinorrhagia (rye-noh-RAY-jee-ah)	rhin/o = nose -rrhagia = abnormal flow condition	Rapid flow of blood from nose
rhinorrhea (rye-noh-REE-ah)	rhin/o = nose -rrhea = discharge	Discharge from nose; commonly called a *runny nose*
rhonchi (RONG-kigh)		Somewhat musical sound during expiration, often found in asthma or infection; caused by spasms of bronchial tubes; also called *wheezing*

Pathology (continued)

Term	Word Parts	Definition
shortness of breath (SOB)		Term used to indicate patient is having some difficulty breathing; also called *dyspnea*; causes can range from mild SOB after exercise to SOB associated with heart disease
sputum (SPYOO-tum)		Mucus or phlegm coughed up from lining of respiratory tract

> **Med Term Tip**
> The term *sputum*, from the Latin word meaning *to spit*, now refers to the material coughed up and spit out from the respiratory system.

Term	Word Parts	Definition
stridor (STRY-der)		Harsh, high-pitched, noisy breathing sound made when there is obstruction of bronchus or larynx; found in conditions such as croup in children
tachypnea (tak-ip-NEE-ah)	tachy- = fast -pnea = breathing	Breathing fast; high respiratory rate
thoracalgia (thor-ah-KAL-jee-ah)	thorac/o = chest -algia = pain	Chest pain; does not refer to angina pectoris
tracheostenosis (tray-kee-oh-steh-NOH-sis)	trache/o = trachea -stenosis = narrowing	Narrowing of trachea
Upper Respiratory System		
croup (KROOP)		Acute respiratory condition found in infants and children characterized by barking type of cough or stridor
diphtheria (dif-THEAR-ee-ah)	-ia = condition	Bacterial upper respiratory infection characterized by formation of thick membranous film across throat and high mortality rate; rare now, due to childhood diphtheria, pertussis, and tetanus (DPT) vaccines
laryngitis (lair-in-JYE-tis)	laryng/o = larynx -itis = inflammation	Inflammation of larynx
nasopharyngitis (nay-zoh-fair-in-JYE-tis)	nas/o = nose pharyng/o = pharynx -itis = inflammation	Inflammation of nasal cavity and pharynx; commonly called *common cold*
pertussis (per-TUH-sis)	tuss/o = cough	Infectious bacterial disease of upper respiratory system that children receive immunization against as part of their DPT shots; commonly called *whooping cough*, due to whoop sound made when coughing
pharyngitis (fair-in-JYE-tis)	pharyng/o = pharynx -itis = inflammation	Inflammation of pharynx; commonly called a *sore throat*
rhinomycosis (rye-noh-my-KOH-sis)	rhin/o = nose myc/o = fungus -osis = abnormal condition	Fungal infection of nasal cavity

Pathology (continued)

Term	Word Parts	Definition
Bronchial Tubes		
asthma (AZ mah) **Med Term Tip** The term *asthma*, from the Greek word meaning *panting*, describes the breathing pattern of a person having an asthma attack.		Disease caused by various conditions, like allergens, and resulting in constriction of bronchial airways, dyspnea, coughing, and wheezing; can cause violent spasms of bronchi (bronchospasms) but generally not life-threatening condition; medication can be very effective
bronchiectasis (brong-kee-EK-tah-sis)	bronchi/o = bronchus -ectasis = dilation	Abnormal enlargement of bronchi; may be result of lung infection; condition can be irreversible and result in destruction of bronchial walls; major symptoms include coughing up large amount of purulent sputum, crackles, and hemoptysis
bronchitis (brong-KIGH-tis)	bronch/o = bronchus -itis = inflammation	Inflammation of a bronchus
bronchogenic carcinoma (brong-koh-JEN-ik / kar-sih-NOH-mah)	bronch/o = bronchus -genic = produced by carcin/o = cancer -oma = tumor	Malignant tumor originating in bronchi; usually associated with history of cigarette smoking

■ **Figure 7-9** Color-enhanced X-ray of large malignant tumor in the right lung. *(Wonderisland/Shutterstock)*

Term	Word Parts	Definition
Lungs		
adult respiratory distress syndrome (ARDS)	re- = again spir/o = breathing -ory = pertaining to	Acute respiratory failure in adults characterized by tachypnea, dyspnea, cyanosis, tachycardia, and hypoxemia; may follow trauma, pneumonia, or septic infections; also called *acute respiratory distress syndrome*
anthracosis (an-thrah-KOH-sis)	anthrac/o = coal -osis = abnormal condition	Type of pneumoconiosis that develops from collection of coal dust in lung; also called *black lung* or *miner's lung*
asbestosis (az-bes-TOH-sis)	-osis = abnormal condition	Type of pneumoconiosis that develops from collection of asbestos fibers in lungs; may lead to development of lung cancer
atelectasis (at-eh-LEK-tah-sis)	atel/o = incomplete -ectasis = dilation	Condition in which alveoli in a portion of the lung collapse, preventing respiratory exchange of oxygen and carbon dioxide; can be caused by variety of conditions, including pressure on lung from tumor or other object; term also used to describe failure of newborn's lungs to expand

Pathology (continued)

Term	Word Parts	Definition
chronic obstructive pulmonary disease (COPD) (PULL-mon-air-ee)	pulmon/o = lung -ary = pertaining to	Progressive, chronic, and usually irreversible group of conditions (often a combination of chronic bronchitis and emphysema) in which lungs have diminished capacity for inhalation and exhalation; person may have dyspnea upon exertion and a cough
cystic fibrosis (CF) (SIS-tik / fye-BROH-sis) **Med Term Tip** Cystic fibrosis received its name from fibrotic cysts that are visible in the pancreas as scarred areas.	cyst/o = sac -ic = pertaining to fibr/o = fibers -osis = abnormal condition	Hereditary condition causing exocrine glands to malfunction; patient produces very thick mucus that causes severe congestion within lungs, pancreas, and intestine; through more advanced treatment, many children are now living into adulthood with this disease
emphysema (em-fih-SEE-mah)		Pulmonary condition characterized by destruction of walls of alveoli, resulting in fewer, overexpanded air sacs; can occur as a result of long-term heavy smoking; air pollution also worsens disease; patient may not be able to breathe except in sitting or standing position
histoplasmosis (his-toh-plaz-MOH-sis)	hist/o = tissue -plasm = formation -osis = abnormal condition	Pulmonary infection caused by fungus *Histoplasma capsulatum*, found in dust and in droppings of pigeons and chickens
infant respiratory distress syndrome (IRDS)	re- = again spir/o = breathing -ory = pertaining to	Lung condition most commonly found in premature infants characterized by tachypnea and respiratory grunting; condition caused by lack of surfactant necessary to keep lungs inflated; also called *hyaline membrane disease* (HMD) and *respiratory distress syndrome of the newborn*
influenza (flu) (in-floo-EN-zah)		Viral infection of respiratory system characterized by chills, fever, body aches, and fatigue; commonly called the *flu*
Legionnaires' disease (lee-jen-AYRZ)		Severe, often fatal bacterial infection characterized by pneumonia and liver and kidney damage; named after people who came down with it at American Legion convention in 1976
Middle East respiratory syndrome (MERS)		Life-threatening viral respiratory illness first reported in Saudi Arabia in September 2012; symptoms include fever, cough, and shortness of breath
***Mycoplasma* pneumonia** (MY-koh-plaz-mah)	myc/o = fungus -plasm = formation	Less severe but longer-lasting form of pneumonia caused by *Mycoplasma pneumoniae* bacteria; also called *walking pneumonia*

Pathology (continued)

Term	Word Parts	Definition
pneumoconiosis (noo-moh-koh-nee-OH-sis)	pneum/o = lung coni/o = dust -osis = abnormal condition	Condition resulting from inhalation of environmental particles that become toxic; can be result of inhaling coal dust (*anthracosis*) or asbestos (*asbestosis*)
pneumonia (noo-MOH-nee-ah)	pneumon/o = lung -ia = condition	Inflammatory condition of lung that can be caused by bacteria, viruses, fungi, and aspirated substances; results in filling of alveoli and air spaces with fluid
pulmonary edema (PULL-mon-air-ee / eh-DEE-mah)	pulmon/o = lung -ary = pertaining to	Condition in which lung tissue retains excessive amount of fluid, especially in alveoli; results in dyspnea
pulmonary embolism (PE) (EM-boh-lizm)	pulmon/o = lung -ary = pertaining to embol/o = plug -ism = state of	Obstruction of pulmonary artery or one of its branches by embolus (often blood clot broken away from another area of body); may cause infarct in lung tissue
pulmonary fibrosis (fye-BROH-sis)	pulmon/o = lung -ary = pertaining to fibr/o = fibers -osis = abnormal condition	Formation of fibrous scar tissue in lungs that leads to decreased ability to expand lungs; may be caused by infections, pneumoconiosis, autoimmune diseases, and toxin exposure
severe acute respiratory syndrome (SARS)	re- = again spir/o = breathing -ory = pertaining to	Acute viral respiratory infection that begins like flu but quickly progresses to severe dyspnea; high fatality rate in persons over age 65; first appeared in China in 2003
silicosis (sil-ih-KOH-sis)	-osis = abnormal condition	Type of pneumoconiosis that develops from inhalation of silica (quartz) dust found in quarrying, glasswork, sandblasting, and ceramics
sleep apnea (AP-nee-ah)	a- = without -pnea = breathing	Condition in which breathing stops repeatedly during sleep long enough to cause drop in oxygen levels in blood
sudden infant death syndrome (SIDS)		Unexpected and unexplained death of apparently well infant under one year of age; child suddenly stops breathing for unknown reasons
tuberculosis (TB) (too-ber-kyoo-LOH-sis)	-osis = abnormal condition	Infectious disease caused by bacteria *Mycobacterium tuberculosis*; most commonly affects respiratory system and causes inflammation and calcification in lungs; tuberculosis incidence is on the increase and is seen in many patients with weakened immune systems; multidrug-resistant tuberculosis is a particularly dangerous form of the disease because some bacteria have developed resistance to standard drug therapy

Pleural Cavity

Term	Word Parts	Definition
empyema (em-pye-EE-mah)	py/o = pus	Pus within pleural space usually associated with bacterial infection; also called *pyothorax*

Pathology (continued)

Term	Word Parts	Definition
pleural effusion (PLOO-ral / eh-FYOO-zhun)	pleur/o = pleura -al = pertaining to	Abnormal accumulation of fluid in pleural cavity preventing lungs from fully expanding; physicians can detect presence of fluid by tapping chest (percussion) or listening with stethoscope (auscultation)
pleurisy (PLOOR-ih-see)	pleur/o = pleura	Inflammation of pleura characterized by sharp chest pain with each breath; also called *pleuritis*
pneumothorax (noo-moh-THOH-raks)	pneum/o = air -thorax = chest	Collection of air or gas in pleural cavity, possibly resulting in collapse of lung

Torn pleura
Outside air entering pleural cavity
Left lung
Diaphragm
Inspiration

■ **Figure 7-10**   Pneumothorax. Figure illustrates how puncture of thoracic wall and tearing of pleural membrane allows air into lung and results in collapsed lung.

PRACTICE AS YOU GO

D. Terminology Matching

Match each term to its definition.

1. _____ inhaling environmental particles
2. _____ whooping cough
3. _____ may result in collapsed lung
4. _____ pus in the pleural space
5. _____ respiratory tract mucus
6. _____ nosebleed
7. _____ cyanosis
8. _____ *Mycoplasma* pneumonia
9. _____ disease with overexpanded air sacs
10. _____ histoplasmosis

a. empyema
b. blue tint to the skin
c. caused by a fungus
d. epistaxis
e. pneumoconiosis
f. emphysema
g. walking pneumonia
h. pneumothorax
i. pertussis
j. phlegm

Diagnostic Procedures

Term	Word Parts	Definition
Clinical Laboratory Tests		
arterial blood gases (ABGs) (ar-TEE-ree-al)	arteri/o = artery -al = pertaining to	Testing for gases present in blood; generally used to assist in determining levels of oxygen and carbon dioxide in blood
sputum culture and sensitivity (C&S) (SPYOO-tum)		Testing sputum by placing it on culture medium and observing any bacterial growth; specimen is then tested to determine antibiotic effectiveness
sputum cytology (SPYOO-tum / sigh-TALL-oh-jee)	cyt/o = cell -logy = study of	Examining sputum for malignant cells
Diagnostic Imaging		
bronchogram (BRONG-koh-gram)	bronch/o = bronchus -gram = record	X-ray record of bronchus produced by bronchography
bronchography (brong-KOG-rah-fee)	bronch/o = bronchus -graphy = process of recording	X-ray of lung after radiopaque substance inserted into trachea or bronchial tube; resulting X-ray is called *bronchogram*
chest X-ray (CXR)		Taking radiographic picture of lungs and heart from back and sides
pulmonary angiography (PULL-mon-air-ee / an-jee-OG-rah-fee)	pulmon/o = lung -ary = pertaining to angi/o = vessel -graphy = process of recording	Injecting dye into blood vessel for purpose of taking X-ray of arteries and veins of lungs
ventilation-perfusion scan (per-FYOO-zhun)		Nuclear medicine diagnostic test especially useful in identifying pulmonary emboli; radioactive air is inhaled for ventilation portion to determine if air is filling entire lung; radioactive intravenous injection shows if blood is flowing to all parts of lung
Endoscopic Procedures		
bronchoscope (BRONG-koh-skohp)	bronch/o = bronchus -scope = instrument for viewing	Instrument used to view inside bronchus during *bronchoscopy*
bronchoscopy (Bronch) (brong-KOSS-koh-pee)	bronch/o = bronchus -scopy = process of visually examining	Visual examination of inside of bronchi; uses instrument called *bronchoscope* (see Figure 7-11 ■)
laryngoscope (lah-RING-goh-skohp)	laryng/o = larynx -scope = instrument for viewing	Instrument used to view inside larynx during *laryngoscopy*
laryngoscopy (lair-in-GOSS-koh-pee)	laryng/o = larynx -scopy = process of visually examining	Examination of interior of larynx with lighted instrument called *laryngoscope*

Diagnostic Procedures (continued)

Term	Word Parts	Definition

■ **Figure 7-11** Bronchoscopy. Figure illustrates physician using a bronchoscope to inspect the patient's bronchial tubes. Advances in technology include using a videoscope, which projects the internal view of the bronchus onto a video screen.

Pulmonary Function Tests

Term	Word Parts	Definition
oximeter (ok-SIM-eh-ter)	ox/i = oxygen -meter = instrument to measure	Instrument that measures amount of oxygen in bloodstream
oximetry (ok-SIM-eh-tree)	ox/i = oxygen -metry = process of measuring	Procedure to measure oxygen level in blood using device, an *oximeter*, placed on patient's fingertip or earlobe
pulmonary function test (PFT) (PULL-mon-air-ee)	pulmon/o = lung -ary = pertaining to	Group of diagnostic tests that give information regarding airflow in and out of lungs, lung volumes, and gas exchange between lungs and bloodstream
spirometer (spy-ROM-eh-ter)	spir/o = breathing -meter = instrument to measure	Instrument to measure lung capacity used for *spirometry*
spirometry (spy-ROM-eh-tree)	spir/o = breathing -metry = process of measuring	Procedure to measure lung capacity using *spirometer*

Additional Diagnostic Procedures

Term	Word Parts	Definition
polysomnography (pol-ee-som-NOG-rah-fee)	poly- = many somn/o = sleep -graphy = process of recording	Monitoring patient while sleeping to identify sleep apnea; also called *sleep apnea study*
sweat test		Test for cystic fibrosis; patients with this disease have abnormally large amount of salt in their sweat
tuberculin skin test (TB test) (too-BER-kyoo-lin)		Procedure in which tuberculin purified protein derivative (PPD) is applied under surface of skin to determine if patient has been exposed to tuberculosis; also called a *Mantoux test*

Therapeutic Procedures

Term	Word Parts	Definition
Respiratory Therapy		
aerosol therapy (AIR-oh-sol)	aer/o = air	Medication suspended in mist intended for inhalation; delivered by *nebulizer*, which provides mist for period of time while patient breathes, or *metered-dose inhaler* (MDI), which delivers single puff of mist
continuous positive airway pressure (CPAP)		Machine that supplies constant and steady air pressure through mask; keeps airways continuously open; common treatment for sleep apnea
endotracheal intubation (en-doh-TRAY-kee-al / in-too-BAY-shun)	endo- = within trache/o = trachea -al = pertaining to	Placing of a tube through mouth, through glottis, and into trachea to create patent airway

Epiglottis   Trachea

Esophagus

■ **Figure 7-12**   Endotracheal intubation. First, a lighted scope is used to distinguish the trachea from the esophagus. Next, the tube is placed through the pharynx and into the trachea. Finally, the scope is removed, leaving the tube in place.

intermittent positive pressure breathing (IPPB)		Method for assisting patients in breathing using mask connected to machine that produces increased positive thoracic pressure
nasal cannula (KAN-yoo-lah)	nas/o = nose -al = pertaining to	Two-pronged plastic device for delivering oxygen into nose; one prong is inserted into each naris
postural drainage	-al = pertaining to	Drainage of secretions from bronchi by placing patient in position that uses gravity to promote drainage; used for treatment of cystic fibrosis and bronchiectasis
supplemental oxygen therapy	-al = pertaining to	Providing patient with additional concentration of oxygen to improve oxygen levels in bloodstream; oxygen may be provided by mask or nasal cannula
ventilator (VEN-tih-lay-ter)		Machine that provides artificial ventilation for patient unable to breathe on his or her own; also called *respirator*
Surgical Procedures		
bronchoplasty (BRONG-koh-plas-tee)	bronch/o = bronchus -plasty = surgical repair	Surgical repair of a bronchus
laryngectomy (lair-in-JEK-toh-mee)	laryng/o = larynx -ectomy = surgical removal	Surgical removal of larynx

Therapeutic Procedures (continued)

Term	Word Parts	Definition
laryngoplasty (lah-RING-goh-plas-tee)	laryng/o = larynx -plasty = surgical repair	Surgical repair of larynx
lobectomy (loh-BEK-toh-mee)	lob/o = lobe -ectomy = surgical removal	Surgical removal of a lobe of a lung
pleurectomy (ploor-EK-toh-mee)	pleur/o = pleura -ectomy = surgical removal	Surgical removal of pleura
pleurocentesis (ploor-oh-sen-TEE-sis)	pleur/o = pleura -centesis = puncture to withdraw fluid	Procedure involving insertion of needle into pleural space to withdraw fluid; may be treatment for excess fluid accumulating or to obtain fluid for diagnostic examination
pneumonectomy (noo-moh-NEK-toh-mee)	pneum/o = lung -ectomy = surgical removal	Surgical removal of entire lung
rhinoplasty (RYE-noh-plas-tee)	rhin/o = nose -plasty = surgical repair	Surgical repair of nose
thoracentesis (thor-ah-sen-TEE-sis)	thorac/o = chest -centesis = puncture to withdraw fluid	Surgical puncture of chest wall for removal of fluids; also called *thoracocentesis*

Needle inserted into pleural space to withdraw fluid

■ **Figure 7-13** Thoracentesis. Insertion of a needle between the ribs to withdraw fluid from the pleural sac at the base of the left lung.

Term	Word Parts	Definition
thoracostomy (thor-ah-KOS-toh-mee)	thorac/o = chest -ostomy = surgically create an opening	Insertion of tube into chest cavity for purpose of draining off fluid or air; also called *chest tube*
thoracotomy (thor-ah-KOT-oh-mee)	thorac/o = chest -otomy = cutting into	To cut into chest cavity

Therapeutic Procedures (continued)

Term	Word Parts	Definition
tracheotomy (tray-kee-OT-oh-mee)	trache/o = trachea -otomy = cutting into	Surgical procedure often performed in emergency that creates opening directly into trachea to allow patient to breathe easier, also called *tracheostomy*

■ **Figure 7-14** A tracheotomy tube in place, inserted through an opening in the front of the neck and anchored within the trachea.

Labels: Epiglottis, Thyroid cartilage, Larynx, Esophagus, Trachea, Tracheotomy tube

Additional Procedures

Term	Word Parts	Definition
cardiopulmonary resuscitation (CPR) (kar-dee-oh-PULL-mon-air-ee / ree-suss-ih-TAY-shun)	cardi/o = heart pulmon/o = lung -ary = pertaining to	Emergency treatment provided by persons trained in CPR and given to patients when their respirations and heart stop; CPR provides oxygen to brain, heart, and other vital organs until medical treatment can restore normal heart and pulmonary function
Heimlich maneuver (HYME-lik)		Technique for removing foreign body from trachea or pharynx by exerting diaphragmatic pressure; named for Henry Heimlich, a U.S. thoracic surgeon
percussion (per-KUH-shun)		Use of fingertips to tap on surface to assess condition beneath; determined in part by feel of surface as it is tapped and sound generated

PRACTICE AS YOU GO

E. Terminology Matching

Match each term to its definition.

1. _____ sweat test
2. _____ measures oxygen levels in blood
3. _____ ventilator
4. _____ test to identify sleep apnea
5. _____ thoracentesis
6. _____ tuberculin test

a. polysomnography
b. Mantoux test
c. oximetry
d. puncture chest wall to remove fluid
e. respirator
f. test for cystic fibrosis

Pharmacology

Vocabulary

Term	Word Parts	Definition
cumulative action		Action that occurs in body when drug is allowed to accumulate or stay in body
prophylaxis (proh-fih-LAK-sis)	pro- = before -phylaxis = protection	Prevention of disease; for example, antibiotic can be used to prevent occurrence of bacterial infection

Drugs

Classification	Word Parts	Action	Examples
antibiotic (an-tih-bye-AW-tik)	anti- = against bi/o = life -tic = pertaining to	Kills bacteria causing respiratory infections	ampicillin; amoxicillin, Amoxil; ciprofloxacin, Cipro
	Med Term Tip There are three accepted pronunciations for the prefix anti-, "an-tih," "an-tee," and "an-tye."		
antihistamine (an-tih-HIST-ah-meen)	anti- = against	Blocks effects of histamine released by body during allergy attack	fexofenadine, Allegra; loratadine, Claritin; diphenhydramine, Benadryl
antitussive (an-tih-TUSS-iv)	anti- = without tuss/o = cough	Relieves urge to cough	hydrocodon, Hycodan; dextromethorphan, Vicks Formula 44
bronchodilator (BRONG-koh-dye-lay-ter)	bronch/o = bronchus	Relaxes muscle spasms in bronchial tubes; used to treat asthma	albuterol, Proventil, Ventolin; salmeterol, Serevent
corticosteroids (kor-tih-koh-STAIR-oydz)	cortic/o = outer layer, cortex	Reduces inflammation and swelling in respiratory tract	fluticasone, Flonase; mometasone, Nasonex; triamcinolone, Azmacort
decongestant (dee-kon-JES-tant)	de- = without	Reduces stuffiness and congestion throughout respiratory system	oxymetazoline, Afrin, Dristan, Sinex; pseudoephedrine, Drixoral, Sudafed
expectorant (ek-SPEK-toh-rent)		Improves ability to cough up mucus from respiratory tract	guaifenesin, Robitussin, Mucinex
mucolytic (myoo-koh-LIT-ik)	muc/o = mucus -lytic = destruction	Liquefies mucus so it is easier to cough and clear from respiratory tract	N-acetyl-cysteine, Mucomyst

Abbreviations

ABGs	arterial blood gases	**MERS**	Middle East respiratory syndrome
ad lib	as desired	**O$_2$**	oxygen
ARDS	adult (or acute) respiratory distress syndrome	**PE**	pulmonary embolism
Bronch	bronchoscopy	**per**	with
CF	cystic fibrosis	**PFT**	pulmonary function test
CO$_2$	carbon dioxide	**po**	by mouth
COPD	chronic obstructive pulmonary disease	**PPD**	purified protein derivative
CPAP	continuous positive airway pressure	**prn**	as needed
CPR	cardiopulmonary resuscitation	**R**	respiration
C&S	culture and sensitivity	**RA**	room air
CTA	clear to auscultation	**RDS**	respiratory distress syndrome
CXR	chest X-ray	**RLL**	right lower lobe
d	day	**RML**	right middle lobe
DOE	dyspnea on exertion	**RRT**	registered respiratory therapist
DPT	diphtheria, pertussis, tetanus injection	**RUL**	right upper lobe
ENT	ear, nose, and throat	**RV**	reserve volume
ERV	expiratory reserve volume	**SARS**	severe acute respiratory syndrome
flu	influenza	**SIDS**	sudden infant death syndrome
FRC	functional residual capacity	**SOB**	shortness of breath
HMD	hyaline membrane disease	**TB**	tuberculosis
IC	inspiratory capacity	**TLC**	total lung capacity
IPPB	intermittent positive pressure breathing	**TPR**	temperature, pulse, and respiration
IRDS	infant respiratory distress syndrome	**TV**	tidal volume
IRV	inspiratory reserve volume	**URI**	upper respiratory infection
LLL	left lower lobe	**VC**	vital capacity
LUL	left upper lobe	**VS**	vital signs
MDI	metered-dose inhaler		

PRACTICE AS YOU GO

F. What's the Abbreviation?

1. upper respiratory infection   _____

2. pulmonary function test   _____

3. oxygen   _____

4. carbon dioxide   _____

5. chronic obstructive pulmonary disease   _____

6. bronchoscopy   _____

7. tuberculosis   _____

8. infant respiratory distress syndrome   _____

Chapter Review

Real-World Applications

Medical Record Analysis

This Pulmonology Consultation Report contains 12 medical terms. Underline each term and write it in the list below the report. Then explain each term as you would to a nonmedical person.

Pulmonology Consultation Report

Reason for Consultation:	Evaluation of increasingly severe asthma
History of Present Illness:	Patient is a 10-year-old male who first presented to the Emergency Room with dyspnea, coughing, and wheezing at seven years of age. Attacks are increasing in frequency, and there do not appear to be any precipitating factors such as exercise. No other family members are asthmatics.
Results of Physical Examination:	Patient is currently in the ER with marked dyspnea, cyanosis around the lips, prolonged expiration, and a hacking cough producing thick phlegm. Auscultation revealed rhonchi throughout lungs. ABGs indicate hypoxemia. Spirometry reveals moderately severe airway obstruction during expiration. This patient responded to Proventil and he is beginning to cough less and breathe with less effort.
Assessment:	Acute asthma attack with severe airway obstruction. There is no evidence of infection. In view of increasing severity and frequency of attacks, all his medications should be reevaluated for effectiveness and all attempts to identify precipitating factors should be made.
Recommendations:	Patient is to continue to use Proventil for relief of bronchospasms. Instructions for taking medications and controlling severity of asthma attacks were carefully reviewed with the patient and his family.

Term **Explanation**

1. _____
2. _____
3. _____
4. _____
5. _____
6. _____
7. _____
8. _____
9. _____
10. _____
11. _____
12. _____

Chart Note Transcription

The chart note below contains 11 phrases that can be reworded with a medical term presented in this chapter. Each phrase is identified with an underline. Determine the medical term and write your answers in the space provided.

Pearson General Hospital Emergency Room Record

Task   Edit   View   Time Scale   Options   Help Download   Archive   Date: 17 May 2017

Current Complaint: A 43-year-old female was brought to the Emergency Room by her family. She complained of painful and labored breathing, **1** rapid breathing, **2** and fever. Symptoms began three days ago, but have become much worse during the past 12 hours.

Past History: Patient is a mother of three and a business executive. She has had no surgeries or previous serious illnesses.

Signs and Symptoms: Temperature is 103°F, respiratory rate is 20 breaths/minute, blood pressure is 165/98, and heart rate is 90 bpm. A blood test to measure the levels of oxygen in the blood **3** indicates a marked low level of oxygen in the blood. **4** The process of listening to body sounds **5** of the lungs revealed abnormal crackling sounds **6** over the left lower chest. She is producing large amounts of pus-filled **7** mucus coughed up from the respiratory tract **8** and a chest X-ray **9** shows a large cloudy patch in the lower lobe of the left lung.

Diagnosis: Left lower lobe inflammatory condition of the lungs caused by bacterial infection **10**

Treatment: Patient was started on intravenous antibiotics. She also required a tube placed through the mouth to create an airway **11** for three days.

1. _____

2. _____

3. _____

4. _____

5. _____

6. _____

7. _____

8. _____

9. _____

10. _____

11. _____

Case Study

Below is a case study presentation of a patient with a condition discussed in this chapter. Read the case study and answer the questions below. Some questions will ask for information not included within this chapter. Use your text, a medical dictionary, or any other reference material you choose to answer these questions.

An 88-year-old female was seen in the physician's office complaining of dyspnea, dizziness, orthopnea, elevated temperature, and a cough. Lung auscultation revealed crackles over the right bronchus. CXR revealed fluid in the RUL. The patient was sent to the hospital with an admitting diagnosis of pneumonia. Vital signs upon admission were temperature 102°F, pulse 100 BPM and rapid, respirations 24 breaths/min and labored, blood pressure 180/110. She was treated with IV antibiotics and IPPB. She responded well to treatment and was released home to her family with oral antibiotics on the third day.

(Real444/E+/Getty Images)

Questions

1. What was this patient's admitting diagnosis? Look up this condition in a reference source and include a short description of it.

   _____

   _____

2. List and define each of the patient's presenting symptoms in your own words.

   _____

   _____

3. Define auscultation and CXR. Describe what each revealed in your own words.

   _____

   _____

4. What does the term *vital signs* mean? Describe this patient's vital signs.

   _____

   _____

5. Describe the treatments this patient received while in the hospital in your own words.

   _____

   _____

6. Explain the change in the patient's medication when she was discharged home.

   _____

   _____

Practice Exercises

A. Complete the Statement

1. The primary function of the respiratory system is _____.

2. The movement of air in and out of the lungs is called _____.

3. *External respiration* is defined as _____.

4. *Internal respiration* is defined as _____.

5. The muscle that divides the thoracic cavity from the abdominal cavity is the _____.

6. Total lung capacity means _____.

7. Tidal volume means _____.

8. Residual volume means _____.

9. The organs of the respiratory system are _____.

10. The four vital signs are _____, _____, _____, and _____.

B. Word Building Practice

The combining form **rhin/o** refers to the *nose*. Use it to write a term that means:

1. inflammation of the nose _____

2. discharge from the nose _____

3. surgical repair of the nose _____

The combining form **laryng/o** refers to the *larynx* or *voice box*. Use it to write a term that means:

4. inflammation of the larynx _____

5. spasm of the larynx _____

6. visual examination of the larynx _____

7. pertaining to the larynx _____

8. removal of the larynx _____

9. surgical repair of the larynx _____

10. paralysis of the larynx _____

The combining form **bronch/o** refers to the *bronchus*. Use it to write a term that means:

11. pertaining to bronchus _____

12. inflammation of the bronchus _____

13. visually examine the interior of the bronchus _____

14. produced by bronchus _____

15. spasm of the bronchus _____

The combining form **thorac/o** refers to the *chest*. Use it to write a term that means:

16. cutting into the chest _____

17. chest pain _____

18. pertaining to chest _____

The combining form **trache/o** refers to the *trachea*. Use it to write a term that means:

19. cutting into the trachea   _____

20. narrowing of the trachea   _____

21. pertaining to inside the trachea _____

The suffix **-pnea** means *breathing*. Use this suffix to write a medical term that means:

22. difficult or labored breathing   _____

23. rapid breathing   _____

24. can breathe only in an upright position _____

25. lack of breathing   _____

C. Complete the Term

For each definition given below, fill in the blank with the word part that completes the term.

Definition	Term
1. lack of sense of smell	an _____
2. breathing too slowly	brady _____
3. paralysis of the larynx	_____plegia
4. to cough up and spit out blood	hemo _____
5. abnormal flow of blood from the nose	rhino _____
6. abnormal voice	dys_____
7. commonly called a *sore throat*	_____itis
8. dilation of bronchi	_____ectasis
9. commonly called *black lung*	_____osis
10. air in the chest	_____thorax
11. instrument to measure oxygen	_____meter
12. process of visually examining the voice box	_____scopy
13. process to withdraw fluid from the pleura	pleuro_____
14. pertaining to heart and lung	_____ary
15. narrowing of the windpipe	_____stenosis

D. Name that Term

1. the process of breathing in   _____

2. spitting up of blood   _____

3. blood clot in the pulmonary artery   _____

4. inflammation of a sinus   _____

5. sore throat   _____

6. air in the pleural cavity   _____

7. whooping cough   _____

8. cutting into the pleura   _____

9. pain in the pleural region   _____

10. common cold   _____

E. Using Abbreviations

Fill in each blank with the appropriate abbreviation.

1. He went to see a(n) _____ for his recurring throat and sinus infections.

2. _____ is a chronic condition with reduced capacity for inhaling and exhaling.

3. It was discovered at birth that the child had _____, a malfunction of the exocrine glands.

4. _____ is also called HMD.

5. A(n) _____ obstructs a pulmonary artery.

6. _____ is the unexpected and unexplained death of a newborn.

7. A(n) _____ tests the amount of oxygen and carbon dioxide in the blood.

8. The area of pneumonia could be seen on the _____.

9. Due to her difficulty breathing, the doctor ordered a(n) _____, a group of diagnostic tests.

10. A(n) _____ machine is a common treatment for sleep apnea.

F. Fill in the Blank

anthracosis	sputum cytology	cardiopulmonary resuscitation	patent
thoracentesis	respirator	ventilation-perfusion scan	rhonchi
supplemental oxygen	hyperventilation		

1. When the patient's breathing and heart stopped, the paramedics began _____.

2. The physician performed a _____ to remove fluid from the chest.

3. A _____ is also called a ventilator.

4. The patient received _____ through a nasal cannula.

5. An endotracheal intubation was performed to establish a _____ airway.

6. A _____ is a particularly useful test to identify a pulmonary embolus.

7. The result of the _____ was negative for cancer.

8. _____ involves tachypnea and hyperpnea.

9. _____ are wheezing lung sounds.

10. Miners are at risk of developing _____.

G. Pharmacology Challenge

Fill in the classification for each drug description, then match the brand name.

Drug Description	Classification	Brand Name
1. _____ Reduces stuffiness and congestion	_____	a. Hycodan
2. _____ Relieves the urge to cough	_____	b. Flonase
3. _____ Kills bacteria	_____	c. Cipro
4. _____ Improves ability to cough up mucus	_____	d. Ventolin
5. _____ Liquefies mucus	_____	e. Allegra
6. _____ Relaxes bronchial muscle spasms	_____	f. Afrin
7. _____ Blocks allergy attack	_____	g. Robitussin
8. _____ Reduces inflammation and swelling	_____	h. Mucomyst

H. Anatomical Adjectives

Fill in the blank with the missing noun or adjective.

Noun	Adjective
1. air sacs	_____
2. _____	pulmonary
3. chest	_____
4. _____	bronchial
5. windpipe	_____
6. _____	epiglottic
7. mucus	_____
8. throat	_____
9. _____	bronchiolar
10. _____	septal

I. Spelling Practice

Some of the following terms are misspelled. Identify the incorrect terms and spell them correctly in the blank provided.

1. nasopharyngial   _____

2. asphyxia   _____

3. canula   _____

4. hemoptosis   _____

5. bronchodilater   _____

6. rhinorrhagia   _____

7. polysomnography   _____

8. bronchiectasis   _____

9. tuberculosis   _____

10. pneumoconosis   _____

MyLab Medical Terminology™

MyLab Medical Terminology is a premium online homework management system that includes a host of features to help you study. Registered users will find:

- A multitude of activities and assignments built within the MyLab platform

- Powerful tools that track and analyze your results—allowing you to create a personalized learning experience

- Videos and audio pronunciations to help enrich your progress

- Streaming lesson presentations (Guided Lectures) and self-paced learning modules

- A space where you and your instructors can check your progress and manage your assignments

Labeling Exercises

Image A

Write the labels for this figure on the numbered lines provided.

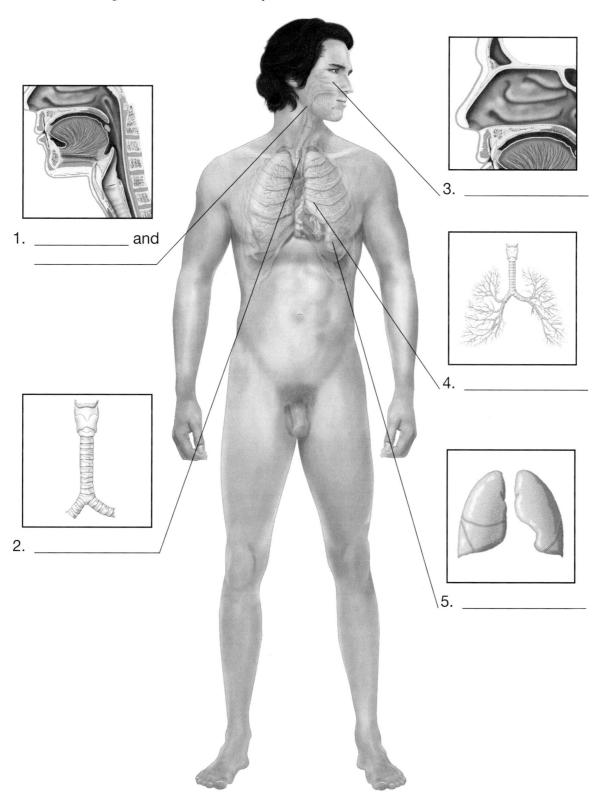

1. _____ and
   _____

2. _____

3. _____

4. _____

5. _____

Image B

Write the labels for this figure on the numbered lines provided.

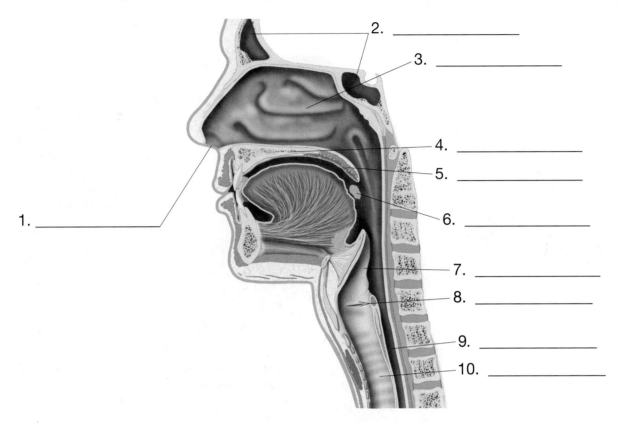

2. _____

3. _____

4. _____

5. _____

6. _____

1. _____

7. _____

8. _____

9. _____

10. _____

Image C

Write the labels for this figure on the numbered lines provided.

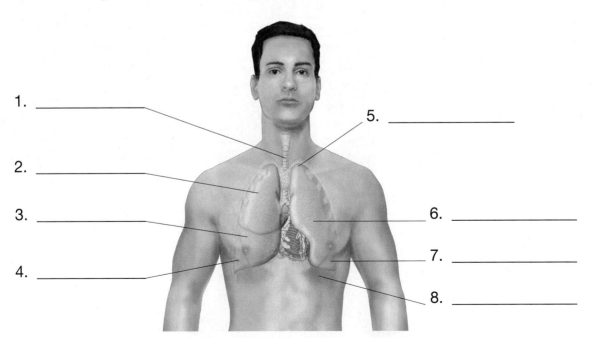

1. _____

2. _____

3. _____

4. _____

5. _____

6. _____

7. _____

8. _____

Chapter 8

Digestive System

Learning Objectives

Upon completion of this chapter, you will be able to

1. Identify and define the combining forms and suffixes introduced in this chapter.
2. Correctly spell and pronounce medical terms and major anatomical structures relating to the digestive system.
3. Locate and describe the major organs of the digestive system and their functions.
4. Identify the shape and function of each type of tooth.
5. Describe the function of the accessory organs of the digestive system.
6. Identify and define digestive system anatomical terms.
7. Identify and define selected digestive system pathology terms.
8. Identify and define selected digestive system diagnostic procedures.
9. Identify and define selected digestive system therapeutic procedures.
10. Identify and define selected medications relating to the digestive system.
11. Define selected abbreviations associated with the digestive system.

(Pearson Education, Inc.)

DIGESTIVE SYSTEM

AT A GLANCE

Function

The digestive system begins breaking down food through mechanical and chemical digestion. After being digested, nutrient molecules are absorbed into the body and enter the blood-stream; any food not digested or absorbed is eliminated as solid waste.

Organs

The primary structures that comprise the digestive system:

anus	oral cavity
esophagus	pancreas
gallbladder (GB)	pharynx
large intestine	salivary glands
liver	small intestine
mouth	stomach

Word Parts

Presented here are the most common word parts (with their meanings) used to build digestive system terms. For a more comprehensive list, refer to the Terminology section of this chapter.

Combining Forms

an/o	anus	gloss/o	tongue
append/o	appendix	hepat/o	liver
appendic/o	appendix	ile/o	ileum
bar/o	weight	jejun/o	jejunum
bucc/o	cheek	labi/o	lip
cec/o	cecum	lapar/o	abdomen
cholangi/o	bile duct	lingu/o	tongue
chol/e	bile, gall	lith/o	stone
cholecyst/o	gallbladder	odont/o	tooth
choledoch/o	common bile duct	or/o	mouth
cirrh/o	yellow	palat/o	palate
col/o	colon	pancreat/o	pancreas
colon/o	colon	pharyng/o	pharynx
dent/o	tooth	polyp/o	polyp
diverticul/o	pouch	proct/o	anus and rectum
duoden/o	duodenum	pylor/o	pylorus
enter/o	small intestine	pyr/o	fire
esophag/o	esophagus	rect/o	rectum
gastr/o	stomach	sialaden/o	salivary gland
gingiv/o	gums	sigmoid/o	sigmoid colon

(continued on page 270)

Digestive System Illustrated

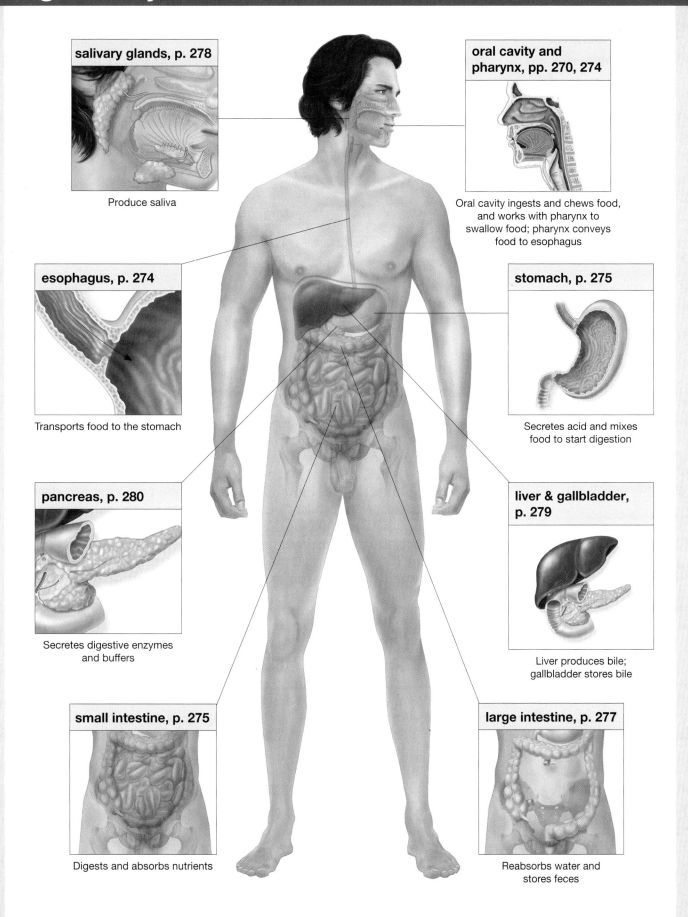

salivary glands, p. 278

Produce saliva

oral cavity and pharynx, pp. 270, 274

Oral cavity ingests and chews food, and works with pharynx to swallow food; pharynx conveys food to esophagus

esophagus, p. 274

Transports food to the stomach

stomach, p. 275

Secretes acid and mixes food to start digestion

pancreas, p. 280

Secretes digestive enzymes and buffers

liver & gallbladder, p. 279

Liver produces bile; gallbladder stores bile

small intestine, p. 275

Digests and absorbs nutrients

large intestine, p. 277

Reabsorbs water and stores feces

(continued from page 268)

Suffixes

-emesis	vomiting	-orexia	appetite
-emetic	pertaining to vomiting	-pepsia	digestion
-iatric	pertaining to medical treatment	-phagia	eat, swallow
-istry	specialty of	-prandial	pertaining to a meal
-lithiasis	condition of stones	-tripsy	surgical crushing

Anatomy and Physiology of the Digestive System

accessory organs
alimentary canal (al-ih-MEN-tah-ree)
anus (AY-nus)
esophagus (eh-SOFF-ah-gus)
gallbladder
gastrointestinal system (gas-troh-in-TESS-tih-nal)
gastrointestinal tract
gut

large intestine
liver
mouth
oral cavity
pancreas (PAN-kree-as)
pharynx (FAIR-inks)
salivary glands (SAL-ih-vair-ee)
small intestine
stomach (STUM-ak)

What's In A Name?
Look for these word parts:
-ary = pertaining to
-ory = pertaining to

Med Term Tip
The term *alimentary* comes from the Latin term *alimentum* meaning *nourishment*.

The digestive system, also known as the **gastrointestinal (GI) system**, includes approximately 30 feet of a continuous muscular tube called the **gut**, **alimentary canal**, or **gastrointestinal tract** that stretches between two external openings, the **mouth** and the **anus**. Most of the organs in this system are actually different sections of this tube. In order, beginning at the mouth and continuing to the anus, these organs are the **oral cavity**, **pharynx**, **esophagus**, **stomach**, **small intestine**, and **large intestine**. The **accessory organs** of digestion are those that participate in the digestion process, but are not part of the continuous alimentary canal. These organs, which are connected to the gut by ducts, are the **liver**, **pancreas**, **gallbladder**, and **salivary glands**.

The digestive system has three main functions: digesting food, absorbing nutrients, and eliminating waste. Digestion includes the physical and chemical breakdown of large food particles into simple nutrient molecules like glucose, triglycerides, and amino acids. These simple nutrient molecules are absorbed from the intestines and circulated throughout the body by the cardiovascular system. They are used for growth and repair of organs and tissues. Any food that cannot be digested or absorbed by the body is eliminated from the gastrointestinal system as solid waste.

Oral Cavity

cheeks
deglutition (dee-gloo-TISH-un)
gingiva (JIN-jih-vah)
gums
lips
mastication (mass-tih-KAY-shun)

palate (PAL-et)
saliva (suh-LYE-vah)
taste buds
teeth
tongue
uvula (YOO-vyoo-lah)

Digestion begins when food enters the mouth and is mechanically broken up by **mastication,** the chewing movements of the **teeth.** The muscular **tongue** moves the food within the mouth and mixes it with **saliva** (see Figure 8-1 ■). Saliva contains digestive enzymes to break down carbohydrates, and slippery lubricants to make food easier for **deglutition** (swallowing). **Taste buds,** found on the surface of the tongue, can distinguish the bitter, sweet, sour, salty, and umami (savory) flavors in food. The roof of the oral cavity is known as the **palate** and is subdivided into the hard palate (the bony anterior portion) and the soft palate (the flexible posterior portion). Hanging down from the posterior edge of the soft palate is the **uvula.** The uvula serves two important functions. First, it has a role in speech production and, second, it is the location of the gag reflex. This reflex is stimulated when food enters the throat without swallowing (e.g., laughing with food in the mouth). It is important because swallowing also results in the epiglottis covering the larynx to prevent food from entering the lungs (see Figure 8-2 ■). The **cheeks** form the lateral walls of this cavity and the **lips** are the anterior opening. The entire oral cavity is lined with mucous membrane, a portion of which forms the **gums,** or **gingiva,** that combine with connective tissue to cover the jawbone and seal off the teeth in their bony sockets.

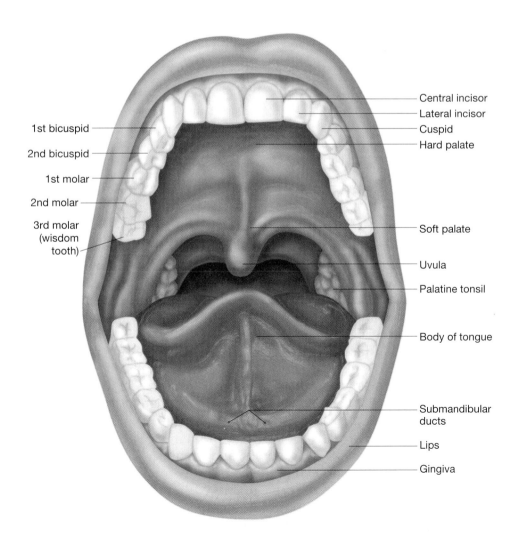

■ **Figure 8-1** Anatomy of structures of the oral cavity.

■ **Figure 8-2** Structures of the oral cavity, pharynx, and esophagus.

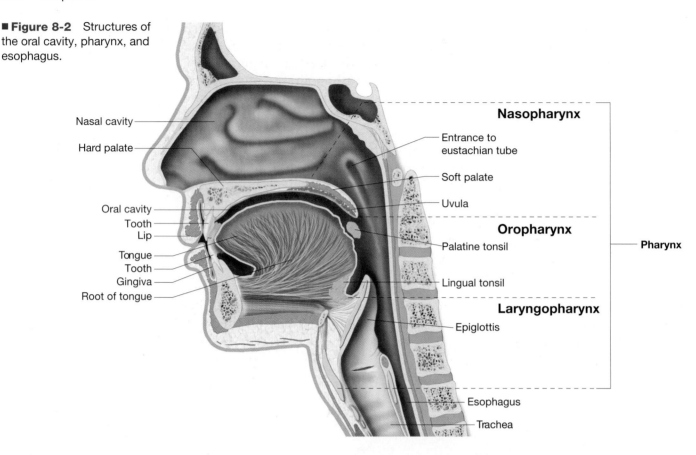

Teeth

bicuspids (bye-KUSS-pids)

canines (KAY-nines)

cementum (seh-MEN-tum)

crown

cuspids (KUSS-pids)

deciduous teeth (dih-SID-joo-us)

dentin (DEN-tin)

enamel

incisors (in-SIGH-zers)

molars (MOH-lars)

periodontal ligaments (pair-ee-oh-DON-tal)

permanent teeth

premolars (pree-MOH-lars)

pulp cavity

root

root canal

Teeth are an important part of the first stage of digestion. The teeth in the front of the mouth bite, tear, or cut food into small pieces. These cutting teeth include the **cuspids** (or **canines**) and the **incisors** (see Figure 8-3 ■). The remaining posterior teeth grind and crush food into even finer pieces. These grinding teeth include the **bicuspids** (or **premolars**) and the **molars**. A tooth can be subdivided into the **crown** and the **root**. The crown is that part of the tooth visible above the gum line; the root is below the gum line. The root is anchored in the bony socket of the jaw by **cementum** and tiny **periodontal ligaments**. The crown of the tooth is covered by a layer of **enamel**, the hardest substance in the body. Under the enamel layer is **dentin**, the substance that makes up the main bulk of the tooth. The hollow interior of a tooth is called the **pulp cavity** in the crown and the **root canal** in the root. These cavities contain soft tissue made up of blood vessels, nerves, and lymph vessels (see Figure 8-4 ■).

Humans have two sets of teeth. The first set, often referred to as *baby teeth*, are **deciduous teeth**. There are 20 teeth in this set that erupt through the gums between the ages of six and 28 months. At approximately six years of age, these teeth begin to fall out and are replaced by the 32 **permanent teeth**. This replacement process continues until about 18–20 years of age.

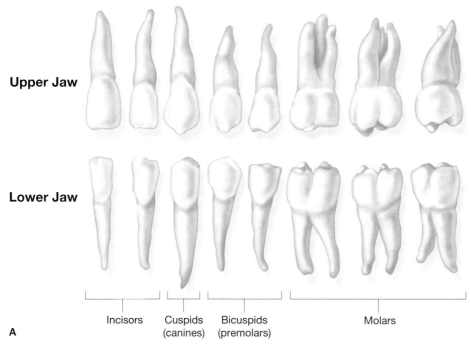

Upper Jaw

Lower Jaw

Incisors   Cuspids   Bicuspids   Molars
(canines) (premolars)

A

■ **Figure 8-3** A) The name and shape of the adult teeth. These teeth represent those found in the right side of the mouth. Those of the left side would be a mirror image. The incisors and cuspids are cutting teeth. The bicuspids and molars are grinding teeth. B) X-ray scan of all teeth. Note the four wisdom teeth (third molars) that have not erupted. *(Mkarco/Shutterstock)*

B

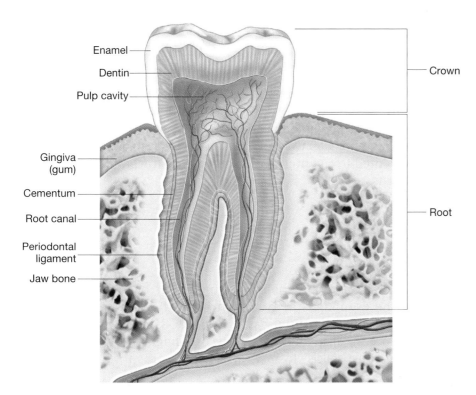

Enamel

Dentin

Pulp cavity

Crown

Gingiva
(gum)

Cementum

Root canal

Root

Periodontal
ligament

Jaw bone

■ **Figure 8-4** An adult tooth, longitudinal view showing internal structures of the crown and root.

PRACTICE AS YOU GO

A. Complete the Statement

1. The digestive system is also known as the _____ system.

2. The continuous muscular tube of the digestive system is called the _____, _____, or _____ and stretches between the _____ and _____.

3. The three main functions of the digestive system are _____, _____, and _____.

4. The cutting teeth are _____ and _____.

5. The grinding teeth are _____ and _____.

6. The _____ of a tooth is above the gum line and the _____ is below the gum line.

7. The hardest substance in the body is _____.

8. There are 20 _____ teeth and 32 _____ teeth.

Pharynx

epiglottis (ep-ih-GLOT-iss)
oropharynx

laryngopharynx (lah-ring-goh-FAIR-inks)

When food is swallowed, it enters the **oropharynx** and then the **laryngopharynx** (see again Figure 8-2). Recall from the discussion of the respiratory system in Chapter 7 that air is also traveling through these portions of the pharynx. The **epiglottis** is a cartilaginous flap that folds down to cover the larynx and trachea so that food is prevented from entering the respiratory tract and instead continues into the esophagus.

Esophagus

peristalsis (pair-ih-STALL-sis)

The esophagus is a muscular tube measuring about 10 inches long in adults. Food entering the esophagus is carried through the thoracic cavity and diaphragm and into the abdominal cavity, where it enters the stomach (see Figure 8-5 ■). Food is propelled along the esophagus by wavelike muscular contractions called **peristalsis**. In fact, peristalsis works to push food through the entire gastrointestinal tract.

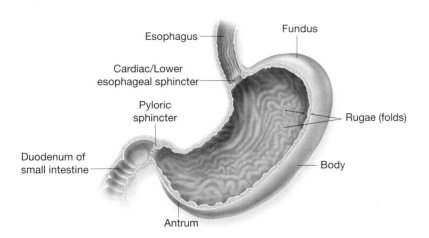

Stomach

antrum (AN-trum)	**hydrochloric acid**
body	**lower esophageal sphincter**
cardiac sphincter (KAR-dee-ak / SFINGK-ter)	(eh-soff-ah-JEE-al / SFINGK-ter)
chyme (KIME)	**pyloric sphincter** (pye-LOR-ik / SFINGK-ter)
fundus (FUN-dus)	**rugae** (ROO-jee)
gastroesophageal sphincter	**sphincters** (SFINGK-ters)
(gas-troh-eh-soff-ah-JEE-al / SFINGK-ter)	

The stomach, a J-shaped muscular organ that acts as a bag or sac to collect and churn food with digestive juices, is composed of three parts: the **fundus** or upper region, the **body** or main portion, and the **antrum** or lower region (see again Figure 8-5). The folds in the lining of the stomach are called **rugae**. When the stomach fills with food, the rugae stretch out and disappear. **Hydro-chloric acid** (HCl) is secreted by glands in the mucous membrane lining of the stomach. Food mixes with hydrochloric acid and other gastric juices to form a liquid mixture called **chyme**, which then passes through the remaining portion of the digestive system.

Entry into and exit from the stomach is controlled by muscular valves called **sphincters**. These valves open and close to ensure that food can only move forward down the gut tube. The **cardiac sphincter**, named for its proximity to the heart, is located between the esophagus and the fundus; also called the **lower esophageal sphincter** (LES) or **gastroesophageal sphincter**, it keeps food from flowing backward into the esophagus. During the processes of regurgitation and vomiting (they are not quite the same), the brain causes both of these sphincters to relax, thereby allowing stomach contents to flow backward.

The antrum tapers off into the **pyloric sphincter**, which regulates the passage of food into the small intestine. Only a small amount of the chyme is allowed to enter the small intestine with each opening of the sphincter for two important reasons. First, the small intestine is much narrower than the stomach and cannot hold as much as can the stomach. Second, the chyme is highly acidic and must be thoroughly neutralized as it leaves the stomach.

> **What's In A Name?**
> Look for these word parts:
> **cardi/o** = heart
> **hydr/o** = water
> **-ac** = pertaining to
> **-ic** = pertaining to

> **Med Term Tip**
> It is easier to remember the function of the pyloric sphincter when you note that **pylor/o** means *gatekeeper*. This gatekeeper controls the forward movement of food. Sphincters are rings of muscle that can be opened and closed to control entry and exit from hollow organs like the stomach, colon, and bladder.

Small Intestine

duodenum (doo-oh-DEE-num/doo-OD-eh-num)	**jejunum** (jeh-JOO-num)
ileocecal valve (il-ee-oh-SEE-kal)	**microvilli** (my-kroh-VILL-eye)
ileum (IL-ee-um)	**villi** (VILL-eye)

■ **Figure 8-6** The small intestine. Anterior view of the abdominopelvic cavity illustrating how the three sections of small intestine—duodenum, jejunum, ileum—begin at the pyloric sphincter and end at the colon, but are not arranged in an orderly fashion.

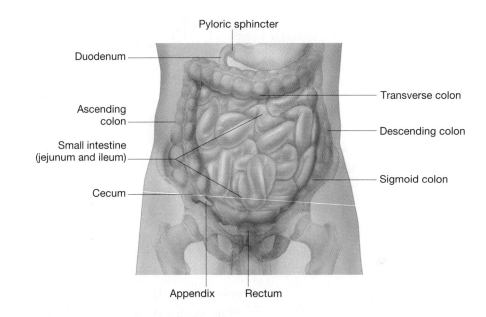

Word Watch

Be careful not to confuse the word root **ile/o** meaning *ileum*, a portion of the small intestine, and **ili/o** meaning *ilium*, a pelvic bone.

The small intestine, or small bowel, is the major site of digestion and absorption of nutrients from food. It is located between the pyloric sphincter and the colon (see Figure 8-6 ■). The small intestine is very efficient at absorbing nutrients due to its structure. First, the lining is highly folded into finger-like projections called **villi** (see Figure 8-7 ■). Then each surface cell of a villus is covered in more projections called **microvilli**. Together, these projections give the small intestine a surface area roughly the size of a tennis court! Because the small intestine is concerned with absorption of food products, an abnormality in this organ may result in malnutrition. The small intestine, with an average length of 20 feet, is the longest portion of the alimentary canal and has three sections: the **duodenum**, the **jejunum**, and the **ileum**.

- The duodenum extends from the pyloric sphincter to the jejunum, and is about 10–12 inches long. Digestion is completed in the duodenum after the liquid chyme from the stomach is mixed with digestive juices from the pancreas and gallbladder.

- The jejunum, or middle portion, extends from the duodenum to the ileum and is about eight feet long.

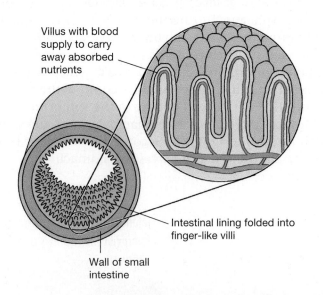

■ **Figure 8-7** Section of small intestine wall illustrating arrangement of villi.

(Mohammed Ali. Pearson India Education Services Pvt. Ltd)

- The ileum is the last portion of the small intestine and extends from the jejunum to the colon. At 12 feet in length, it is the longest portion of the small intestine. The ileum connects to the colon with a sphincter called the **ileocecal valve**.

Large Intestine

anal canal (AY-nal)

anal sphincter (AY-nal / SFINGK-ter)

ascending colon

cecum (SEE-kum)

colon (KOH-lon)

defecation

descending colon

feces (FEE-seez)

rectum (REK-tum)

sigmoid colon (SIG-moyd)

transverse colon

vermiform appendix (VER-mih-form / ah-PEN-diks)

Fluid that remains after the complete digestion and absorption of nutrients in the small intestine enters the large intestine (see Figure 8-8 ■). Most of this fluid is water that is reabsorbed into the body. The material that remains after absorption is solid waste called **feces** (or stool). This is the product evacuated in a bowel movement (BM).

The large intestine is approximately 5 feet long and extends from the ileocecal valve to the anus; this includes the **cecum**, **colon**, **rectum**, and **anal canal**. The cecum is a pouch or saclike area in the first 2–3 inches at the beginning of the colon. The **vermiform appendix** is a small worm-shaped outgrowth at the end of the cecum. The colon consists of the **ascending colon**, **transverse colon**, **descending colon**, and **sigmoid colon**. The ascending colon on the right side extends from the cecum to the lower border of the liver. The transverse colon moves horizontally across the upper abdomen toward the spleen. The descending colon then travels down the left side of the body to where the sigmoid colon begins. The sigmoid colon curves in an S-shape back to the midline of the body and ends at the rectum. The rectum, where feces are stored, leads into the anal canal, which contains the **anal sphincter**. This sphincter consists of rings of voluntary and involuntary muscles to control the evacuation of feces or **defecation**.

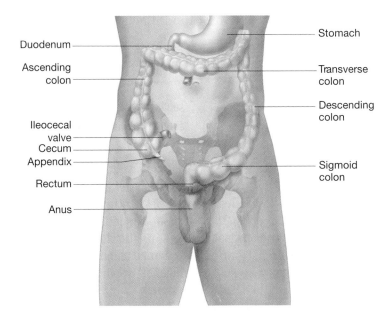

■ Figure 8-8 The regions of the colon beginning with the cecum and ending at the anus.

PRACTICE AS YOU GO

B. Complete the Statement

1. When food is swallowed, it enters the _____.

2. Food is propelled through the gut by wavelike muscular contractions called
   _____.

3. Food in the stomach is mixed with _____ and other gastric juices to form a
   watery mixture called _____.

4. The three sections of small intestine, in order, are the _____,
   _____, and _____.

5. Structures called _____ greatly increase the surface area of the small
   intestine.

6. The large intestine extends from the _____ to the _____, and
   includes the _____, _____, and _____.

7. The S-shaped section of colon that curves back toward the rectum is called the
   _____ colon.

8. The evacuation of feces is called _____.

Med Term Tip

In anatomy, the term *accessory* generally means that the structure is auxiliary to a more important structure. This is not true for these organs. Digestion would not be possible without the digestive juices produced by these organs.

Accessory Organs of the Digestive System

As described earlier, the accessory organs of the digestive system are the salivary glands, the liver, the pancreas, and the gallbladder. In general, these organs function by producing much of the digestive fluids and enzymes necessary for the chemical breakdown of food. Each is attached to the gut tube by a duct.

Salivary Glands

amylase (AM-il-ace)   sublingual glands (sub-LING-gwal)
bolus   submandibular glands (sub-man-DIB-yoo-lar)
parotid glands (pah-ROT-id)

Salivary glands in the oral cavity produce saliva. This very watery and slick fluid allows food to be swallowed with less danger of choking. Saliva mixed with food in the mouth forms a **bolus**, chewed food that is ready to swallow. Saliva also contains the digestive enzyme **amylase** that begins the digestion of carbohydrates. There are three pairs of salivary glands. The **parotid glands** are in front of the ears, and the **submandibular glands** and **sublingual glands** are in the floor of the mouth (see Figure 8-9 ■).

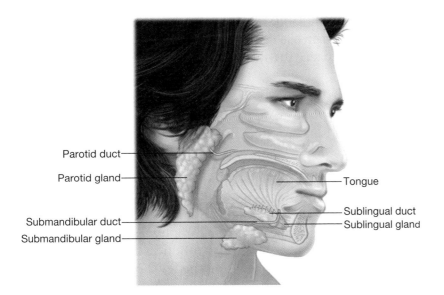

Parotid duct
Parotid gland
Submandibular duct
Submandibular gland
Tongue
Sublingual duct
Sublingual gland

■ **Figure 8-9** The salivary glands: parotid, sublingual, and submandibular. This image shows the position of each gland and its duct emptying into the oral cavity.

Liver

bile (BYE-al)   **emulsification** (ee-mull-sih-fih-KAY-shun)

The liver, a large organ located in the right upper quadrant of the abdomen, has several functions including processing the nutrients absorbed by the intestines, detoxifying harmful substances in the body, and producing **bile** (see Figure 8-10 ■). Bile is important for the digestion of fats and lipids because it breaks up large fat globules into much smaller droplets, making them easier to digest in the watery environment inside the intestines. This process is called **emulsification**.

Gallbladder

common bile duct   **cystic duct** (SIS-tik)
hepatic duct (heh-PAT-ik)

Bile produced by the liver is stored in the gallbladder (GB). As the liver produces bile, it travels down the **hepatic duct** and up the **cystic duct** into the gallbladder (see again Figure 8-10). In response to the presence of fat in the chyme, the

> **Med Term Tip**
>
> The liver weighs about four pounds and has so many important functions that people cannot live without it. It has become a major transplant organ. The liver is also able to regenerate itself. You can lose more than half of your liver, and it will regrow.

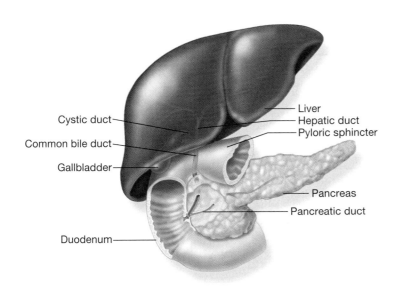

Cystic duct
Common bile duct
Gallbladder
Duodenum
Liver
Hepatic duct
Pyloric sphincter
Pancreas
Pancreatic duct

■ **Figure 8-10** The liver, gallbladder, and pancreas. Image shows the relationship of these three organs and their ducts to the duodenum.

Combining Forms (continued)

duoden/o	duodenum		**jejun/o**	jejunum		**pancreat/o**	pancreas
enter/o	small intestine		**labi/o**	lip		**pharyng/o**	pharynx
esophag/o	esophagus		**lapar/o**	abdomen		**polyp/o**	polyp
gastr/o	stomach		**lingu/o**	tongue		**proct/o**	anus and rectum
gingiv/o	gums		**lith/o**	stone		**pylor/o**	pylorus
gloss/o	tongue		**mandibul/o**	mandible		**pyr/o**	fire
hem/o	blood		**nas/o**	nose		**rect/o**	rectum
hemat/o	blood		**odont/o**	tooth		**sialaden/o**	salivary gland
hepat/o	liver		**or/o**	mouth		**sigmoid/o**	sigmoid colon
ile/o	ileum		**orth/o**	straight		**ven/o**	vein
inguin/o	groin		**palat/o**	palate			

Suffixes

-ac	pertaining to		**-ic**	pertaining to		**-pexy**	surgical fixation
-al	pertaining to		**-istry**	specialty of		**-phagia**	eat, swallow
-algia	pain		**-itis**	inflammation		**-plasty**	surgical repair
-ar	pertaining to		**-lithiasis**	condition of stones		**-plegia**	paralysis
-centesis	process of removing fluid		**-logy**	study of		**-prandial**	pertaining to a meal
			-oma	tumor			
-eal	pertaining to		**-orexia**	appetite		**-ptosis**	drooping
-ectomy	surgical removal		**-osis**	abnormal condition		**-scope**	instrument to view
-emesis	vomiting		**-ostomy**	surgically create an opening		**-scopic**	pertaining to visually examining
-emetic	pertaining to vomiting						
-gram	record		**-otomy**	cutting into		**-scopy**	process of viewing
-graphy	process of recording		**-ous**	pertaining to		**-tripsy**	surgical crushing
-iatric	pertaining to medical treatment		**-pepsia**	digestion			

Prefixes

a-	without		**hyper-**	excessive		**post-**	after
an-	without		**hypo-**	below		**re-**	again
anti-	against		**in-**	inward		**retro-**	backward
brady-	slow		**intra-**	within		**sub-**	under
dys-	abnormal, painful, difficult		**per-**	through		**trans-**	across
			peri-	around			
endo-	within		**poly-**	many			
ex-	outward						

Adjective Forms of Anatomical Terms

Term	Word Parts	Definition
anal	an/o = anus -al = pertaining to	Pertaining to anus
	Word Watch Be careful when using the combining form **an/o** meaning *anus* and the prefix **an-** meaning *without*.	
buccal (BUK-al)	bucc/o = cheek -al = pertaining to	Pertaining to cheeks
buccolabial (buk-oh-LAY-bee-al)	bucc/o = cheek labi/o = lip -al = pertaining to	Pertaining to cheeks and lips
cecal (SEE-kal)	cec/o = cecum -al = pertaining to	Pertaining to cecum
cholecystic (koh-lee-SIS-tik)	cholecyst/o = gallbladder -ic = pertaining to	Pertaining to gallbladder
colonic (koh-LON-ik)	colon/o = colon -ic = pertaining to	Pertaining to colon
colorectal (kohl-oh-REK-tal)	col/o = colon rect/o = rectum -al = pertaining to	Pertaining to colon and rectum
cystic (SIS-tik)	cyst/o = sac -ic = pertaining to	Pertaining to gallbladder
	Med Term Tip The combining form **cyst/o** refers to the sac-like shape of the gallbladder.	
dental (DEN-tal)	dent/o = tooth -al = pertaining to	Pertaining to teeth
duodenal (doo-oh-DEE-nal / doo-OD-eh-nal)	duoden/o = duodenum -al = pertaining to	Pertaining to duodenum
enteric (en-TAIR-ik)	enter/o = small intestine -ic = pertaining to	Pertaining to small intestine
esophageal (eh-soff-ah-JEE-al)	esophag/o = esophagus -eal = pertaining to	Pertaining to esophagus
gastric (GAS-trik)	gastr/o = stomach -ic = pertaining to	Pertaining to stomach
gastrointestinal (GI) (gas-troh-in-TESS-tih-nal)	gastr/o = stomach -al = pertaining to	Pertaining to stomach and intestines
gingival (JIN-jih-vul)	gingiv/o = gums -al = pertaining to	Pertaining to gums
glossal (GLOSS-al)	gloss/o = tongue -al = pertaining to	Pertaining to tongue
hepatic (heh-PAT-ik)	hepat/o = liver -ic = pertaining to	Pertaining to liver
hypoglossal (high-poh-GLOSS-al)	hypo- = under gloss/o = tongue -al = pertaining to	Pertaining to under tongue
ileal (IL-ee-al)	ile/o = ileum -al = pertaining to	Pertaining to ileum
ileocecal (il-ee-oh-SEE-kal)	ile/o = ileum cec/o = cecum -al = pertaining to	Pertaining to ileum and cecum

Adjective Forms of Anatomical Terms (continued)

Term	Word Parts	Definition
jejunal (jeh-JOO-nal)	jejun/o = jejunum -al = pertaining to	Pertaining to jejunum
labial (LAY-bee-al)	labi/o = lips -al = pertaining to	Pertaining to lips
lingual (LING-gwal)	lingu/o = tongue -al = pertaining to	Pertaining to tongue
nasogastric (nay-zoh-GAS-trik)	nas/o = nose gastr/o = stomach -ic = pertaining to	Pertaining to nose and stomach
oral (OR-al)	or/o = mouth -al = pertaining to	Pertaining to mouth
pancreatic (pan-kree-AT-ik)	pancreat/o = pancreas -ic = pertaining to	Pertaining to pancreas
periodontal (pair-ee-oh-DON-tal)	peri- = around odont/o = tooth -al = pertaining to	Pertaining to around teeth
pharyngeal (fair-IN-jee-al)	pharyng/o = pharynx -eal = pertaining to	Pertaining to pharynx
pyloric (pye-LOR-ik)	pylor/o = pylorus -ic = pertaining to	Pertaining to pylorus
rectal (REK-tal)	rect/o = rectum -al = pertaining to	Pertaining to rectum
sigmoidal (sig-MOYD-al)	sigmoid/o = sigmoid colon -al = pertaining to	Pertaining to sigmoid colon
sublingual (sub-LING-gwal)	sub- = under lingu/o = tongue -al = pertaining to	Pertaining to under tongue
submandibular (sub-man-DIB-yoo-lar)	sub- = under mandibul/o = mandible -ar = pertaining to	Pertaining to under mandible

PRACTICE AS YOU GO

D. Give the adjective form for each anatomical structure.

1. The duodenum _____
2. Nose and stomach _____
3. The liver _____
4. The pancreas _____
5. The gallbladder _____
   or _____
6. Under the tongue _____
7. The esophagus _____
8. The sigmoid colon _____

Pathology

Term	Word Parts	Definition
Medical Specialties		
dentistry	dent/o = tooth -istry = specialty of	Branch of healthcare involved with prevention, diagnosis, and treatment of conditions involving teeth, jaw, and mouth; practitioner is a *dentist*
gastroenterology (gas-troh-en-ter-ALL-oh-jee)	gastr/o = stomach enter/o = small intestine -logy = study of	Branch of medicine involved in diagnosis and treatment of diseases and disorders of digestive system; physician is a *gastroenterologist*
oral surgery	or/o = mouth -al = pertaining to	Branch of dentistry that uses surgical means to treat dental conditions; specialist is an *oral surgeon*
orthodontics (or-thoh-DON-tiks)	orth/o = straight odont/o = tooth -ic = pertaining to	Branch of dentistry concerned with correction of problems with tooth alignment; specialist is an *orthodontist*
periodontics (pair-ee-oh-DON-tiks)	peri- = around odont/o = tooth -ic = pertaining to	Branch of dentistry concerned with treating conditions involving gums and tissues surrounding the teeth; specialist is a *periodontist*
proctology (prok-TALL-oh-jee)	proct/o = anus and rectum -logy = study of	Branch of medicine involved in diagnosis and treatment of diseases and disorders of anus and rectum; physician is a *proctologist*
Signs and Symptoms		
anorexia (an-oh-REK-see-ah)	an- = without -orexia = appetite	General term meaning loss of appetite that may accompany other conditions; also used to refer to *anorexia nervosa*, which is characterized by severe weight loss from excessive dieting
aphagia (ah-FAY-jee-ah)	a- = without -phagia = eat, swallow	Being unable to swallow or eat
ascites (ah-SIGH-teez)		Collection or accumulation of fluid in the peritoneal cavity
bradypepsia (brad-ee-PEP-see-ah)	brady- = slow -pepsia = digestion	Having a slow digestive system
cachexia (kuh-KEK-see-ah)		Loss of weight and generalized wasting that occurs during a chronic disease
cholecystalgia (koh-lee-sis-TAL-jee-ah)	cholecyst/o = gallbladder -algia = pain	Having gallbladder pain
constipation (kon-stih-PAY-shun)		Experiencing difficulty in defecation or infrequent defecation
dentalgia (den-TAL-jee-ah)	dent/o = tooth -algia = pain	Tooth pain
diarrhea (dye-ah-REE-ah)		Passing of frequent, watery, or bloody bowel movements; usually accompanies gastrointestinal (GI) disorders
dysorexia (dis-oh-REK-see-ah)	dys- = abnormal -orexia = appetite	Abnormal appetite; usually a diminished appetite

Pathology (continued)

Term	Word Parts	Definition
dyspepsia (dis-PEP-see-ah)	dys- = painful -pepsia = digestion	Indigestion; commonly called an *upset stomach*
dysphagia (dis-FAY-jee-ah)	dys- = difficult -phagia = eat, swallow	Having difficulty swallowing or eating
emesis (EM-eh-sis)	*Emesis* is the Latin term meaning *to vomit*	Vomiting; the expulsion of stomach contents through the mouth
eructation (ee-ruk-TAY-shun)		Burping of gas or stomach acid into the mouth; belching
flatulence (FLAT-choo-lents)	**Med Term Tip** The term *flatulence* comes from the Latin word *flatus*, meaning *to blow.*	Presence of excess gas in stomach or intestines; may be passed through the anus
gastralgia (gas-TRAL-jee-ah)	gastr/o = stomach -algia = pain	Stomach pain
hematemesis (hee-mah-TEM-eh-sis)	hemat/o = blood -emesis = vomiting	Vomiting blood
hematochezia (hee-mat-oh-KEE-zee-ah)	hemat/o = blood	Passing bright red blood in the stool
hyperemesis (high-per-EM-eh-sis)	hyper- = excessive -emesis = vomiting	Excessive vomiting
jaundice (JAWN-dis)		Yellow cast to the skin, mucous membranes, and whites of the eyes caused by deposit of bile pigment from too much bilirubin in the blood; bilirubin is a waste product produced when worn-out red blood cells are broken down; may be symptom of a disorder such as gallstones blocking the common bile duct or carcinoma of the liver; also called *icterus*
melena (meh-LEE-nah)		Passage of dark tarry stool; color is result of digestive enzymes working on blood in the gastrointestinal tract
nausea (NAW-zee-ah)	**Med Term Tip** The term *nausea* comes from the Greek word for *seasickness.*	Urge to vomit
obesity		Having too much body fat leading to a body weight that is above a healthy level; person whose weight interferes with normal activity and body function has *morbid obesity*
polyphagia (pol-ee-FAY-jee-ah)	poly- = many -phagia = eat, swallow	Excessive eating; eating too much
postprandial (pp) (post-PRAN-dee-al)	post- = after -prandial = pertaining to a meal	After a meal

Pathology (continued)

Term	Word Parts	Definition
pyrosis (pye-ROH-sis)	pyr/o = fire -osis = abnormal condition	Pain and burning sensation usually caused by stomach acid splashing up into the esophagus; commonly called *heartburn*
regurgitation (ree-ger-jih-TAY-shun)	re- = again	Return of fluids and solids from the stomach into the mouth
Oral Cavity		
aphthous ulcers (AF-thus)		Painful ulcers in the mouth of unknown cause; commonly called *canker sores*
cleft lip (KLEFT)		Congenital anomaly in which upper lip and jawbone fail to fuse in the midline, leaving an open gap; often seen along with cleft palate; corrected with surgery
cleft palate (KLEFT / PAL-et)		Congenital anomaly in which roof of the mouth has a split or fissure; corrected with surgery
dental caries (KAIR-eez)	dent/o = tooth -al = pertaining to	Gradual decay and disintegration of teeth caused by bacteria; may lead to abscessed teeth; commonly called a *tooth cavity*
gingivitis (jin-jih-VIGH-tis)	gingiv/o = gums -itis = inflammation	Inflammation of the gums
herpes labialis (HER-peez / lay-bee-AL-iss)	labi/o = lip	Infection of the lip by herpes simplex virus type 1 (HSV-1); also called *fever blisters* or *cold sores*
periodontal disease (pair-ee-oh-DON-tal)	peri- = around odont/o = tooth -al = pertaining to	Disease of supporting structures of the teeth, including gums and bones; most common cause of tooth loss
sialadenitis (sigh-al-ad-eh-NIGH-tis)	sialaden/o = salivary gland -itis = inflammation	Inflammation of a salivary gland
Pharynx and Esophagus		
esophageal varices (eh-soff-ah-JEE-al / VAIR-ih-seez)	esophag/o = esophagus -eal = pertaining to	Enlarged and swollen varicose veins in lower end of the esophagus; if these rupture, serious hemorrhage results; often related to liver disease
gastroesophageal reflux disease (GERD) (gas-troh-eh-soff-ah-JEE-al / REE-fluks)	gastr/o = stomach esophag/o = esophagus -eal = pertaining to	Acid from the stomach flows backward up into the esophagus, causing inflammation and pain
pharyngoplegia (fah-ring-oh-PLEE-jee-ah)	pharyng/o = pharynx -plegia = paralysis	Paralysis of throat muscles
Stomach		
gastric carcinoma (GAS-trik / kar-sih-NOH-mah)	gastr/o = stomach -ic = pertaining to	Cancerous tumor in the stomach
gastritis (gas-TRYE-tis)	gastr/o = stomach -itis = inflammation	Stomach inflammation
gastroenteritis (gas-troh-en-ter-EYE-tis)	gastr/o = stomach enter/o = small intestine -itis = inflammation	Inflammation of stomach and small intestine

Term	Word Parts	Definition
hiatal hernia (high-AY-tal / HER-nee-ah)	-al = pertaining to	Protrusion of the stomach through the diaphragm (also called a *diaphragmatocele*) and extending into the thoracic cavity; gastroesophageal reflux disease is a common symptom

■ **Figure 8-11** A hiatal hernia or diaphragmatocele. A portion of the stomach protrudes through the diaphragm into the thoracic cavity.

Term	Word Parts	Definition
peptic ulcer disease (PUD) (PEP-tik / UL-ser)	-ic = pertaining to	Ulcer occurring in lower portion of esophagus, stomach, and/or duodenum; thought to be caused by acid of gastric juices; initial damage to protective lining of the stomach may be caused by *Helicobacter pylori* (*H. pylori*) bacterial infection; if ulcer extends all the way through the wall of the stomach, it is called a *perforated ulcer*, which requires immediate surgery to repair

A B

■ **Figure 8-12** A) Figure illustrating the location and appearance of a peptic ulcer in both the stomach and the duodenum. B) Photomicrograph illustrating a gastric ulcer. *(Dr. E. Walker/Science Source)*

Pathology (continued)

Term	Word Parts	Definition
Small Intestine and Large Intestine		
anal fistula (FIS-tyoo-lah)	an/o = anus -al = pertaining to	Abnormal tube-like passage from surface around anal opening directly into the rectum
appendicitis (ah-pen-dih-SIGH-tis)	appendic/o = appendix -itis = inflammation	Inflammation of the appendix; may require an *appendectomy*
bowel incontinence (in-KON-tih-nens)		Inability to control defecation
celiac disease (SEE-lee-ak)	-ac = pertaining to	Autoimmune condition affecting the small intestine; caused by reaction to eating gluten (protein found in wheat, rye, and barley); symptoms may include abdominal bloating and pain, diarrhea, and nutritional deficiencies
colorectal carcinoma (kohl-oh-REK-tal / kar-sih-NOH-mah)	col/o = colon rect/o = rectum -al = pertaining to carcin/o = cancer -oma = tumor	Cancerous tumor originating in colon or rectum
Crohn's disease (KROHNZ)		Form of chronic inflammatory bowel disease affecting primarily ileum and/or colon; also called *regional ileitis*; auto-immune condition affects all layers of bowel wall and results in scarring and thickening of the gut wall
diverticulitis (dye-ver-tik-yoo-LYE-tis)	diverticul/o = pouch -itis = inflammation	Inflammation of a *diverticulum* (out-pouching off the gut), especially in the colon; inflammation often results when food becomes trapped within the pouch

■ **Figure 8-13** Diverticulosis. Figure illustrates external and internal appearance of diverticula.

Term	Word Parts	Definition
diverticulosis (dye-ver-tik-yoo-LOH-sis)	diverticul/o = pouch -osis = abnormal condition	Condition of having diverticula (out-pouches off the gut); may lead to *diverticulitis* if one becomes inflamed
dysentery (DIS-en-tair-ee)		Disease characterized by diarrhea, often with mucus and blood, severe abdominal pain, fever, and dehydration; caused by ingesting food or water contaminated by chemicals, bacteria, protozoans, or parasites
enteritis (en-ter-EYE-tis)	enter/o = small intestine -itis = inflammation	Inflammation of the small intestine

Pathology (continued)

Term	Word Parts	Definition
hemorrhoids (HEM-oh-roydz)	hem/o = blood	Varicose veins in rectum and anus
ileus (IL-ee-us)		Severe abdominal pain, inability to pass stool, vomiting, and abdominal distension as a result of intestinal blockage; blockage can be a physical block such as a tumor or failure of bowel contents to move forward due to loss of peristalsis (nonmechanical blockage); may require surgery to reverse blockage
inguinal hernia (ING-gwih-nal / HER-nee-ah)	inguin/o = groin -al = pertaining to	Hernia or protrusion of a loop of small intestine into inguinal (groin) region through a weak spot in abdominal muscle wall that develops into a hole; may become *incarcerated* or *strangulated* if muscle tightens down around loop of intestine and cuts off its blood flow

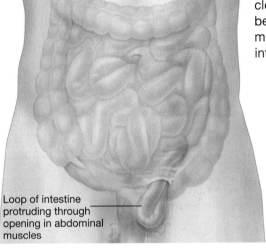

Loop of intestine protruding through opening in abdominal muscles

■ **Figure 8-14** An inguinal hernia. A portion of the small intestine is protruding through the abdominal muscles into the groin region.

Term	Word Parts	Definition
intussusception (in-tuh-suh-SEP-shun)	in- = inward	Result of the intestine slipping or telescoping into another section of intestine just below it; more common in children

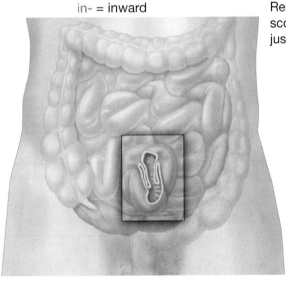

■ **Figure 8-15** Intussusception. A short length of small intestine has telescoped into itself.

Term	Word Parts	Definition
irritable bowel syndrome (IBS)		Disturbance in functions of the intestine from unknown causes; symptoms generally include abdominal discomfort and alteration in bowel activity; also called *spastic colon* or *functional bowel disorder*

Pathology (continued)

Term	Word Parts	Definition
polyposis (pol-ee-POH-sis)	polyp/o = polyp -osis = abnormal condition	Presence of small tumors, called **polyps**, containing a pedicle or stemlike attachment in mucous membranes of the large intestine (colon); may be precancerous

■ **Figure 8-16** Endoscopic view of a polyp in the colon. Note the mushroom-like shape, an enlarged top growing at the end of a stem. It is being removed by means of a wire loop slipped over the polyp and then tightened to cut it off. *(David M. Martin, M.D./Science Source)*

Term	Word Parts	Definition
proctoptosis (prok-top-TOH-sis)	proct/o = rectum and anus -ptosis = drooping	Prolapsed or drooping rectum and anus
ulcerative colitis (UL-ser-ah-tiv / koh-LYE-tis)	col/o = colon -itis = inflammation	Chronic inflammatory condition resulting in numerous ulcers formed on mucous membrane lining of the colon; cause is unknown; also known as *inflammatory bowel disease* (IBD)
volvulus (VOL-vyoo-lus)		Condition in which the bowel twists upon itself, causing an obstruction; painful and requires immediate surgery

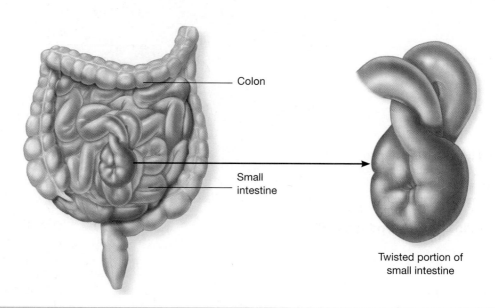

Colon

Small intestine

Twisted portion of small intestine

■ **Figure 8-17** Volvulus. A length of small intestine has twisted around itself, cutting off blood circulation to the twisted loop.

Pathology (continued)

Term	Word Parts	Definition
Accessory Organs		
cholecystitis (koh-lee-sis-TYE-tis)	cholecyst/o = gallbladder -itis = inflammation	Inflammation of the gallbladder; most commonly caused by gallstones in gallbladder or common bile duct that block flow of bile
cholelithiasis (koh-lee-lih-THIGH-ah-sis)	chol/e = bile -lithiasis = condition of stones	Presence of gallstones; may or may not cause symptoms such as *cholecystalgia*

■ **Figure 8-18**   A) Common sites for cholelithiasis. B) A gallbladder specimen with multiple gallstones., *(Clinical Photography, Central Manchester University Hospitals NHS Foundation Trust, UK/Science Source)*

Term	Word Parts	Definition
cirrhosis (sih-ROH-sis)	cirrh/o = yellow -osis = abnormal condition	Chronic disease of the liver associated with failure of the liver to function properly
hepatitis (hep-ah-TYE-tis)	hepat/o = liver -itis = inflammation	Inflammation of the liver, usually due to viral infection; different viruses are transmitted by different routes, such as sexual contact or from exposure to blood or fecally contaminated water or food
hepatoma (hep-ah-TOH-mah)	hepat/o = liver -oma = tumor	Liver tumor
pancreatitis (pan-kree-ah-TYE-tis)	pancreat/o = pancreas -itis = inflammation	Inflammation of the pancreas

PRACTICE AS YOU GO

E. Terminology Matching

Match each term to its definition.

1. _____ anorexia
2. _____ hematemesis
3. _____ pyrosis
4. _____ obesity
5. _____ constipation
6. _____ melena
7. _____ ascites
8. _____ cirrhosis
9. _____ spastic colon
10. _____ polyposis
11. _____ volvulus
12. _____ hiatal hernia
13. _____ ulcerative colitis
14. _____ dysentery
15. _____ jaundice

a. excess body weight
b. chronic liver disease
c. heartburn
d. small colon tumors
e. fluid accumulation in abdominal cavity
f. vomit blood
g. bowel twists upon itself
h. inflammatory bowel disease
i. loss of appetite
j. difficulty having BM
k. irritable bowel syndrome
l. dark tarry stool
m. yellow skin color
n. bloody diarrhea
o. diaphragmatocele

Diagnostic Procedures

Term	Word Parts	Definition
Clinical Laboratory Tests		
alanine transaminase (ALT) (AL-ah-neen / trans-AM-ih-nase)		Enzyme normally present in the blood; blood levels are increased in persons with liver disease
aspartate transaminase (AST) (as-PAR-tate / trans-AM-ih-nase)		Enzyme normally present in the blood; blood levels are increased in persons with liver disease
fecal occult blood test (FOBT) (uh-CULT)	-al = pertaining to	Laboratory test on feces to determine if microscopic amounts of blood are present; also called *hemoccult* or *stool guaiac*
***H. pylori* antibody test** (pye-LOR-ee)	anti- = against	Laboratory test used to diagnose *H. pylori* infection that may be associated with peptic ulcer disease; may be performed on stool, breath, or tissue sample

Diagnostic Procedures (continued)

Term	Word Parts	Definition
ova and parasites (O&P) (OH-vah / PAIR-ah-sights)		Laboratory examination of feces with a microscope for presence of parasites or their eggs
serum bilirubin (SEER-um / bil-ih-ROO-bin)		Blood test to determine amount of waste product bilirubin in bloodstream; elevated levels indicate liver disease
stool culture		Laboratory test of feces to determine if any pathogenic bacteria are present
tissue transglutaminase (tTG) **antibody test** (trans-GLOO-tah-mih-nays)		Laboratory blood test for celiac disease; tests for presence of antibodies formed in autoimmune response to gluten

Diagnostic Imaging

Term	Word Parts	Definition
bitewing X-ray		X-ray taken with a part of film holder held between the teeth and parallel to the teeth
cholecystogram (koh-lee-SIS-toh-gram)	cholecyst/o = gallbladder -gram = record	X-ray image of the gallbladder
intravenous cholecystography (in-trah-VEE-nus / koh-lee-sis-TOG-rah-fee)	intra- = within ven/o = vein -ous = pertaining to cholecyst/o = gallbladder -graphy = process of recording	Dye is administered intravenously to patient allowing for X-ray visualization of gallbladder and bile ducts
lower gastrointestinal series (lower GI series)	gastr/o = stomach -al = pertaining to	X-ray image of colon and rectum is taken after administration of barium (Ba), a radiopaque dye, by enema; also called a *barium enema* (BE, BaE)

■ **Figure 8-19** X-ray of the colon taken during a barium enema. *(Kaling2100/Shutterstock)*

Term	Word Parts	Definition
percutaneous transhepatic cholangiography (PTC) (per-kyoo-TAY-nee-us / trans-heh-PAT-ik / koh-lan-jee-OG-rah-fee)	per- = through cutane/o = skin -ous = pertaining to trans- = across hepat/o = liver -ic = pertaining to cholangi/o = bile duct -graphy = process of recording	Procedure in which contrast medium is injected directly into the liver to visualize the bile ducts; used to detect obstructions such as gallstones in the common bile duct

Diagnostic Procedures (continued)

Term	Word Parts	Definition
upper gastrointestinal (UGI) **series**	gastr/o = stomach -al = pertaining to	Patient is administered a barium (Ba) contrast material orally and then X-rays are taken to visualize esophagus, stomach, and duodenum; also called a *barium swallow*

Endoscopic Procedures

Term	Word Parts	Definition
colonoscope (koh-LON-oh-skohp)	colon/o = colon -scope = instrument to view	Instrument used to view the colon
colonoscopy (koh-lon-OSS-koh-pee)	colon/o = colon -scopy = process of viewing	Flexible fiberscope called a *colonoscope* is passed through anus, rectum, and colon; used to examine upper portion of the colon; polyps and small growths can be removed during this procedure (see again Figure 8-16)
endoscopic retrograde cholangiopancreatography (ERCP) (en-doh-SKOP-ik / RET-roh-grayd / koh-lan-jee-oh-pan-kree-ah-TOG-rah-fee)	endo- = within -scopic = pertaining to visually examining retro- = backward cholangi/o = bile duct pancreat/o = pancreas -graphy = process of recording	Procedure using an endoscope to visually examine hepatic duct, common bile duct, and pancreatic duct; first an endoscope is passed through patient's mouth, esophagus, and stomach until it reaches the duodenum, where the pancreatic and common bile ducts empty; then a thin catheter is passed through the endoscope and into ducts (in retrograde direction); contrast dye is then used to visualize these ducts on an X-ray
esophagogastroduodenoscopy (EGD) (eh-soff-ah-goh-gas-troh-doo-od-eh-NOSS-koh-pee)	esophag/o = esophagus gastr/o = stomach duoden/o = duodenum -scopy = process of viewing	Use of flexible fiberoptic endoscope to visually examine esophagus, stomach, and beginning of the duodenum
gastroscope (GAS-troh-skohp)	gastr/o = stomach -scope = instrument to view	Instrument used to view inside the stomach
gastroscopy (gas-TROSS-koh-pee)	gastr/o = stomach -scopy = process of viewing	Procedure in which flexible *gastroscope* is passed through the mouth and down the esophagus in order to visualize inside the stomach; used to diagnose peptic ulcers and gastric carcinoma
laparoscope (LAP-ah-roh-skohp)	lapar/o = abdomen -scope = instrument to view	Instrument used to view inside the abdomen
laparoscopy (lap-ar-OSS-koh-pee)	lapar/o = abdomen -scopy = process of viewing	*Laparoscope* is passed into abdominal wall through a small incision; abdominal cavity is then visually examined for tumors and other conditions with this lighted instrument; also called *peritoneoscopy*
sigmoidoscope (sig-MOYD-oh-skohp)	sigmoid/o = sigmoid colon -scope = instrument to view	Instrument used to view inside the sigmoid colon

Diagnostic Procedures (continued)

Term	Word Parts	Definition
sigmoidoscopy (sig-moy-DOSS-koh-pee)	sigmoid/o = sigmoid colon -scopy = process of viewing	Procedure using flexible *sigmoido-scope* to visually examine the sigmoid colon; commonly done to diagnose cancer and polyps
Additional Diagnostic Procedures		
body mass index (BMI)		Method of determining if person's weight is healthy (neither under, nor overweight); calculated by dividing person's weight in kilograms by his or her height in square meters; there are many online calculators; a BMI below 18.5 is underweight, 18.5–24.9 is healthy, 25.0–29.9 is overweight, 30.0–39.9 is obese, and over 40 is morbid obesity
paracentesis (pair-ah-sen-TEE-sis)	-centesis = process of removing fluid	Insertion of a needle into abdominal cavity to withdraw fluid; tests to diagnose diseases may be conducted on the fluid

Therapeutic Procedures

Term	Word Parts	Definition
Dental Procedures		
bridge		Dental appliance to replace missing teeth; attached to adjacent teeth for support
crown		Artificial covering for a tooth that is created to replace original enamel covering of the tooth
denture (DEN-chur)	dent/o = tooth	Partial or complete set of artificial teeth that are set in plastic materials; acts as substitute for natural teeth and related structures
extraction	ex- = outward	Removing or "pulling" of teeth
gingivectomy (jin-jih-VEK-toh-mee)	gingiv/o = gums -ectomy = surgical removal	Surgical removal of gum tissue that has pulled away from the teeth and may lead to periodontal disease
implant (IM-plant)		Prosthetic device placed in the jaw to which a tooth or denture may be anchored
root canal	-al = pertaining to	Dental treatment involving pulp cavity of the root of a tooth; procedure is used to save a tooth that is badly infected or abscessed
Medical Procedures		
enema (EN-eh-mah)		Injection of fluid through the rectum and into the large intestine for purpose of cleansing bowel for testing, treating constipation, or administering drugs
gavage (guh-VAHZH)		Use of nasogastric (NG) tube to place liquid nourishment directly into the stomach

Therapeutic Procedures (continued)

Term	Word Parts	Definition
lavage (lah-VAHZH)		Use of nasogastric (NG) tube to wash out the stomach, for example, after ingestion of dangerous substances
nasogastric intubation (NG tube) (nay-zoh-GAS-trik / in-too-BAY-shun)	nas/o = nose gastr/o = stomach -ic = pertaining to in- = inward	Procedure in which a flexible catheter is inserted into the nose and down the esophagus to the stomach; may be used for feeding or to suction out stomach fluids
total parenteral nutrition (TPN) (pah-REN-ter-al)	-al = pertaining to	Providing 100% of patient's nutrition intravenously; used when patient is unable to eat

Surgical Procedures

Term	Word Parts	Definition
anastomosis (ah-nas-toh-MOH-sis)		To surgically create a connection between two organs or vessels; for example, joining together two cut ends of the intestines after a section is removed
appendectomy (ap-en-DEK-toh-mee)	append/o = appendix -ectomy = surgical removal	Surgical removal of the appendix
bariatric surgery (bare-ee-AT-rik)	bar/o = weight -iatric = pertaining to medical treatment	Group of surgical procedures designed to treat morbid (extreme) obesity by reducing size of the stomach or diverting food from passing through a portion of the alimentary canal
cholecystectomy (koh-lee-sis-TEK-toh-mee)	cholecyst/o = gallbladder -ectomy = surgical removal	Surgical removal of the gallbladder
choledocholithotripsy (koh-led-oh-koh-LITH-oh-trip-see)	choledoch/o = common bile duct lith/o = stone -tripsy = surgical crushing	Crushing of a gallstone in the common bile duct
colectomy (koh-LEK-toh-mee)	col/o = colon -ectomy = surgical removal	Surgical removal of the colon
colostomy (koh-LOSS-toh-mee)	col/o = colon -ostomy = surgically create an opening	Surgical creation of an opening of some portion of the colon through the abdominal wall to the outside surface; fecal material (stool) drains into a bag worn on the abdomen

Transverse colostomy
Ascending colostomy
Descending colostomy
Ileostomy
Cecostomy
Sigmoid colostomy

A

B
Functioning stoma
Nonfunctioning remaining colon

■ **Figure 8-20** A) The colon illustrating various ostomy sites. B) Colostomy in the descending colon, illustrating functioning stoma and nonfunctioning distal sigmoid colon and rectum.

Therapeutic Procedures (continued)

Term	Word Parts	Definition
diverticulectomy (dye-ver-tik-yoo-LEK-toh-mee)	diverticul/o = pouch -ectomy = surgical removal	Surgical removal of a diverticulum
exploratory laparotomy (ek-SPLOR-ah-tor-ee / lap-ah-ROT-oh-mee)	lapar/o = abdomen -otomy = cutting into	Abdominal operation for purpose of examining abdominal organs and tissues for signs of disease or other abnormalities
fistulectomy (fis-tyoo-LEK-toh-mee)	-ectomy = surgical removal	Removal of an anal fistula
gastric banding	gastr/o = stomach -ic = pertaining to	Laparoscopic bariatric surgical procedure that places a restrictive band (commonly called a *lap-band*) around top portion of the stomach; leads to eating smaller meals and less food by reducing ability of the stomach to expand and hold food
gastric bypass	gastr/o = stomach -ic = pertaining to	Bariatric surgical procedure that divides the stomach into small upper portion and larger lower portion; small intestine is then connected to small upper portion; food bypasses most of the stomach and duodenum; small stomach seriously limits amount of food eaten and bypassing the duodenum reduces fat absorption
gastrectomy (gas-TREK-toh-mee)	gastr/o = stomach -ectomy = surgical removal	Surgical removal of the stomach
gastric stapling	gastr/o = stomach -ic = pertaining to	Procedure that closes off a large section of the stomach with rows of staples; results in much smaller stomach to assist very obese patients to lose weight
gastrostomy (gas-TROSS-toh-mee)	gastr/o = stomach -ostomy = surgically create an opening	Surgical procedure to create opening in the stomach
hemorrhoidectomy (hem-oh-royd-EK-toh-mee)	-ectomy = surgical removal	Surgical removal of hemorrhoids from anorectal area
hernioplasty (her-nee-oh-PLAS-tee)	-plasty = surgical repair	Surgical repair of a hernia; also called *herniorrhaphy*
ileostomy (il-ee-OSS-toh-mee)	ile/o = ileum -ostomy = surgically create an opening	Surgical creation of an opening in the ileum
laparoscopic cholecystectomy (lap-ar-oh-SKOP-ik / koh-lee-sis-TEK-toh-mee)	lapar/o = abdomen -scopic = pertaining to visually examining cholecyst/o = gallbladder -ectomy = surgical removal	Surgical removal of the gallbladder through a very small abdominal incision with assistance of a laparoscope
laparotomy (lap-ah-ROT-oh-mee)	lapar/o = abdomen -otomy = cutting into	Surgical incision into the abdomen
liver transplant		Transplant of a liver from a donor
palatoplasty (PAL-ah-toh-plas-tee)	palat/o = palate -plasty = surgical repair	Surgical repair of the palate

Therapeutic Procedures (continued)

Term	Word Parts	Definition
pharyngoplasty (fah-RING-oh-plas-tee)	pharyng/o = pharynx -plasty = surgical repair	Surgical repair of the throat
proctopexy (PROK-toh-pek-see)	proct/o = rectum and anus -pexy = surgical fixation	Surgical fixation of the rectum and anus

PRACTICE AS YOU GO

F. Procedure Matching

Match each procedure term with its definition.

1. _____ serum bilirubin
2. _____ lavage
3. _____ bariatric surgery
4. _____ proctopexy
5. _____ lower GI series
6. _____ paracentesis
7. _____ fecal occult blood test
8. _____ laparoscopy

a. withdraws fluid from abdominal cavity
b. barium enema
c. visually examines abdominal cavity
d. stool guaiac
e. treatment for obesity
f. elevated levels indicate liver disease
g. to wash out the stomach
h. surgical fixation of rectum and anus

Pharmacology

Classification	Word Parts	Action	Examples
anorexiant (an-oh-REKS-ee-ant)	an- = without -orexia = appetite	Treats obesity by suppressing appetite	phendimetrazine, Adipost, Obezine; phentermine, Zantryl, Adipex
antacid	anti- = against	Used to neutralize stomach acids	calcium carbonate, Tums; aluminum hydroxide and magnesium hydroxide, Maalox, Mylanta
antidiarrheal (an-tee-dye-ah-REE-al)	anti- = against -al = pertaining to	Used to control diarrhea	loperamide, Imodium; diphenoxylate and atropine, Lomotil; kaolin/pectin, Kaopectate
antiemetic (an-tye-ee-MEH-tik)	anti- = against -emetic = pertaining to vomiting	Treats nausea and vomiting and motion sickness	prochlorperazine, Compazine; promethazine, Phenergan
herpes antivirals	anti- = against	Treat herpes simplex infection	valacyclovir, Valtrex; famcyclovir, Famvir; acyclovir, Zovirax

Pharmacology (continued)

Classification	Word Parts	Action	Examples
H$_2$-receptor antagonist	anti- = against	Used to treat peptic ulcers and gastroesophageal reflux disease; when stimulated, H$_2$-receptors increase production of stomach acid; using an antagonist to block these receptors results in low acid level in the stomach	ranitidine, Zantac; cimetidine, Tagamet; famotidine, Pepcid
laxative		Treats constipation by stimulating a bowel movement	senosides, Senokot; psyllium, Metamucil
proton pump inhibitors		Used to treat peptic ulcers and gastroesophageal reflux disease; blocks the stomach's ability to secrete acid	esomeprazole, Nexium; omeprazole, Prilosec

Med Term Tip

The term *laxative* comes from the Latin term meaning *to relax*.

Abbreviations

ac	before meals	HDV	hepatitis D virus
ALT	alanine transaminase	HEV	hepatitis E virus
AST	aspartate transaminase	HSV-1	herpes simplex virus type 1
Ba	barium	IBD	inflammatory bowel disease
BaE	barium enema	IBS	irritable bowel syndrome
BE	barium enema	IVC	intravenous cholangiography
BM	bowel movement	N&V	nausea and vomiting
BMI	body mass index	NG	nasogastric (tube)
BS	bowel sounds	NPO	nothing by mouth
CBD	common bile duct	O&P	ova and parasites
EGD	esophagogastroduodenoscopy	pc	after meals
ERCP	endoscopic retrograde cholangiopancreatography	PO	by mouth
FOBT	fecal occult blood test	pp	postprandial
GB	gallbladder	PTC	percutaneous transhepatic cholangiography
GERD	gastroesophageal reflux disease	PUD	peptic ulcer disease
GI	gastrointestinal	q	every
H. pylori	*Helicobacter pylori*	qam	every morning
HAV	hepatitis A virus	qh	every hour
HBV	hepatitis B virus	TPN	total parenteral nutrition
HCl	hydrochloric acid	tTG	tissue transglutaminase
HCV	hepatitis C virus	UGI	upper gastrointestinal series

PRACTICE AS YOU GO

G. What's the Abbreviation?

1. nasogastric _____

2. gastrointestinal _____

3. hepatitis B virus _____

4. fecal occult blood test _____

5. inflammatory bowel disease _____

6. herpes simplex virus type 1 _____

7. aspartate transaminase _____

8. after meals _____

9. peptic ulcer disease _____

10. gastroesophageal reflux disease _____

Chapter Review

Real-World Applications

Medical Record Analysis
This Gastroenterology Consultation Report contains 12 medical terms. Underline each term and write it in the list below the report. Then explain each term as you would to a nonmedical person.

Gastroenterology Consultation Report

Reason for Consultation:	Evaluation of recurrent epigastric pain with anemia and melena.
History of Present Illness:	Patient is a 56-year-old male. He reports a long history of mild dyspepsia characterized by burning epigastric pain, especially when his stomach is empty. This pain has been temporarily relieved by over-the-counter antacids. Approximately two weeks ago, the pain became significantly worse and he noted that his stool was dark and tarry.
Results of Physical Examination:	CBC indicates anemia, and a fecal occult blood test is positive for blood. A blood test for *Helicobacter pylori* is positive. Gastroscopy located an ulcer in the lining of the stomach. This ulcer is 1.5 cm in diameter and deep. There is evidence of active bleeding from the ulcer.
Assessment:	Peptic ulcer disease
Recommendations:	A gastrectomy to remove the ulcerated portion of the stomach is indicated because the ulcer is already bleeding.

Term   **Explanation**

1. _____   _____
2. _____   _____
3. _____   _____
4. _____   _____
5. _____   _____
6. _____   _____
7. _____   _____
8. _____   _____
9. _____   _____
10. _____   _____
11. _____   _____
12. _____   _____

Chart Note Transcription

The chart note below contains 12 phrases that can be reworded with a medical term presented in this chapter. Each phrase is identified with an underline. Determine the medical term and write your answers in the space provided.

Pearson General Hospital Consultation Report

Task   Edit   View   Time Scale   Options   Help Download   Archive   Date: 17 May 2017

Current Complaint: Patient is a 74-year-old female seen by a <u>physician who specializes in the treatment of the gastrointestinal tract</u> **1** with complaints of severe lower abdominal pain and extreme <u>difficulty with having a bowel movement</u>. **2**

Past History: Patient has a history of the <u>presence of gallstones</u> **3** requiring <u>surgical removal of the gallbladder</u> **4** 10 years ago and chronic <u>acid backing up from the stomach into the esophagus</u>. **5**

Signs and Symptoms: The patient's abdomen is distended with <u>fluid collecting in the abdominal cavity</u>. **6** <u>X-ray of the colon after inserting barium dye with an enema</u> **7** revealed <u>the presence of multiple small tumors growing on a stalk</u> **8** throughout the colon. <u>Visual examination of the colon by a scope inserted through the rectum</u> **9** was performed, and biopsies taken for microscopic examination located a tumor.

Diagnosis: Carcinoma of the section of colon between <u>the descending colon and the rectum</u> **10**

Treatment: <u>Surgical removal of the colon</u> **11** between the descending colon and the rectum with <u>the surgical creation of an opening of the colon through the abdominal wall</u>. **12**

1. _____
2. _____
3. _____
4. _____
5. _____
6. _____
7. _____
8. _____
9. _____
10. _____
11. _____
12. _____

Case Study

Below is a case study presentation of a patient with a condition discussed in this chapter. Read the case study and answer the questions below. Some questions will ask for information not included within this chapter. Use your text, a medical dictionary, or any other reference material you choose to answer these questions.

A 60-year-old obese female has come into the ER due to severe RUQ pain for the past two hours. Patient also reports increasing nausea but denies emesis. Patient states she has been told she has cholelithiasis by her family physician following a milder episode of this pain two years ago. In addition to severe pain, patient displays a moderate degree of scleral jaundice. Abdominal ultrasound identified acute cholecystitis and a large number of gallstones. Because of the jaundice, a PTC was performed and confirmed choledocholithiasis. Patient was sent to surgery for laparoscopic cholecystectomy to remove the gallbladder and all gallstones. She recovered without incident.

(Rob Marmion/Shutterstock)

Questions

1. Define each of the patient's symptoms.

   _____

   _____

2. The patient has severe RUQ pain. What organs are located in the RUQ?

   _____

   _____

3. After reading the definition of jaundice, what is most likely causing this patient to have it?

   _____

   _____

4. Describe the diagnostic imaging procedures this patient received.

   _____

   _____

5. What is the difference between *cholelithiasis* and *cholecystitis?*

   _____

   _____

6. The patient's gallbladder was removed laparoscopically. What does that mean?

   _____

   _____

Practice Exercises

A. Word Building Practice

The combining form **gastr/o** refers to the *stomach*. Use it to write a term that means:

1. inflammation of the stomach _____
2. study of the stomach and small intestine _____
3. removal of the stomach _____
4. visual exam of the stomach _____
5. stomach pain _____
6. enlargement of the stomach _____
7. cutting into the stomach _____

The combining form **esophag/o** refers to the *esophagus*. Use it to write a term that means:

8. inflammation of the esophagus _____
9. visual examination of the esophagus _____
10. surgical repair of the esophagus _____
11. pertaining to the esophagus _____
12. surgical removal (of part) of esophagus _____

The combining form **proct/o** refers to the *rectum* and *anus*. Use it to write a term that means:

13. surgical fixation of the rectum and anus _____
14. drooping of the rectum and anus _____
15. inflammation of the rectum and anus _____
16. specialist in the study of the rectum and anus _____

The combining form **cholecyst/o** refers to the *gallbladder*. Use it to write a term that means:

17. removal of the gallbladder _____
18. condition of having gallbladder stones _____
19. gallbladder stone surgical crushing _____
20. gallbladder inflammation _____

The combining form **lapar/o** refers to the *abdomen*. Use it to write a term that means:

21. instrument to view inside the abdomen _____
22. cutting into the abdomen _____
23. visual examination of the abdomen _____

The combining form **hepat/o** refers to the *liver*. Use it to write a term that means:

24. liver tumor _____
25. enlargement of the liver _____
26. pertaining to the liver _____
27. inflammation of the liver _____

The combining form **pancreat/o** refers to the *pancreas*. Use it to write a term that means:

28. inflammation of the pancreas _____

29. pertaining to the pancreas   _____

The combining form **col/o** refers to the *colon*. Use it to write a term that means:

30. surgically create an opening in the colon _____

31. inflammation of the colon   _____

B. Complete the Term

For each definition given below, fill in the blank with the word part that completes the term.

Definition	Term
1. surgical repair of the throat	_____plasty
2. liver tumor	_____oma
3. surgical removal of the stomach	_____ectomy
4. abnormal condition of polyps	_____osis
5. instrument to view inside sigmoid colon	_____scope
6. after a meal	post _____
7. record of the gallbladder	_____gram
8. inflammation of the pancreas	_____itis
9. salivary gland inflammation	_____itis
10. without appetite	_____
11. vomiting blood	hemat_____
12. slow digestion	brady_____
13. study of stomach and small intestine	_____logy
14. difficult eating/swallowing	dys_____
15. pertaining to around the tooth	peri_____al

C. Using Abbreviations

Fill in each blank with the appropriate abbreviation.

1. As the colon was no longer functioning, _____ was given via a(n) _____ tube.

2. Peter had to drink barium to have a(n) _____ series.

3. The physician thought the patient may have intestinal parasites, so a(n) _____ was ordered.

4. _____ is commonly called *spastic colon*.

5. The diagnosis of _____ was confirmed after the ulcer was observed during a gastroscopy.

6. Stomach acid splashing up into the esophagus resulted in the development of _____.

7. The child complained of severe _____ because of having the stomach flu.

8. Persons with liver disease may have increased levels of _____ and _____ in the blood.

9. The _____ is also called a *hemoccult*.

10. After colon surgery, the nurses watched for the first _____ to know that the colon was functioning properly.

D. Define the Term

1. colonoscopy _____

2. bitewing X-ray _____

3. hematochezia _____

4. serum bilirubin _____

5. cachexia _____

6. lavage _____

7. hernioplasty _____

8. extraction _____

9. choledocholithotripsy _____

10. anastomosis _____

E. Fill in the Blank

colonoscopy	barium swallow	lower GI series
gastric stapling	colostomy	colectomy
total parenteral nutrition	choledocholithotripsy	liver biopsy
ileostomy	fecal occult blood test	intravenous cholecystography

1. Excising a small piece of hepatic tissue for microscopic examination is called a(n) _____.

2. When a surgeon performs a total or partial colectomy for cancer, she may have to create an opening on the surface of the skin for fecal matter to leave the body. This procedure is called a(n) _____.

3. Another name for an upper GI series is a(n) _____.

4. Mr. White has had a radiopaque material placed into his colon by means of an enema for the purpose of viewing his colon. This procedure is called a(n) _____.

5. A(n) _____ is the surgical removal of the colon.

6. Jessica has been on a red meat–free diet in preparation for a test of her feces for the presence of hidden blood. This test is called a(n) _____.

7. Dr. Mendez uses equipment to crush gallstones in the common bile duct. This procedure is called a(n) _____.

8. Mrs. Alcazar required _____ because she could not eat following her intestinal surgery.

9. Mr. Bright had a(n) _____ to treat his morbid obesity.

10. Visualizing the gallbladder and bile ducts by injecting a dye into the patient's arm is called a(n) _____.

11. Passing an instrument into the anus and rectum in order to see the colon is called a(n) _____.

12. Ms. Fayne suffers from Crohn's disease, which has necessitated the removal of much of her small intestine. She has had a surgical passage created for the external disposal of waste material from the ileum. This is called a(n) _____.

F. Terminology Matching

Match each term to its definition.

1. _____ denture

2. _____ cementum

3. _____ root canal

4. _____ crown

5. _____ bridge

6. _____ implant

7. _____ gingivitis

8. _____ dental caries

a. tooth decay

b. prosthetic device used to anchor a tooth

c. inflammation of the gums

d. full set of artificial teeth

e. portion of the tooth covered by enamel

f. replacement for missing teeth

g. anchors root in bony socket of jaw

h. surgery on the tooth pulp

G. Pharmacology Challenge

Fill in the classification for each drug description, then match the brand name.

Drug Description	Classification	Brand Name
1. _____ Controls diarrhea	_____	a. Pepcid
2. _____ Blocks stomach's ability to secrete acid	_____	b. Obezine
3. _____ Treats motion sickness	_____	c. Metamucil
4. _____ Blocks acid-producing receptors	_____	d. Compazine
5. _____ Suppresses appetite	_____	e. Maalox
6. _____ Stimulates a bowel movement	_____	f. Imodium
7. _____ Neutralizes stomach acid	_____	g. Valtrex
8. _____ Treats herpes simplex infection	_____	h. Nexium

H. Spelling Practice

Some of the following terms are misspelled. Identify the incorrect terms and spell them correctly in the blank provided.

1. gastrointestinal _____

2. salivery _____

3. ileoceccal _____

4. submandibuler _____

5. cachexia _____

6. cholecystalgia _____

7. diverticulosis _____

8. proctoptisis _____

9. laparoscopy _____

10. antidiarheal _____

I. Anatomical Adjectives

Fill in the blank with the missing noun or adjective.

Noun	Adjective
1. cheek	_____
2. gallbladder	_____
3. _____	jejunal
4. _____	colorectal
5. under the tongue	_____
6. _____	enteric
7. _____	pancreatic
8. tooth	_____
9. _____	labial
10. _____	sigmoidal
11. throat	_____
12. stomach	_____
13. _____	duodenal
14. liver	_____
15. mouth	_____

J. Complete the Statement

1. The pancreas secretes _____ and _____ to aid in digestion.
2. The gallbladder stores _____ produced by the _____.
3. Saliva contains the digestive enzyme _____.
4. The colon extends from the _____ to the _____.
5. The major site for digestion and absorption of nutrients is the _____.
6. The _____ regulates the passage of food into the small intestine.
7. _____ is the wavelike muscular contractions that move food through the esophagus.
8. The _____ prevents food from entering the respiratory tract.
9. The biting teeth are the _____ and _____. The grinding teeth are the _____ and _____.
10. Another term for the gums is _____.

MyLab Medical Terminology™

MyLab Medical Terminology is a premium online homework management system that includes a host of features to help you study. Registered users will find:

- A multitude of activities and assignments built within the MyLab platform
- Powerful tools that track and analyze your results—allowing you to create a personalized learning experience
- Videos and audio pronunciations to help enrich your progress
- Streaming lesson presentations (Guided Lectures) and self-paced learning modules
- A space where you and your instructors can check your progress and manage your assignments

Labeling Exercises

Image A

Write the labels for this figure on the numbered lines provided.

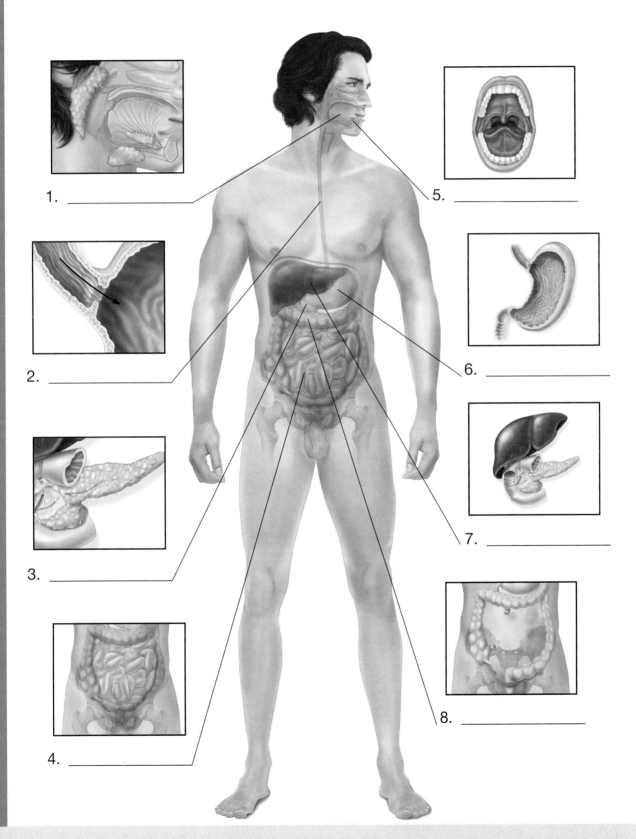

1. _____

2. _____

3. _____

4. _____

5. _____

6. _____

7. _____

8. _____

Image B

Write the labels for this figure on the numbered lines provided.

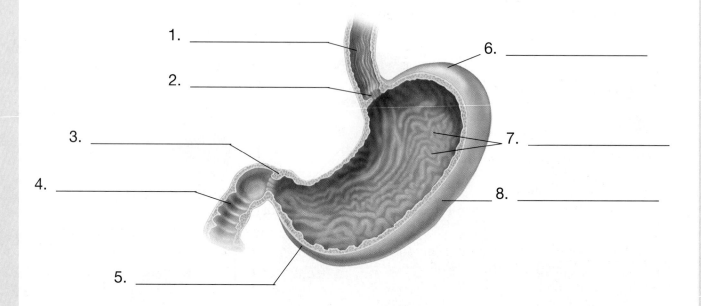

1. _____

2. _____

3. _____

4. _____

5. _____

6. _____

7. _____

8. _____

Image C

Write the labels for this figure on the numbered lines provided.

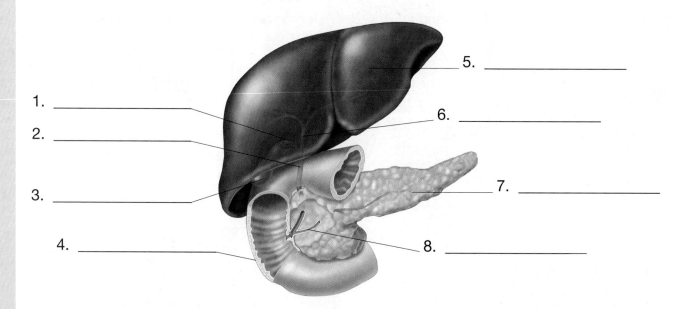

1. _____

2. _____

3. _____

4. _____

5. _____

6. _____

7. _____

8. _____

Chapter 9

Urinary System

Learning Objectives

Upon completion of this chapter, you will be able to

1. Identify and define the combining forms and suffixes introduced in this chapter.

2. Correctly spell and pronounce medical terms and major anatomical structures relating to the urinary system.

3. Locate and describe the major organs of the urinary system and their functions.

4. Describe the nephron and the mechanisms of urine production.

5. Identify the characteristics of urine and a urinalysis.

6. Identify and define urinary system anatomical terms.

7. Identify and define selected urinary system pathology terms.

8. Identify and define selected urinary system diagnostic procedures.

9. Identify and define selected urinary system therapeutic procedures.

10. Identify and define selected medications relating to the urinary system.

11. Define selected abbreviations associated with the urinary system.

AT A GLANCE

Function

The urinary system is responsible for maintaining a stable internal environment for the body. In order to achieve this state, the urinary system removes waste products, adjusts water and electrolyte levels, and maintains the correct pH.

Organs

The primary structures that comprise the urinary system:

kidneys   **ureters**

urethra   **urinary bladder**

Word Parts

Presented here are the most common word parts (with their meanings) used to build urinary system terms. For a more comprehensive list, refer to the Terminology section of this chapter.

Combining Forms

azot/o	nitrogenous waste	**meat/o**	meatus
bacteri/o	bacteria	**nephr/o**	kidney
corpor/o	body	**noct/i**	night
cyst/o	urinary bladder	**olig/o**	scanty
genit/o	genitals	**protein/o**	protein
glomerul/o	glomerulus	**pyel/o**	renal pelvis
glycos/o	sugar, glucose	**ren/o**	kidney
home/o	sameness	**tox/o**	poison
hydr/o	water	**ureter/o**	ureter
iatr/o	physician, medicine, treatment	**urethr/o**	urethra
		urin/o	urine
idi/o	distinctive	**ur/o**	urine
keton/o	ketones		

Suffixes

-lith	stone	**-ptosis**	drooping
-lysis	to destroy	**-uria**	urine condition

Urinary System Illustrated

kidney, p. 314

Filters blood and produces urine

urinary bladder, p. 316

Stores urine

female urethra, p. 317

Transports urine to exterior

ureter, p. 315

Transports urine to the bladder

male urethra, p. 317

Transports urine to exterior

Anatomy and Physiology of the Urinary System

genitourinary system
(jen-ih-toh-YOO-rih-nair-ee)

kidneys

nephrons (NEF-ronz)

uremia (yoo-REE-mee-ah)

ureters (YOO-reh-ters)

urethra (yoo-REE-thrah)

urinary bladder (YOO-rih-nair-ee)

urine (YOO-rin)

Think of the urinary system, sometimes referred to as the **genitourinary** (GU) **system**, as similar to a water filtration plant. Its main function is to filter and remove waste products from the blood. These waste materials result in the production and excretion of **urine** from the body.

The urinary system is one of the hardest working systems of the body. All the body's metabolic processes result in the production of waste products. These waste products are a natural part of life but quickly become toxic if they are allowed to build up in the blood, resulting in a condition called **uremia**. Waste products in the body are removed through a very complicated system of blood vessels and kidney tubules. The actual filtration of wastes from the blood takes place in millions of **nephrons**, which make up each of the **kidneys**. As urine drains from each kidney, the **ureters** transport it to the **urinary bladder**. The body is constantly producing urine, and the bladder can collect up to one quart of this liquid during the night. When the urinary bladder empties, urine moves from the bladder down the **urethra** to the outside of the body.

Kidneys

calyx (KAY-liks)

cortex (KOR-teks)

hilum (HYE-lum)

medulla (meh-DULL-ah)

renal artery

renal papilla (pah-PILL-ah)

renal pelvis

renal pyramids

renal vein

retroperitoneal (ret-roh-pair-ih-toh-NEE-al)

The body has two kidneys located in the lumbar region of the back above the waist, with one on either side of the vertebral column. They are not inside the peritoneal sac, a location referred to as **retroperitoneal**. Each kidney has a concave or indented area on the edge toward the center that gives the kidney its bean shape. The center of this concave area is called the **hilum**. The hilum is where the **renal artery** enters and the **renal vein** leaves the kidney (see Figure 9-1 ■). The renal artery delivers blood that is full of waste products to the kidney and the renal vein returns the now cleansed blood to general circulation. Narrow tubes called *ureters* also leave the kidneys at the hilum and lead to the bladder.

When a surgeon cuts into a kidney, several structures or areas are visible. The outer portion, called the **cortex**, is much like a shell for the kidney. The inner area called the **medulla**, contains a dozen or so triangular-shaped areas, the **renal pyramids**, which resemble their namesake, the Egyptian pyramids. The tip of each pyramid points inward toward the hilum. At its tip, called the **renal papilla**, each pyramid opens into a **calyx** (plural is *calyces*), which is continuous with the **renal pelvis**. The calyces and ultimately the renal pelvis collect urine as it is formed. The ureter for each kidney arises from the renal pelvis (see Figure 9-2 ■).

Cortex

Medulla

Renal artery

Renal vein

Ureter

■ **Figure 9-1**   Kidney structure. Longitudinal section showing the renal artery entering and the renal vein and ureter exiting at the hilum of the kidney.

Cortex

Medulla

Hilum

Calyx

Renal papilla

Renal pyramid

Renal pelvis

Ureter

■ **Figure 9-2**   Longitudinal section of a kidney illustrating the internal structures.

Nephrons

afferent arteriole (AF-er-ent)	**glomerulus** (gloh-MAIR-yoo-lus)
Bowman's capsule	**loop of Henle**
collecting tubule	**nephron loop**
distal convoluted tubule (DIS-tal / kon-voh-LOOT-ed)	**proximal convoluted tubule** (PROK-sim-al / kon-voh-LOOT-ed)
efferent arteriole (EF-er-ent)	**renal corpuscle** (KOR-pus-el)
glomerular capsule (gloh-MAIR-yoo-ler)	**renal tubule**

The functional or working unit of the kidney is the nephron. There are more than one million of these microscopic structures in each human kidney. Each nephron consists of the **renal corpuscle** and the **renal tubule** (see Figure 9-3 ■). The renal corpuscle is the blood-filtering portion of the nephron. It has a double-walled cuplike structure called the **glomerular capsule** (also known as **Bowman's capsule**) that encases a ball of capillaries called the **glomerulus**. An **afferent arteriole** carries blood to the glomerulus, and an **efferent arteriole** carries blood away from the glomerulus.

Water and substances that were removed from the bloodstream in the renal corpuscle flow into the renal tubules to finish the urine production process. This continuous tubule is divided into four sections: the **proximal convoluted tubule**, followed by the narrow **nephron loop** (also known as the **loop of Henle**), then the **distal convoluted tubule**, and finally the **collecting tubule**.

Ureters

As urine drains out of the renal pelvis it enters the ureter, which carries it down to the urinary bladder (see Figure 9-4 ■). Ureters are very narrow tubes measuring less than ¼-inch wide and 10–12 inches long that extend from the renal pelvis to the urinary bladder. Mucous membrane lines the ureters just as it lines most passages that open to the external environment.

Med Term Tip

The kidney bean is so named because it resembles a kidney in shape. Each organ weighs four to six ounces, is two to three inches wide, and approximately one inch thick, and is about the size of your fist. In most people, the left kidney is slightly higher and larger than the right kidney. Functioning kidneys are necessary for life, but it is possible to live with only one working kidney.

What's In A Name?

Look for these word parts:
dist/o = away from
proxim/o = near to
-al = pertaining to

Med Term Tip

Afferent, meaning *moving toward*, and *efferent*, meaning *moving away from*, are terms used when discussing moving either toward or away from the central point in many systems. For example, there are afferent and efferent nerves in the nervous system.

What's In A Name?

Look for these word parts:

ex- = outward
in- = inward
-al = pertaining to

Word Watch

The terms *ureter* and *urethra* are frequently confused. Remember that there are two ureters carrying urine from the kidneys into the bladder. There is only one urethra, and it carries urine from the bladder to the outside of the body.

Med Term Tip

Terms such as *micturition*, *voiding*, and *urination* all mean basically the same thing—the process of releasing urine from the body.

Urinary Bladder

external sphincter (SFINGK-ter)	**rugae** (ROO-jee)
internal sphincter	**urination**

The urinary bladder is an elastic muscular sac that lies in the base of the pelvis just behind the pubic symphysis (see Figure 9-5 ■). It is composed of three layers of smooth muscle tissue lined with mucous membrane containing **rugae**, or folds, that allow it to stretch. The bladder receives the urine directly from the ureters, stores it, and excretes it by **urination** through the urethra.

Generally, an adult bladder signals the urge to void (or empty the bladder) when it contains 300–400 mL of urine. Involuntary muscle action causes the bladder to contract and the **internal sphincter** to relax. The internal sphincter prevents the bladder from emptying at the wrong time. Voluntary action controls

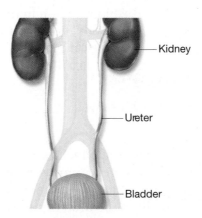

■ **Figure 9-4** The ureters extend from the kidneys to the urinary bladder.

■ **Figure 9-5** The structure of the urinary bladder. (Note the prostate gland.)

the **external sphincter**, which opens on demand to allow the intentional emptying of the bladder. The act of controlling the emptying of urine is developed sometime after a child is two years of age.

Urethra

urinary meatus (mee-AY-tus)

The urethra is a tubular canal that carries the flow of urine from the bladder to the outside of the body (see Figure 9-6 ■). The external opening through which urine passes out of the body is called the **urinary meatus**. Mucous membrane also lines the urethra as it does other structures of the urinary system. This is one of the reasons that bladder infections may spread up the urinary tract. The urethra is one to two inches long in the female and eight inches long in the male. In a woman it functions only as the outlet for urine and is located in front of the vagina. In the male, however, it has two functions: an outlet for urine and the passageway for semen to leave the body.

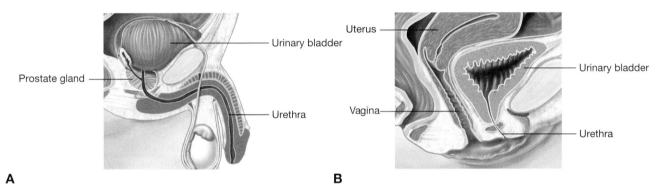

A   **B**

■ **Figure 9-6**   A) The male urethra extends from the urinary bladder in the floor of the pelvis through the penis to the urinary meatus. B) The much shorter female urethra extends from the urinary bladder to the floor of the pelvis and exits just in front of the vaginal opening.

PRACTICE AS YOU GO

A. Complete the Statement

1. The functional or working units of the kidneys are the _____.

2. The glomerular capsule is also called _____ and the nephron loop is also called the _____.

3. The urinary bladder is composed of three layers of _____ tissue.

4. The term that describes the location of the kidneys is _____.

5. The glomerular capsule surrounds the _____.

6. The tip of each renal pyramid opens into a(n) _____.

7. There are _____ ureters and _____ urethra.

8. Urination can also be referred to as _____ or _____.

Role of Kidneys in Homeostasis

electrolytes (ee-LEK-troh-lites)   **homeostasis** (hoh-mee-oh-STAY-sis)

The kidneys are responsible for **homeostasis** or balance in the body. They continually adjust the chemical conditions in the body, allowing humans to survive. Because of its interaction with the bloodstream and its ability to excrete substances from the body, the urinary system maintains the body's proper balance of water (H_2O) and chemicals. If the body is low on water, the kidneys conserve it, or in the opposite case, if there is excess water in the body, the kidneys excrete the excess. In addition to water, the kidneys regulate the level of **electrolytes**— small biologically important molecules such as sodium (Na^+), potassium (K^+), chloride (Cl^-), and bicarbonate (HCO_3^-). Finally, the kidneys play an important role in maintaining the correct pH range within the body, making sure it does not become too acidic or too alkaline. The kidneys accomplish these important tasks through the production of urine.

Stages of Urine Production

filtration   **reabsorption**

glomerular filtrate (gloh-MAIR-yoo-ler)   **secretion**

peritubular capillaries (pair-ih-TOO-byoo-lar)

As wastes and unnecessary substances are removed from the bloodstream by the nephrons, many desirable molecules are also removed initially. Waste products are eliminated from the body, but other substances such as water, electrolytes, and nutrients must be returned to the bloodstream. Urine, in its final form ready for elimination from the body, is the ultimate product of this entire process.

Urine production occurs in three stages: **filtration**, **reabsorption**, and **secretion**. Each of these steps is performed by a different section of the nephrons (see Figure 9-7 ■).

■ Figure 9-7 The three stages of urine production: filtration, reabsorption, and secretion.

1. **Filtration.**   The first stage is the filtering of particles, which occurs in the renal corpuscle. The pressure of blood flowing through the glomerulus forces material out of the bloodstream, through the wall of the glomerular capsule, and into the renal tubules. This fluid in the tubules is called the **glomerular filtrate** and consists of water, electrolytes, nutrients such as glucose and amino acids, wastes, and toxins.

2. **Reabsorption.**   After filtration, the filtrate passes through the four sections of the tubule. As the filtrate moves along its twisted journey, most of the water and much of the electrolytes and nutrients are reabsorbed into the **peritubular capillaries**, a capillary bed that surrounds the renal tubules. They can then reenter the circulating blood.

3. **Secretion.**   The final stage of urine production occurs when the special cells of the renal tubules secrete ammonia, uric acid, and other waste substances directly into the renal tubule. Urine formation is now finished; it passes into the collecting tubules, renal papilla, calyx, renal pelvis, and ultimately into the ureter.

Urine

albumin (al-BYOO-min)   **specific gravity**

nitrogenous wastes (nigh-TROJ-eh-nus)   **urinalysis** (yoo-rih-NAL-ih-sis)

Normal urine color may vary from almost clear, pale yellow, to deep gold, depending on how dilute it is. As it is being produced and collecting in the bladder, it is sterile. However, as it passes through the urethra to the outside, it may become contaminated by bacteria. Although it is 95% water, it also contains many dissolved substances, such as electrolytes, toxins, and **nitrogenous wastes**, the by-products of muscle metabolism. At times the urine also contains substances that should not be there, such as glucose, blood, or **albumin**, a protein that should remain in the blood. This is the reason for performing a **urinalysis**, a physical and chemical analysis of urine, which gives medical personnel important information regarding disease processes occurring in a patient. Normally, during a 24-hour period the output of urine will be 1,000–2,000 mL, depending on the amount of fluid consumed and the general health of the person. Normal urine is acidic because this is one way the body disposes of excess acids. **Specific gravity** indicates the amount of dissolved substances in urine. The specific gravity of pure water is 1.000. The specific gravity of urine varies from 1.001 to 1.030. Highly concentrated urine has a higher specific gravity, while the specific gravity of very dilute urine is close to that of water. See Table 9-1 ■ for the normal values for urine testing and Table 9-2 ■ for abnormal findings.

What's In A Name?

Look for these word parts:
urin/o = urine
-lysis = to destroy
-ous = pertaining to

Med Term Tip

The color, odor, volume, and sugar content of urine have been examined for centuries. Color charts for urine were developed by 1140, and "taste testing" was common in the late 17th century. By the 19th century, urinalysis was a routine part of a physical examination.

■ TABLE 9-1   Normal Values for Urinalysis Testing

Element	Normal Findings
Color	Straw-colored, pale yellow to deep gold
Odor	Aromatic
Appearance	Clear
Specific gravity	1.001–1.030
pH	5.0–8.0
Protein	Negative to trace
Glucose	None
Ketones	None
Blood	Negative

■ **TABLE 9-2**   Abnormal Urinalysis Findings

Element	Implications
Color	Color varies depending on patient's fluid intake and output or medication; brown or black urine color indicates a serious disease process
Odor	Fetid or foul odor may indicate infection, while fruity odor may be found in diabetes mellitus, dehydration, or starvation; other odors may be due to medication or foods
Appearance	Cloudiness may mean that infection is present
Specific gravity	Concentrated urine has a higher specific gravity; dilute urine, such as can be found with diabetes insipidus, acute tubular necrosis, or salt-restricted diets, has a lower specific gravity
pH	pH value below 7.0 (acidic) is common in urinary tract infections, metabolic or respiratory acidosis, diets high in fruits or vegetables, or administration of some drugs; pH higher than 7.0 (basic or alkaline) is common in metabolic or respiratory alkalosis, fever, high-protein diets, and taking ascorbic acid
Protein	Protein may indicate glomerulonephritis or preeclampsia in a pregnant woman
Glucose	Small amounts of glucose may be present as result of eating a high-carbohydrate meal, stress, pregnancy, and taking some medications, such as aspirin or corticosteroids; higher levels may indicate poorly controlled diabetes, Cushing's syndrome, or infection
Ketones	Presence of ketones may indicate poorly controlled diabetes, dehydration, starvation, or ingestion of large amounts of aspirin
Blood	Blood may indicate glomerulonephritis, cancer of urinary tract, some types of anemia, taking of some medications (such as blood thinners), arsenic poisoning, reactions to transfusion, trauma, burns, and convulsions

PRACTICE AS YOU GO

B. Complete the Statement

1. The kidneys are responsible for _____ or the balance in the body.

2. The three stages of urine production are _____, _____, and _____.

3. Na⁺, K⁺, and Cl⁻ are collectively known as _____.

4. The capillary bed surrounding the renal tubules is called the _____ capillaries.

5. _____ indicates the amount of dissolved substances in urine.

6. Nitrogenous wastes are the by-products of _____ metabolism.

Terminology

Word Parts Used to Build Urinary System Terms

The following lists contain the combining forms, suffixes, and prefixes used to build terms in the remaining sections of this chapter.

Combining Forms

azot/o	nitrogenous waste		**corpor/o**	body		**hem/o**	blood
bacteri/o	bacteria		**cyst/o**	bladder, pouch		**hemat/o**	blood
bi/o	life		**glomerul/o**	glomerulus		**hydr/o**	water
carcin/o	cancer		**glycos/o**	sugar		**iatr/o**	medicine

Combining Forms (continued)

idi/o	distinctive		**noct/i**	night		**tox/o**	poison
keton/o	ketones		**olig/o**	scanty		**ur/o**	urine
lith/o	stone		**peritone/o**	peritoneum		**ureter/o**	ureter
meat/o	meatus		**protein/o**	protein		**urethr/o**	urethra
necr/o	death		**py/o**	pus		**urin/o**	urine
nephr/o	kidney		**pyel/o**	renal pelvis		**ven/o**	vein
neur/o	nerve		**ren/o**	kidney			

Suffixes

-al	pertaining to		**-lith**	stone		**-pathy**	disease
-algia	pain		**-lithiasis**	condition of stones		**-pexy**	surgical fixation
-ar	pertaining to		**-logy**	study of		**-plasty**	surgical repair
-ary	pertaining to		**-lysis**	to destroy (to break down)		**-ptosis**	drooping
-cele	protrusion		**-malacia**	abnormal softening		**-rrhagia**	abnormal flow condition
-eal	pertaining to		**-megaly**	enlarged		**-sclerosis**	hardening
-ectasis	dilated		**-meter**	instrument to measure		**-scope**	instrument to visually examine
-ectomy	surgical removal		**-oma**	tumor		**-scopy**	process of visually examining
-emia	blood condition		**-ory**	pertaining to		**-stenosis**	narrowing
-genic	producing		**-osis**	abnormal condition		**-tic**	pertaining to
-gram	record		**-ostomy**	surgically create an opening		**-tripsy**	surgical crushing
-graphy	process of recording		**-otomy**	cutting into		**-uria**	urine condition
-ic	pertaining to		**-ous**	pertaining to			
-itis	inflammation						

Prefixes

an-	without		**extra-**	outside of		**poly-**	many
anti-	against		**intra-**	within		**retro-**	backward
dys-	painful, difficult						

Adjective Forms of Anatomical Terms

Term	Word Parts	Definition
cystic (SIS-tik)	cyst/o = bladder -ic = pertaining to	Pertaining to bladder
	Word Watch The adjective *cystic* may be used to refer to the urinary bladder, the gallbladder, or a cyst.	
glomerular (gloh-MAIR-yoo-ler)	glomerul/o = glomerulus -ar = pertaining to	Pertaining to a glomerulus
meatal (mee-AY-tal)	meat/o = meatus -al = pertaining to	Pertaining to meatus
pyelitic (pye-eh-LIT-ik)	pyel/o = renal pelvis -tic = pertaining to	Pertaining to renal pelvis
renal (REE-nal)	ren/o = kidney -al = pertaining to	Pertaining to kidney
ureteral (yoo-REE-ter-al)	ureter/o = ureter -al = pertaining to	Pertaining to ureter
	Word Watch Be particularly careful when using the three very similar combining forms: **uter/o** meaning *uterus*, **ureter/o** meaning *ureter*, and **urethr/o** meaning *urethra*.	
urethral (yoo-REE-thral)	urethr/o = urethra -al = pertaining to	Pertaining to urethra
urinary (YOO-rih-nair-ee)	urin/o = urine -ary = pertaining to	Pertaining to urine

PRACTICE AS YOU GO

C. Give the adjective form for each term.

1. The ureter _____

2. The kidney _____

3. A glomerulus _____

4. Urine _____

5. The urethra _____

Pathology

Term	Word Parts	Definition
Medical Specialties		
nephrology (neh-FROL-oh-jee)	nephr/o = kidney -logy = study of	Branch of medicine involved in diagnosis and treatment of diseases and disorders of the kidney; physician is a *nephrologist*
urology (yoo-RALL-oh-jee)	ur/o = urine -logy = study of	Branch of medicine involved in diagnosis and treatment of diseases and disorders of the urinary system (and male reproductive system); physician is a *urologist*
Signs and Symptoms		
anuria (an-YOO-ree-ah)	an- = without -uria = urine condition	Complete suppression of urine formed by the kidneys and a complete lack of urine excretion
azotemia (az-oh-TEE-mee-ah)	azot/o = nitrogenous waste -emia = blood condition	Accumulation of nitrogenous waste in bloodstream; occurs when the kidney fails to filter these wastes from the blood
bacteriuria (bak-teer-ee-YOO-ree-ah)	bacteri/o = bacteria -uria = urine condition	Presence of bacteria in the urine
calculus (KAL-kyoo-lus)		Stone formed within an organ by accumulation of mineral salts; found in kidney, renal pelvis, ureters, bladder, or urethra; plural is *calculi*

■ **Figure 9-8** Photograph of sectioned kidney specimen illustrating extensive renal calculi. *(Dr. E. Walker/Science Source)*

Term	Word Parts	Definition
cystalgia (sis-TAL-jee-ah)	cyst/o = bladder -algia = pain	Urinary bladder pain

> **Word Watch**
> Be careful using the combining forms **cyst/o** meaning *bladder* and **cyt/o** meaning *cell*.

Term	Word Parts	Definition
cystolith (SIS-toh-lith)	cyst/o = bladder -lith = stone	Bladder stone
cystorrhagia (sis-toh-RAY-jee-ah)	cyst/o = bladder -rrhagia = abnormal flow condition	Abnormal bleeding from the urinary bladder
diuresis (dye-yoo-REE-sis)		Increased formation and excretion of urine
dysuria (dis-YOOR-ee-ah)	dys- = painful, difficult -uria = urine condition	Difficult or painful urination

Pathology (continued)

Term	Word Parts	Definition
enuresis (en-yoo-REE-sis)		Involuntary discharge of urine after age by which bladder control should have been established; usually occurs by age five; *nocturnal enuresis* refers to bed-wetting at night
frequency		Greater-than-normal occurrence in urge to urinate, without increase in total daily volume of urine; frequency is indication of inflammation of bladder or urethra
glycosuria (gly-koh-SOO-ree-ah)	glycos/o = sugar -uria = urine condition	Presence of sugar in the urine
hematuria (hee-mah-TOO-ree-ah)	hemat/o = blood -uria = urine condition	Presence of blood in the urine
hesitancy		Decrease in force of urine stream, often with difficulty initiating flow; often a symptom of blockage along the urethra, such as enlarged prostate gland
ketonuria (kee-toh-NYOOR-ee-ah)	keton/o = ketones -uria = urine condition	Presence of ketones in urine; occurs when body burns fat instead of glucose for energy, such as in uncontrolled diabetes mellitus
nephrolith (NEF-roh-lith)	nephr/o = kidney -lith = stone	Kidney stone
nephromalacia (nef-roh-mah-LAY-shee-ah)	nephr/o = kidney -malacia = abnormal softening	Kidney is abnormally soft
nephromegaly (nef-roh-MEG-ah-lee)	nephr/o = kidney -megaly = enlarged	Kidney is enlarged
nephrosclerosis (nef-roh-skleh-ROH-sis)	nephr/o = kidney -sclerosis = hardening	Kidney tissue has become hardened
nocturia (nok-TOO-ree-ah)	noct/i = night -uria = urine condition	Having to urinate frequently during the night
oliguria (ol-ig-YOO-ree-ah)	olig/o = scanty -uria = urine condition	Producing too little urine
polyuria (pol-ee-YOO-ree-ah)	poly- = many -uria = urine condition	Producing unusually large volume of urine
proteinuria (proh-teen-YOO-ree-ah)	protein/o = protein -uria = urine condition	Presence of protein in urine
pyuria (pye-YOO-ree-ah)	py/o = pus -uria = urine condition	Presence of pus in urine
renal colic (KOL-ik)	ren/o = kidney -al = pertaining to -ic = pertaining to	Pain caused by kidney stone; can be excruciating pain and generally requires medical treatment
stricture (STRIK-chur)		Narrowing of passageway in the urinary system
uremia (yoo-REE-mee-ah)	ur/o = urine -emia = blood condition	Accumulation of waste products (especially nitrogenous wastes) in bloodstream; associated with renal failure

Pathology (continued)

Term	Word Parts	Definition
ureterectasis (yoo-ree-ter-EK-tah-sis)	ureter/o = ureter -ectasis = dilated	Ureter is stretched out or dilated
ureterolith (yoo-REE-teh-roh-lith)	ureter/o = ureter -lith = stone	Stone in the ureter
ureterostenosis (yoo-ree-ter-oh-steh-NOH-sis)	ureter/o = ureter -stenosis = narrowing	Ureter has become narrow
urethralgia (yoo-ree-THRAL-jee-ah)	urethr/o = urethra -algia = pain	Urethral pain
urethrorrhagia (yoo-ree-throh-RAY-jee-ah)	urethr/o = urethra -rrhagia = abnormal flow condition	Abnormal bleeding from the urethra
urethrostenosis (yoo-ree-throh-steh-NOH-sis)	urethr/o = urethra -stenosis = narrowing	Urethra has become narrow
urgency (ER-jen-see)		Feeling need to urinate immediately
urinary incontinence (in-KON-tih-nens)	urin/o = urine -ary = pertaining to	Involuntary release of urine; in some patients, indwelling catheter is inserted into the bladder for continuous urine drainage

■ **Figure 9-9** Healthcare worker draining urine from a bladder catheter bag. *(Michal Heron/Pearson Education, Inc.)*

Term	Word Parts	Definition
urinary retention	urin/o = urine -ary = pertaining to	Inability to fully empty the bladder; often indicates blockage in the urethra

Kidney

Term	Word Parts	Definition
acute tubular necrosis (ATN) (neh-KROH-sis)	-ar = pertaining to necr/o = death -osis = abnormal condition	Damage to and potential death of the renal tubules due to presence of toxins in urine or to ischemia; results in oliguria
diabetic nephropathy (neh-FROP-ah-thee)	-ic = pertaining to nephr/o = kidney -pathy = disease	Accumulation of damage to the glomerulus capillaries due to chronic high blood sugars of diabetes mellitus
glomerulonephritis (gloh-mair-yoo-loh-neh-FRYE-tis)	glomerul/o = glomerulus nephr/o = kidney -itis = inflammation	Inflammation of the kidney (primarily of the glomerulus); since the glomerular membrane is inflamed, it becomes more permeable and will allow protein and blood cells to enter the filtrate; results in protein in urine (proteinuria) and hematuria

Pathology (continued)

Term	Word Parts	Definition
hydronephrosis (high-droh-neh-FROH-sis)	hydr/o = water nephr/o = kidney -osis = abnormal condition	Distention of the renal pelvis due to urine collecting in the kidney; often result of obstruction of a ureter
nephritis (neh-FRYE-tis)	nephr/o = kidney -itis = inflammation	Kidney inflammation
nephrolithiasis (nef-roh-lith-EYE-ah-sis)	nephr/o = kidney -lithiasis = condition of stones	Presence of calculi in the kidney; usually begins with solidification of salts present in urine
nephroma (neh-FROH-mah)	nephr/o = kidney -oma = tumor	Kidney tumor
nephropathy (neh-FROP-ah-thee)	nephr/o = kidney -pathy = disease	General term describing presence of kidney disease
nephroptosis (nef-rop-TOH-sis)	nephr/o = kidney -ptosis = drooping	Downward displacement of the kidney out of its normal location; commonly called a *floating kidney*
nephrotic syndrome (NS)	nephr/o = kidney -tic = pertaining to	Damage to the glomerulus resulting in protein appearing in urine, proteinuria, and corresponding decrease in protein in bloodstream; also called *nephrosis*
polycystic kidneys (pol-ee-SIS-tik)	poly- = many cyst/o = pouch -ic = pertaining to	Formation of multiple cysts (pouches) within kidney tissue; results in destruction of normal kidney tissue and uremia

■ **Figure 9-10** Photograph of a polycystic kidney on the left compared to a normal kidney on the right. *(Arthur Glauberman/ Science Source)*

Term	Word Parts	Definition
pyelitis (pye-eh-LYE-tis)	pyel/o = renal pelvis -itis = inflammation	Renal pelvis inflammation
pyelonephritis (pye-eh-loh-neh-FRYE-tis)	pyel/o = renal pelvis nephr/o = kidney -itis = inflammation	Inflammation of the renal pelvis and the kidney; one of most common types of kidney disease; may be result of lower urinary tract infection that moved up to the kidney by way of the ureter; large quantities of white blood cells and bacteria in urine are possible; blood (hematuria) may even be present in urine in this condition; can occur with any untreated or persistent case of cystitis
renal cell carcinoma	ren/o = kidney -al = pertaining to carcin/o = cancer -oma = tumor	Cancerous tumor that arises from kidney tubule cells

Pathology (continued)

Term	Word Parts	Definition
renal failure	ren/o = kidney -al = pertaining to	Inability of the kidneys to filter wastes from the blood, resulting in uremia; may be acute or chronic; major reason for patient being placed on dialysis
Wilms' tumor (VILMZ)		Malignant kidney tumor found most often in children; also called *nephroblastoma*
Urinary Bladder		
bladder cancer		Cancerous tumor that arises from cells lining the bladder; major sign is hematuria
bladder neck obstruction (BNO)		Blockage of the bladder outlet; often caused by enlarged prostate gland in males
cystitis (sis-TYE-tis)	cyst/o = bladder -itis = inflammation	Urinary bladder inflammation
cystocele (SIS-toh-seel)	cyst/o = bladder -cele = protrusion	Protrusion (or herniation) of the urinary bladder into wall of the vagina
interstitial cystitis (in-ter-STISH-al / sis-TYE-tis)	-al = pertaining to cyst/o = bladder -itis = inflammation	Disease of unknown cause in which there is inflammation and irritation of the bladder; most commonly seen in middle-aged women
neurogenic bladder (noo-roh-JEN-ik)	neur/o = nerve -genic = producing	Loss of nervous control that leads to retention; may be caused by spinal cord injury or multiple sclerosis
urinary tract infection (UTI)	urin/o = urine -ary = pertaining to	Infection, usually from bacteria, of any organ of the urinary system; most often begins with cystitis and may ascend into ureters and kidneys; most common in women because of shorter urethra

PRACTICE AS YOU GO

D. Terminology Matching

Match each term to its definition.

1. _____ Wilms' tumor
2. _____ azotemia
3. _____ urinary retention
4. _____ nephroptosis
5. _____ nocturia
6. _____ incontinence
7. _____ hydronephrosis
8. _____ urgency
9. _____ nephrolithiasis
10. _____ polycystic kidney disease

a. kidney stones
b. feeling need to urinate immediately
c. childhood malignant kidney tumor
d. swelling of kidney due to urine collecting in renal pelvis
e. involuntary release of urine
f. frequent urination at night
g. excess nitrogenous waste in bloodstream
h. inability to fully empty bladder
i. a floating kidney
j. multiple cysts in the kidneys

Diagnostic Procedures

Term	Word Parts	Definition
Clinical Laboratory Tests		
albumin/creatinine ratio (ACR)		Screening test for persons at risk (e.g., diabetics) for developing kidney disease; measures amount of albumin and creatinine in urine; there is a high level of albumin in the blood, but almost none is excreted in urine; creatinine, a waste product of muscle metabolism, is excreted into urine at a relatively constant rate; if ratio of these two substances increases, it is an early warning sign of kidney disease
blood urea nitrogen (BUN) (yoo-REE-ah / NIGH-troh-jen)		Blood test to measure kidney function by level of nitrogenous waste (urea) in the blood
clean catch specimen (CC) **Word Watch** Note that the abbreviation for clean catch uses capital letters. Lower case, cc, is the abbreviation for chief complaint.		Urine sample obtained after cleaning off urinary opening and catching or collecting a urine sample in midstream (halfway through urination process) to minimize contamination from genitalia
creatinine clearance (kree-AT-in-in)		Test of kidney function; creatinine is a waste product cleared from bloodstream by the kidneys; for this test, urine is collected for 24 hours, and amount of creatinine in urine is compared to amount of creatinine that remains in bloodstream
estimated glomerular filtration rate (eGFR) (gloh-MAIR-yoo-ler)	glomerul/o = glomerulus -ar = pertaining to	Test to measure kidney function; measures level of creatinine, a waste product of muscle metabolism, in urine and uses this in a formula that estimates how well glomeruli are filtering water out of bloodstream
urinalysis (U/A, UA) (yoo-rih-NAL-ih-sis)	urin/o = urine -lysis = to destroy (to break down)	Laboratory test consisting of physical, chemical, and microscopic examination of urine
urine culture and sensitivity (C&S)		Laboratory test of urine for bacterial infection; attempt to grow bacteria on culture medium in order to identify it and determine to which antibiotics it is sensitive
urinometer (yoor-ih-NOM-eh-ter)	urin/o = urine -meter = instrument to measure	Instrument to measure specific gravity of urine; part of urinalysis
Diagnostic Imaging		
cystogram (SIS-toh-gram)	cyst/o = bladder -gram = record	X-ray record of the urinary bladder
cystography (sis-TOG-rah-fee)	cyst/o = bladder -graphy = process of recording	Process of instilling contrast material or dye into the bladder by catheter to visualize the urinary bladder on X-ray

Diagnostic Procedures (continued)

Term	Word Parts	Definition
excretory urography (EU) (EKS-kreh-tor-ee / yoo-ROG-rah-fee)	-ory = pertaining to ur/o = urine -graphy = process of recording	Injecting dye into bloodstream and then taking X-ray to trace action of the kidney as it excretes dye in the urine
intravenous pyelography (IVP) (in-trah-VEE-nus / pye-eh-LOG-rah-fee)	intra- = within ven/o = vein -ous = pertaining to pyel/o = renal pelvis -graphy = process of recording	Diagnostic X-ray procedure in which dye is injected into a vein and then X-rays are taken to visualize the renal pelvis as dye is removed by the kidney
kidneys, ureters, bladder (KUB)		X-ray taken of the abdomen demonstrating kidneys, ureters, and bladder without using any contrast dye; also called *flat-plate abdomen*
nephrogram (NEF-roh-gram)	nephr/o = kidney -gram = record	X-ray record of the kidney
pyelogram (PYE-eh-loh-gram)	pyel/o = renal pelvis -gram = record	X-ray record of the renal pelvis
retrograde pyelography (RP) (RET-roh-grayd / pye-eh-LOG-rah-fee)	retro- = backward pyel/o = renal pelvis -graphy = process of recording	Diagnostic X-ray procedure in which dye is inserted through the urethra to outline bladder, ureters, and renal pelvis

■ **Figure 9-11** Retrograde pyelogram X-ray. Radiopaque dye outlines urinary bladder, ureters, and renal pelvis. Bladder, right kidney, and both ureters appear normal. Left kidney appears abnormal. *(Jarva Jar/ Shutterstock)*

Term	Word Parts	Definition
voiding cystourethrography (VCUG) (sis-toh-yoo-ree-THROG-rah-fee)	cyst/o = bladder urethr/o = urethra -graphy = process of recording	X-ray taken to visualize the urethra while patient is voiding after contrast dye is placed in the bladder

Endoscopic Procedure

Term	Word Parts	Definition
cystoscope (SIS-toh-skohp)	cyst/o = bladder -scope = instrument to visually examine	Instrument used to visually examine inside of the urinary bladder
cystoscopy (cysto) (sis-TOSS-koh-pee)	cyst/o = bladder -scopy = process of visually examining	Visual examination of the urinary bladder using instrument called *cystoscope*
urethroscope (yoo-REE-throh-skohp)	urethr/o = urethra -scope = instrument to visually examine	Instrument to visually examine inside of the urethra

Therapeutic Procedures

Term	Word Parts	Definition
Medical Treatments		
catheter (KATH-eh-ter)		Flexible tube inserted into body for purpose of moving fluids into or out of body; most commonly refers to tube threaded through the urethra into the bladder to withdraw urine (see again Figure 9-9)
catheterization (cath) (kath-eh-ter-ih-ZAY-shun)		Insertion of tube through the urethra and into the urinary bladder for purpose of withdrawing urine or inserting dye
extracorporeal shockwave lithotripsy (ESWL) (eks-trah-kor-POR-ee-al / shockwave / LITH-oh-trip-see)	extra- = outside of corpor/o = body -eal = pertaining to lith/o = stone -tripsy = surgical crushing	Use of ultrasound waves from outside the body to break up stones; process does not require invasive surgery

— Beam focused on kidney stones

— Shockwave generator

— Reflector

■ **Figure 9-12** Extracorporeal shockwave lithotripsy, a noninvasive procedure using high-frequency sound waves to shatter kidney stones.

Term	Word Parts	Definition
hemodialysis (HD) (hee-moh-dye-AL-ih-sis)	hem/o = blood	Use of artificial kidney machine that filters the blood of a person to remove waste products; use of this technique in patients who have defective kidneys is lifesaving

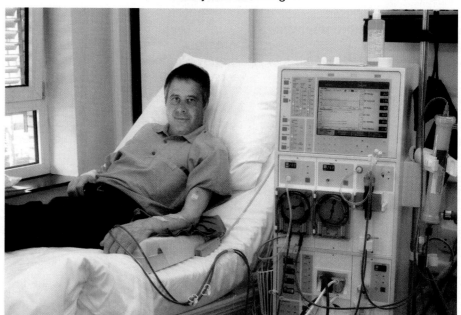

■ **Figure 9-13** Patient undergoing hemodialysis. Patient's blood passes through hemodialysis machine for cleansing and is then returned to the body. *(Gopixa/Shutterstock)*

Therapeutic Procedures (continued)

Term	Word Parts	Definition
peritoneal dialysis (pair-ih-toh-NEE-al / dye-AL-ih-sis)	peritone/o = peritoneum -al = pertaining to	Removal of toxic waste substances from body by placing warm, chemically balanced solutions into peritoneal cavity; wastes are filtered out of blood across peritoneum; used in treating renal failure and certain poisonings

Collecting tube

Peritoneal cavity

Position of bag to receive used dialysis fluid

■ **Figure 9-14** Peritoneal dialysis. Chemically balanced solution is placed into the abdominal cavity to draw impurities out of the bloodstream. It is removed after several hours.

Surgical Treatments

Term	Word Parts	Definition
cystectomy (sis-TEK-toh-mee)	cyst/o = bladder -ectomy = surgical removal	Surgical removal of the urinary bladder
cystopexy (SIS-toh-pek-see)	cyst/o = bladder -pexy = surgical fixation	Surgical fixation of the urinary bladder; performed to correct cystocele
cystoplasty (SIS-toh-plas-tee)	cyst/o = bladder -plasty = surgical repair	To repair a defect in the urinary bladder by surgical means
cystostomy (sis-TOSS-toh-mee)	cyst/o = bladder -ostomy = surgically create an opening	To surgically create opening into the urinary bladder through the abdominal wall
cystotomy (sis-TOT-oh-mee)	cyst/o = bladder -otomy = cutting into	To cut into the urinary bladder
lithotomy (lith-OT-oh-mee)	lith/o = stone -otomy = cutting into	To cut into an organ for purpose of removing a stone
lithotripsy (LITH-oh-trip-see)	lith/o = stone -tripsy = surgical crushing	Physical destruction of a stone in urinary system by crushing or sound waves
meatotomy (mee-ah-TOT-oh-mee)	meat/o = meatus -otomy = cutting into	To cut into the meatus in order to enlarge opening of the urethra
nephrectomy (neh-FREK-toh-mee)	nephr/o = kidney -ectomy = surgical removal	Surgical removal of a kidney

Therapeutic Procedures (continued)

Term	Word Parts	Definition
nephrolithotomy (nef-roh-lith-OT-oh-mee)	nephr/o = kidney lith/o = stone -otomy = cutting into	To cut into the kidney in order to remove stones
nephropexy (NEF-roh-pek-see)	nephr/o = kidney -pexy = surgical fixation	Surgical fixation of a kidney to anchor it in its normal anatomical position
nephrostomy (neh-FROS-toh-mee)	nephr/o = kidney -ostomy = surgically create an opening	To surgically create an opening into the kidney through the abdominal wall
nephrotomy (neh-FROT-oh-mee)	nephr/o = kidney -otomy = cutting into	To cut into the kidney
pyeloplasty (PYE-eh-loh-plas-tee)	pyel/o = renal pelvis -plasty = surgical repair	To repair the renal pelvis by surgical means
renal transplant	ren/o = kidney -al = pertaining to	Surgical placement of a donor kidney

Transplanted kidney

Internal iliac artery and vein

Grafted ureter

External iliac artery and vein

■ **Figure 9-15** Figure illustrates location utilized for implantation of donor kidney.

PRACTICE AS YOU GO

E. Procedure Matching

Match each procedure term with its definition.

1. _____ clean catch specimen
2. _____ hemodialysis
3. _____ pyeloplasty
4. _____ urinometer
5. _____ lithotripsy
6. _____ cystoscopy
7. _____ catheter
8. _____ kidneys, ureters, bladder

a. measures specific gravity

b. abdominal X-ray

c. visual examination of the bladder

d. a flexible tube inserted into the body

e. removes waste products from blood

f. method of obtaining urine sample

g. crushing of a stone

h. surgical repair of the renal pelvis

Pharmacology

Vocabulary

Term	Word Parts	Definition
antidote (AN-tih-doht)	anti- = against	Substance that will neutralize poisons or their side effects
iatrogenic (eye-ah-troh-JEN-ik)	iatr/o = physician, medicine, treatment -genic = producing	Usually unfavorable response resulting from physician's actions, taking of medication, or a treatment
idiosyncrasy (id-ee-oh-SIN-krah-see)	idi/o = distinctive	Unusual or abnormal response to drug or food
side effect		Response to drug other than effect desired; also called *adverse reaction*
toxicity (tok-SISS-ih-tee)	tox/o = poison	Extent or degree to which a substance is poisonous

Drugs

Classification	Word Parts	Action	Examples
antibiotic	anti- = against bi/o = life -tic = pertaining to	Used to treat bacterial infections of the urinary tract	ciprofloxacin, Cipro; nitrofurantoin, Macrobid
antispasmodic (an-tye-spaz-MOD-ik)	anti- = against -ic = pertaining to	Used to prevent or reduce bladder muscle spasms	oxybutynin, Ditropan; neostigmine, Prostigmine
diuretic (dye-yoo-REH-tik)	-tic = pertaining to	Increases volume of urine produced by the kidneys; useful in treatment of edema, kidney failure, heart failure, and hypertension	furosemide, Lasix; spironolactone, Aldactone

Abbreviations

ACR	albumin/creatinine ratio	**C&S**	culture and sensitivity
AGN	acute glomerulonephritis	**cysto**	cystoscopy
AKI	acute kidney injury	**eGFR**	estimated glomerular filtration rate
ARF	acute renal failure	**ESRD**	end-stage renal disease
ATN	acute tubular necrosis	**ESWL**	extracorporeal shockwave lithotripsy
BNO	bladder neck obstruction	**EU**	excretory urography
BUN	blood urea nitrogen	**GU**	genitourinary
CAPD	continuous ambulatory peritoneal dialysis	**HCO_3^-**	bicarbonate
cath	catheterization	**HD**	hemodialysis
CC	clean catch urine specimen	**H_2O**	water
Cl⁻	chloride	**I&O**	intake and output
CRF	chronic renal failure	**IPD**	intermittent peritoneal dialysis

Abbreviations (continued)

IVP	intravenous pyelogram	**NS**	nephrotic syndrome
K⁺	potassium	**pH**	acidity or alkalinity of urine
KUB	kidneys, ureters, bladder	**RP**	retrograde pyelogram
mcg	microgram	**SG, sp. gr.**	specific gravity
mEq	milliequivalent	**U/A, UA**	urinalysis
mg	milligram	**UC**	urine culture
mL	milliliter	**UTI**	urinary tract infection
Na⁺	sodium	**VCUG**	voiding cystourethrography

PRACTICE AS YOU GO

F. What Does it Stand For?

1. KUB _____

2. cath _____

3. cysto _____

4. GU _____

5. ESWL _____

6. UTI _____

7. UC _____

8. RP _____

9. ARF _____

10. BUN _____

11. CRF _____

12. H₂O _____

Chapter Review

Real-World Applications

Medical Record Analysis

This Discharge Summary contains 13 medical terms. Underline each term and write it in the list below the report. Then explain each term as you would to a nonmedical person.

Discharge Summary

Admitting Diagnosis:	Severe right side pain and hematuria
Final Diagnosis:	Pyelonephritis right kidney, complicated by chronic cystitis
History of Present Illness:	Patient has long history of frequent bladder infections, but denies any recent lower pelvic pain or dysuria. Earlier today he had rapid onset of severe right side pain and is unable to stand fully erect. His temperature was 101°F, and his skin was sweaty and flushed. He was admitted from the ER for further testing and diagnosis.
Summary of Hospital Course:	Clean catch urinalysis revealed gross hematuria and pyuria, but no albuminuria. A culture and sensitivity was ordered to identify the pathogen and an antibiotic was started. Cystoscopy showed evidence of chronic cystitis, bladder irritation, and a bladder neck obstruction. The obstruction appears to be congenital and the probable cause of the chronic cystitis. The patient was catheterized to ensure complete emptying of the bladder, and fluids were encouraged. Patient responded well to the antibiotic therapy and fluids, and his symptoms improved.
Discharge Plans:	Patient was discharged home after three days in the hospital. He was switched to an oral antibiotic for the pyelonephritis and chronic cystitis. A repeat urinalysis is scheduled for next week. After all inflammation is corrected, will repeat cystoscopy to reevaluate bladder neck obstruction.

Term	Explanation
1. _____	_____
2. _____	_____
3. _____	_____
4. _____	_____
5. _____	_____
6. _____	_____
7. _____	_____
8. _____	_____
9. _____	_____
10. _____	_____
11. _____	_____
12. _____	_____
13. _____	_____

Chart Note Transcription

The chart note below contains 11 phrases that can be reworded with a medical term presented in this chapter. Each phrase is identified with an underline. Determine the medical term and write your answers in the space provided.

Pearson General Hospital Consultation Report

Task   Edit   View   Time Scale   Options   Help Download   Archive   Date: 17 May 2017

Current Complaint: A 36-year-old male was seen by the <u>specialist in the treatment of diseases of the urinary system</u> **1** because of right flank pain and <u>blood in the urine</u>. **2**

Past History: Patient has a history of <u>bladder infection</u>; **3** denies experiencing any symptoms for two years.

Signs and Symptoms: <u>A technique used to obtain an uncontaminated urine sample</u> **4** obtained for <u>laboratory analysis of the urine</u> **5** revealed blood in the urine, but no <u>pus in the urine</u>. **6** A <u>kidney X-ray made after inserting dye into the bladder</u> **7** was normal on the left, but dye was seen filling the right <u>tube between the kidney and bladder</u> **8** only halfway to the kidney.

Diagnosis: <u>Stone in the tube between the kidney and the bladder</u> **9** on the right

Treatment: Patient underwent <u>the use of ultrasound waves to break up stones</u>. **10** Pieces of dissolved <u>kidney stones</u> **11** were flushed out, after which symptoms resolved.

1. _____

2. _____

3. _____

4. _____

5. _____

6. _____

7. _____

8. _____

9. _____

10. _____

11. _____

Case Study

Below is a case study presentation of a patient with a condition discussed in this chapter. Read the case study and answer the questions below. Some questions will ask for information not included within this chapter. Use your text, a medical dictionary, or any other reference material you choose to answer these questions.

(Gina Smith/Shutterstock)

A 32-year-old female is seen in the urologist's office because of a fever, chills, and generalized fatigue. She also reported urgency, frequency, dysuria, and hematuria. In addition, she noticed that her urine was cloudy with a fishy odor. The physician ordered the following tests: a clean catch specimen for a U/A, a urine C&S, and a KUB. The U/A revealed pyuria, bacteriuria, and a slightly acidic pH. A common type of bacteria was grown in the culture. X-rays reveal acute pyelonephritis resulting from cystitis, which has spread up to the kidney from the bladder. The patient was placed on an antibiotic and encouraged to "push fluids" by drinking two liters of water a day.

Questions

1. This patient has two urinary system infections in different locations; name them. Which one caused the other and how?

2. List and define each of the patient's presenting symptoms in your own words.

3. What diagnostic tests did the urologist order? Describe them in your own words.

4. Explain the results of each diagnostic test in your own words.

5. What were the physician's treatment instructions for this patient? Explain the purpose of each treatment.

6. Describe the normal appearance of urine.

Practice Exercises

A. Word Building Practice

The combining form **nephr/o** refers to *kidney*. Use it to write a term that means:

1. surgical fixation of the kidney _____

2. X-ray record of the kidney _____

3. condition of kidney stones _____

4. removal of a kidney _____

5. inflammation of the kidney _____

6. kidney disease _____

7. hardening of the kidney _____

The combining form **cyst/o** refers to the *urinary bladder*. Use it to write a term that means:

8. inflammation of the bladder _____

9. abnormal flow condition from the bladder _____

10. surgical repair of the bladder _____

11. instrument to view inside the bladder _____

12. bladder pain _____

The combining form **pyel/o** refers to the *renal pelvis*. Use it to write a term that means:

13. surgical repair of the renal pelvis _____

14. inflammation of the renal pelvis _____

15. X-ray record of the renal pelvis _____

The combining form **ureter/o** refers to one or both of the *ureters*. Use it to write a term that means:

16. a ureteral stone _____

17. ureter dilation _____

18. ureter narrowing _____

The combining form **urethr/o** refers to the *urethra*. Use it to write a term that means:

19. urethra inflammation _____

20. instrument to view inside the urethra _____

The suffix **-uria** refers to a *urine condition*. Use it to write a term that means:

21. condition of scanty urine _____

22. condition of blood in the urine _____

23. condition of protein in the urine _____

24. condition of sugar in the urine _____

25. condition of pus in the urine _____

B. Complete the Term

For each definition given below, fill in the blank with the word part that completes the term.

Definition	Term
1. surgical fixation of the bladder	_____ pexy
2. surgical crushing of a stone	_____ tripsy
3. surgical repair of renal pelvis	_____ plasty
4. to destroy (break down) urine	_____ lysis
5. drooping kidney	nephro _____
6. pus urine condition	py _____
7. dilated ureter	_____ ectasis
8. inflammation of kidney glomerulus	_____ nephritis
9. cutting into the meatus	_____ otomy
10. pain in the urethra	_____ algia

C. Pharmacology Challenge

Fill in the classification for each drug description, then match the brand name.

Drug Description	Classification	Brand Name
1. _____ Reduces bladder muscle spasms	_____	a. Lasix
2. _____ Treats bacterial infections	_____	b. Ditropan
3. _____ Increases volume of urine produced	_____	c. Cipro

D. Define the Term

1. micturition _____

2. diuretic _____

3. renal colic _____

4. catheterization _____

5. pyelitis _____

6. glomerulonephritis _____

7. lithotomy _____

8. enuresis _____

9. meatotomy _____

10. diabetic nephropathy _____

11. urinalysis _____

12. hesitancy _____

E. Name that Term

1. absence of urine _____

2. blood in the urine _____

3. kidney stone _____

4. crushing a stone _____

5. inflammation of the urethra _____

6. pus in the urine _____

7. bacteria in the urine _____

8. painful urination _____

9. ketones in the urine _____

10. protein in the urine _____

11. (too) much urine _____

F. Using Abbreviations

Fill in each blank with the appropriate abbreviation.

1. During _____ an artificial kidney machine filters waste from the blood.

2. _____ breaks up kidney stones without surgery.

3. A(n) _____ was performed to look for the source of bladder bleeding.

4. Manuel was concerned about having a(n) _____ because he is allergic to the dye injected into a vein.

5. A(n) _____ is an X-ray also called a flat-plate abdomen.

6. The _____ showed no bacteria growing in the urine.

7. The _____ was caused by an enlarged prostate gland.

8. Her _____ began as simple cystitis, but ascended the ureters and infected her kidneys.

G. Fill in the Blank

renal transplant	ureterectomy	intravenous pyelogram (IVP)
cystostomy	pyelolithectomy	nephropexy
renal biopsy	cystoscopy	urinary tract infection

1. Juan suffered from chronic renal failure. His sister, Maria, donated one of her normal kidneys to him, and he

   had a(n) _____.

2. Anesha's floating kidney needed surgical fixation. Her physician performed a surgical procedure

   known as _____.

3. Kenya's physician stated that she had a general infection that he referred to as a UTI. The full name for this infection is _____.

4. Surgeons operated on Robert to remove calculi from his renal pelvis. The name of this surgery is _____.

5. Charles had to have a small piece of his kidney tissue removed so that the physician could perform a microscopic evaluation. This procedure is called a(n) _____.

6. Naomi had to have one of her ureters removed due to a stricture. This procedure is called _____.

7. The physician had to create a temporary opening between Eric's bladder and his abdominal wall. This procedure is called _____.

8. Sally's bladder was visually examined using a special instrument. This procedure is called a(n) _____.

9. The doctors believe that Jacob has a tumor of the right kidney. They are going to do a test called a(n) _____ that requires them to inject a radiopaque contrast medium intravenously so that they can see the kidney on X-ray.

H. Anatomical Adjectives

Fill in the blank with the missing noun or adjective.

Noun	Adjective
1. _____	cystic
2. ureter	_____
3. _____	urinary
4. kidney	_____
5. _____	glomerular
6. _____	pyelitic
7. meatus	_____
8. urethra	_____

I. Spelling Practice

Some of the following terms are misspelled. Identify the incorrect terms and spell them correctly in the blank provided.

1. glycosuria   _____
2. nephrosklerosis   _____
3. cystorrhagia   _____
4. ureterectasis   _____
5. incontinance   _____

6. hydronephrosis _____

7. cystoseal _____

8. cathaterization _____

9. hemodialysis _____

10. lithotripsey _____

J. Complete the Statement

1. The by-products of muscle metabolism, _____, are removed from the body in urine.

2. The filtration stage of urine production takes place in the _____.

3. The kidneys regulate the levels of _____, such as sodium and potassium.

4. The folds in the lining of the bladder are called _____.

5. The nephron loop is also known as the _____.

6. There is one _____ leading away from the urinary bladder and two _____ leading into it.

7. In the kidney, the renal artery enters and the renal vein and ureter exit at the _____.

8. The outer portion of the kidney is the _____ and the inner area is the

   _____.

MyLab Medical Terminology™

MyLab Medical Terminology is a premium online homework management system that includes a host of features to help you study. Registered users will find:

- A multitude of activities and assignments built within the MyLab platform

- Powerful tools that track and analyze your results—allowing you to create a personalized learning experience

- Videos and audio pronunciations to help enrich your progress

- Streaming lesson presentations (Guided Lectures) and self-paced learning modules

- A space where you and your instructors can check your progress and manage your assignments

Labeling Exercises

Image A

Write the labels for this figure on the numbered lines provided.

1. _____

2. _____

3. _____

4. _____

5. _____

Image B

Write the labels for this figure on the numbered lines provided.

1. _____

2. _____

3. _____

4. _____

5. _____

6. _____

7. _____

Image C

Write the labels for this figure on the numbered lines provided.

7. _____

1. _____

2. _____

3. _____

4. _____

5. _____

6. _____

8. _____

9. _____

10. _____

Chapter 10

Reproductive System

Learning Objectives

Upon completion of this chapter, you will be able to

1. Identify and define the combining forms, suffixes, and prefixes introduced in this chapter.

2. Correctly spell and pronounce medical terms and major anatomical structures relating to the reproductive systems.

3. Locate and describe the major organs of the reproductive systems and their functions.

4. Use medical terms to describe circumstances relating to pregnancy.

5. Identify and define reproductive system anatomical terms.

6. Identify and define selected reproductive system pathology terms.

7. Identify the symptoms and origin of sexually transmitted diseases.

8. Identify and define selected reproductive system diagnostic procedures.

9. Identify and define selected reproductive system therapeutic procedures.

10. Identify and define selected medications relating to the reproductive systems.

11. Define selected abbreviations associated with the reproductive systems.

(Pearson Education, Inc.)

AT A GLANCE

Function

The female reproductive system produces ova (the female reproductive cells), provides a location for fertilization and growth of a baby, and secretes female sex hormones. In addition, the breasts produce milk to nourish the newborn.

Organs

The primary structures that comprise the female reproductive system:

ovaries	vagina
uterine tubes	vulva
uterus	breasts

Word Parts

Presented here are the most common word parts (with their meanings) used to build female reproductive system terms. For a more comprehensive list, refer to the Terminology section of this chapter.

Combining Forms

amni/o	amnion	mast/o	breast
cervic/o	neck, cervix	men/o	menses, menstruation
chori/o	chorion	metr/o	uterus
colp/o	vagina	nat/o	birth
culd/o	cul-de-sac	o/o	egg
dilat/o	to widen	oophor/o	ovary
embry/o	embryo	ov/o, ov/i	ovum
episi/o	vulva	ovari/o	ovary
estr/o	female	pareun/o	sexual intercourse
fet/o	fetus	perine/o	perineum
gynec/o	female	radic/o	root
hymen/o	hymen	salping/o	uterine (fallopian) tubes
hyster/o	uterus	uter/o	uterus
lact/o	milk	vagin/o	vagina
mamm/o	breast	vulv/o	vulva

Suffixes

-arche	beginning	-para	to bear (offspring)
-cyesis	state of pregnancy	-partum	childbirth
-genesis	produces	-salpinx	uterine tube
-gravida	pregnant woman	-tocia	labor, childbirth

Prefixes

ante-	before, in front of	primi-	first
contra-	against		

Female Reproductive System Illustrated

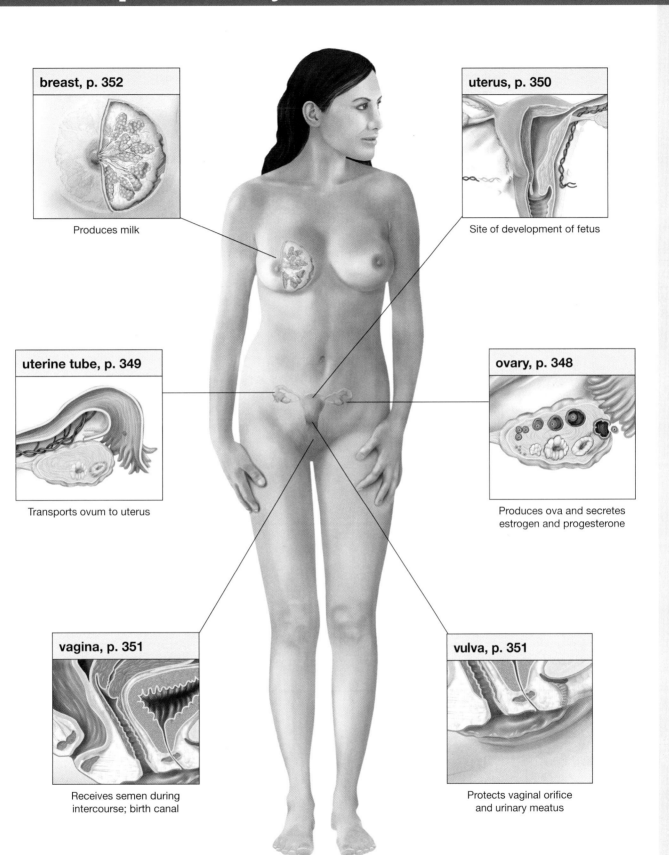

breast, p. 352

Produces milk

uterus, p. 350

Site of development of fetus

uterine tube, p. 349

Transports ovum to uterus

ovary, p. 348

Produces ova and secretes estrogen and progesterone

vagina, p. 351

Receives semen during intercourse; birth canal

vulva, p. 351

Protects vaginal orifice and urinary meatus

Anatomy and Physiology of the Female Reproductive System

breasts	sex hormones
fertilization	uterine tubes (YOO-ter-in)
genitalia (jen-ih-TAY-lee-ah)	uterus (YOO-ter-us)
ova (OH-vah)	vagina (vah-JIGH-nah)
ovaries (OH-vah-reez)	vulva (VUL-vah)
pregnancy	

The female reproductive system plays many vital functions that ensure the continuation of the human race. First, it produces **ova**, the female reproductive cells. It then provides a place for **fertilization** to occur and for a baby to grow during **pregnancy**. The **breasts** provide nourishment for the newborn. Finally, this system secretes the female **sex hormones**.

This system consists of both internal and external **genitalia**, or reproductive organs (see Figure 10-1 ■). The internal genitalia are located in the pelvic cavity and consist of the **uterus**, two **ovaries**, two **uterine tubes**, and the **vagina**, which extends to the external surface of the body. The external genitalia are collectively referred to as the **vulva**.

What's In A Name?

Look for these word parts:
genit/o = genitals
-al = pertaining to

Corpus (body) of uterus
Cervix
Vagina
Rectum

Uterine (fallopian) tube
Ovary
Fundus of uterus
Urinary bladder
Symphysis pubis
Clitoris
Urethra
Labium majora
Labium minora

■ **Figure 10-1**   The female reproductive system, sagittal view showing organs of the system in relation to the urinary bladder and rectum.

Med Term Tip

The singular for egg is *ovum*. The plural term for many eggs is *ova*. The term *ova* is not used exclusively when discussing the human reproductive system. For instance, testing the stool for ova and parasites is used to detect the presence of parasites or their ova in the digestive tract, a common cause for severe diarrhea. Ova are produced in the ovary by a process called *oogenesis* (**o/o** = egg and **-genesis** = produces).

Internal Genitalia

Ovaries

estrogen (ESS-troh-jen)	oocyte (OH-oh-sight)
follicle-stimulating hormone (FALL-ih-kl)	ovulation (ov-yoo-LAY-shun)
luteinizing hormone (LOO-teh-nigh-zing)	progesterone (proh-JES-ter-ohn)

There are two ovaries, one located on each side of the uterus within the pelvic cavity (see again Figure 10-1). These are small almond-shaped glands that produce ova (singular is *ovum*) and the female sex hormones (see Figure 10-2 ■). In humans approximately every 28 days hormones from the anterior pituitary,

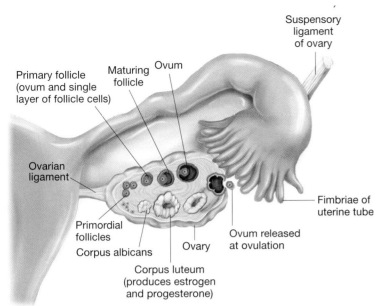

Suspensory ligament of ovary

Primary follicle (ovum and single layer of follicle cells)

Maturing follicle

Ovum

Ovarian ligament

Primordial follicles

Corpus albicans

Ovary

Ovum released at ovulation

Corpus luteum (produces estrogen and progesterone)

Fimbriae of uterine tube

■ **Figure 10-3** Photomicrograph of human ovary showing ovum in its follicle prior to ovulation.
(Anna Jurkovska/Shutterstock)

■ **Figure 10-2** Structure of the ovary and uterine (fallopian) tube. Figure illustrates stages of ovum development and the relationship of the ovary to the uterine tube.

follicle-stimulating hormone (FSH) and **luteinizing hormone** (LH), stimulate maturation of an ovum and trigger **ovulation**, the process by which one ovary releases an ovum (or **oocyte**) (see Figure 10-3 ■). The principal female sex hormones produced by the ovaries, **estrogen** and **progesterone**, stimulate the lining of the uterus to be prepared to receive a fertilized ovum. These hormones are also responsible for the female secondary sexual characteristics.

Uterine Tubes

conception (kon-SEP-shun)

fallopian tubes (fah-LOH-pee-an)

fimbriae (FIM-bree-ee)

oviducts (OH-vih-dukts)

The uterine tubes, also called the **fallopian tubes** or **oviducts**, are approximately 4 inches (10 cm) long and run from the area around each ovary to either side of the upper portion of the uterus (see Figure 10-4 ■ and Figure 10-5 ■). As they near the ovaries, the unattached ends of these two tubes expand into finger-like projections called **fimbriae**. The fimbriae catch an ovum after ovulation and direct it into

> **What's In A Name?**
>
> Look for these word parts:
> **estr/o** = female
> **o/o** = egg
> **ov/o** = ovum
> **-cyte** = cell
> **-gen** = that which produces
> **pro-** = before

> **What's In A Name?**
>
> Look for this word part:
> **ov/i** = ovum

> **Med Term Tip**
>
> When the fertilized egg adheres or implants to the uterine tube instead of moving into the uterus, a condition called *tubal pregnancy* exists. There is not enough room in the uterine tube for the fetus to grow normally. Implantation of the fertilized egg in any location other than the uterus is called an *ectopic pregnancy. Ectopic* is a general term meaning *in the wrong place.*

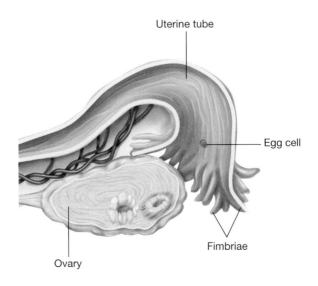

Uterine tube

Egg cell

Fimbriae

Ovary

■ **Figure 10-4** Uterine (fallopian) tube, showing released ovum within the uterine tube.

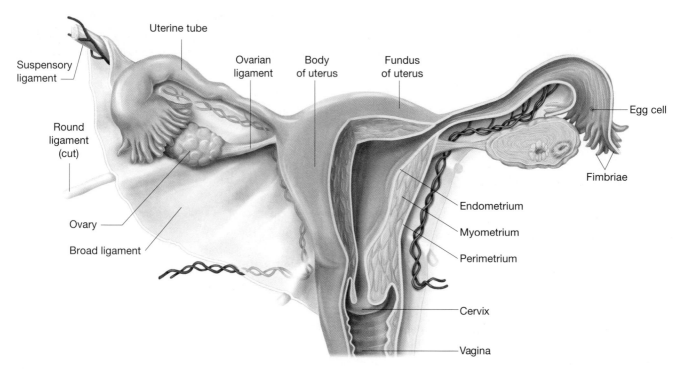

Figure 10-5 The uterus. Cutaway view shows regions of the uterus and cervix and its relationship to the uterine (fallopian) tubes and vagina.

the uterine tube. The uterine tube can then propel the ovum from the ovary to the uterus so that it can implant. The meeting of the egg and sperm, called fertilization or **conception**, normally takes place within the upper one-half of the uterine tubes.

Uterus

anteflexion (an-tee-FLEK-shun)
cervix (SER-viks)
corpus (KOR-pus)
endometrium (en-doh-MEE-tree-um)
fundus (FUN-dus)
menarche (men-AR-kee)

menopause (MEN-oh-pawz)
menstrual period (MEN-stroo-al)
menstruation (men-stroo-AY-shun)
myometrium (my-oh-MEE-tree-um)
perimetrium (pair-ih-MEE-tree-um)
puberty (PYOO-ber-tee)

The uterus is a hollow, pear-shaped organ that contains a thick muscular wall, a mucous membrane lining, and a rich supply of blood (see again Figure 10-5). Located in the center of the pelvic cavity between the bladder and the rectum, it is normally bent slightly forward, which is called **anteflexion**, and is held in position by strong fibrous ligaments anchored in the outer layer of the uterus, called the **perimetrium** (see again Figure 10-5). The uterus has three sections: the **fundus** or upper portion, between where the uterine tubes connect to the uterus; **corpus** or body, which is the central portion; and **cervix** (Cx), or lower portion, also called the neck of the uterus, which opens into the vagina.

The inner layer, or **endometrium**, of the uterine wall contains a rich blood supply. The endometrium reacts to hormonal changes every month that prepare it to receive a fertilized ovum. In a normal pregnancy the fertilized ovum implants in the endometrium, which can then provide nourishment and protection for the developing fetus. Contractions of the thick muscular walls of the uterus, called the **myometrium**, assist in propelling the fetus through the birth canal at delivery.

If a pregnancy is not established, most of the endometrium is sloughed off, resulting in **menstruation** or the **menstrual period**. During a pregnancy, the lining of the uterus does not leave the body but remains to nourish the fetus. A girl's first menstrual period occurs during **puberty** (the sequence of events by which

What's In A Name?

Look for these word parts:
flex/o = to bend
men/o = menses
metr/o = uterus
my/o = muscle
-al = pertaining to
-arche = beginning
-ion = action
ante- = in front of
endo- = inner
peri- = around

Med Term Tip

During pregnancy, the height of the fundus is an important measurement for estimating the stage of pregnancy and the size of the fetus. Following birth, massaging the fundus with pressure applied in a circular pattern stimulates the uterine muscle to contract to help stop bleeding. Patients may be more familiar with a common term for uterus, *womb.* However, the correct medical term is *uterus.*

a child becomes a young adult capable of reproduction) and is called **menarche**. In the United States, the average age for menarche is 12½ years. The ending of menstrual activity and childbearing years is called **menopause**. This generally occurs between the ages of 40 and 55.

Vagina

Bartholin's glands (BAR-toh-linz)   vaginal orifice (VAJ-in-al / OR-ih-fis)
hymen (HIGH-men)

The vagina is a muscular tube lined with mucous membrane that extends from the cervix of the uterus to the outside of the body (see Figure 10-6 ■). The vagina allows for the passage of the menstrual flow. In addition, during intercourse, it receives the male's penis and semen, which is the fluid containing sperm. The vagina also serves as the birth canal through which the baby passes during a normal vaginal birth.

The **hymen** is a thin membranous tissue that partially covers the external vaginal opening or **vaginal orifice**. This membrane may be broken by the use of tampons, during physical activity, or during sexual intercourse. A pair of glands (called **Bartholin's glands**) are located on either side of the vaginal orifice and secrete mucus for lubrication during intercourse.

Vulva

clitoris (KLIT-oh-ris)   labia minora (LAY-bee-ah / mih-NOR-ah)
erectile tissue (ee-REK-tile)   perineum (pair-ih-NEE-um)
labia majora (LAY-bee-ah / mah-JOR-ah)   urinary meatus (YOO-rih-nair-ee / mee-AY-tus)

The vulva is a general term that refers to the group of structures that make up the female external genitalia. The **labia majora** and **labia minora** are paired folds of skin (each side of the pair would use the singular labium majora or labium minora) that serve as protection for the genitalia, the vaginal orifice, and the **urinary meatus** (see Figure 10-7 ■). Since the urinary tract and the reproductive organs are located in proximity to one another and each contains mucous membranes that can transport infection, there is a danger of infection entering the urinary tract. The **clitoris** is a small organ containing sensitive **erectile tissue** that is aroused during sexual stimulation and corresponds to the glans penis in the male. The region between the vaginal orifice and the anus is referred to as the **perineum**.

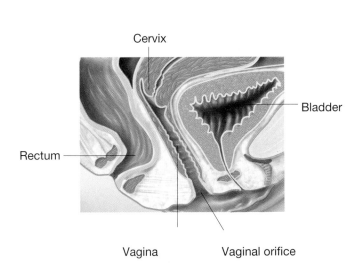

■ **Figure 10-6** The vagina, sagittal section showing the location of the vagina and its relationship to the cervix, uterus, rectum, and bladder.

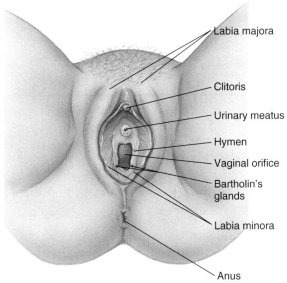

■ **Figure 10-7** The vulva, illustrating how the labia majora and labia minora cover and protect the vaginal orifice, clitoris, and urinary meatus.

Breast

areola (ah-REE-oh-lah)   mammary glands (MAM-ah-ree)

lactation (lak-TAY-shun)   nipple

lactiferous ducts (lak-TIF-er-us)   nurse

lactiferous glands (lak-TIF-er-us)

<table>
<tr><td>What's In A Name?</td></tr>
<tr><td>Look for these word parts:
lact/o = milk
mamm/o = breast
-ous = pertaining to
-ary = pertaining to</td></tr>
</table>

The breasts, or **mammary glands**, play a vital role in the reproductive process because they produce milk, a process called **lactation**, to nourish the newborn. The size of the breasts, which varies greatly from woman to woman, has no bearing on the ability to **nurse** or feed a baby. Milk is produced by the **lactiferous glands** and is carried to the **nipple** by the **lactiferous ducts** (see Figure 10-8 ■). The **areola** is the pigmented area around the nipple. As long as the breast is stimulated by the nursing infant, the breast will continue to secrete milk.

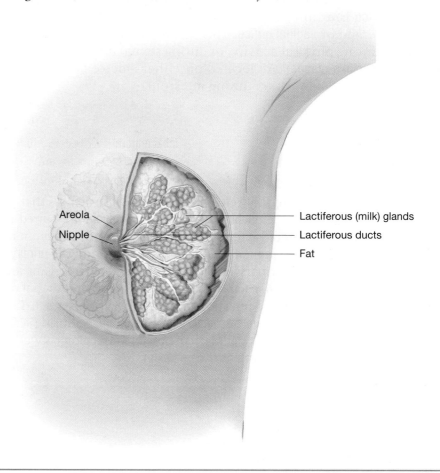

Areola
Nipple
Lactiferous (milk) glands
Lactiferous ducts
Fat

■ **Figure 10-8** The breast, cutaway view showing both internal and external features.

PRACTICE AS YOU GO

A. Complete the Statement

1. The tubes that extend from the outer edges of the uterus and assist in transporting the ova and sperm are called _____.

2. The external genitalia of the female reproductive system are collectively called the _____.

3. The principal sex hormones secreted by the ovaries are _____ and _____.

4. The cessation of menstruation is called _____.

5. The female sex cell is a(n) _____.

6. The inner lining of the uterus is called the _____.

7. The _____ is a membrane that may be broken by the use of tampons.

8. The process of _____ produces milk to nourish the infant.

Pregnancy

amnion (AM-nee-on)
amniotic fluid (am-nee-OT-ik)
chorion (KOH-ree-on)
embryo (EM-bree-oh)
fetus (FEE-tus)

gestation (jess-TAY-shun)
placenta (plah-SEN-tah)
premature
umbilical cord (um-BIL-ih-kal)

Pregnancy refers to the period of time during which a fetus grows and develops in its mother's uterus (see Figure 10-9 ■). The normal length of time for a pregnancy (**gestation**) is 40 weeks. If a baby is born before completing at least 37 weeks of gestation, it is considered **premature**.

During pregnancy, the female body undergoes many changes. In fact, all of the body systems become involved in the development of a healthy infant. From

What's In A Name?
Look for these word parts:
-al = pertaining to
pre- = before

■ **Figure 10-9** A full-term pregnancy. Image illustrates position of the fetus and the structures associated with pregnancy.

■ **Figure 10-10** Computer rendering illustrating the development of an embryo. *(u3d/Shutterstock)*

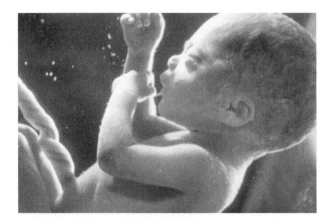

■ **Figure 10-11** Photograph illustrating the development of a fetus. *(Petit Format/Science Source)*

the time the fertilized egg implants in the uterus until approximately the end of the eighth week, the infant is referred to as an **embryo** (see Figure 10-10 ■). During this period all the major organs and body systems are formed. Following the embryo stage and lasting until birth, the infant is called a **fetus** (see Figure 10-11 ■). During this time, the longest period of gestation, the organs mature and begin to function.

The fetus receives nourishment from its mother by way of the **placenta**, which is a spongy, blood-filled organ that forms in the uterus next to the fetus. The placenta is commonly referred to as the afterbirth because it is delivered through the birth canal after the birth of a baby. The fetus is attached to the placenta by way of the **umbilical cord** and is surrounded by two membranous sacs, the **amnion** and the **chorion**. The amnion is the innermost sac, and it holds the **amniotic fluid** in which the fetus floats. The chorion is an outer, protective sac and also forms part of the placenta.

Labor and Delivery

breech presentation
crowning
delivery
dilation stage (dye-LAY-shun)
effacement (eh-FAYS-ment)

expulsion stage (eks-PUL-shun)
labor
parturition (par-tyoo-RISH-un)
placental stage (plah-SEN-tal)

Labor and **delivery**, or **parturition**, is the actual process of expelling the fetus from the uterus and through the vagina. The first stage is referred to as the **dilation stage**, in which the uterine muscle contracts strongly to expel the fetus (see Figure 10-12A ■). During this process the fetus presses on the cervix and causes it to dilate or expand. As the cervix dilates, it also becomes thinner, referred to as **effacement**. When the cervix is completely dilated to 10 centimeters, the second stage of labor begins (see Figure 10-12B ■). This is the **expulsion stage** and ends with delivery of the baby. Generally, the head of the baby appears first, which is referred to as **crowning**. In some cases, the baby's buttocks will appear first, and this is referred to as a **breech presentation** (see Figure 10-13 ■). The last stage of labor is the **placental stage** (see Figure 10-12C ■). Immediately after childbirth, the uterus continues to contract, causing the placenta to be expelled through the vagina.

A

DILATION STAGE:
Uterine contractions dilate cervix

B

EXPULSION STAGE:
Birth of baby or expulsion

■ **Figure 10-12**   The stages of labor and delivery. A) During the dilation stage the cervix thins and dilates to 10 cm. B) During the expulsion stage the infant is delivered. C) During the placental stage the placenta is delivered.

C

PLACENTAL STAGE:
Delivery of placenta

■ **Figure 10-13**   A breech birth. This image illustrates a newborn that has been delivered buttocks first.

PRACTICE AS YOU GO

B. Complete the Statement

1. The organ that provides nourishment to the fetus is the _____. The fetus is attached to it by the _____.

2. The time required for the development of a fetus is called _____.

3. The three stages of labor and delivery are the _____ stage, the _____ stage, and the _____ stage.

4. _____ refers to the head of the infant appearing in the birth canal.

5. In a(n) _____ presentation, the buttocks of the infant appear first.

6. The two membranous sacs surrounding the fetus are the _____ and _____.

Terminology

Word Parts Used to Build Female Reproductive System Terms

The following lists contain the combining forms, suffixes, and prefixes used to build terms in the remaining sections of this chapter.

Combining Forms

abdomin/o	abdomen	**hem/o**	blood	**or/o**	mouth
amni/o	amnion	**hemat/o**	blood	**ovari/o**	ovary
bi/o	life	**hymen/o**	hymen	**pareun/o**	sexual intercourse
carcin/o	cancer	**hyster/o**	uterus	**pelv/o**	pelvis
cervic/o	cervix	**lact/o**	milk	**perine/o**	perineum
chori/o	chorion	**lapar/o**	abdomen	**py/o**	pus
colp/o	vagina	**later/o**	side	**radic/o**	root
culd/o	cul-de-sac	**leuk/o**	white	**rect/o**	rectum
cyst/o	urinary bladder	**mamm/o**	breast	**salping/o**	uterine tube
dilat/o	to widen	**mast/o**	breast	**son/o**	sound
embry/o	embryo	**men/o**	menstruation	**tox/o**	poison
episi/o	vulva	**metr/o**	uterus	**uter/o**	uterus
fet/o	fetus	**nat/o**	birth	**vagin/o**	vagina
fibr/o	fibers	**olig/o**	scanty	**vulv/o**	vulva
gynec/o	female	**oophor/o**	ovary		

Suffixes

-al	pertaining to	**-ar**	pertaining to	**-centesis**	puncture to withdraw fluid
-algia	pain	**-ary**	pertaining to		
-an	pertaining to	**-cele**	protrusion	**-cyesis**	pregnancy

Suffixes (continued)

-ectomy	surgical removal	**-lytic**	destruction	**-rrhagia**	abnormal flow condition
-emesis	vomiting	**-nic**	pertaining to	**-rrhaphy**	suture
-gram	record	**-oid**	resembling	**-rrhea**	discharge
-graphy	process of recording	**-oma**	tumor	**-rrhexis**	rupture
		-opsy	view of	**-salpinx**	uterine tube
-gravida	pregnant woman	**-osis**	abnormal condition	**-scope**	instrument for viewing
-ia	condition	**-otomy**	cutting into		
-iasis	abnormal condition	**-ous**	pertaining to	**-scopy**	process of viewing
		-para	to bear	**-tic**	pertaining to
-ic	pertaining to	**-partum**	childbirth	**-tocia**	labor and childbirth
-ine	pertaining to	**-pexy**	surgical fixation		
-itis	inflammation	**-plasty**	surgical repair		
-logy	study of				

Prefixes

a-	without	hyper-	excessive	peri-	around
ante-	before	in-	not	post-	after
bi-	two	intra-	within	pre-	before
contra-	against	multi-	many	primi-	first
dys-	painful	neo-	new	pseudo-	false
endo-	inner, within	nulli-	none	ultra-	beyond

Adjective Forms of Anatomical Terms

Term	Word Parts	Definition
amniotic (am-nee-OT-ik)	amni/o = amnion -tic = pertaining to	Pertaining to amnion
cervical (SER-vih-kal)	cervic/o = cervix -al = pertaining to	Pertaining to cervix
chorionic (kor-ee-ON-ik)	chori/o = chorion -nic = pertaining to	Pertaining to chorion
embryonic (em-bree-ON-ik)	embry/o = embryo -nic = pertaining to	Pertaining to embryo
endometrial (en-doh-MEE-tree-al)	endo- = inner metr/o = uterus -al = pertaining to	Pertaining to inner lining of uterus

> **Word Watch**
>
> Extra caution must be used in spelling terms containing **metr/o**. This combining form often uses an "**i**" for its combining vowel instead of the more common "**o**."

Term	Word Parts	Definition
fetal (FEE-tal)	fet/o = fetus -al = pertaining to	Pertaining to fetus
fibrous (FYE-bruss)	fibr/o = fibers -ous = pertaining to	Pertaining to having fibers

Adjective Forms of Anatomical Terms (continued)

Term	Word Parts	Definition
lactic (LAK-tik)	lact/o = milk -ic = pertaining to	Pertaining to milk
mammary (MAM-ah-ree)	mamm/o = breast -ary = pertaining to	Pertaining to breast
ovarian (oh-VAIR-ee-an)	ovari/o = ovary -an = pertaining to	Pertaining to ovary
perineal (pair-ih-NEE-al)	perine/o = perineum -al = pertaining to	Pertaining to perineum
uterine (YOO-ter-in)	uter/o = uterus -ine = pertaining to	Pertaining to uterus
vaginal (VAJ-in-al)	vagin/o = vagina -al = pertaining to	Pertaining to vagina
vulvar (VUL-var)	vulv/o = vulva -ar = pertaining to	Pertaining to vulva

PRACTICE AS YOU GO

C. Give the adjective form for each anatomical structure.

1. The embryo _____

2. The fetus _____

3. The uterus _____

4. An ovary _____

5. A breast _____

6. The vagina _____

Pregnancy Terms

Term	Word Parts	Definition
antepartum (an-tee-PAR-tum)	ante- = before -partum = childbirth	Period of time before birth
colostrum (kuh-LOS-trum)		Thin fluid first secreted by the breast after delivery; does not contain much protein, but is rich in antibodies
fraternal twins	-al = pertaining to	Twins that develop from two different ova fertilized by two different sperm; although twins, these siblings do not have identical DNA
identical twins	-al = pertaining to	Twins that develop from splitting of one fertilized ovum, these siblings have exactly the same DNA
meconium (meh-KOH-nee-um)		First bowel movement of newborn; greenish-black in color and consists of mucus and bile

Pregnancy Terms (continued)

Term	Word Parts	Definition
multigravida (mull-tih-GRAV-ih-dah)	multi- = many -gravida = pregnant woman	Woman who has been pregnant many (two or more) times
multipara (mull-TIP-ah-rah)	multi- = many -para = to bear	Woman who has given birth to live infant many (two or more) times
neonate (NEE-oh-nayt)	neo- = new nat/o = birth	Term for newborn baby
nulligravida (null-ih-GRAV-ih-dah)	nulli- = none -gravida = pregnant woman	Woman who has not been pregnant
nullipara (null-IP-ah-rah)	nulli- = none -para = to bear	Woman who has not given birth to a live infant
postpartum (post-PAR-tum)	post- = after -partum = childbirth	Period of time shortly after birth
primigravida (GI, grav I) (prye-mih-GRAV-ih-dah)	primi- = first -gravida = pregnant woman	Woman who is pregnant for the first time
primipara (PI, para I) (prye-MIP-ah-rah)	primi- = first -para = to bear	Woman who has given birth to a live infant once

Pathology

Term	Word Parts	Definition
Medical Specialties		
gynecology (GYN, gyn) (gigh-neh-KALL-oh-jee)	gynec/o = female -logy = study of	Branch of medicine specializing in diagnosis and treatment of conditions of the female reproductive system; physician is called a *gynecologist*
neonatology (nee-oh-nay-TALL-oh-jee)	neo- = new nat/o = birth -logy = study of	Branch of medicine specializing in diagnosis and treatment of conditions involving newborns; physician is called a *neonatologist*
obstetrics (OB) (ob-STET-riks)		Branch of medicine specializing in diagnosis and treatment of women during pregnancy and childbirth and immediately after childbirth; physician is called an *obstetrician*
Signs and Symptoms		
amenorrhea (ah-men-oh-REE-ah)	a- = without men/o = menstruation -rrhea = flow	Condition of having no menstrual flow
amniorrhea (am-nee-oh-REE-ah)	amni/o = amnion -rrhea = flow	Flow of amniotic fluid when amnion ruptures
dysmenorrhea (dis-men-oh-REE-ah)	dys- = painful men/o = menstruation -rrhea = flow	Condition of having painful menstrual flow
dyspareunia (dis-pah-ROO-nee-ah)	dys- = painful pareun/o = sexual intercourse -ia = condition	Condition of having painful sexual intercourse
dystocia (dis-TOH-see-ah)	dys- = abnormal, difficult -tocia = labor and childbirth	Difficult labor and childbirth

Pathology (continued)

Term	Word Parts	Definition
hematosalpinx (hee-mah-toh-SAL-pinks)	hemat/o = blood -salpinx = uterine tube	Presence of blood in a uterine tube
leukorrhea (loo-koh-REE-ah)	leuk/o = white -rrhea = discharge	Whitish or yellowish vaginal discharge; may be caused by vaginal infection
mastalgia (mas-TAL-jee-ah)	mast/o = breast -algia = pain	Breast pain
menorrhagia (men-oh-RAY-jee-ah)	men/o = menstruation -rrhagia = abnormal flow condition	Condition of having abnormally heavy menstrual flow during normal menstruation time
metrorrhagia (mee-troh-RAY-jee-ah)	metr/o = uterus -rrhagia = abnormal flow condition	Term used to describe uterine bleeding between menstrual periods
metrorrhea (mee-troh-REE-ah)	metr/o = uterus -rrhea = discharge	Having discharge (such as mucus or pus) from the uterus that is not the menstrual flow
oligomenorrhea (ol-ih-goh-men-oh-REE-ah)	olig/o = scanty men/o = menstruation -rrhea = flow	Condition of having light menstrual flow
Ovary		
oophoritis (oh-of-or-EYE-tis)	oophor/o = ovary -itis = inflammation	Inflammation of the ovary
ovarian carcinoma (oh-VAIR-ee-an / kar-sih-NOH-mah)	ovari/o = ovary -an = pertaining to carcin/o = cancer -oma = tumor	Cancer of the ovary
ovarian cyst (oh-VAIR-ee-an / SIST)	ovari/o = ovary -an = pertaining to	Cyst that develops within the ovary; may be multiple cysts and may rupture, causing pain and bleeding
Uterine Tubes		
pyosalpinx (pye-oh-SAL-pinks)	py/o = pus -salpinx = uterine tube	Presence of pus in a uterine tube
salpingitis (sal-pin-JIGH-tis)	salping/o = uterine tube -itis = inflammation	Inflammation of a uterine tube
Uterus		
cervical cancer (SER-vih-kal)	cervic/o = cervix -al = pertaining to	Malignant growth in the cervix; main cause is infection by *human papillomavirus* (HPV), a sexually transmitted virus for which there is now a vaccine; Pap smear tests have helped to detect early cervical cancer
endocervicitis (en-doh-ser-vih-SIGH-tis)	endo- = within cervic/o = cervix -itis = inflammation	Inflammation that occurs within the cervix
endometrial cancer (en-doh-MEE-tree-al)	endo- = inner metr/o = uterus -al = pertaining to	Cancer of endometrial lining of the uterus
endometritis (en-doh-meh-TRYE-tis)	endo- = inner metr/o = uterus -itis = inflammation	Inflammation of endometrium (inner layer of the uterine wall)

Word Watch

Be careful when using the combining form **metr/o** meaning *uterus* and the suffix **-metry** meaning *process of measuring*.

Pathology (continued)

Term	Word Parts	Definition
fibroid tumor (FIGH-broyd / TOO-mer)	fibr/o = fibers -oid = resembling	Benign tumor or growth that contains fiberlike tissue; uterine fibroid tumors are the most common benign tumors in women of childbearing age

Under the perimetrium

Within the myometrium

Under the endometrium

■ **Figure 10-14** Common sites for the development of fibroid tumors.

Term	Word Parts	Definition
hysterorrhexis (hiss-ter-oh-REK-sis)	hyster/o = uterus -rrhexis = rupture	Rupture of the uterus; may occur during labor
menometrorrhagia (men-oh-mee-troh-RAY-jee-ah)	men/o = menstruation metr/o = uterus -rrhagia = abnormal flow condition	Excessive bleeding during menstrual period and at intervals between menstrual periods
premenstrual syndrome (PMS) (pree-MEN-stroo-al / SIN-drohm)	pre- = before men/o = menstruation -al = pertaining to	Symptoms that develop just prior to onset of a menstrual period, which can include irritability, headache, tender breasts, and anxiety
prolapsed uterus (proh-LAPST / YOO-ter-us)		Fallen uterus that can cause the cervix to protrude through the vaginal opening; generally caused by weakened muscles from vaginal delivery or as a result of pelvic tumors pressing down

Vagina

Term	Word Parts	Definition
candidiasis (kan-dih-DYE-ah-sis)	-iasis = abnormal condition	Yeast infection of the skin and mucous membranes that can result in white plaques on tongue and vagina

> **Med Term Tip**
> The term *candida* comes from a Latin term meaning *dazzling white*. Candida is the scientific name for yeast and refers to the very white discharge that is the hallmark of a yeast infection.

Term	Word Parts	Definition
cystocele (SIS-toh-seel)	cyst/o = urinary bladder -cele = protrusion	Hernia or outpouching of the bladder that protrudes into the vagina; may cause urinary frequency and urgency
rectocele (REK-toh-seel)	rect/o = rectum -cele = protrusion	Protrusion or herniation of the rectum into the vagina
toxic shock syndrome (TSS)	tox/o = poison -ic = pertaining to	Rare and sometimes fatal staphylococcus infection that generally occurs in menstruating women; initial infection occurs in vagina and associated with prolonged wearing of super-absorbent tampon; toxins secreted by bacteria then enter bloodstream

Pathology (continued)

Term	Word Parts	Definition
vaginitis (vaj-ih-NIGH-tis)	vagin/o = vagina -itis = inflammation	Inflammation of the vagina
Pelvic Cavity		
endometriosis (en-doh-mee-tree-OH-sis)	endo- = within metr/o = uterus -osis = abnormal condition	Abnormal condition of endometrium tissue appearing throughout pelvis or on abdominal wall; tissue normally found within the uterus
pelvic inflammatory disease (PID) (PEL-vik / in-FLAM-ah-tor-ee)	pelv/o = pelvis -ic = pertaining to	Chronic or acute infection, usually bacterial, that has ascended through female reproductive organs and out into pelvic cavity; may result in scarring that interferes with fertility
perimetritis (pair-ih-meh-TRYE-tis)	peri- = around metr/o = uterus -itis = inflammation	Inflammation in pelvic cavity around outside of the uterus
Breast		
breast cancer		Malignant tumor of the breast; usually forms in milk-producing gland tissue or lining of the milk ducts

Adipose

Cysts

Lactiferous glands

Tumor

Lactiferous glands

A

B

■ **Figure 10-15** Comparison of breast cancer and fibrocystic disease. A) Breast with a malignant tumor growing in the lactiferous gland and duct. B) The location of a fibrocystic lump in the adipose tissue covering the breast.

Term	Word Parts	Definition
fibrocystic breast disease (figh-broh-SIS-tik)	fibr/o = fibers cyst/o = pouch -ic = pertaining to	Benign cysts forming in the breast (see Figure 10-15B ■)
lactorrhea (lak-toh-REE-ah)	lact/o = milk -rrhea = discharge	Discharge of milk from the breast other than normal lactation; any white discharge from a nipple
mastitis (mas-TYE-tis)	mast/o = breast -itis = inflammation	Inflammation of the breast
Pregnancy		
abruptio placentae (ah-BRUP-shee-oh / plah-SEN-tee)		Emergency condition in which the placenta tears away from uterine wall prior to delivery of infant; requires immediate delivery of baby
eclampsia (eh-KLAMP-see-ah)	-ia = condition	Further worsening of preeclampsia symptoms with addition of seizures and coma; may occur between 20th week of pregnancy and up to six weeks postpartum

Pathology (continued)

Term	Word Parts	Definition
hemolytic disease of the newborn (HDN) (hee-moh-LIT-ik)	hem/o = blood -lytic = destruction	Condition developing in baby when mother's blood type is Rh-negative and baby's blood is Rh-positive; antibodies in mother's blood enter fetus' bloodstream through placenta and destroy fetus' red blood cells, causing anemia, jaundice, and enlargement of liver and spleen; treatment is early diagnosis and blood transfusion; also called *erythroblastosis fetalis*
hyperemesis gravidarum (high-per-EM-eh-sis / grav-ih-DAIR-um)	hyper- = excessive -emesis = vomiting	Severe nausea and vomiting during pregnancy; may cause dangerous level of dehydration and weight loss; may require hospitalization

> **Med Term Tip**
> This term uses *gravidarum* as a free-standing word rather than a suffix. It also uses the plural form meaning *pregnant women* (rather than the singular *gravida*).

Term	Word Parts	Definition
infertility	in- = not	Inability to produce children; generally defined as no pregnancy after properly timed intercourse for one year
placenta previa (plah-SEN-tah / PREE-vee-ah)		A placenta that is implanted in lower portion of the uterus and, in turn, blocks birth canal

Figure 10-16 Placenta previa, longitudinal section showing the placenta growing over the opening into the cervix.

Umbilical cord
Fetus
Placenta
Severe bleeding

Term	Word Parts	Definition
preeclampsia (pree-eh-KLAMP-see-ah)	pre- = before	Metabolic disease of pregnancy; if untreated, may progress to eclampsia; symptoms include hypertension, headaches, albumin in urine, and edema; may occur between 20th week of pregnancy and up to six weeks postpartum; also called *toxemia* or *pregnancy-induced hypertension* (PIH)
prolapsed umbilical cord (proh-LAPST / um-BIL-ih-kal)		When the umbilical cord of baby is expelled first during delivery and is squeezed between baby's head and vaginal wall; presents emergency situation since baby's circulation is compromised
pseudocyesis (soo-doh-sigh-EE-sis)	pseudo- = false -cyesis = pregnancy	Condition in which body reacts as if there is a pregnancy (especially hormonal changes), but there is no pregnancy

Pathology (continued)

Term	Word Parts	Definition
salpingocyesis (sal-ping-goh-sigh-EE-sis)	salping/o = uterine tube -cyesis = pregnancy	Pregnancy that occurs in the uterine tube instead of in the uterus
spontaneous abortion **Med Term Tip** The term *abortion* (AB) has different meanings for medical professionals and the general population. The general population equates the term *abortion* specifically with the planned termination of a pregnancy. However, to the medical community, *abortion* is a broader medical term meaning that a pregnancy has ended before a fetus is *viable*, meaning before it can live on its own.		Unplanned loss of a pregnancy due to death of embryo or fetus before time it is viable, commonly referred to as *miscarriage*
stillbirth		Birth in which a viable-aged fetus dies shortly before or at the time of delivery

PRACTICE AS YOU GO

D. Terminology Matching

Match each term to its definition.

1. _____ hemolytic disease of the newborn
2. _____ dysmenorrhea
3. _____ breech presentation
4. _____ abruptio placentae
5. _____ eclampsia
6. _____ pyosalpinx
7. _____ fibroid
8. _____ candidiasis
9. _____ lactorrhea
10. _____ neonate

a. seizures and coma during pregnancy
b. erythroblastosis fetalis
c. detached placenta
d. yeast infection
e. abnormal discharge from breast
f. newborn
g. buttocks first to appear in birth canal
h. painful menstruation
i. pus in the uterine tube
j. benign tumor

Diagnostic Procedures

Term	Word Parts	Definition
Clinical Laboratory Tests		
human papillomavirus (HPV) DNA test (pap-ih-LOH-mah-vigh-russ)		Examination of sample of cervical tissue, obtained by swabbing or scraping cervix, to determine infection by virus responsible for cervical cancer

Diagnostic Procedures (continued)

Term	Word Parts	Definition
Pap (Papanicolaou) **smear** (pap-ah-NIK-oh-lao)		Test for early detection of cancer of the cervix named after developer of test, George Papanicolaou, a Greek physician; a scraping of cells is removed from the cervix for examination under microscope
pregnancy test (PREG-nan-see)		Chemical test that can determine pregnancy during first few weeks; can be performed in physician's office or with home-testing kit
vaginal smear wet mount (VAJ-in-al)	vagin/o = vagina -al = pertaining to	Microscopic examination of cells obtained by swabbing vaginal wall; used to diagnose candidiasis
Diagnostic Imaging		
hysterosalpingography (HSG) (hiss-ter-oh-sal-pin-GOG-rah-fee)	hyster/o = uterus salping/o = uterine tube -graphy = process of recording	Taking of X-ray after injecting radiopaque material into uterus and uterine tubes
mammogram (MAM-oh-gram)	mamm/o = breast -gram = record	X-ray record of the breast
mammography (mam-OG-rah-fee)	mamm/o = breast -graphy = process of recording	X-ray to diagnose breast disease, especially breast cancer
pelvic ultrasonography (PEL-vik / ul-trah-son-OG-rah-fee)	pelv/o = pelvis -ic = pertaining to ultra- = beyond son/o = sound -graphy = process of recording	Use of high-frequency sound waves to produce image or photograph of an organ, such as uterus, ovaries, or fetus
Endoscopic Procedures		
colposcope (KOL-poh-skohp)	colp/o = vagina -scope = instrument for viewing	Instrument used to view inside the vagina
colposcopy (kol-POS-koh-pee)	colp/o = vagina -scopy = process of viewing	Examination of vagina using instrument called *colposcope*
culdoscopy (kul-DOS-koh-pee)	culd/o = cul-de-sac -scopy = process of viewing	Examination of a blind pouch-like area of the female pelvic cavity located posterior to the uterus, by introducing endoscope through wall of the vagina
laparoscope (LAP-ah-roh-skohp)	lapar/o = abdomen -scope = instrument for viewing	Instrument used to view inside abdomen
laparoscopy (lap-ar-OSS-koh-pee)	lapar/o = abdomen -scopy = process of viewing	Examination of peritoneal cavity using an instrument called a *laparoscope*; instrument is passed through small incision made by surgeon into abdominopelvic cavity

■ **Figure 10-17** Illustration depicting a laparoscopic examination of the uterus, ovaries, and uterine tubes. *(Medical Art Inc/Shutterstock)*

Diagnostic Procedures (continued)

Term	Word Parts	Definition
Obstetrical Diagnostic Procedures		
amniocentesis (am-nee-oh-sen-TEE-sis)	amni/o = amnion -centesis = puncture to withdraw fluid	Puncturing of amniotic sac using needle and syringe for purpose of withdrawing amniotic fluid for testing; can assist in determining fetal maturity, development, and genetic disorders
Apgar score (AP-gar)		Evaluation of neonate's adjustment to outside world; observes color, heart rate, muscle tone, respiratory rate, and response to stimulus at one minute and five minutes after birth
chorionic villus sampling (CVS) (kor-ee-ON-ik / VILL-us)	chori/o = chorion -nic = pertaining to	Removal of a small piece of chorion for genetic analysis; may be done at earlier stage of pregnancy than amniocentesis
fetal monitoring (FEE-tal)	fet/o = fetus -al = pertaining to	Using electronic equipment placed on mother's abdomen or fetus' scalp to check fetal heart rate (FHR) (also called fetal heart tone [FHT]) during labor; normal heart rate of fetus is rapid, ranging from 120 to 160 beats per minute; a drop in fetal heart rate indicates fetus is in distress
Additional Diagnostic Procedures		
cervical biopsy (SER-vih-kal / BYE-op-see)	cervic/o = cervix -al = pertaining to bi/o = life -opsy = view of	Taking a sample of tissue from the cervix to test for presence of cancer cells
endometrial biopsy (EMB) (en-doh-MEE-tree-al / BYE-op-see)	endo- = inner metr/o = uterus -al = pertaining to bi/o = life -opsy = view of	Taking a sample of tissue from lining of the uterus to test for abnormalities
pelvic examination (PEL-vik)	pelv/o = pelvis -ic = pertaining to	Physical examination of the vagina and adjacent organs performed by physician placing fingers of one hand into the vagina in order to visually examine vagina and cervix and to obtain cervical cells for Pap smear; instrument called *speculum* is used to open the vagina

■ **Figure 10-18** A speculum used to hold the vagina open in order to visualize the cervix. *(Patrick Watson/Pearson Education, Inc.)*

Therapeutic Procedures

Term	Word Parts	Definition
Medical Procedures		
barrier contraception (kon-trah-SEP-shun)	contra- = against	Prevention of pregnancy using a device to prevent sperm from meeting an ovum; examples include condoms, diaphragms, and cervical caps
hormonal contraception	-al = pertaining to contra- = against	Use of hormones to block ovulation and prevent conception; may be in form of a pill, a patch, an implant under the skin, or an injection
intrauterine device (IUD) (in-trah-YOO-ter-in)	intra- = within uter/o = uterus -ine = pertaining to	Device inserted into the uterus by physician for purpose of contraception

■ **Figure 10-19** Photograph illustrating the shape of two different intrauterine devices (IUDs). The intrauterine portion is approximately 1–1/4 inches long. The thin thread attached to the end of the device extends through the cervix into the vagina. This allows a woman to check that the IUD remains properly in place. *(Jules Selmes and Debi Treloar/Dorling Kindersley Media Library)*

Term	Word Parts	Definition
Surgical Procedures		
amniotomy (am-nee-OT-oh-mee)	amni/o = amnion -otomy = cutting into	Surgically cutting open the amnion; commonly referred to as *breaking the water*
cervicectomy (ser-vih-SEK-toh-mee)	cervic/o = cervix -ectomy = surgical removal	Surgical removal of the cervix
cesarean section (CS, C-section) (seh-SAIR-ee-an)		Surgical delivery of baby through incision into abdominal and uterine walls; legend has it that Roman emperor Julius Caesar was first person born by this method
conization (kon-ih-ZAY-shun)		Surgical removal of a core of cervical tissue; also refers to partial removal of the cervix
dilation and curettage (D&C) (dye-LAY-shun / kyoo-reh-TAZH)	dilat/o = to widen	Surgical procedure in which opening of the cervix is dilated and the uterus is scraped or suctioned of its lining or tissue; often performed after spontaneous abortion and to stop excessive bleeding from other causes
elective abortion		Legal termination of a pregnancy for nonmedical reasons
episiorrhaphy (eh-peez-ee-OR-ah-fee)	episi/o = vulva -rrhaphy = suture	To suture the perineum; postpartum procedure to repair episiotomy or any tearing of the perineum that occurred during birth; note that combining form **episi/o** is used even though the perineum is not part of the vulva
episiotomy (eh-peez-ee-OT-oh-mee)	episi/o = vulva -otomy = cutting into	Surgical incision of the perineum to facilitate delivery process; can prevent irregular tearing of tissue during birth; note that combining form **episi/o** is used even though the perineum is not part of the vulva

Therapeutic Procedures (continued)

Term	Word Parts	Definition
hymenectomy (high-men-EK-toh-mee)	hymen/o = hymen -ectomy = surgical removal	Surgical removal of the hymen
hysterectomy (hiss-ter-EK-toh-mee)	hyster/o = uterus -ectomy = surgical removal	Surgical removal of the uterus
hysteropexy (HISS-ter-oh-pek-see)	hyster/o = uterus -pexy = surgical fixation	To surgically anchor the uterus to its proper location in pelvic cavity; treatment for prolapsed uterus
laparotomy (lap-ah-ROT-oh-mee)	lapar/o = abdomen -otomy = cutting into	To cut open abdomen; performed in order to complete other surgical procedures inside abdomen or performed during a C-section
lumpectomy (lum-PEK-toh-mee)	-ectomy = surgical removal	Removal of only a breast tumor and tissue immediately surrounding it
mammoplasty (MAM-oh-plas-tee)	mamm/o = breast -plasty = surgical repair	Surgical repair or reconstruction of the breast
mastectomy (mas-TEK-toh-mee)	mast/o = breast -ectomy = surgical removal	Surgical removal of the breast
oophorectomy (oh-of-or-EK-toh-mee)	oophor/o = ovary -ectomy = surgical removal	Surgical removal of the ovary
radical mastectomy (mas-TEK-toh-mee)	radic/o = root -al = pertaining to mast/o = breast -ectomy = surgical removal	Surgical removal of breast tissue plus chest muscles and axillary lymph nodes; term *radical* is used to describe extensive surgical procedures designed to remove root cause of disease
salpingectomy (sal-pin-JEK-toh-mee)	salping/o = uterine tube -ectomy = surgical removal	Surgical removal of a uterine tube
simple mastectomy (mas-TEK-toh-mee)	mast/o = breast -ectomy = surgical removal	Surgical removal of only breast tissue; all underlying tissue is left intact
therapeutic abortion		Termination of a pregnancy for health of mother or another medical reason
total abdominal hysterectomy—bilateral salpingo-oophorectomy (TAH-BSO) (hiss-ter-EK-toh-mee / sal-ping-goh / oh-of-or-EK-toh-mee)	abdomin/o = abdomen -al = pertaining to hyster/o = uterus -ectomy = surgical removal bi- = two later/o = side -al = pertaining to salping/o = uterine tube oophor/o = ovary -ectomy = surgical removal	Removal of entire uterus, cervix, both ovaries, and both uterine tubes
tubal ligation (TOO-bal / lye-GAY-shun)	-al = pertaining to	Surgical tying-off of uterine tubes to prevent conception from taking place; results in sterilization of female
vaginal hysterectomy (VAJ-in-al / hiss-ter-EK-toh-mee)	vagin/o = vagina -al = pertaining to hyster/o = uterus -ectomy = surgical removal	Removal of the uterus through the vagina rather than through abdominal incision

PRACTICE AS YOU GO

E. Terminology Matching

Match each term to its definition.

1. _____ Pap smear
2. _____ intrauterine device
3. _____ colposcopy
4. _____ Apgar
5. _____ chorionic villus sampling
6. _____ lumpectomy
7. _____ episiotomy
8. _____ tubal ligation

a. measures newborn's adjustment to outside world
b. widens birth canal; facilitates delivery
c. removes only tumor and tissue around it
d. visually examines vagina
e. test for cervical cancer
f. sterilization procedure
g. birth control method
h. obtains cells for genetic testing

Pharmacology

Classification	Word Parts	Action	Examples
abortifacient (ah-bor-tih-FAY-shent)		Terminates a pregnancy	mifepristone, Mifeprex; dinoprostone, Prostin E2
fertility drug		Triggers ovulation; also called *ovulation stimulant*	clomiphene, Clomid; follitropin alfa, Gonal-F
hormone replacement therapy (HRT)		Replaces hormones missing from menopause or lost ovaries, which can result in lack of estrogen production; replacing this hormone may prevent some consequences of menopause, especially in younger women who have surgically lost their ovaries	conjugated estrogens, Cenestin, Premarin
oral contraceptive pills (OCPs) (kon-trah-SEP-tiv)	or/o = mouth -al = pertaining to contra- = against	Form of birth control that uses low doses of female hormones to prevent conception by blocking ovulation	desogestrel/ethinyl estradiol, Ortho-Cept; ethinyl estradiol/norgestrel, Lo/Ovral
oxytocin (ok-see-TOH-sin)		Natural hormone that begins or improves uterine contractions during labor and delivery	oxytocin, Pitocin, Syntocinon

Abbreviations

AB	abortion	**HPV**	human papillomavirus
AI	artificial insemination	**HRT**	hormone replacement therapy
BSE	breast self-examination	**HSG**	hysterosalpingography
CS, C-section	cesarean section	**IUD**	intrauterine device
CVS	chorionic villus sampling	**IVF**	*in vitro* fertilization
Cx	cervix	**LBW**	low birth weight
D&C	dilation and curettage	**LH**	luteinizing hormone
EDD	estimated date of delivery	**LMP**	last menstrual period
EMB	endometrial biopsy	**NB**	newborn
ERT	estrogen replacement therapy	**OB**	obstetrics
FEKG	fetal electrocardiogram	**OCPs**	oral contraceptive pills
FHR	fetal heart rate	**Pap**	Papanicolaou test
FHT	fetal heart tone	**PI, para I**	first delivery
FSH	follicle-stimulating hormone	**PID**	pelvic inflammatory disease
FTND	full-term normal delivery	**PIH**	pregnancy-induced hypertension
GI, grav I	first pregnancy	**PMS**	premenstrual syndrome
GYN, gyn	gynecology	**TAH-BSO**	total abdominal hysterectomy–bilateral salpingo-oophorectomy
HCG, hCG	human chorionic gonadotropin	**TSS**	toxic shock syndrome
HDN	hemolytic disease of the newborn	**UC**	uterine contractions

PRACTICE AS YOU GO

F. What's the Abbreviation?

1. first pregnancy _____

2. artificial insemination _____

3. uterine contractions _____

4. full-term normal delivery _____

5. intrauterine device _____

6. dilation and curettage _____

7. hormone replacement therapy _____

8. gynecology _____

9. abortion _____

10. oral contraceptive pills _____

AT A GLANCE

Function

Similar to the female reproductive system, the male reproductive system is responsible for producing sperm, the male reproductive cell, secreting the male sex hormones, and delivering sperm to the female reproductive tract.

Organs

The primary structures that comprise the male reproductive system:

testes	seminal vesicles
epididymis	prostate gland
penis	bulbourethral glands
vas deferens	

Word Parts

Presented here are the most common word parts (with their meanings) used to build male reproductive system terms. For a more comprehensive list, refer to the Terminology section of this chapter.

Combining Forms

andr/o	male	pen/o	penis
balan/o	glans penis	prostat/o	prostate gland
crypt/o	hidden	spermat/o	sperm
epididym/o	epididymis	testicul/o	testes
orch/o	testes	vas/o	vas deferens
orchi/o	testes	vesicul/o	seminal vesicle
orchid/o	testes		

Suffixes

-cide	to kill
-plasia	formation of cells
-spermia	condition of sperm

Male Reproductive System Illustrated

testes, p. 373

Produce sperm and secrete testosterone

epididymis, p. 374

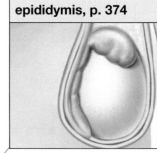

Stores sperm

vas deferens, p. 374

Transports sperm to urethra

seminal vesicles, p. 374

Secrete fluid for semen

prostate gland, p. 375

Secretes fluid for semen

penis, p. 374

Delivers semen during intercourse

bulbourethral gland, p. 375

Secretes fluid for semen

Anatomy and Physiology of the Male Reproductive System

bulbourethral glands
(buhl-boh-yoo-REE-thral)

epididymis (ep-ih-DID-ih-mis)

genitourinary system
(jen-ih-toh-YOO-rih-nair-ee)

penis (PEE-nis)

prostate gland (PROSS-tayt)

semen (SEE-men)

seminal vesicles (SEM-ih-nal / VES-ih-kls)

sex hormones

sperm

testes (TESS-teez)

vas deferens (VAS / DEF-er-enz)

The male reproductive system has two main functions. The first is to produce **sperm**, the male reproductive cell; the second is to secrete the male **sex hormones**. In the male, the major organs of reproduction are located outside the body: the **penis** and the two **testes**, each with an **epididymis** (see Figure 10-20 ■). The penis contains the urethra, which carries both urine and **semen** to the outside of the body. For this reason, this system is sometimes referred to as the **genitourinary (GU) system**.

The internal organs of reproduction include two **seminal vesicles**, two **vas deferens**, the **prostate gland**, and two **bulbourethral glands**.

> **What's In A Name?**
> Look for these word parts:
> **genit/o** = genitals
> **urethr/o** = urethra
> **urin/o** = urine
> **-al** = pertaining to
> **-ary** = pertaining to

External Organs of Reproduction

Testes

androgen (AN-droh-jen)

perineum

scrotum (SKROH-tum)

seminiferous tubules (sem-ih-NIF-er-us / TOO-byools)

spermatogenesis (sper-mat-oh-JEN-eh-sis)

testicles (TESS-tih-kls)

testosterone (tess-TAHS-ter-ohn)

> **What's In A Name?**
> Look for these word parts:
> **andr/o** = male
> **spermat/o** = sperm
> **-gen** = that which produces
> **-genesis** = produces
> **-ous** = pertaining to

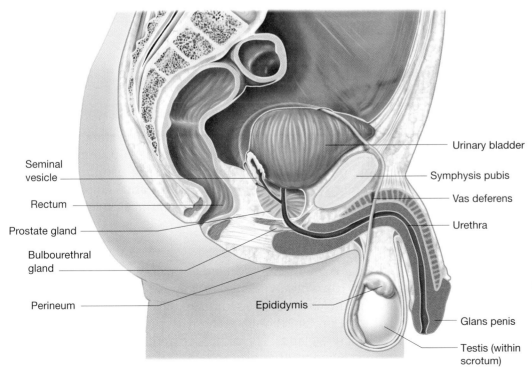

Seminal vesicle

Rectum

Prostate gland

Bulbourethral gland

Perineum

Epididymis

Urinary bladder

Symphysis pubis

Vas deferens

Urethra

Glans penis

Testis (within scrotum)

■ **Figure 10-20** The male reproductive system, sagittal section showing the organs of the system and their relation to the urinary bladder and rectum.

■ **Figure 10-21**
Illustration of human sperm structure. *(Sebastian Kaulitzki/Shutterstock)*

The testes (singular is *testis*) or **testicles** are oval in shape and are responsible for the production of sperm (see again Figure 10-20). This process, called **spermatogenesis**, takes place within the **seminiferous tubules** that make up the insides of the testes (see Figure 10-21 ■). The testes must be maintained at the proper temperature for the sperm to survive. This lower temperature level is achieved by the placement of the testes suspended in the **scrotum**, a sac outside the body. The **perineum** of the male is similar to that in the female and is the area between the scrotum and the anus. The chief **androgen** (male sex hormone) is **testosterone**, which is responsible for the development of the male reproductive organs, sperm, and secondary sex characteristics, and is also produced by the testes.

Epididymis

Each epididymis is a coiled tubule that lies on top of the testes within the scrotum (see again Figure 10-20). This elongated structure serves as the location for sperm maturation and storage until they are ready to be released into the vas deferens.

Penis

circumcision (ser-kum-SIH-zhun)   prepuce (PREE-pyoos)
ejaculation (ee-jak-yoo-LAY-shun)   sphincter (SFINGK-ter)
erectile tissue (ee-REK-tile)   urinary meatus (YOO-rih-nair-ee /
glans penis (GLANS / PEE-nis)   mee-AY-tus)

The penis is the male sex organ containing **erectile tissue** that is encased in skin (see again Figure 10-20). This organ delivers semen into the female vagina. The soft tip of the penis is referred to as the **glans penis**. It is protected by a covering called the **prepuce** or foreskin. It is this covering of skin that is removed during the procedure known as **circumcision**. The penis becomes erect during sexual stimulation, which allows it to be placed within the female for the **ejaculation** of semen. The male urethra extends from the urinary bladder to the external opening in the penis, the **urinary meatus**, and serves a dual function: the elimination of urine and the ejaculation of semen. During the ejaculation process, a **sphincter** closes to keep urine from escaping.

Internal Organs of Reproduction

Vas Deferens

spermatic cord (sper-MAT-ik)

Each vas deferens carries sperm from the epididymis up into the pelvic cavity. They travel up in front of the urinary bladder, over the top, and then back down the posterior side of the bladder to empty into the urethra (see again Figure 10-20). They, along with nerves, arteries, veins, and lymphatic vessels running between the pelvic cavity and the testes, form the **spermatic cord**.

Seminal Vesicles

The two seminal vesicles are small glands located at the base of the urinary bladder (see again Figure 10-20). These vesicles are connected to the vas deferens just before it empties into the urethra. The seminal vesicles secrete a glucose-rich fluid that nourishes the sperm. This liquid, along with the sperm and secretions from other male reproductive glands, constitutes semen, the fluid that is eventually ejaculated during sexual intercourse.

Prostate Gland

The single prostate gland is located just below the urinary bladder (see again Figure 10-20). It surrounds the urethra and when enlarged can cause difficulty in urination. The prostate is important for the reproductive process as it secretes an alkaline fluid that assists in keeping the sperm alive by neutralizing the pH of the urethra and female vagina.

Bulbourethral Glands

Cowper's glands (KOW-perz)

The bulbourethral glands, also known as **Cowper's glands**, are two small glands located on either side of the urethra just below the prostate (see again Figure 10-20). They produce a mucuslike lubricating fluid that joins with semen to become a part of the ejaculate.

PRACTICE AS YOU GO

G. Complete the Statement

1. The male reproductive system is a combination of the _____ and _____ systems.

2. The male's external organs of reproduction consist of the _____, _____, and _____.

3. Another term for the prepuce is the _____.

4. The organs responsible for developing the sperm cells are the _____.

5. The glands of lubrication and fluid production at each side of the male urethra are the _____.

6. The male sex hormone is _____.

7. The area between the scrotum and the anus is called the _____.

Terminology

Word Parts Used to Build Male Reproductive System Terms

The following lists contain the combining forms, suffixes, and prefixes used to build terms in the remaining sections of this chapter.

Combining Forms					
andr/o	male	**genit/o**	genital	**orchi/o**	testes
balan/o	glans penis	**hydr/o**	water	**orchid/o**	testes
carcin/o	cancer	**immun/o**	protection	**pen/o**	penis
crypt/o	hidden	**olig/o**	scanty	**prostat/o**	prostate gland
epididym/o	epididymis	**orch/o**	testes	**rect/o**	rectum

Combining Forms (continued)

spermat/o	sperm	**urethr/o**	urethra	**vas/o**	vas deferens
testicul/o	testes	**varic/o**	dilated vein	**vesicul/o**	seminal vesicle
ur/o	urine				

Suffixes

-al	pertaining to	**-ile**	pertaining to	**-ostomy**	surgically create an opening
-ar	pertaining to	**-ism**	state of	**-otomy**	cutting into
-cele	protrusion	**-itis**	inflammation	**-pexy**	surgical fixation
-cide	to kill	**-logy**	study of	**-plasia**	formation of cells
-ectomy	surgical removal	**-lysis**	to destroy	**-plasty**	surgical repair
-gen	that which produces	**-oid**	resembling	**-rrhea**	discharge
-iasis	abnormal condition	**-oma**	tumor	**-spermia**	sperm condition
-ic	pertaining to	**-osis**	abnormal condition		

Prefixes

a-	without	**dys-**	abnormal	**hypo-**	below
an-	without	**epi-**	above	**trans-**	across
anti-	against	**hyper-**	excessive		

Adjective Forms of Anatomical Terms

Term	Word Parts	Definition
balanic (buh-LAN-ik)	balan/o = glans penis -ic = pertaining to	Pertaining to the glans penis
epididymal (ep-ih-DID-ih-mal)	epididym/o = epididymis -al = pertaining to	Pertaining to the epididymis
penile (PEE-nile)	pen/o = penis -ile = pertaining to	Pertaining to the penis
prostatic (pross-TAT-ik)	prostat/o = prostate gland -ic = pertaining to	Pertaining to the prostate gland
spermatic (sper-MAT-ik)	spermat/o = sperm -ic = pertaining to	Pertaining to sperm
testicular (tess-TIK-yoo-lar)	testicul/o = testes -ar = pertaining to	Pertaining to the testes
vasal (VAY-sal)	vas/o = vas deferens -al = pertaining to	Pertaining to the vas deferens
vesicular (veh-SIK-yoo-lar)	vesicul/o = seminal vesicle -ar = pertaining to	Pertaining to the seminal vesicle

Word Watch

Be careful using the combining forms **vesic/o** meaning *bladder* and **vesicul/o** meaning *seminal vesicle*.

PRACTICE AS YOU GO

H. Give the adjective form for each anatomical structure.

1. A testis _____
2. Sperm _____
3. A seminal vesicle _____
4. The penis _____
5. The prostate gland _____

Pathology

Term	Word Parts	Definition
Medical Specialties		
urology (yoo-RALL-oh-jee)	ur/o = urine -logy = study of	Branch of medicine involved in diagnosis and treatment of diseases and disorders of urinary system and male reproductive system; physician is a *urologist*
Signs and Symptoms		
aspermia (ah-SPER-mee-ah)	a- = without -spermia = sperm condition	Condition of having no sperm
balanorrhea (bah-lah-noh-REE-ah)	balan/o = glans penis -rrhea = discharge	Discharge from the glans penis
oligospermia (ol-ih-goh-SPER-mee-ah)	olig/o = scanty -spermia = sperm condition	Condition of having too few sperm, making chances of fertilization very low
spermatolysis (sper-mah-TALL-ih-sis)	spermat/o = sperm -lysis = to destroy	Term that refers to anything that destroys sperm
Testes		
anorchism (an-OR-kizm)	an- = without orch/o = testes -ism = state of	Absence of testes; may be congenital or as result of accident or surgery
cryptorchidism (kript-OR-kid-izm)	crypt/o = hidden orchid/o = testes -ism = state of	Failure of the testes to descend into scrotal sac before birth; usually, the testes will descend before birth; surgical procedure called *orchidopexy* may be required to bring the testes down into the scrotum permanently; failure of the testes to descend could result in sterility in male or increased risk of testicular cancer
hydrocele (HIGH-droh-seel)	hydr/o = water -cele = protrusion	Accumulation of fluid around the testes or along the spermatic cord; common in infants
orchitis (or-KIGH-tis)	orch/o = testes -itis = inflammation	Inflammation of one or both testes
sterility		Inability to father children due to problem with spermatogenesis
testicular carcinoma (kar-sih-NOH-mah)	testicul/o = testes -ar = pertaining to carcin/o = cancer -oma = tumor	Cancer of one or both testicles; most common cancer in men under age 40
testicular torsion	testicul/o = testes -ar = pertaining to	Twisting of the spermatic cord

Pathology (continued)

Term	Word Parts	Definition
varicocele (VAIR-ih-koh-seel)	varic/o = dilated vein -cele = protrusion	Enlargement of veins of the spermatic cord that commonly occurs on left side of adolescent males
Epididymis		
epididymitis (ep-ih-did-ih-MY-tis)	epididym/o = epididymis -itis = inflammation	Inflammation of the epididymis
Prostate Gland		
benign prostatic hyperplasia (BPH) (bee-NINE / pross-TAT-ik / high-per-PLAY-zha)	prostat/o = prostate gland -ic = pertaining to hyper- = excessive -plasia = formation of cells	Noncancerous enlargement of the prostate gland commonly seen in males over age 50; formerly called *benign prostatic hypertrophy*
prostate cancer (PROSS-tayt)		Slow-growing cancer that affects a large number of males after age 50; prostate-specific antigen (PSA) test is used to assist in early detection of disease
prostatitis (pross-tah-TYE-tis)	prostat/o = prostate gland -itis = inflammation	Inflammation of the prostate gland
Penis		
balanitis (bal-ah-NYE-tis)	balan/o = glans penis -itis = inflammation	Inflammation of the glans penis
epispadias (ep-ih-SPAY-dee-as)	epi- = above	Congenital opening of the urethra on dorsal surface of the penis
erectile dysfunction (ED) (ee-REK-tile)	-ile = pertaining to dys- = abnormal, difficult	Inability to engage in sexual intercourse due to inability to maintain erection; also called *impotence*
hypospadias (high-poh-SPAY-dee-as)	hypo- = below	Congenital opening of male urethra on underside of the penis
phimosis (fye-MOH-sis)	-osis = abnormal condition	Narrowing of foreskin over the glans penis resulting in difficulty with hygiene; condition can lead to infection or difficulty with urination; treated with circumcision, surgical removal of the foreskin
priapism (PRYE-ah-pizm)	-ism = state of	Persistent and painful erection due to pathological causes, not sexual arousal
Sexually Transmitted Diseases		
chancroid (SHANG-kroyd)	-oid = resembling	Highly infectious nonsyphilitic venereal ulcer

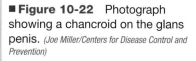

■ **Figure 10-22** Photograph showing a chancroid on the glans penis. *(Joe Miller/Centers for Disease Control and Prevention)*

Pathology (continued)

Term	Word Parts	Definition
chlamydia (klah-MID-ee-ah)		Bacterial infection causing genital inflammation in males and females; can lead to pelvic inflammatory disease in females and eventual infertility
genital herpes (JEN-ih-tal / HER-peez)	genit/o = genital -al = pertaining to	Spreading skin disease that can appear like a blister or vesicle on genital region of males and females; may spread to other areas of body; caused by sexually transmitted virus
genital warts (JEN-ih-tal)	genit/o = genital -al = pertaining to	Growth of warts on genitalia of both males and females that can lead to cancer of the cervix in females; caused by sexual transmission of human papillomavirus (HPV)
gonorrhea (GC) (gon-oh-REE-ah)	-rrhea = discharge	Sexually transmitted bacterial infection of mucous membranes of either sex; can be passed on to infant during birth process
human immunodeficiency virus (HIV)	immun/o = protection	Sexually transmitted virus that attacks immune system
sexually transmitted disease		Disease usually acquired as result of sexual intercourse; also called *sexually transmitted infection* (STI); formerly referred to as *venereal disease* (VD)
syphilis (SIF-ih-lis)		Infectious, chronic, bacterial sexually transmitted infection that can involve any organ; may exist for years without symptoms, but is fatal if untreated; treated with antibiotic penicillin
trichomoniasis (trik-oh-moh-NYE-ah-sis)	-iasis = abnormal condition	Genitourinary infection caused by single-cell protozoan parasite that is usually without symptoms (asymptomatic) in both males and females; in women disease can produce itching and/or burning, foul-smelling discharge, and result in vaginitis

PRACTICE AS YOU GO

I. Terminology Matching

Match each term to its definition.

1. _____ aspermia
2. _____ phimosis
3. _____ balanitis
4. _____ chancroid
5. _____ varicocele
6. _____ oligospermia

a. inflammation of glans penis

b. having no sperm

c. venereal ulcer

d. having too few sperm

e. narrowing of foreskin

f. enlarged spermatic cord veins

Diagnostic Procedures

Term	Word Parts	Definition
Clinical Laboratory Tests		
prostate-specific antigen (PSA) (PROSS-tayt-specific / AN-tih-jen)	anti- = against -gen = that which produces	Blood test to screen for prostate cancer; elevated blood levels of PSA are associated with prostate cancer
semen analysis (SEE-men / ah-NAL-ih-sis)		Procedure used when performing fertility workup to determine if male is able to produce sperm; semen is collected by patient after abstaining from sexual intercourse for a period of three to five days; sperm in semen are analyzed for number, swimming strength, and shape; also used to determine if vasectomy has been successful; after a period of six weeks, no further sperm should be present in a sample from patient
Additional Diagnostic Procedures		
digital rectal exam (DRE) (DIJ-ih-tal / REK-tal)	rect/o = rectum -al = pertaining to	Manual examination for an enlarged prostate gland performed by palpating (feeling) the prostate gland through wall of the rectum

Therapeutic Procedures

Term	Word Parts	Definition
Surgical Procedures		
balanoplasty (BAL-ah-noh-plas-tee)	balan/o = glans penis -plasty = surgical repair	Surgical repair of the glans penis
castration (kass-TRAY-shun)		Removal of the testicles in male or the ovaries in female
circumcision (ser-kum-SIH-zhun)		Surgical removal of the prepuce, or foreskin, of the penis; generally performed on newborn male at request of parents; primary reason is for ease of hygiene; circumcision is also a ritual practice in some religions
epididymectomy (ep-ih-did-ih-MEK-toh-mee)	epididym/o = epididymis -ectomy = surgical removal	Surgical removal of the epididymis
orchidectomy (or-kih-DEK-toh-mee)	orchid/o = testes -ectomy = surgical removal	Surgical removal of one or both testes
orchidopexy (OR-kid-oh-pek-see)	orchid/o = testes -pexy = surgical fixation	Surgical fixation to move undescended testes into the scrotum and to attach them to prevent retraction; used to treat cryptorchidism
orchiectomy (or-kee-EK-toh-mee)	orchi/o = testes -ectomy = surgical removal	Surgical removal of one or both testes
orchiotomy (or-kee-OT-oh-mee)	orchi/o = testes -otomy = cutting into	To cut into the testes
orchioplasty (OR-kee-oh-plas-tee)	orchi/o = testes -plasty = surgical repair	Surgical repair of the testes
prostatectomy (pross-tah-TEK-toh-mee)	prostat/o = prostate gland -ectomy = surgical removal	Surgical removal of the prostate gland
sterilization (stair-ih-lih-ZAY-shun)		Process of rendering a male or female sterile or unable to conceive children
transurethral resection of the prostate (TUR, TURP) (trans-yoo-REE-thral / ree-SEK-shun / PROSS-tayt)	trans- = across urethr/o = urethra -al = pertaining to	Surgical removal of part of the prostate gland that is blocking urine flow by inserting a device through the urethra and removing prostate tissue

Therapeutic Procedures (continued)

Term	Word Parts	Definition
vasectomy (vah-SEK-toh-mee)	vas/o = vas deferens -ectomy = surgical removal	Removal of a segment or all of the vas deferens to prevent sperm from leaving male body; used for contraception purposes

Med Term Tip

The vas deferens is the tubing that is severed during a procedure called a *vasectomy.* A vasectomy results in the sterilization of the male since the sperm are no longer able to travel into the urethra and out of the penis during sexual intercourse. The surgical procedure to reverse a vasectomy is a *vasovasostomy.* A new opening is created in order to reconnect one section of the vas deferens to another section of the vas deferens, thereby reestablishing an open tube for sperm to travel through.

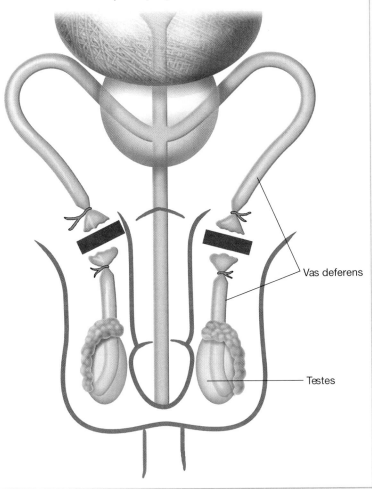

■ **Figure 10-23** A vasectomy, showing how each vas deferens is tied off in two places and then a section is removed from the middle. This prevents sperm from traveling through the vas deferens during ejaculation.

Term	Word Parts	Definition
vasovasostomy (vay-soh-vah-SOS-tah-mee)	vas/o = vas deferens -ostomy = surgically create an opening	Surgical procedure to reconnect the vas deferens to reverse a vasectomy

PRACTICE AS YOU GO

J. Procedure Matching

Match each procedure to its definition.

1. _____ digital rectal exam
2. _____ circumcision
3. _____ vasectomy
4. _____ orchidopexy
5. _____ semen analysis

a. removes prepuce

b. surgical fixation of testis

c. examination for enlarged prostate

d. sterilization procedure

e. part of a fertility workup

Pharmacology

Classification	Word Parts	Action	Examples
androgen therapy (AN-droh-jen)	andr/o = male -gen = that which produces	Replaces male hormones to treat patients who produce insufficient hormone naturally	testosterone cypionate, Andronate, depAndro
antiprostatic agents (an-tye-pross-TAT-ik)	anti- = against prostat/o = prostate gland -ic = pertaining to	Treat early cases of benign prostatic hyperplasia; may prevent surgery for mild cases	finasteride, Proscar; dutasteride, Avodart
erectile dysfunction agents (ee-REK-tile)	-ile = pertaining to dys- = abnormal	Temporarily produce erection in patients with erectile dysfunction	sildenafil citrate, Viagra; tadalafil, Cialis
spermatocide (sper-MAH-toh-side)	spermat/o = sperm -cide = to kill	Destroys sperm; one form of birth control is use of spermatolytic creams	octoxynol 9, Semicid, Ortho-Gynol

Abbreviations

BPH	benign prostatic hyperplasia	**SPP**	suprapubic prostatectomy
DRE	digital rectal exam	**STD**	sexually transmitted disease
ED	erectile dysfunction	**STI**	sexually transmitted infection
GC	gonorrhea	**TUR**	transurethral resection
GU	genitourinary	**TURP**	transurethral resection of the prostate
PSA	prostate-specific antigen	**VD**	venereal disease
RPR	rapid plasma reagin (test for syphilis)		

PRACTICE AS YOU GO

K. What's the Abbreviation?

1. erectile dysfunction _____
2. gonorrhea _____
3. digital rectal exam _____
4. transurethral resection of the prostate _____
5. sexually transmitted infection _____

Chapter Review

Real-World Applications

Medical Record Analysis

This High-Risk Obstetrics Consultation Report contains 12 medical terms. Underline each term and write it in the list below the report. Then explain each term as you would to a nonmedical person.

High-Risk Obstetrics Consultation Report

Reason for Consultation:	High-risk pregnancy with late-term bleeding
History of Present Illness:	Patient is 23 years old. She is currently estimated to be at 175 days' gestation. Amniocentesis at 20 weeks shows a normally developing male fetus. She noticed a moderate degree of bleeding this morning but denies any cramping or pelvic pain. She immediately saw her obstetrician who referred her for high-risk evaluation.
Past Medical History:	This patient is multigravida but nullipara with three early miscarriages without obvious cause.
Results of Physical Examination:	Patient appears well nourished and abdominal girth appears consistent with length of gestation. Pelvic ultrasound indicates placenta previa with placenta almost completely overlying cervix. However, there is no evidence of abruptio placentae at this time. Fetal size estimate is consistent with 25 weeks' gestation. The fetal heartbeat is strong with a rate of 130 beats/minute.
Recommendations:	Fetus appears to be developing well and in no distress at this time. The placenta appears to be well attached on ultrasound, but the bleeding is cause for concern. With the extremely low position of the placenta, this patient is at very high risk for abruptio placentae. She will require C-section at onset of labor.

Term	Explanation
1. _____	_____
2. _____	_____
3. _____	_____
4. _____	_____
5. _____	_____
6. _____	_____
7. _____	_____
8. _____	_____
9. _____	_____
10. _____	_____
11. _____	_____
12. _____	_____

Chart Note Transcription

The chart note below contains 10 phrases that can be reworded with a medical term presented in this chapter. Each phrase is identified with an underline. Determine the medical term and write your answers in the space provided.

Current Complaint: Patient is a 77-year-old male seen by the urologist with complaints of nocturia and difficulty with <u>the release of semen from the urethra</u>. **1**

Past History: Medical history revealed that the patient had <u>failure of the testes to descend into the scrotum</u> **2** at birth, which was repaired by <u>surgical fixation of the testes</u>. **3** He had also undergone elective sterilization <u>by removal of a segment of the vas deferens</u> **4** at the age of 41.

Signs and Symptoms: Patient states he first noted these symptoms about five years ago. They have become increasingly severe and now he is not able to sleep without waking to urinate up to 20 times a night. He has difficulty with <u>release of semen</u>. **5** <u>Palpation of the prostate gland through the rectum</u> **6** revealed multiple round, firm nodules in prostate gland. A needle biopsy was negative for <u>slow-growing cancer that frequently affects males over age 50</u> **7** and a <u>blood test for prostate cancer</u> **8** was normal.

Diagnosis: <u>Noncancerous enlargement of the prostate gland</u> **9**

Treatment: Patient was scheduled for a <u>surgical removal of prostate tissue through the urethra</u>. **10**

1. _____
2. _____
3. _____
4. _____
5. _____
6. _____
7. _____
8. _____
9. _____
10. _____

Case Study

Below is a case study presentation of a patient with a condition discussed in this chapter. Read the case study and answer the questions below. Some questions will ask for information not included within this chapter. Use your text, a medical dictionary, or any other reference material you choose to answer these questions.

(Jason Stitt/Shutterstock)

A 22-year-old female has come into the gynecologist's office complaining of fever, malaise, dysuria, and vaginal leukorrhea. Upon examination the physician observes fluid-filled vesicles on her cervix, vulva, and perineum. Several have ruptured into ulcers with marked erythema and edema. Palpation revealed painful and enlarged inguinal lymph nodes. She also has an extragenital lesion on her mouth.

Her diagnosis is genital herpes.

Questions

1. What pathological condition does this patient have? Look this condition up in a reference source and include a short description of it.

   _____

   _____

2. List and define each of the patient's presenting symptoms in your own words.

   _____

   _____

3. Describe the results of the physician's examination in your own words.

   _____

   _____

4. Explain what *extragenital lesion* means.

   _____

   _____

5. Explain what *palpation* means.

   _____

   _____

6. What is the potential effect of having this virus present in open genital lesions on the patient's future pregnancy and childbirth?

   _____

   _____

Practice Exercises

A. Using Abbreviations

Fill in each blank with the appropriate abbreviation.

1. A(n) _____ specializes in treating conditions of the female reproductive system and a(n) _____ specializes in treating pregnant women.

2. _____ always develops symptoms just prior to the menstrual period.

3. _____ is also called erythroblastosis fetalis.

4. A(n) _____ can be performed at an earlier stage of the pregnancy than an amniocentesis.

5. When she stopped taking _____, Natasha had a(n) _____ inserted into her uterus for contraception.

6. Some cases of cervical cancer are caused by a(n) _____ infection.

7. _____ were formerly referred to as VD.

8. The _____ is an important screening tool for prostate cancer.

9. A(n) _____ is performed when the prostate gland is blocking urine flow from the bladder.

10. _____ is associated with prolonged wearing of a super-absorbent tampon.

B. Define the Term

1. spermatogenesis _____

2. hydrocele _____

3. transurethral resection of the prostate (TURP) _____

4. sterility _____

5. orchiectomy _____

6. vasectomy _____

7. castration _____

8. gestation _____

9. meconium _____

10. nulligravida _____

11. dystocia _____

12. metrorrhea _____

13. fibroid tumor _____

14. fibrocystic disease _____

15. placenta previa _____

C. Word Building Practice

The combining form **colp/o** refers to the *vagina*. Use it to write a term that means:

1. visual examination of the vagina _____

2. instrument used to examine the vagina _____

The combining form **cervic/o** refers to the *cervix*. Use it to write a term that means:

3. removal of the cervix _____

4. inflammation of the cervix _____

The combining form **hyster/o** also refers to the *uterus*. Use it to write a term that means:

5. surgical fixation of the uterus _____

6. removal of the uterus _____

7. rupture of the uterus _____

The combining form **oophor/o** refers to the *ovaries*. Use it to write a term that means:

8. inflammation of an ovary _____

9. removal of an ovary _____

The combining form **mamm/o** refers to the *breasts*. Use it to write a term that means:

10. record of breast _____

11. surgical repair of breast _____

The combining form **amni/o** refers to the *amnion*. Use it to write a term that means:

12. cutting into amnion _____

13. flow from amnion _____

The combining form **prostat/o** refers to the *prostate*. Use this to write a term that means:

14. removal of prostate _____

15. inflammation of the prostate _____

The combining form **orchi/o** refers to the *testes*. Use this to write a term that means:

16. removal of the testes _____

17. surgical repair of the testes _____

18. incision into the testes _____

The suffix **-spermia** refers to a *sperm condition*. Use this to write a term that means:

19. condition of being without sperm _____

20. condition of having too few (scanty) sperm _____

The combining form **spermat/o** refers to *sperm*. Use this to write a term that means:

21. sperm forming _____

22. to destroy sperm _____

D. Complete the Term

For each definition given below, fill in the blank with the word part that completes the term.

Definition	Term
1. surgical repair of glans penis	_____plasty
2. excessive formation of cells	hyper_____
3. state of hidden testes	_____ism
4. dilated vein protrusion	_____cele
5. scanty sperm condition	oligo_____

Definition	Term
6. surgical removal of ovary	_____ectomy
7. instrument for viewing vagina	_____scope
8. tubal pregnancy	_____cyesis
9. milk flow	_____rrhea
10. abnormal condition within the uterus	endo_____osis
11. pus in the uterine tube	pyo_____
12. study of new birth	neo_____logy
13. menstruation abnormal flow condition	_____rrhagia
14. first pregnancy	primi_____
15. uterus rupture	_____rrhexis

E. Fill in the Blank

premenstrual syndrome	stillbirth	conization	laparoscopy
D&C	puberty	endometriosis	eclampsia
fibroid tumor	cesarean section		

1. Kesha had a core of tissue from her cervix removed for testing. This is called _____.

2. Joan delivered a baby that had died while still in the uterus. She had a(n) _____.

3. Ashley has just started her first menstrual cycle. She is said to have entered _____.

4. Kimberly is experiencing tender breasts, headaches, and some irritability just prior to her monthly menstrual cycle. This may be _____.

5. Ana has been scheduled for an examination in which her physician will use an instrument to observe her abdominal cavity to rule out the diagnosis of severe endometriosis. The physician will insert the instrument through a small incision. This procedure is called a(n) _____.

6. Lenora is scheduled to have a hysterectomy as a result of a long history of large benign growths in her uterus that have caused pain and bleeding. Lenora has a(n) _____.

7. Tiffany's physician has recommended that she have a uterine scraping to stop excessive bleeding after a miscarriage. She will be scheduled for a(n) _____.

8. Stacey is having frequent prenatal checkups to prevent the serious condition of pregnancy called _____.

9. Marion has experienced painful menstrual periods as a result of the lining of her uterus being displaced into her pelvic cavity. This is called _____.

10. Because her cervix was not dilating, Shataundra was informed that she will probably require a(n) _____ for her baby's delivery.

F. Terminology Matching

Match each term to its definition.

1. _____ gonorrhea

2. _____ genital herpes

3. _____ human immunodeficiency virus

a. also called STD

b. may lead to pelvic inflammatory disease in females

c. treated with penicillin

4. _____ syphilis

5. _____ venereal disease

6. _____ genital warts

7. _____ chancroid

8. _____ chlamydia

9. _____ trichomoniasis

d. caused by human papillomavirus

e. can pass to infant during birth

f. caused by protozoan parasite

g. venereal ulcer

h. attacks the immune system

i. skin disease with vesicles

G. Pharmacology Challenge

Fill in the classification for each drug description, then match the brand name.

Drug Description	Classification	Brand Name
1. _____ replacement male hormone	_____	a. Pitocin
2. _____ improves uterine contractions	_____	b. Avodart
3. _____ treats early BPH	_____	c. Clomid
4. _____ blocks ovulation	_____	d. Semicid
5. _____ kills sperm	_____	e. Mifeprex
6. _____ produces an erection	_____	f. Andronate
7. _____ replaces estrogen	_____	g. Ortho-Cept
8. _____ terminates a pregnancy	_____	h. Viagra
9. _____ triggers ovulation	_____	i. Premarin

H. Anatomical Adjectives

Fill in the blank with the missing noun or adjective.

Noun	Adjective
1. amnion	_____
2. cervix	_____
3. embryo	_____
4. _____	endometrial
5. breast	_____
6. _____	ovarian
7. _____	uterine
8. _____	fetal
9. seminal vesicle	_____
10. _____	spermatic
11. testes	_____
12. _____	balanic
13. epididymis	_____
14. _____	prostatic
15. penis	_____

I. Spelling Practice

Some of the following terms are misspelled. Identify the incorrect terms and spell them correctly in the blank provided.

1. spermatolysis _____
2. epispadius _____
3. chlamydia _____
4. circumsicion _____
5. salpingectomy _____
6. cesarean _____
7. mamogram _____
8. preclampsia _____
9. menometrorrhagia _____
10. premenstral _____

J. Complete the Statement

1. The two anterior pituitary hormones that target the ovaries are _____ and _____.

   The two ovarian hormones that target the uterus are _____ and _____.
2. During _____, an ovum is released from an ovary.
3. Fertilization typically occurs in the _____.
4. The process that produces milk is called _____.
5. The major organs are formed during the _____ period of gestation.
6. The infant is delivered during the _____ stage of labor and delivery.
7. _____ takes place in the seminiferous tubules.
8. The _____ is located at the base of the urinary bladder.

MyLab Medical Terminology™

MyLab Medical Terminology is a premium online homework management system that includes a host of features to help you study. Registered users will find:

- A multitude of activities and assignments built within the MyLab platform
- Powerful tools that track and analyze your results—allowing you to create a personalized learning experience
- Videos and audio pronunciations to help enrich your progress
- Streaming lesson presentations (Guided Lectures) and self-paced learning modules
- A space where you and your instructors can check your progress and manage your assignments

Labeling Exercises

Image A

Write the labels for this figure on the numbered lines provided.

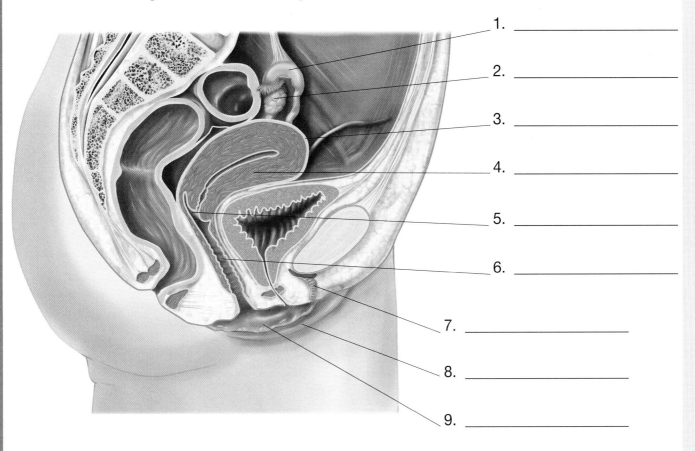

1. _____

2. _____

3. _____

4. _____

5. _____

6. _____

7. _____

8. _____

9. _____

Image B

Write the labels for this figure on the numbered lines provided.

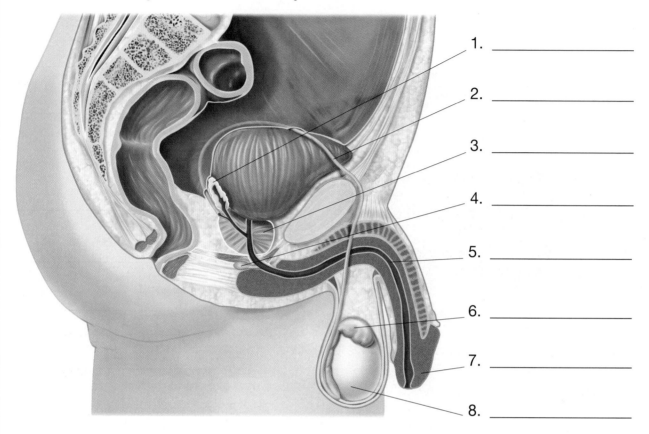

1. _____

2. _____

3. _____

4. _____

5. _____

6. _____

7. _____

8. _____

Image C

Write the labels for this figure on the numbered lines provided.

1. _____

2. _____

3. _____

4. _____

5. _____

Chapter 11

Endocrine System

Learning Objectives

Upon completion of this chapter, you will be able to

1. Identify and define the combining forms and suffixes introduced in this chapter.

2. Correctly spell and pronounce medical terms and major anatomical structures relating to the endocrine system.

3. Locate and describe the major organs of the endocrine system and their functions.

4. List the major hormones secreted by each endocrine gland and describe their functions.

5. Identify and define endocrine system anatomical terms.

6. Identify and define selected endocrine system pathology terms.

7. Identify and define selected endocrine system diagnostic procedures.

8. Identify and define selected endocrine system therapeutic procedures.

9. Identify and define selected medications relating to the endocrine system.

10. Define selected abbreviations associated with the endocrine system.

(Pearson Education, Inc.)

AT A GLANCE

Function

Endocrine glands secrete hormones that regulate many body activities such as metabolic rate, water and mineral balance, immune system reactions, and sexual functioning.

Organs

The primary structures that comprise the endocrine system:

adrenal glands	pituitary gland
ovaries	testes
pancreas (islets of Langerhans)	thymus gland
parathyroid glands	thyroid gland
pineal gland	

Word Parts

Presented here are the most common word parts used to build endocrine system terms. For a more comprehensive list, refer to the Terminology section of this chapter.

Combining Forms

acr/o	extremities	natr/o	sodium
aden/o	gland	ovari/o	ovary
adren/o	adrenal glands	pancreat/o	pancreas
adrenal/o	adrenal glands	parathyroid/o	parathyroid gland
andr/o	male	pineal/o	pineal gland
calc/o	calcium	pituit/o	pituitary gland
crin/o	to secrete	pituitar/o	pituitary gland
estr/o	female	radi/o	ray
gluc/o	glucose	somat/o	body
glyc/o	sugar	testicul/o	testes
gonad/o	sex glands	thym/o	thymus gland
iod/o	iodine	thyr/o	thyroid gland
kal/i	potassium	thyroid/o	thyroid gland
ket/o	ketones	toxic/o	poison
mineral/o	minerals, electrolytes		

Suffixes

-dipsia	thirst	-tropic	pertaining to stimulating
-emic	pertaining to a blood condition	-tropin	to stimulate

Endocrine System Illustrated

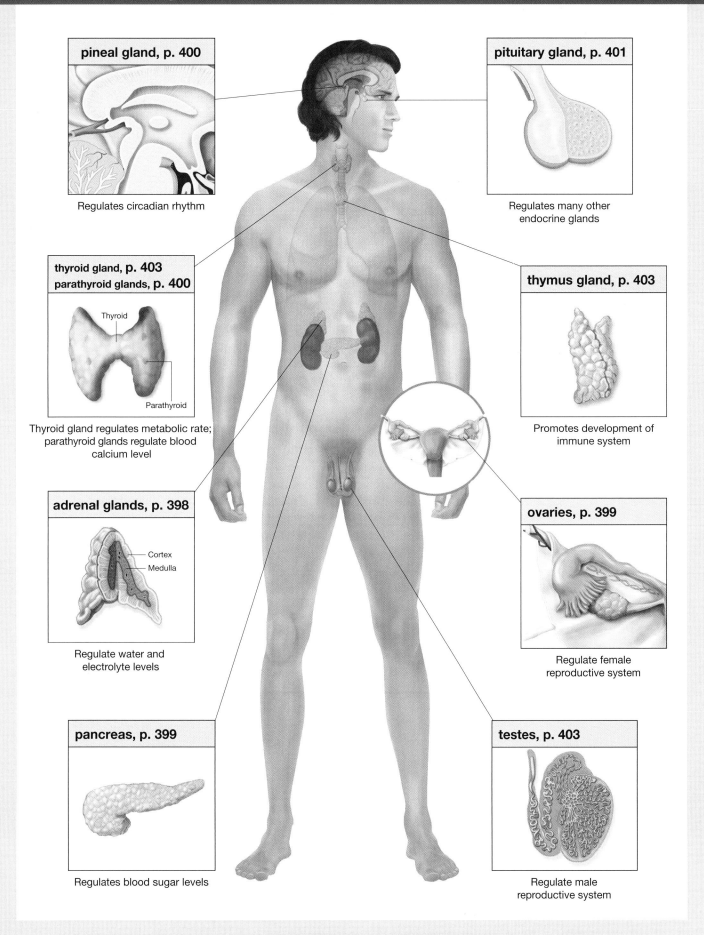

pineal gland, p. 400

Regulates circadian rhythm

pituitary gland, p. 401

Regulates many other
endocrine glands

thyroid gland, p. 403
parathyroid glands, p. 400

Thyroid

Parathyroid

Thyroid gland regulates metabolic rate;
parathyroid glands regulate blood
calcium level

thymus gland, p. 403

Promotes development of
immune system

adrenal glands, p. 398

Cortex
Medulla

Regulate water and
electrolyte levels

ovaries, p. 399

Regulate female
reproductive system

pancreas, p. 399

Regulates blood sugar levels

testes, p. 403

Regulate male
reproductive system

Anatomy and Physiology of the Endocrine System

adrenal glands (ah-DREE-nal)

endocrine glands (EN-doh-krin)

endocrine system

exocrine glands (EKS-oh-krin)

glands

homeostasis (hoh-mee-oh-STAY-sis)

hormones (HOR-mohnz)

ovaries (OH-vah-reez)

pancreas (PAN-kree-as)

parathyroid glands (pair-ah-THIGH-royd)

pineal gland (PIN-ee-al)

pituitary gland (pih-TOO-ih-tair-ee)

target organs

testes (TESS-teez)

thymus gland (THIGH-mus)

thyroid gland (THIGH-royd)

What's In A Name?

Look for these word parts:

home/o = sameness

-stasis = standing still

Med Term Tip

The terms *endocrine* and *exocrine* were constructed to reflect the function of each type of gland. As glands, they both secrete, indicated by the combining form **crin/o**. The prefix **exo-**, meaning *external* or *outward*, tells us that exocrine gland secretions are carried to the outside of the body or to a passageway connected to the outside of the body. However, the prefix **endo-**, meaning *within* or *internal*, indicates that endocrine gland secretions are carried to other internal body structures by the bloodstream.

The **endocrine system** is a collection of **glands** that secrete **hormones** directly into the bloodstream. Hormones are chemicals that act on their **target organs** to either increase or decrease the target's activity level. In this way the endocrine system is instrumental in maintaining **homeostasis** (**home/o** = sameness; **-stasis** = standing still)—that is, adjusting the activity level of most of the tissues and organs of the body to maintain a stable internal environment.

The body actually has two distinct types of glands: **exocrine glands** and **endocrine glands**. Exocrine glands release their secretions into a duct that carries them to the outside of the body or to a passageway connected to the outside of the body. For example, sweat glands release sweat into a sweat duct that travels to the surface of the body. Endocrine glands, however, release hormones directly into the bloodstream. For example, the thyroid gland secretes its hormones directly into the bloodstream. Because endocrine glands have no ducts, they are also referred to as *ductless glands*.

The endocrine system consists of the following glands: two **adrenal glands**, two **ovaries** in the female, four **parathyroid glands**, the **pancreas**, the **pineal gland**, the **pituitary gland**, two **testes** in the male, the **thymus gland**, and the **thyroid gland**. The endocrine glands as a whole affect the functions of the entire body. Table 11-1 ■ presents a description of the endocrine glands, their hormones, and their functions.

■ TABLE 11-1   Endocrine Glands and Their Hormones

Gland and Hormone	Word Parts	Function
Adrenal cortex	**adren/o** = adrenal gland **-al** = pertaining to	
Glucocorticoids such as cortisol	**gluc/o** = glucose **cortic/o** = outer layer	Regulate carbohydrate levels in body
Mineralocorticoids such as aldosterone	**mineral/o** = minerals, electrolytes **cortic/o** = outer layer	Regulate electrolytes and fluid volume in body
Steroid sex hormones such as androgen	**andr/o** = male **-gen** = that which produces	Male sex hormones from adrenal cortex may be converted to estrogens in the bloodstream; responsible for reproduction and secondary sexual characteristics
Adrenal medulla	**adren/o** = adrenal gland **-al** = pertaining to	
Epinephrine (adrenaline)	**epi-** = above **nephr/o** = kidney **-ine** = pertaining to	Intensifies response during stress; "fight-or-flight" response
Norepinephrine	**epi-** = above **nephr/o** = kidney **-ine** = pertaining to	Chiefly a vasoconstrictor
Ovaries		
Estrogen	**estr/o** = female **-gen** = that which produces	Stimulates development of secondary sex characteristics in females; regulates menstrual cycle

■ **TABLE 11-1**   Endocrine Glands and Their Hormones (continued)

Gland and Hormone	Word Parts	Function
Progesterone	pro- = before estr/o = female	Prepares for conditions of pregnancy
Pancreas		
Glucagon		Stimulates liver to release glucose into the blood
Insulin		Regulates and promotes entry of glucose into cells
Parathyroid glands	para- = beside	
Parathyroid hormone (PTH)	para- = beside	Stimulates bone breakdown; regulates calcium level in the blood
Pineal gland	pineal/o = pineal gland -al = pertaining to	
Melatonin		Regulates circadian rhythm
Pituitary anterior lobe	pituit/o = pituitary gland -ary = pertaining to anter/o = front -ior = pertaining to	
Adrenocorticotropic hormone (ACTH)	adren/o = adrenal gland cortic/o = outer layer -tropic = pertaining to stimulating	Regulates secretion of some adrenal cortex hormones
Gonadotropins	gonad/o = gonads -tropin = to stimulate	Consists of two hormones, follicle-stimulating hormone and luteinizing hormone
Follicle-stimulating hormone (FSH)		Stimulates growth of eggs in females and sperm in males
Luteinizing hormone (LH)		Regulates function of male and female gonads and plays role in releasing ova in females
Growth hormone (GH)		Stimulates growth of body
Melanocyte-stimulating hormone (MSH)	melan/o = black -cyte = cell	Stimulates pigment production in skin
Prolactin (PRL)	pro- = before lact/o = milk	Stimulates milk production
Thyroid-stimulating hormone (TSH)		Regulates function of thyroid gland
Pituitary posterior lobe	pituit/o = pituitary gland -ary = pertaining to poster/o = back -ior = pertaining to	
Antidiuretic hormone (ADH)	anti- = against -tic = pertaining to	Stimulates reabsorption of water by the kidneys
Oxytocin		Stimulates uterine contractions and releases milk into ducts
Testes		
Testosterone		Promotes sperm production and development of secondary sex characteristics in males
Thymus		
Thymosin	thym/o = thymus gland	Promotes development of cells in immune system
Thyroid gland		
Calcitonin (CT)		Stimulates deposition of calcium into bone
Thyroxine (T$_4$)	thyr/o = thyroid gland -ine = pertaining to	Stimulates metabolism in cells
Triiodothyronine (T$_3$)	tri- = three iod/o = iodine thyr/o = thyroid gland -ine = pertaining to	Stimulates metabolism in cells

PRACTICE AS YOU GO

A. Match Glands and Hormones

_____	1. epinephrine	**a.**	pancreas
_____	2. oxytocin	**b.**	pineal gland
_____	3. testosterone	**c.**	thyroid gland
_____	4. insulin	**d.**	adrenal medulla
_____	5. cortisol	**e.**	ovaries
_____	6. melatonin	**f.**	anterior pituitary gland
_____	7. estrogen	**g.**	posterior pituitary gland
_____	8. growth hormone	**h.**	thymus gland
_____	9. thymosin	**i.**	testes
_____	10. thyroxine	**j.**	adrenal cortex

Adrenal Glands

adrenal cortex (KOR-teks)
adrenal medulla (meh-DULL-ah)
adrenaline (ah-DREN-ah-lin)
aldosterone (al-DOSS-ter-ohn)
androgens (AN-droh-jenz)
corticosteroids (kor-tih-koh-STAIR-oydz)
cortisol (KOR-tih-zawl)

epinephrine (ep-ih-NEF-rin)
glucocorticoids (gloo-koh-KOR-tih-koydz)
mineralocorticoids
(min-er-al-oh-KOR-tih-koydz)
norepinephrine (nor-ep-ih-NEF-rin)
steroid sex hormones (STAIR-oyd)

The two adrenal glands are located above each of the kidneys (see Figure 11-1 ■). Each gland is composed of two sections: **adrenal cortex** and **adrenal medulla**.

The outer adrenal cortex manufactures several different families of hormones: **mineralocorticoids**, **glucocorticoids**, and **steroid sex hormones** (see again Table 11-1). However, because they are all produced by the cortex, they are collectively referred to as **corticosteroids**. The mineralocorticoid hormone, **aldosterone**, regulates sodium (Na⁺) and potassium (K⁺) levels in the body. The glucocorticoid

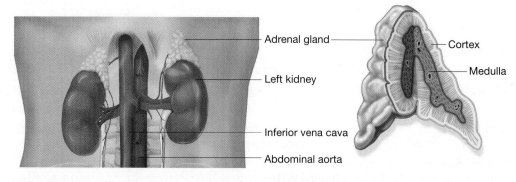

■ **Figure 11-1**   The adrenal glands. These glands sit on top of each kidney. Each adrenal is subdivided into an outer cortex and an inner medulla. Each region secretes different hormones.

hormone, **cortisol**, regulates carbohydrates in the body. The adrenal cortex of both men and women secretes steroid sex hormones, **androgens** (which may be converted to estrogen once released into the bloodstream). These hormones regulate secondary sexual characteristics. All hormones secreted by the adrenal cortex are steroid hormones.

The inner adrenal medulla is responsible for secreting the hormones **epinephrine**, also called **adrenaline**, and **norepinephrine**. These hormones are critical during emergency situations because they increase blood pressure, heart rate, and respiration levels. This helps the body perform better during emergencies or otherwise stressful times.

Ovaries

estrogen (ESS-troh-gen)

gametes (GAM-eets)

gonads (GOH-nadz)

menstrual cycle (MEN-stroo-al)

ova

progesterone (proh-JES-ter-ohn)

The two ovaries are located in the lower abdominopelvic cavity of the female (see Figure 11-2 ■). They are the female **gonads**. Gonads are organs that produce **gametes** or the reproductive sex cells. In the case of females, the gametes are the **ova**. Of importance to the endocrine system, the ovaries produce the female sex hormones, **estrogen** and **progesterone** (see again Table 11-1). Estrogen is responsible for the appearance of the female sexual characteristics and regulation of the **menstrual cycle**. Progesterone helps to maintain a suitable uterine environment for pregnancy.

> **What's In A Name?**
> Look for these word parts:
> **men/o** = menses, menstruation
> **-al** = pertaining to

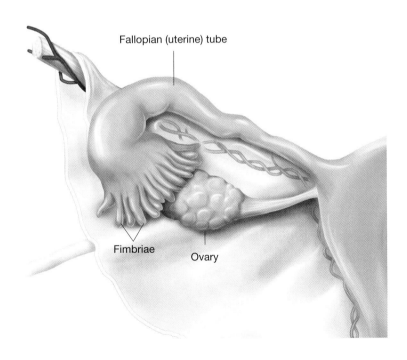

Fallopian (uterine) tube

Fimbriae

Ovary

■ **Figure 11-2** The right ovary. In addition to producing ova, each ovary secretes the female sex hormones, estrogen and progesterone.

Pancreas

glucagon (GLOO-kuh-gon)

insulin (IN-suh-lin)

islets of Langerhans (EYE-lets / of / LAHNG-er-hahnz)

pancreatic islets (pan-kree-AT-ik / EYE-lets)

The pancreas is located along the lower curvature of the stomach (see Figure 11-3A ■). It is the only organ in the body that has both endocrine and

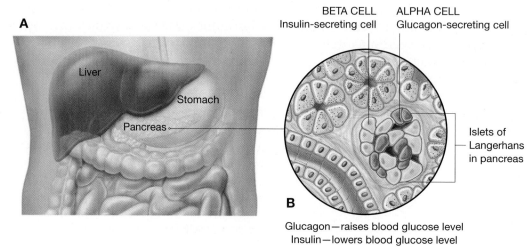

A

B

BETA CELL
Insulin-secreting cell

ALPHA CELL
Glucagon-secreting cell

Liver

Stomach

Pancreas

Islets of
Langerhans
in pancreas

Glucagon—raises blood glucose level
Insulin—lowers blood glucose level

exocrine functions. The exocrine portion of the pancreas releases digestive enzymes through a duct into the duodenum of the small intestine. The endocrine sections of the pancreas are the **pancreatic islets** or **islets of Langerhans** (see Figure 11-3B ■). The islets cells produce two different hormones: **insulin** and **glucagon** (see again Table 11-1). Insulin, produced by beta (β) islet cells, stimulates the cells of the body to take in glucose from the bloodstream, lowering the body's blood sugar level. This occurs after a meal has been eaten and the carbohydrates are absorbed into the bloodstream. In this way the cells obtain the glucose they need for cellular respiration.

Another set of islet cells, the alpha (α) cells, secrete a different hormone, glucagon, which stimulates the liver to release glucose, thereby raising the blood glucose level. Glucagon is released when the body needs more sugar, such as at the beginning of strenuous activity or several hours after the last meal has been digested. Insulin and glucagon have opposite effects on blood sugar level. Insulin will reduce the blood sugar level, while glucagon will increase it.

Parathyroid Glands

calcium

parathyroid hormone (pair-ah-THIGH-royd / HOR-mohn)

The four tiny parathyroid glands are located on the dorsal surface of the thyroid gland (see Figure 11-4 ■). The **parathyroid hormone** (PTH) secreted by these glands regulates the amount of **calcium** in the blood (see again Table 11-1). If blood calcium levels fall too low, parathyroid hormone levels in the blood are increased and will stimulate bone breakdown to release more calcium into the blood.

Pineal Gland

circadian rhythm (ser-KAY-dee-an)
thalamus (THAL-ah-mus)

melatonin (mel-ah-TOH-nin)

The pineal gland is a small pine cone–shaped organ that is part of the **thalamus** region of the brain (see Figure 11-5 ■). The pineal gland secretes **melatonin**, which plays a role in regulating the body's **circadian rhythm** (see again Table 11-1). This is the 24-hour clock that governs periods of wakefulness and sleepiness.

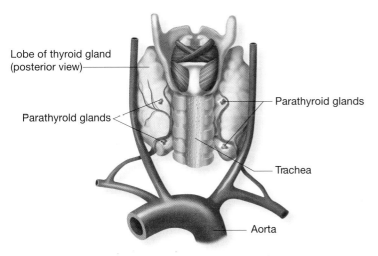

Lobe of thyroid gland
(posterior view)

Parathyroid glands

Parathyrold glands

Parathyroid glands

Trachea

Aorta

■ **Figure 11-4** The parathyroid glands. These four glands are located on the posterior side of the thyroid gland. They secrete parathyroid hormone.

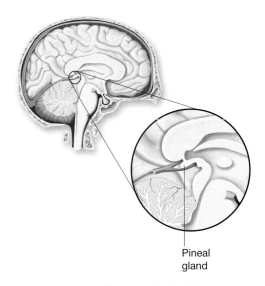

Pineal
gland

■ **Figure 11-5** The pineal gland is a part of the thalamus region of the brain. It secretes melatonin.

Pituitary Gland

adrenocorticotropic hormone
(ah-dree-noh-kor-tih-koh-TROH-pik)

anterior lobe

antidiuretic hormone (an-tye-dye-yoo-RET-ik)

follicle-stimulating hormone (FALL-ih-kl /
STIM-yoo-lay-ting)

gonadotropins (goh-nad-oh-TROH-pins)

growth hormone

hypothalamus (high-poh-THAL-ah-mus)

luteinizing hormone (LOO-teh-nigh-zing)

melanocyte-stimulating hormone

oxytocin (ok-see-TOH-sin)

posterior lobe

prolactin (proh-LAK-tin)

somatotropin (soh-mat-oh-TROH-pin)

thyroid-stimulating hormone

> **What's In A Name?**
> Look for these word parts:
> **somat/o** = body
> **-tropin** = to stimulate
> **hypo-** = below

The pituitary gland is located underneath the brain (see Figure 11-6 ■). The small marble-shaped organ is divided into an **anterior lobe** and a **posterior lobe**.

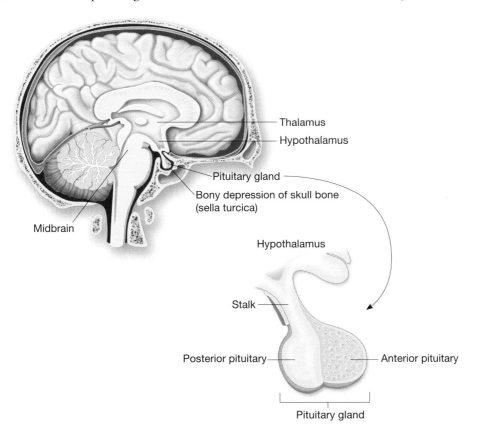

Thalamus

Hypothalamus

Pituitary gland

Bony depression of skull bone
(sella turcica)

Midbrain

Hypothalamus

Stalk

Posterior pituitary

Anterior pituitary

Pituitary gland

■ **Figure 11-6** The pituitary gland lies just underneath the brain. It is subdivided into anterior and posterior lobes. Each lobe secretes different hormones.

Med Term Tip

The pituitary gland is sometimes referred to as the *master gland* because several of its secretions regulate other endocrine glands.

Med Term Tip

Many people use the term *diabetes* to refer to diabetes mellitus (DM). But there is another type of diabetes, called *diabetes insipidus* (DI), that is a result of the inadequate secretion of the antidiuretic hormone (ADH) from the pituitary gland.

Both lobes are controlled by the **hypothalamus**, a region of the brain active in regulating automatic body responses.

The anterior pituitary secretes several different hormones (see again Table 11-1 and Figure 11-7 ■). **Growth hormone** (GH), also called **somatotropin**, promotes growth of the body by stimulating cells to rapidly increase in size and divide. **Thyroid-stimulating hormone** (TSH) regulates the function of the thyroid gland. **Adrenocorticotropic hormone** (ACTH) regulates the function of the adrenal cortex. **Prolactin** (PRL) stimulates milk production in the breast following pregnancy and birth. **Follicle-stimulating hormone** (FSH) and **luteinizing hormone** (LH) both exert their influence on the male and female gonads. Therefore, these two hormones together are referred to as the **gonadotropins**. Follicle-stimulating hormone is responsible for the development of ova in ovaries and sperm in testes. It also stimulates the ovary to secrete estrogen. Luteinizing hormone stimulates the secretion of sex hormones in both males and females and plays a role in releasing ova in females. **Melanocyte-stimulating hormone** (MSH) stimulates melanocytes to produce more melanin, thereby darkening the skin.

The posterior pituitary secretes two hormones, **antidiuretic hormone** (ADH) and **oxytocin** (see again Table 11-1). Antidiuretic hormone promotes water reabsorption by the kidney tubules. Oxytocin stimulates uterine contractions during labor and delivery and, after birth, the release of milk from the mammary glands.

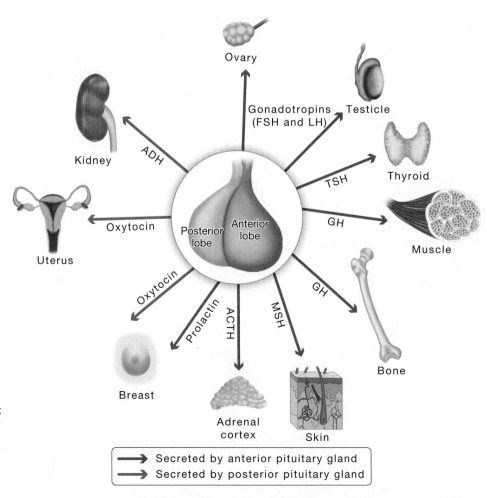

■ **Figure 11-7** The pituitary gland is sometimes called the master gland because it secretes many hormones that regulate other glands. This figure illustrates the different hormones and target tissues for the pituitary gland. *(Pearson Education, Inc.)*

Testes

sperm   **testosterone** (tess-TAHS-ter-ohn)

The testes are two oval glands located in the scrotal sac of the male (see Figure 11-8 ■). They are the male gonads, which produce the male gametes, **sperm**, and the male sex hormone, **testosterone** (see again Table 11-1). Testosterone produces the male secondary sexual characteristics and regulates sperm production.

Thymus Gland

T cells   **thymosin** (THIGH-moh-sin)

In addition to its role as part of the immune system, the thymus is also one of the endocrine glands because it secretes the hormone **thymosin** (see again Table 11-1). Thymosin, like the rest of the thymus gland, is important for proper development of the immune system. The thymus gland is located in the mediastinal cavity anterior and superior to the heart (see Figure 11-9 ■). The thymus is present at birth and grows to its largest size during puberty. At puberty it begins to shrink and eventually is replaced with connective and adipose tissue.

The most important function of the thymus is its role in the development of the immune system in the newborn. It is essential to the growth and development of thymic lymphocytes or **T cells**, which are critical for the body's immune system.

Thyroid Gland

basal metabolic rate	**thyroxine** (thigh-ROKS-in)
calcitonin (kal-sih-TOH-nin)	**triiodothyronine**
iodine (EYE-oh-dine)	(trye-eye-oh-doh-THIGH-roh-neen)

> **What's In A Name?**
> Look for these word parts:
> **bas/o** = base
> **-al** = pertaining to
> **-ic** = pertaining to

The thyroid gland, which resembles a butterfly in shape, has right and left lobes (see Figure 11-10 ■). It is located on either side of the trachea and larynx. The

■ **Figure 11-8**   A testis. In addition to producing sperm, each testis secretes the male sex hormones, primarily testosterone.

■ Figure 11-9 The thymus gland. This gland lies in the mediastinum of the thoracic cavity, just above the heart. It secretes thymosin.

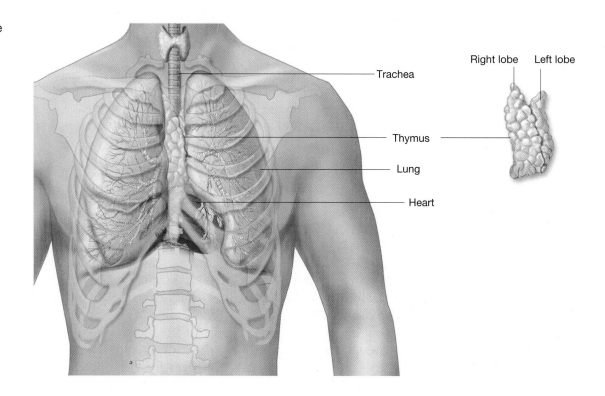

Right lobe Left lobe

Trachea

Thymus

Lung

Heart

Med Term Tip

Iodine is found in many foods, including vegetables and seafood. It is also present in iodized salt, which is one of the best sources of iodine for people living in the Goiter Belt, composed of states located away from saltwater. A lack of iodine in the diet can lead to thyroid disorders, including *goiter*.

thyroid cartilage, or Adam's apple, is located just above the thyroid gland. This gland produces the hormones **thyroxine** (T_4) and **triiodothyronine** (T_3) (see again Table 11-1). These hormones are produced in the thyroid gland using the mineral **iodine**. Thyroxine and triiodothyronine help to regulate the production of energy and heat in the body to adjust the body's metabolic rate. The minimum rate of metabolism necessary to support the function of the body at rest is called the **basal metabolic rate** (BMR).

The thyroid gland also secretes **calcitonin** (CT) in response to hypercalcemia (too high blood calcium level). Its action is the opposite of the parathyroid hormone and stimulates the increased deposition of calcium into bone, thereby lowering blood levels of calcium.

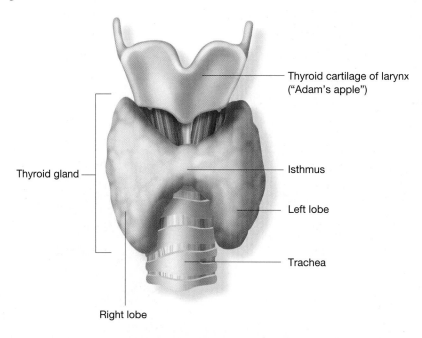

Thyroid cartilage of larynx ("Adam's apple")

Thyroid gland

Isthmus

Left lobe

Trachea

Right lobe

■ Figure 11-10 The thyroid gland is subdivided into two lobes, one on each side of the trachea.

PRACTICE AS YOU GO

B. Complete the Statement

1. The study of the endocrine system is called _____.

2. The master endocrine gland is the _____.

3. _____ is a general term for the sexual organs that produce gametes.

4. The term for the hormones produced by the outer layer of the adrenal cortex is _____.

5. The _____ is the body's 24-hour clock that governs periods of wakefulness and sleepiness.

6. Thyroxine and triiodothyronine are produced using the mineral _____.

7. _____ and _____ work to regulate the level of glucose in the bloodstream.

8. The endocrine gland associated with the immune system is the _____.

Terminology

Word Parts Used to Build Endocrine System Terms

The following lists contain the combining forms, suffixes, and prefixes used to build terms in the remaining sections of this chapter.

Combining Forms

acr/o	extremities	gynec/o	female	parathyroid/o	parathyroid gland
aden/o	gland	immun/o	protection	pineal/o	pineal gland
adren/o	adrenal gland	kal/i	potassium	pituit/o	pituitary gland
adrenal/o	adrenal gland	ket/o	ketones	pituitar/o	pituitary gland
calc/o	calcium	lapar/o	abdomen	radi/o	radiation
carcin/o	cancer	lob/o	lobe	retin/o (see Chapter 13)	retina
chem/o	drug	mast/o	breast	testicul/o	testes
cortic/o	outer layer	natr/o	sodium	thym/o	thymus gland
crin/o	to secrete	neur/o	nerve	thyr/o	thyroid gland
cyt/o	cell	ophthalm/o	eye	thyroid/o	thyroid gland
gluc/o	glucose	or/o	mouth	toxic/o	poison
glyc/o	sugar	ovari/o	ovary		
glycos/o	sugar	pancreat/o	pancreas		

Suffixes

-al	pertaining to
-an	pertaining to
-ar	pertaining to
-ary	pertaining to
-dipsia	thirst
-ectomy	surgical removal
-edema	swelling
-emia	blood condition
-emic	pertaining to a blood condition

-graphy	process of recording
-ia	condition
-ic	pertaining to
-ism	state of
-itis	inflammation
-logy	study of
-megaly	enlarged
-meter	instrument to measure

-oma	tumor
-osis	abnormal condition
-pathy	disease
-prandial	pertaining to a meal
-scopic	pertaining to visually examining
-tic	pertaining to
-uria	urine condition

Prefixes

anti-	against
endo-	within
ex-	outward

hyper-	excessive
hypo-	insufficient
pan-	all

poly-	many
post-	after

Adjective Forms of Anatomical Terms

Term	Word Parts	Definition
adrenal (ah-DREE-nal)	adren/o = adrenal gland -al = pertaining to	Pertaining to adrenal glands
ovarian (oh-VAIR-ee-an)	ovari/o = ovary -an = pertaining to	Pertaining to ovary
pancreatic (pan-kree-AT-ik)	pancreat/o = pancreas -ic = pertaining to	Pertaining to pancreas
parathyroidal (pair-ah-thigh-ROYD-al)	parathyroid/o = parathyroid gland -al = pertaining to	Pertaining to parathyroid gland
pineal (PIN-ee-al)	pineal/o = pineal gland -al = pertaining to	Pertaining to pineal gland

Word Watch

Note the atypical way in which the term *pineal* is formed. More of the letters from the combining form are dropped before adding the suffix.

Term	Word Parts	Definition
pituitary (pih-TOO-ih-tair-ee)	pituit/o = pituitary gland -ary = pertaining to	Pertaining to pituitary gland
testicular (tess-TIK-yoo-lar)	testicul/o = testes -ar = pertaining to	Pertaining to testes
thymic (THIGH-mik)	thym/o = thymus gland -ic = pertaining to	Pertaining to thymus gland
thyroidal (thigh-ROYD-al)	thyroid/o = thyroid gland -al = pertaining to	Pertaining to thyroid gland

PRACTICE AS YOU GO

C. Give the adjective form for each anatomical structure.

1. The thymus gland   _____

2. The pancreas   _____

3. The thyroid gland   _____

4. An ovary   _____

5. A testis   _____

Pathology

Term	Word Parts	Definition
Medical Specialties		
endocrinology (en-doh-krin-ALL-oh-jee)	endo- = within crin/o = to secrete -logy = study of	Branch of medicine involving diagnosis and treatment of conditions and diseases of endocrine glands; physician is *endocrinologist*
Signs and Symptoms		
adrenomegaly (ah-dree-noh-MEG-ah-lee)	adren/o = adrenal gland -megaly = enlarged	Having one or both adrenal glands enlarged
adrenopathy (ad-ren-OP-ah-thee)	adren/o = adrenal gland -pathy = disease	General term for adrenal gland disease
edema (eh-DEE-mah)	**Word Watch** Watch how the term *edema* is used in this condition. It may also appear as the suffix **-edema**.	Condition in which body tissues contain excessive amounts of fluid
endocrinopathy (en-doh-krin-OP-ah-thee)	endo- = within crin/o = to secrete -pathy = disease	General term for diseases of the endocrine system
exophthalmos (eks-off-THAL-muss)	ex- = outward ophthalm/o = eye	Condition in which the eyeballs protrude, such as in Graves' disease; generally caused by overproduction of thyroid hormone
glycosuria (gly-kohs-YOO-ree-ah)	glycos/o = sugar -uria = urine condition	Having a high level of sugar excreted in urine
gynecomastia (gigh-neh-koh-MAST-ee-ah)	gynec/o = female mast/o = breast -ia = condition	Development of breast tissue in males; may be symptom of adrenal feminization
hirsutism (HER-soo-tizm)	-ism = state of	Condition of having excessive amount of hair; generally used to describe females who have adult male pattern of hair growth; can be result of hormonal imbalance

Pathology (continued)

Term	Word Parts	Definition
hypercalcemia (high-per-kal-SEE-mee-ah)	hyper- = excessive calc/o = calcium -emia = blood condition	Condition of having high level of calcium in the blood; associated with hypersecretion of parathyroid hormone
hyperglycemia (high-per-gly-SEE-mee-ah)	hyper- = excessive glyc/o = sugar -emia = blood condition	Condition of having high level of sugar in the blood; associated with diabetes mellitus
hyperkalemia (high-per-kuh-LEE-mee-ah)	hyper- = excessive kal/i = potassium -emia = blood condition	Condition of having high level of potassium in the blood
hypersecretion	hyper- = excessive	Excessive hormone production by an endocrine gland
hypocalcemia (high-poh-kal-SEE-mee-ah)	hypo- = insufficient calc/o = calcium -emia = blood condition	Condition of having low level of calcium in the blood; associated with hyposecretion of parathyroid hormone; hypocalcemia may result in tetany
hypoglycemia (high-poh-gly-SEE-mee-ah)	hypo- = insufficient glyc/o = sugar -emia = blood condition	Condition of having low level of sugar in the blood
hyponatremia (high-poh-nuh-TREE-mee-ah)	hypo- = insufficient natr/o = sodium -emia = blood condition	Condition of having low level of sodium in the blood
hyposecretion	hypo- = insufficient	Deficient hormone production by an endocrine gland
obesity (oh-BEE-sih-tee)		Having abnormal amount of fat in the body
polydipsia (pol-ee-DIP-see-ah)	poly- = many -dipsia = thirst	Excessive feeling of thirst
polyuria (pol-ee-YOO-ree-ah)	poly- = many -uria = urine condition	Condition of producing excessive amount of urine
syndrome (SIN-drohm)		Group of symptoms and signs that, when combined, present clinical picture of disease or condition
thyromegaly (thigh-roh-MEG-ah-lee)	thyr/o = thyroid gland -megaly = enlarged	Having enlarged thyroid gland
Adrenal Glands		
Addison's disease (AD-ih-sons)		Disease named for British physician Thomas Addison; results from deficiency in adrenocortical hormones; there may be increased pigmentation of skin, generalized weakness, and weight loss
adrenal feminization (ah-DREE-nal / fem-ih-nih-ZAY-shun)	adren/o = adrenal gland -al = pertaining to	Development of female secondary sexual characteristics (such as breasts) in a male; often as result of increased estrogen secretion by the adrenal cortex
adrenal virilism (ah-DREE-nal / VIR-ill-izm)	adren/o = adrenal gland -al = pertaining to -ism = state of	Development of male secondary sexual characteristics (such as deeper voice and facial hair) in a female; often as result of increased androgen secretion by the adrenal cortex

Pathology (continued)

Term	Word Parts	Definition
adrenalitis (ah-dree-nal-EYE-tis)	adrenal/o = adrenal gland -itis = inflammation	Inflammation of one or both adrenal glands
Cushing's syndrome (KUSH-ings / SIN-drohm)		Set of symptoms caused by excessive levels of cortisol due to high doses of corticosteroid drugs and adrenal tumors; syndrome may present symptoms of weakness, edema, excess hair growth, skin discoloration, and osteoporosis
pheochromocytoma (fee-oh-kroh-moh-sigh-TOH-mah)	cyt/o = cell -oma = tumor	Usually benign tumor of the adrenal medulla that secretes epinephrine; symptoms include anxiety, heart palpitations, dyspnea, profuse sweating, headache, and nausea
Pancreas		
diabetes mellitus (DM) (dye-ah-BEE-teez / MEL-ih-tus)		Chronic disorder of carbohydrate metabolism resulting in hyperglycemia and glycosuria; there are two distinct forms of diabetes mellitus: *insulin-dependent diabetes mellitus* (IDDM) or *type 1*, and *non-insulin-dependent diabetes mellitus* (NIDDM) or *type 2*
diabetic retinopathy (dye-ah-BET-ik / ret-in-OP-ah-thee)	-tic = pertaining to retin/o = retina -pathy = disease	Secondary complication of diabetes that affects blood vessels of the retina, resulting in visual changes and even blindness
insulin-dependent diabetes mellitus (IDDM) (dye-ah-BEE-teez / MEL-ih-tus)		Also called *type 1 diabetes mellitus*; develops early in life when the pancreas stops insulin production; patient must take daily insulin injections
insulinoma (in-soo-lin-OH-mah)	-oma = tumor	Tumor of the islets of Langerhans cells of the pancreas that secretes excessive amount of insulin
ketoacidosis (kee-toh-ass-ih-DOH-sis)	ket/o = ketones -osis = abnormal condition	Acidosis due to excess of acidic ketone bodies (waste products); serious condition requiring immediate treatment as it may result in death for diabetic patient if not reversed; also called *diabetic acidosis*
non-insulin-dependent diabetes mellitus (NIDDM) (dye-ah-BEE-teez / MEL-ih-tus)		Also called *type 2 diabetes mellitus*; typically develops later in life; the pancreas produces normal to high levels of insulin, but cells fail to respond to it; patients may take oral hypoglycemics to improve insulin function or may eventually have to take insulin
peripheral neuropathy (per-IF-eh-ral / noo-ROP-ah-thee)	-al = pertaining to neur/o = nerve -pathy = disease	Damage to nerves in lower legs and hands as result of diabetes mellitus; symptoms include either extreme sensitivity or numbness and tingling
Parathyroid Glands		
hyperparathyroidism (high-per-pair-ah-THIGH-royd-izm)	hyper- = excessive parathyroid/o = parathyroid gland -ism = state of	Hypersecretion of parathyroid hormone; may result in hypercalcemia and Recklinghausen disease
hypoparathyroidism (high-poh-pair-ah-THIGH-royd-izm)	hypo- = insufficient parathyroid/o = parathyroid gland -ism = state of	Hyposecretion of parathyroid hormone; may result in hypocalcemia and tetany

Pathology (continued)

Term	Word Parts	Definition
Recklinghausen disease (REK-ling-how-zen)		Excessive production of parathyroid hormone resulting in degeneration of bones
tetany (TET-ah-nee)		Nerve irritability and painful muscle cramps resulting from hypocalcemia; hypoparathyroidism is one cause of tetany

Pituitary Gland

Term	Word Parts	Definition
acromegaly (ak-roh-MEG-ah-lee)	acr/o = extremities -megaly = enlarged	Chronic disease of adults that results in elongation and enlargement of bones of head and extremities; can also be mood changes; due to excessive amount of growth hormone in adult

■ **Figure 11-11** Skull X-ray (lateral view) of person with acromegaly showing abnormally enlarged mandible. *(Zephyr/Science Source)*

Term	Word Parts	Definition
diabetes insipidus (DI) (dye-ah-BEE-teez / in-SIP-ih-dus)		Disorder caused by inadequate secretion of antidiuretic hormone by posterior lobe of the pituitary gland; may be polyuria and polydipsia
dwarfism (DWARF-izm)	-ism = state of	Condition of being abnormally short in height; may be result of hereditary condition or lack of growth hormone
gigantism (JYE-gan-tizm)	-ism = state of	Excessive development of body due to overproduction of growth hormone by the pituitary gland in child or teenager; opposite of *dwarfism*
hyperpituitarism (high-per-pih-TOO-ih-tuh-rizm)	hyper- = excessive pituitar/o = pituitary gland -ism = state of	Hypersecretion of one or more pituitary gland hormones
hypopituitarism (high-poh-pih-TOO-ih-tuh-rizm)	hypo- = insufficient pituitar/o = pituitary gland -ism = state of	Hyposecretion of one or more pituitary gland hormones
panhypopituitarism (pan-high-poh-pih-TOO-ih-tuh-rizm)	pan- = all hypo- = insufficient pituitar/o = pituitary gland -ism = state of	Deficiency in all hormones secreted by the pituitary gland; often recognized because of problems with glands regulated by the pituitary—adrenal cortex, thyroid, ovaries, and testes

Thymus Gland

Term	Word Parts	Definition
thymitis (thigh-MY-tis)	thym/o = thymus gland -itis = inflammation	Inflammation of the thymus gland

Pathology (continued)

Term	Word Parts	Definition
thymoma (thigh-MOH-mah)	thym/o = thymus gland -oma = tumor	Tumor in the thymus gland
Thyroid Gland		
congenital hypothyroidism (high-poh-THIGH-royd-izm)	hypo- = insufficient thyroid/o = thyroid gland -ism = state of	Congenital condition in which lack of thyroid hormones may result in arrested physical and mental development; formerly called *cretinism*
goiter (GOY-ter)		Enlargement of the thyroid gland

■ **Figure 11-12** Goiter. A photograph of a male with an extreme goiter or enlarged thyroid gland. *(Eugene Gordon/ Pearson Education, Inc.)*

Term	Word Parts	Definition
Graves' disease		Condition named for Irish physician Robert Graves that results in overactivity of the thyroid gland and can cause a crisis situation; symptoms include exophthalmos and goiter; a type of *hyperthyroidism*
Hashimoto's thyroiditis (hash-ee-MOH-tohz / thigh-roy-DYE-tis)	thyroid/o = thyroid gland -itis = inflammation	Chronic autoimmune form of thyroiditis; results in hyposecretion of thyroid hormones
hyperthyroidism (high-per-THIGH-royd-izm)	hyper- = excessive thyroid/o = thyroid gland -ism = state of	Hypersecretion of thyroid gland hormones
hypothyroidism (high-poh-THIGH-royd-izm)	hypo- = insufficient thyroid/o = thyroid gland -ism = state of	Hyposecretion of thyroid gland hormones
myxedema (miks-eh-DEE-mah)	-edema = swelling	Condition resulting from hyposecretion of the thyroid gland in adult; symptoms can include swollen facial features, edematous skin, anemia, slow speech, drowsiness, and mental lethargy
thyrotoxicosis (thigh-roh-tok-sih-KOH-sis)	thyr/o = thyroid gland toxic/o = poison -osis = abnormal condition	Condition resulting from marked overproduction of the thyroid gland; symptoms include rapid heart action, tremors, enlarged thyroid gland, exophthalmos, and weight loss
All Glands		
adenocarcinoma (ad-eh-noh-kar-sih-NOH-mah)	aden/o = gland carcin/o = cancer -oma = tumor	Cancerous tumor in gland that is capable of producing hormones secreted by that gland; one cause of hypersecretion pathologies

PRACTICE AS YOU GO

D. Terminology Matching

Match each term to its definition.

1. _____ Cushing's syndrome
2. _____ goiter
3. _____ acromegaly
4. _____ gigantism
5. _____ myxedema
6. _____ diabetes mellitus
7. _____ diabetes insipidus
8. _____ Hashimoto's thyroiditis
9. _____ Graves' disease
10. _____ Addison's disease

a. enlarged thyroid
b. overactive adrenal cortex
c. hyperthyroidism
d. underactive adrenal cortex
e. enlarged bones of head and extremities
f. may cause polyuria and polydipsia
g. an autoimmune disease
h. excessive growth hormone in a child
i. disorder of carbohydrate metabolism
j. insufficient thyroid hormone in an adult

Diagnostic Procedures

Term	Word Parts	Definition
Clinical Laboratory Tests		
blood serum test		Blood test to measure level of substances such as calcium, electrolytes, testosterone, insulin, and glucose; used to assist in determining function of various endocrine glands
fasting blood sugar (FBS)		Blood test to measure amount of sugar circulating throughout body after 12-hour fast
glucose tolerance test (GTT) (GLOO-kohs)		Test to determine blood sugar level; measured dose of glucose is given to a patient either orally or intravenously; blood samples are then drawn at certain intervals to determine ability of patient to use glucose; used for diabetic patients to determine insulin response to glucose
protein-bound iodine (PBI) **test**		Blood test to measure concentration of thyroxine (T_4) circulating in bloodstream; iodine becomes bound to protein in blood and can be measured; useful in establishing thyroid function
radioimmunoassay (RIA) (ray-dee-oh-im-yoo-noh-ASS-ay)	radi/o = ray immun/o = protection	Blood test that uses radioactively tagged hormones and antibodies to measure quantity of hormone in the plasma
thyroid function test (TFT) (THIGH-royd)		Blood test used to measure levels of thyroxine, triiodothyronine, and thyroid-stimulating hormone in bloodstream to assist in determining thyroid function

Diagnostic Procedures (continued)

Term	Word Parts	Definition
total calcium		Blood test to measure total amount of calcium to assist in detecting parathyroid and bone disorders
two-hour postprandial glucose tolerance test (post-PRAN-dee-al)	post- = after -prandial = pertaining to a meal	Blood test to assist in evaluating glucose metabolism; patient eats high-carbohydrate diet and then fasts overnight before test; then blood sample is taken two hours after a meal
Diagnostic Imaging		
thyroid echography (THIGH-royd / eh-KOG-rah-fee)	-graphy = process of recording	Ultrasound examination of thyroid that can assist in distinguishing a thyroid nodule from a cyst
thyroid scan (THIGH-royd)		Test in which radioactive iodine is administered that localizes in the thyroid gland; gland can then be visualized with scanning device to detect pathology such as tumors

Therapeutic Procedures

Term	Word Parts	Definition
Medical Procedures		
adrenalectomy (ah-dree-nal-EK-toh-mee)	adrenal/o = adrenal gland -ectomy = surgical removal	Surgical removal of one or both adrenal glands
chemical thyroidectomy (thigh-royd-EK-toh-mee)	chem/o = drug -al = pertaining to thyroid/o = thyroid gland -ectomy = surgical removal	Large dose of radioactive iodine (RAI) is given in order to kill thyroid gland cells without having to actually do surgery
glucometer (gloo-KOM-eh-ter)	gluc/o = glucose -meter = instrument to measure	Device designed for diabetic to use at home to measure level of glucose in bloodstream
hormone replacement therapy (HRT)		Artificial replacement of hormones in patients with hyposecretion disorders; may be oral pills, injections, or adhesive skin patches
laparoscopic adrenalectomy (lap-ar-oh-SKOP-ik / ah-dree-nal-EK-toh-mee)	lapar/o = abdomen -scopic = pertaining to visually examining adrenal/o = adrenal gland -ectomy = surgical removal	Removal of the adrenal gland through small incision in abdomen and using endoscopic instruments
lobectomy (loh-BEK-toh-mee)	lob/o = lobe -ectomy = surgical removal	Removal of a lobe from an organ; for example, one lobe of the thyroid gland
parathyroidectomy (pair-ah-thigh-royd-EK-toh-mee)	parathyroid/o = parathyroid gland -ectomy = surgical removal	Surgical removal of one or more of the parathyroid glands
pinealectomy (pin-ee-ah-LEK-toh-mee)	pineal/o = pineal gland -ectomy = surgical removal	Surgical removal of the pineal gland
thymectomy (thigh-MEK-toh-mee)	thym/o = thymus gland -ectomy = surgical removal	Surgical removal of the thymus gland
thyroidectomy (thigh-royd-EK-toh-mee)	thyroid/o = thyroid gland -ectomy = surgical removal	Surgical removal of the thyroid gland

PRACTICE AS YOU GO

E. Procedure Matching

Match each procedure term with its definition.

1. _____ protein-bound iodine test
2. _____ fasting blood sugar
3. _____ radioimmunoassay
4. _____ thyroid scan
5. _____ two-hour postprandial glucose tolerance test
6. _____ glucose tolerance test
7. _____ glucometer
8. _____ chemical thyroidectomy

a. measures levels of hormones in the blood
b. determines glucose metabolism after patient receives a measured dose of glucose
c. test of glucose metabolism two hours after eating a meal
d. measures blood sugar level after 12-hour fast
e. measures T_4 concentration in the blood
f. uses radioactive iodine
g. used instead of a surgical procedure
h. instrument to measure blood glucose

Pharmacology

Classification	Word Parts	Action	Examples
antithyroid agents	anti- = against	Block production of thyroid hormones in patients with hypersecretion disorders	methimazole, Tapazole; propylthiouracil
aquaretics (ak-wuh-RET-iks)	Aqua is the Latin term for water	Inserts aquaporins (water channels) in the nephron to treat hyponatremia; increases water excretion by kidney without increasing sodium excretion	conivaptan, Vaprisol; tolvaptan, Samsca
corticosteroids (kor-tih-koh-STAIR-oydz)	cortic/o = outer layer	Although function of these hormones in body is to regulate carbohydrate metabolism, they also have strong anti-inflammatory action; therefore are used to treat severe chronic inflammatory diseases such as rheumatoid arthritis; long-term use has adverse side effects such as osteoporosis and symptoms of Cushing's syndrome; also used to treat adrenal cortex hyposecretion disorders such as Addison's disease	prednisone, Deltasone
human growth hormone therapy		Hormone replacement therapy with human growth hormone in order to stimulate skeletal growth; used to treat children with abnormally short stature	somatropin, Genotropin; somatrem, Protropin
insulin (IN-suh-lin)		Replaces insulin for type 1 diabetics or treats severe type 2 diabetics	human insulin, Humulin
oral hypoglycemic agents (high-poh-gly-SEE-mik)	or/o = mouth -al = pertaining to hypo- = insufficient glyc/o = sugar -emic = pertaining to a blood condition	Taken by mouth to cause decrease in blood sugar; not used for insulin-dependent patients	metformin, Glucophage; glipizide, Glucotrol

Pharmacology (continued)

Classification	Word Parts	Action	Examples
thyroid replacement hormone		Hormone replacement therapy for patients with hypothyroidism or who have had a thyroidectomy	levothyroxine, Levo-T; liothyronine, Cytomel

Abbreviations

α	alpha	**MSH**	melanocyte-stimulating hormone
ACTH	adrenocorticotropic hormone	**Na⁺**	sodium
ADH	antidiuretic hormone	**NIDDM**	non-insulin-dependent diabetes mellitus
aq	aqueous	**NPH**	neutral protamine Hagedorn (insulin)
β	beta	**od**	overdose
BMR	basal metabolic rate	**PBI**	protein-bound iodine
cap(s)	capsule(s)	**PRL**	prolactin
CT	calcitonin	**PTH**	parathyroid hormone
DI	diabetes insipidus	**RAI**	radioactive iodine
DM	diabetes mellitus	**RIA**	radioimmunoassay
FBS	fasting blood sugar	**sol**	solution
FSH	follicle-stimulating hormone	**susp**	suspension
GH	growth hormone	**syr**	syrup
GTT	glucose tolerance test	**T₃**	triiodothyronine
HRT	hormone replacement therapy	**T₄**	thyroxine
IDDM	insulin-dependent diabetes mellitus	**tab(s)**	tablet(s)
inj	injection	**TFT**	thyroid function test
K⁺	potassium	**TSH**	thyroid-stimulating hormone
LH	luteinizing hormone		

PRACTICE AS YOU GO

F. What's the Abbreviation?

1. non-insulin-dependent diabetes mellitus _____

2. insulin-dependent diabetes mellitus _____

3. adrenocorticotropic hormone _____

4. parathyroid hormone _____

5. triiodothyronine _____

6. thyroid-stimulating hormone _____

7. fasting blood sugar _____

8. prolactin _____

Chapter Review

Real-World Applications

Medical Record Analysis
This Discharge Summary below contains 10 medical terms. Underline each term and write it in the list below the report. Then explain each term as you would to a nonmedical person.

Discharge Summary

Admitting Diagnosis:	Hyperglycemia, ketoacidosis, glycosuria
Final Diagnosis:	New-onset type 1 diabetes mellitus
History of Present Illness:	A 12-year-old female patient presented to her physician's office with a two-month history of weight loss, fatigue, polyuria, and polydipsia. Her family history is significant for a grandfather, mother, and older brother with type 1 diabetes mellitus. The pediatrician found hyperglycemia with a fasting blood sugar and glycosuria with a urine dipstick. She is being admitted at this time for management of new-onset diabetes mellitus.
Summary of Hospital Course:	At the time of admission, the FBS was 300 mg/100 mL and she was in ketoacidosis. She rapidly improved after receiving insulin; her blood glucose level normalized. The next day a glucose tolerance test confirmed the diagnosis of diabetes mellitus. The patient was started on insulin injections. Patient and family were instructed on diabetes mellitus, insulin, diet, exercise, and long-term complications.
Discharge Plans:	Patient was discharged to home with her parents. Her parents are to check her blood glucose levels twice daily and call the office for insulin dosage. She is to return to the office in two weeks.

Term   **Explanation**

1. _____   _____
2. _____   _____
3. _____   _____
4. _____   _____
5. _____   _____
6. _____   _____
7. _____   _____
8. _____   _____
9. _____   _____
10. _____   _____

Chart Note Transcription

The chart note below contains 11 phrases that can be reworded with a medical term presented in this chapter. Each phrase is identified with an underline. Determine the medical term and write your answers in the space provided.

Pearson General Hospital Consultation Report

Task   Edit   View   Time Scale   Options   Help Download   Archive   Date: 17 May 2017

Current Complaint: A 56-year-old female was referred to the specialist in the treatment of diseases of the endocrine glands **1** for evaluation of weakness, edema, an abnormal amount of fat in the body, **2** and an excessive amount of hair for a female. **3**

Past History: Patient reports she has been overweight most of her life in spite of a healthy diet and regular exercise. She was diagnosed with osteoporosis after incurring a pathological rib fracture following a coughing attack.

Signs and Symptoms: Patient has moderate edema in bilateral feet and lower legs as well as a puffy face and an upper lip moustache. She is 100 lbs. over normal body weight for her age and height. She moves slowly and appears generally lethargic. A test to measure the hormone levels in the blood plasma **4** reports increased steroid hormone that regulates carbohydrates in the body. **5** A CT scan demonstrates a gland tumor **6** in the right outer layer of the adrenal gland. **7**

Diagnosis: A group of symptoms associated with hypersecretion of the adrenal cortex **8** secondary to a gland tumor **9** in the right outer layer of the adrenal gland **10**

Treatment: Surgical removal of the right adrenal gland **11**

1. _____

2. _____

3. _____

4. _____

5. _____

6. _____

7. _____

8. _____

9. _____

10. _____

11. _____

Case Study

Below is a case study presentation of a patient with a condition discussed in this chapter. Read the case study and answer the questions below. Some questions will ask for information not included within this chapter. Use your text, a medical dictionary, or any other reference material you choose to answer these questions.

A 22-year-old college student was admitted to the emergency room after his friends called an ambulance when he passed out in a bar. He had become confused, developed slurred speech, and had difficulty walking after having only consumed one beer. In the ER he was noted to have diaphoresis, rapid respirations and pulse, and was disoriented. Upon examination, needle marks were found on his abdomen and outer thighs. The physician ordered blood serum tests that revealed hyperglycemia and ketoacidosis. Unknown to his friends, this young man has had diabetes mellitus since early childhood. The patient quickly recovered following an insulin injection.

(Flashon Studio/Shutterstock)

Questions

1. What pathological condition has this patient had since childhood? Look this condition up in a reference source and include a short description of it.

   _____

   _____

2. List and define each symptom noted in the ER in your own words.

   _____

   _____

3. What diagnostic test was performed? Describe it in your own words.

   _____

   _____

4. Explain the results of the test.

   _____

   _____

5. What specific type of diabetes does this young man probably have? Justify your answer.

   _____

   _____

6. Describe the other type of diabetes mellitus that this young man did not have.

   _____

   _____

Practice Exercises

A. Word Building Practice

The combining form **thyroid/o** refers to the *thyroid*. Use it to write a term that means:

1. removal of the thyroid _____
2. pertaining to the thyroid _____
3. state of excessive thyroid _____

The combining form **pancreat/o** refers to the *pancreas*. Use it to write a term that means:

4. pertaining to the pancreas _____
5. inflammation of the pancreas _____
6. removal of the pancreas _____
7. cutting into the pancreas _____

The combining form **adren/o** refers to the *adrenal glands*. Use it to write a term that means:

8. pertaining to the adrenal glands _____
9. enlargement of an adrenal gland _____
10. adrenal gland disease _____

The combining form **thym/o** refers to the *thymus gland*. Use it to write a term that means:

11. tumor of the thymus gland _____
12. removal of the thymus gland _____
13. pertaining to the thymus gland _____
14. inflammation of the thymus gland _____

B. Complete the Term

For each definition given below, fill in the blank with the word part that completes the term.

Definition	Term
1. surgical removal of thyroid gland	_____ectomy
2. instrument to measure glucose	_____meter
3. relating to after a meal	post_____
4. state of insufficient thyroid gland	hypo_____ism
5. state of excessive pituitary gland	hyper_____ism
6. enlarged extremities	_____megaly
7. blood condition of insufficient sodium	hypo_____emia
8. many (abnormally great) thirst	poly_____
9. inflammation of adrenal gland	_____itis
10. blood condition of excessive calcium	hyper_____emia
11. sugar urine condition	_____uria
12. tumor of thymus gland	_____oma

C. Using Abbreviations

Fill in each blank with the appropriate abbreviation.

1. Due to low estrogen levels following early menopause, she received _____.

2. _____ is a test using radioactively tagged hormones and antibodies to measure hormone levels.

3. A(n) _____ measures the level of glucose in the blood after a 12-hour fast.

4. _____ may be either insulin-dependent or non-insulin-dependent.

5. The two gonadotropins are _____ and _____.

6. _____ is the only hormone secreted by the parathyroid gland.

7. _____ is secreted by the anterior pituitary and regulates secretion of some adrenal cortex hormones.

8. _____ regulates function of the thyroid gland.

9. _____ stimulates reabsorption of water by the kidneys.

10. _____ and _____ are secreted by the thyroid gland and stimulate metabolism in the cells.

D. Define the Term

1. corticosteroid _____

2. hirsutism _____

3. tetany _____

4. diabetic retinopathy _____

5. hyperglycemia _____

6. hypoglycemia _____

7. adrenaline _____

8. insulin _____

9. thyrotoxicosis _____

10. hypersecretion _____

E. Fill in the Blank

insulinoma	ketoacidosis	pheochromocytoma
gynecomastia	panhypopituitarism	Hashimoto's thyroiditis

1. The doctor found that Marsha's high level of insulin and hypoglycemia were caused by a(n) _____.

2. Kevin developed _____ as a result of his diabetes mellitus and required emergency treatment.

3. It was determined that Karen had _____ when doctors realized she had problems with her thyroid gland, adrenal cortex, and ovaries.

4. Luke's high epinephrine level was caused by a(n) _____.

5. When it was determined that Carl's thyroiditis was an autoimmune condition, it became obvious that he had _____.

6. Excessive sex hormones caused Jack to develop _____.

F. Pharmacology Challenge

Fill in the classification for each drug description, then match the brand name.

Drug Description	Classification	Brand Name
1. _____ strong anti-inflammatory	_____	a. Genotropin
2. _____ stimulates skeletal growth	_____	b. Levo-T
3. _____ treats type 2 diabetes mellitus	_____	c. Tapazole
4. _____ blocks production of thyroid hormone	_____	d. Glucophage
5. _____ treats type 1 diabetes mellitus	_____	e. Deltasone
6. _____ treatment for hypothyroidism	_____	f. Humulin

G. Terminology Matching

Match each term to its definition.

1. _____ calcitonin
2. _____ exophthalmos
3. _____ ketoacidosis
4. _____ Cushing's syndrome
5. _____ tetany
6. _____ goiter
7. _____ acromegaly
8. _____ MSH
9. _____ melatonin
10. _____ GTT

a. a severe condition for diabetics
b. elongation and enlargement of bones of head and limbs
c. caused by excessive levels of cortisol
d. regulates circadian rhythm
e. enlarged thyroid gland
f. secreted by thyroid gland
g. stimulates pigment in the skin
h. determines blood sugar level
i. bulging eyeballs
j. nerve irritability

H. Spelling Practice

Some of the following terms are misspelled. Identify the incorrect terms and spell them correctly in the blank provided.

1. endocrinopathy _____
2. glycouria _____
3. hypocalcemia _____
4. adrenallitis _____
5. pheochromocytoma _____
6. ketoacidosis _____
7. Reklinghausen _____
8. hyperpituitarianism _____
9. myxedema _____
10. radioimunoassay _____

I. Anatomical Adjectives

Fill in the blank with the adjective for each anatomical structure.

Noun	Adjective
1. ovary	_____
2. pancreas	_____
3. testes	_____
4. thymus gland	_____
5. thyroid gland	_____
6. parathyroid gland	_____

J. Complete the Statement

1. The endocrine system is instrumental in maintaining _____ to maintain a stable internal environment.

2. _____ glands release their secretions into a duct; _____ glands release their secretions into the bloodstream.

3. The _____ glands are located above each kidney.

4. The pancreatic _____ cells secrete _____ and _____.

5. Parathyroid hormone regulates the level of _____ in the bloodstream.

6. The _____ gland is sometimes called the "master gland."

7. _____ is a hormone instrumental in the proper development of the immune system.

8. The minimum rate of metabolism necessary to support the function of the body is the _____.

MyLab Medical Terminology™

MyLab Medical Terminology is a premium online homework management system that includes a host of features to help you study. Registered users will find:

- A multitude of activities and assignments built within the MyLab platform

- Powerful tools that track and analyze your results—allowing you to create a personalized learning experience

- Videos and audio pronunciations to help enrich your progress

- Streaming lesson presentations (Guided Lectures) and self-paced learning modules

- A space where you and your instructors can check your progress and manage your assignments

Labeling Exercises

Image A

Write the labels for this figure on the numbered lines provided.

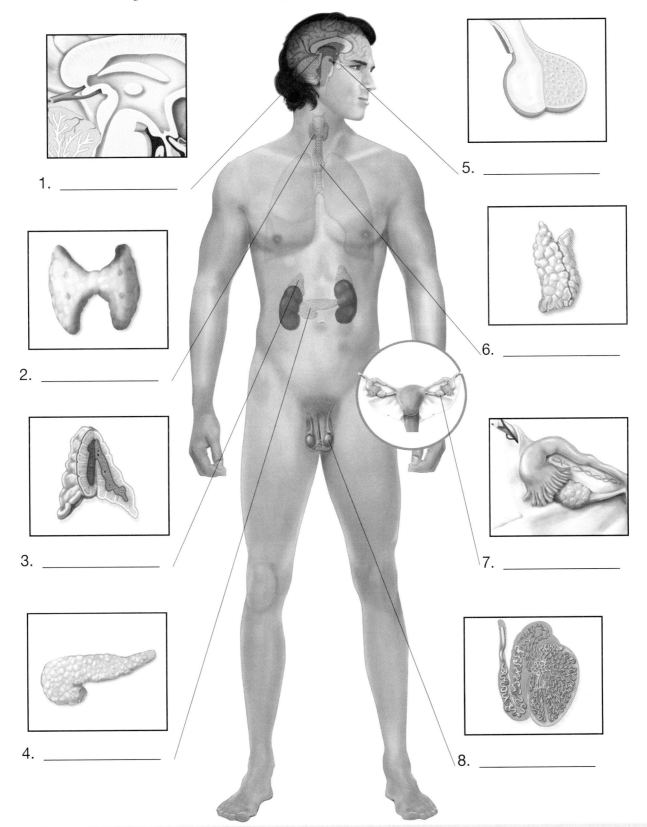

1. _____

2. _____

3. _____

4. _____

5. _____

6. _____

7. _____

8. _____

Image B

Write the labels for this figure on the numbered lines provided.

2. (target)_____

3. (hormone)_____

1. _____

8. (target)_____

9. (hormone)_____

4. (target)_____

5. (hormones)_____,

_____

10. (target)_____

11. (hormone)_____

6. (target)_____

7. (hormones)_____,

_____

12. (target)_____

13. (hormone)_____

Image C

Write the labels for this figure on the numbered lines provided.

1. _____

2. _____

4. Insulin-secreting cell

_____

5. Glucagon-secreting cell

_____

3. _____

6. _____

Chapter 12

Nervous System and Mental Health

Learning Objectives

Upon completion of this chapter, you will be able to

1. Identify and define the combining forms and suffixes introduced in this chapter.

2. Correctly spell and pronounce medical terms and major anatomical structures relating to the nervous system.

3. Locate and describe the major organs of the nervous system and their functions.

4. Describe the components of a neuron.

5. Distinguish between the central nervous system, peripheral nervous system, and autonomic nervous system.

6. Identify and define nervous system anatomical terms.

7. Identify and define selected nervous system pathology terms.

8. Identify and define selected nervous system diagnostic procedures.

9. Identify and define selected nervous system therapeutic procedures.

10. Identify and define selected medications relating to the nervous system.

11. Define selected abbreviations associated with the nervous system.

12. Define the classifications of mental disorders as defined in the *Diagnostic and Statistical Manual of Mental Disorders*, 5th edition.

13. Describe examples of each classification of mental disorders.

14. Identify and define selected mental health therapeutic procedures.

15. Define selected abbreviations associated with mental health.

(Pearson Education, Inc.)

AT A GLANCE

Function

The nervous system coordinates and controls body functions. It receives sensory input, makes decisions, and then orders body responses.

Organs

The primary structures that comprise the nervous system:

brain

spinal cord

nerves

Word Parts

Presented here are the most common word parts (with their meanings) used to build nervous system terms. For a more comprehensive list, refer to the Terminology section of this chapter.

Combining Forms

alges/o	sense of pain	**meningi/o**	meninges
astr/o	star	**ment/o**	mind
centr/o	center	**myel/o**	spinal cord
cerebell/o	cerebellum	**neur/o**	nerve
cerebr/o	cerebrum	**peripher/o**	away from center
clon/o	rapid contracting and relaxing	**poli/o**	gray matter
concuss/o	to shake violently	**pont/o**	pons
dur/o	dura mater	**radicul/o**	nerve root
encephal/o	brain	**thalam/o**	thalamus
esthesi/o	sensation, feeling	**thec/o**	sheath (meninges)
gli/o	glue	**tom/o**	to cut
medull/o	medulla oblongata	**ton/o**	tone
mening/o	meninges	**ventricul/o**	ventricle

Suffixes

-paresis	weakness
-phasia	speech
-taxia	muscle coordination

Nervous System Illustrated

brain, p. 429

Coordinates body functions

spinal cord, p. 432

Transmits messages to and
from the brain

nerves, p. 433

Transmit messages to and
from the central nervous
system

Anatomy and Physiology of the Nervous System

brain	nerves
central nervous system	peripheral nervous system (per-IF-eh-ral)
cranial nerves (KRAY-nee-al)	sensory receptors
glands	spinal cord
muscles	spinal nerves

The nervous system is responsible for coordinating all the activity of the body. To do this, it first receives information from both external and internal **sensory receptors** and then uses that information to adjust the activity of **muscles** and **glands** to match the needs of the body.

The nervous system can be subdivided into the **central nervous system** (CNS) and the **peripheral nervous system** (PNS). The central nervous system consists of the **brain** and **spinal cord**. Sensory information comes into the central nervous system, where it is processed. Motor messages then exit the central nervous system carrying commands to muscles and glands. The **nerves** of the peripheral nervous system are **cranial nerves** and **spinal nerves**. Sensory nerves carry information to the central nervous system, and motor nerves carry commands away from the central nervous system. All portions of the nervous system are composed of nervous tissue.

Nervous Tissue

axon (AK-son)	neuron (NOO-ron)
dendrites (DEN-drights)	neurotransmitter (noo-roh-TRANS-mit-ter)
myelin (MY-eh-lin)	synapse (SIN-aps)
nerve cell body	synaptic cleft (sih-NAP-tik)
neuroglial cells (noo-ROG-lee-al)	

Nervous tissue consists of two basic types of cells: **neurons** and **neuroglial cells**. Neurons are individual nerve cells. These are the cells that are capable of conducting electrical impulses in response to a stimulus. Neurons have three basic parts: **dendrites**, a **nerve cell body**, and an **axon** (see Figure 12-1A ■). Dendrites are highly branched projections that receive impulses. The nerve cell body contains the nucleus and many of the other organelles of the cell (see Figure 12-1B ■). A neuron has only a single axon, a projection from the nerve cell body that conducts the electrical impulse toward its destination. The point at which the axon of one neuron meets the dendrite of the next neuron is called a **synapse**. Electrical impulses cannot pass directly across the gap between two neurons, called the **synaptic cleft**. They instead require the help of a chemical messenger, called a **neurotransmitter**.

A variety of neuroglial cells are found in nervous tissue. Each has a different support function for the neurons. For example, some neuroglial cells produce **myelin**, a fatty substance that acts as insulation for many axons so that they conduct electrical impulses faster. Neuroglial cells *do not* conduct electrical impulses.

Central Nervous System

gray matter	tracts
meninges (men-IN-jeez)	white matter
myelinated (MY-eh-lih-nayt-ed)	

Because the central nervous system is a combination of the brain and spinal cord, it is able to receive impulses from all over the body, process this information, and

■ **Figure 12-1**   A) The structure of a neuron, showing the dendrites, nerve cell body, and axon. B) Photomicrograph of typical neuron showing the nerve cell body, nucleus, and dendrites. *(Christopher Meade/Shutterstock)*

then respond with an action. This system consists of both **gray matter** and **white matter**. Gray matter is comprised of unsheathed or uncovered cell bodies and dendrites. White matter is **myelinated** nerve fibers. The myelin sheath makes the nervous tissue appear white. Bundles of nerve fibers interconnecting different parts of the central nervous system are called **tracts**. The central nervous system is encased and protected by three membranes known as the **meninges**.

> **Med Term Tip**
>
> *Myelin* is a lipid and a very white molecule. This is why myelinated neurons are called *white matter*.

Brain

brainstem
cerebellum (sair-eh-BELL-um)
cerebral cortex (seh-REE-bral / KOR-teks)
cerebral hemisphere
cerebrospinal fluid (seh-ree-broh-SPY-nal)
cerebrum (seh-REE-brum)
diencephalon (dye-en-SEFF-ah-lon)
frontal lobe
gyri (JYE-rye)
hypothalamus (high-poh-THAL-ah-mus)

medulla oblongata
(meh-DULL-ah / ob-long-GAH-tah)
midbrain
occipital lobe (ok-SIP-ih-tal)
parietal lobe (pah-RYE-eh-tal)
pons (PONZ)
sulci (SULL-sigh)
temporal lobe (TEM-por-al)
thalamus (THAL-ah-mus)
ventricles (VEN-trih-kulz)

> **What's In A Name?**
>
> Look for these word parts:
> **encephal/o** = brain
> **-al** = pertaining to
> **hypo-** = below

The brain is one of the largest organs in the body and coordinates most body activities. It is the center for all thought, memory, judgment, and emotion. Each part of the brain is responsible for controlling different body functions, such as temperature regulation, blood pressure, and breathing. There are four sections to the brain: the **cerebrum**, **cerebellum**, **diencephalon**, and **brainstem** (see Figure 12-2 ■).

Located in the upper portion of the brain is the largest section called the cerebrum. It is this area that processes thoughts, judgment, memory, problem solving, and language. The outer layer of the cerebrum is the **cerebral cortex**, which is composed of folds of gray matter. The elevated portions of the cerebrum, or

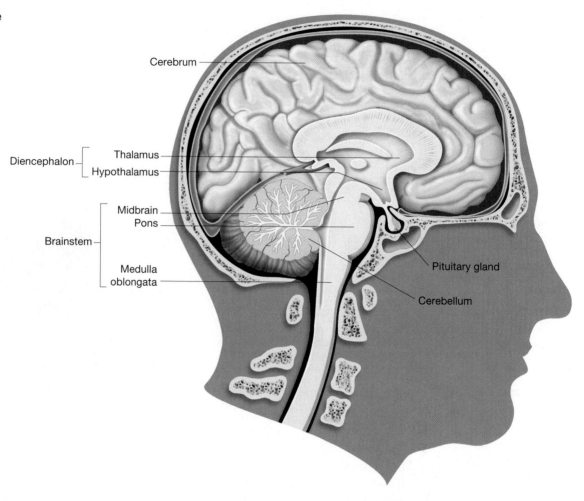

convolutions, are called **gyri** and are separated by fissures, or valleys, called **sulci**.
The cerebrum is subdivided into left and right halves called **cerebral hemispheres**.
Each hemisphere has four lobes. The lobes and their locations and functions are
(see Figure 12-3 ■):

1. **Frontal lobe:** Most anterior portion of the cerebrum; controls motor function, personality, and speech
2. **Parietal lobe:** Most superior portion of the cerebrum; receives and interprets
   nerve impulses from sensory receptors and interprets language
3. **Occipital lobe:** Most posterior portion of the cerebrum; controls vision
4. **Temporal lobe:** Left and right lateral portion of the cerebrum; controls hearing and smell

The diencephalon, located below the cerebrum, contains two of the most
critical areas of the brain, the **thalamus** and the **hypothalamus**. The thalamus is
composed of gray matter and acts as a center for relaying impulses from the eyes,
ears, and skin to the cerebrum. Pain perception is controlled by the thalamus.
The hypothalamus, located just below the thalamus, controls body temperature, appetite, sleep, sexual desire, and emotions. The hypothalamus is actually
responsible for controlling the autonomic nervous system, cardiovascular system,
digestive system, and the release of hormones from the pituitary gland.

The cerebellum, the second largest portion of the brain, is located beneath
the posterior part of the cerebrum. This part of the brain aids in coordinating
voluntary body movements and maintaining balance and equilibrium. The cerebellum refines the muscular movement that is initiated in the cerebrum.

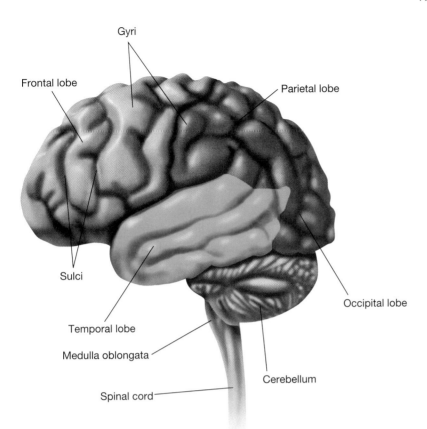

Gyri

Frontal lobe

Parietal lobe

Sulci

Occipital lobe

Temporal lobe

Medulla oblongata

Cerebellum

Spinal cord

■ **Figure 12-3**   The brain; colors indicate the different cerebral lobes. *(Lightspring/ Shutterstock)*

The final portion of the brain is the brainstem, which has three components: **midbrain, pons**, and **medulla oblongata**. The midbrain acts as a pathway for impulses to be conducted between the brain and the spinal cord. The pons—a term meaning *bridge*—connects the cerebellum to the rest of the brain. The medulla oblongata is the most inferior positioned portion of the brain; it connects the brain to the spinal cord. However, this vital area contains the centers that control respiration, heart rate, temperature, and blood pressure. Additionally, this is the site where nerve tracts cross from one side of the brain to control functions and movement on the other side of the body. In other words, with few exceptions, the left side of the brain controls the right side of the body and vice versa.

The brain has four interconnected cavities called **ventricles**: one in each cerebral hemisphere, one in the thalamus, and one in front of the cerebellum. These contain **cerebrospinal fluid** (CSF), which is the watery, clear fluid that provides protection from shock or sudden motion to the brain and spinal cord.

PRACTICE AS YOU GO

A. Complete the Statement

1. The organs of the central nervous system are the _____ and _____.

2. The nerves of the peripheral nervous system are either _____ nerves or _____ nerves.

3. The three basic parts of a neuron are _____, _____, and _____.

4. _____ is a fatty substance that insulates some axons.

5. The largest portion of the brain is the _____.

6. The second largest portion of the brain is the _____.

7. The occipital lobe controls _____.

8. The temporal lobe controls _____ and _____.

Spinal Cord

ascending tracts

central canal

descending tracts

spinal cavity

vertebral canal

vertebral column

Med Term Tip

Certain disease processes attack the gray matter and the white matter of the central nervous system. For instance, *poliomyelitis* is a viral infection of the gray matter of the spinal cord. The combining term **poli/o** means *gray matter*. This disease has almost been eradicated, due to the polio vaccine.

The function of the spinal cord is to provide a pathway for impulses traveling to and from the brain. The spinal cord is actually a column of nervous tissue extending from the medulla oblongata of the brain down to the level of the second lumbar vertebra within the **vertebral column**. The 33 vertebrae of the backbone line up to form a continuous canal for the spinal cord called the **spinal cavity** or **vertebral canal** (see Figure 12-4 ■).

Similar to the brain, the spinal cord is also protected by cerebrospinal fluid. It flows down the center of the spinal cord within the **central canal**. The inner core of the spinal cord consists of cell bodies and dendrites of peripheral nerves and therefore is gray matter. The outer portion of the spinal cord is myelinated white

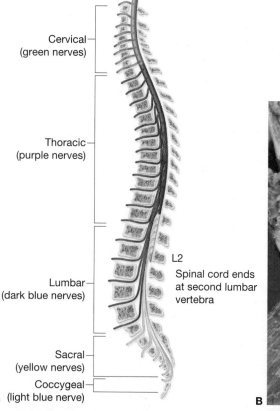

Cervical (green nerves)

Thoracic (purple nerves)

L2
Spinal cord ends at second lumbar vertebra

Lumbar (dark blue nerves)

Sacral (yellow nerves)

Coccygeal (light blue nerve)

A

B

■ **Figure 12-4**   A) The levels of the spinal cord and spinal nerves. B) Photograph of the spinal cord as it descends from the brain. The spinal nerve roots are clearly visible branching off from the spinal cord. *(VideoSurgery/Science Source)*

matter. The white matter is either **ascending tracts** carrying sensory information up to the brain or **descending tracts** carrying motor commands down from the brain to a peripheral nerve.

Meninges

arachnoid layer (ah-RAK-noyd)

dura mater (DOO-rah / MAH-ter)

pia mater (PEE-ah / MAH-ter)

subarachnoid space (sub-ah-RAK-noyd)

subdural space (sub-DOO-ral)

The meninges are three layers of connective tissue membranes surrounding the brain and spinal cord (see Figure 12-5 ∎). Moving from external to internal, the meninges are:

1. **Dura mater:** Meaning *tough mother*; it forms a tough, fibrous sac around the central nervous system
2. **Subdural space:** Actual space between the dura mater and arachnoid layer
3. **Arachnoid layer:** Meaning *spiderlike*; it is a thin, delicate layer attached to the pia mater by weblike filaments
4. **Subarachnoid space:** Space between the arachnoid layer and the pia mater; it contains cerebrospinal fluid that cushions the brain from the outside
5. **Pia mater:** Meaning *soft mother*; it is the innermost membrane layer and is applied directly to the surface of the brain and spinal cord

Peripheral Nervous System

afferent neurons (AF-er-ent)

autonomic nervous system (aw-toh-NOM-ik)

efferent neurons (EF-er-ent)

ganglion (GANG-lee-on)

motor neurons

nerve root

sensory neurons

somatic nerves

The peripheral nervous system (PNS) includes both the 12 pairs of cranial nerves and the 31 pairs of spinal nerves. A nerve is a group or bundle of axon fibers located outside the central nervous system that carries messages between the central nervous system and the various parts of the body. Whether a nerve is

Skin

Bone of skull
Epidural space
Dura mater
Subdural space
Arachnoid layer

Subarachnoid space

Pia mater

Brain

∎ **Figure 12-5** The meninges. This figure illustrates the location and structure of each layer of the meninges and their relationship to the skull and brain.

cranial or spinal is determined by where the nerve originates. Cranial nerves arise from the brain, mainly at the medulla oblongata. Spinal nerves split off from the spinal cord, and one pair (a left and a right) exits between each pair of vertebrae. The point where either type of nerve is attached to the central nervous system is called the **nerve root**. The names of most nerves reflect either the organ the nerve serves or the portion of the body the nerve is traveling through. The entire list of cranial nerves is found in Table 12-1 ■. Figure 12-6 ■ illustrates some of the major spinal nerves in the human body.

Although most nerves carry information to and from the central nervous system, individual neurons carry information in only one direction. **Afferent neurons**, also called **sensory neurons**, carry sensory information from a sensory receptor to the central nervous system. **Efferent neurons**, also called **motor neurons**, carry activity instructions from the central nervous system to muscles or glands out in the body (see Figure 12-7 ■). The nerve cell bodies of the neurons forming the nerve are grouped together in a knot-like mass, called a **ganglion**, located outside the central nervous system.

The nerves of the peripheral nervous system are subdivided into two divisions, the **autonomic nervous system** (ANS) and **somatic nerves**, each serving a different area of the body.

Autonomic Nervous System

parasympathetic branch
(pair-ah-sim-pah-THET-ik)

sympathetic branch (sim-pah-THET-ik)

The autonomic nervous system is involved with the control of involuntary or unconscious bodily functions. It may increase or decrease the activity of the smooth muscle found in viscera and blood vessels, cardiac muscle, and glands. The autonomic nervous system is divided into two branches: **sympathetic branch** and **parasympathetic branch**. The sympathetic nerves control the "fight-or-flight" reaction during times of stress and crisis. These nerves increase heart rate, dilate airways, increase blood pressure, inhibit digestion, and stimulate the production of adrenaline during a crisis. The parasympathetic nerves serve as a counterbalance for the sympathetic nerves, the "rest-and-digest" reaction. Therefore, they cause heart rate to slow down, lower blood pressure, and stimulate digestion.

■ **TABLE 12-1** Cranial Nerves

Number	Name	Function
I	Olfactory	Transports impulses for sense of smell
II	Optic	Carries impulses for sense of sight
III	Oculomotor	Motor impulses for eye muscle movement and the pupil of the eye
IV	Trochlear	Controls superior oblique muscle of eye on each side
V	Trigeminal	Carries sensory facial impulses and controls muscles for chewing; branches into eyes, forehead, upper and lower jaw
VI	Abducens	Controls eyeball muscle to turn eye to side
VII	Facial	Controls facial muscles for expression, salivation, and taste on two-thirds of tongue (anterior)
VIII	Vestibulocochlear	Responsible for impulses of equilibrium and hearing; also called *auditory nerve*
IX	Glossopharyngeal	Carries sensory impulses from pharynx (swallowing) and taste on one-third of tongue
X	Vagus	Supplies most organs in abdominal and thoracic cavities
XI	Accessory	Controls neck and shoulder muscles
XII	Hypoglossal	Controls tongue muscles

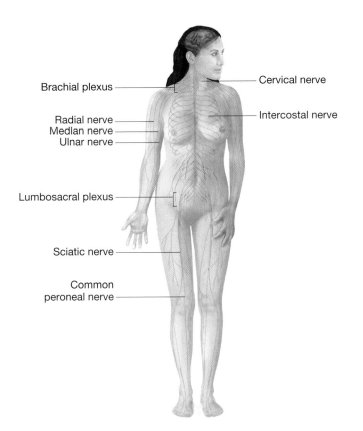

Brachial plexus
Cervical nerve
Radial nerve
Medlan nerve
Ulnar nerve
Intercostal nerve
Lumbosacral plexus
Sciatic nerve
Common
peroneal nerve

■ **Figure 12-6**   The major spinal nerves.

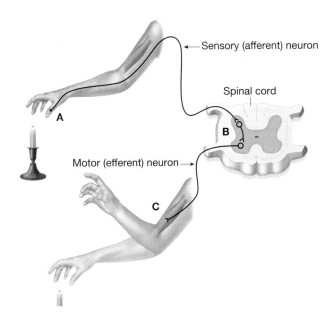

Sensory (afferent) neuron
Spinal cord
A
B
Motor (efferent) neuron
C

■ **Figure 12-7**   The functional structure of the peripheral nervous system. A) Afferent or sensory neurons carry sensory information to the spinal cord. B) The spinal cord receives incoming sensory information and delivers motor messages. C) Efferent or motor neurons deliver motor commands to muscles and glands.

Somatic Nerves

Somatic nerves serve the skin and skeletal muscles and are mainly involved with the conscious and voluntary activities of the body. The large variety of sensory receptors found in the dermis layer of the skin use somatic nerves to send their information, such as touch, temperature, pressure, and pain, to the brain. These are also the nerves that carry motor commands to skeletal muscles.

PRACTICE AS YOU GO

B. Complete the Statement

1. _____tracts of the spinal cord carry sensory information. _____ tracts carry motor commands.

2. The neurons that carry impulses away from the brain and spinal cord are called _____ neurons and the neurons that carry impulses to the brain and spinal cord are called _____ neurons.

3. The tough outer meninges is the _____. The spiderlike middle meninges is the _____. The delicate inner meninges is the _____.

4. The two divisions of the autonomic nervous system are the _____ and _____.

5. _____ nerves serve the skin and skeletal muscles.

Terminology

Word Parts Used to Build Nervous System Terms

The following lists contain the combining forms, suffixes, and prefixes used to build terms in the remaining sections of this chapter.

Combining Forms

alges/o	sense of pain	encephal/o	brain	neur/o	nerve
angi/o	vessel	esthesi/o	sensation, feeling	poli/o	gray matter
arteri/o	artery	gli/o	glue	pont/o	pons
astr/o	star	hal/o	to breathe	radicul/o	nerve root
cephal/o	head	hemat/o	blood	scler/o	hard
cerebell/o	cerebellum	hydr/o	water	spin/o	spine
cerebr/o	cerebrum	isch/o	to hold back	thalam/o	thalamus
clon/o	rapid contracting and relaxing	later/o	side	thec/o	sheath
		lumb/o	low back	tom/o	to cut
concuss/o	to shake violently	medull/o	medulla oblongata	ton/o	tone
crani/o	skull	mening/o	meninges	topic/o	a specific area
cutane/o	skin	meningi/o	meninges	vascul/o	blood vessel
cyt/o	cell	ment/o	mind	ven/o	vein
dur/o	dura mater	my/o	muscle	ventricul/o	ventricle
electr/o	electricity	myel/o	spinal cord	vertebr/o	vertebra

Suffixes

-al	pertaining to	-ia	condition	-ous	pertaining to
-algia	pain	-ic	pertaining to	-paresis	weakness
-ar	pertaining to	-ical	pertaining to	-pathy	disease
-ary	pertaining to	-ine	pertaining to	-phasia	speech
-asthenia	weakness	-ion	action	-plasty	surgical repair
-cele	protrusion	-itis	inflammation	-plegia	paralysis
-eal	pertaining to	-logy	study of	-rrhaphy	suture
-ectomy	surgical removal	-nic	pertaining to	-taxia	muscle coordination
-emic	pertaining to a blood condition	-oma	tumor, mass	-tic	pertaining to
		-osis	abnormal condition	-trophic	pertaining to development
-gram	record	-otomy	cutting into		
-graphy	process of recording				

Prefixes

a-	without	dys-	abnormal, difficult	in-	inward
an-	without	endo-	within	intra-	within
anti-	against	epi-	above	mono-	one
bi-	two	hemi-	half	para-	abnormal, two like parts of a pair
de-	without	hyper-	excessive		

Prefixes (continued)

poly-	many	sub-	under	tri-	three
quadri-	four	trans-	across	un-	not
semi-	partial				

Adjective Forms of Anatomical Terms

Term	Word Parts	Definition
cephalic (seh-FAL-ik)	cephal/o = head -ic = pertaining to	Pertaining to head
cerebellar (sair-eh-BELL-ar)	cerebell/o = cerebellum -ar = pertaining to	Pertaining to cerebellum
cerebral (seh-REE-bral)	cerebr/o = cerebrum -al = pertaining to	Pertaining to cerebrum
cerebrospinal (seh-ree-broh-SPY-nal)	cerebr/o = cerebrum spin/o = spine -al = pertaining to	Pertaining to cerebrum and spine
cranial (KRAY-nee-al)	crani/o = skull -al = pertaining to	Pertaining to skull
encephalic (en-seh-FAL-ik)	encephal/o = brain -ic = pertaining to	Pertaining to brain
intracranial (in-trah-KRAY-nee-al)	intra- = within crani/o = skull -al = pertaining to	Pertaining to within the skull
intrathecal (in-trah-THEE-kal)	intra- = within thec/o = sheath -al = pertaining to	Pertaining to within the meninges (sheath encasing central nervous system), specifically the subdural or subarachnoid space
medullary (MED-yoo-lair-ee)	medull/o = medulla oblongata -ary = pertaining to	Pertaining to medulla oblongata
meningeal (meh-NIN-jee-al)	mening/o = meninges -eal = pertaining to	Pertaining to meninges
myelonic (my-eh-LON-ik)	myel/o = spinal cord -nic = pertaining to	Pertaining to spinal cord
neural (NOO-ral)	neur/o = nerve -al = pertaining to	Pertaining to nerves
neuroglial (noo-ROG-lee-al)	neur/o = nerve gli/o = glue -al = pertaining to	Pertaining to glial cells that surround and support neurons
pontine (PON-teen)	pont/o = pons -ine = pertaining to	Pertaining to pons
spinal (SPY-nal)	spin/o = spine -al = pertaining to	Pertaining to spine
subdural (sub-DOO-ral)	sub- = under dur/o = dura mater -al = pertaining to	Pertaining to under dura mater
thalamic (thah-LAM-ik)	thalam/o = thalamus -ic = pertaining to	Pertaining to thalamus
ventricular (ven-TRIK-yoo-lar)	ventricul/o = ventricle -ar = pertaining to	Pertaining to ventricles
vertebral (VER-teh-bral)	vertebr/o = vertebra -al = pertaining to	Pertaining to vertebrae

PRACTICE AS YOU GO

C. Give the adjective form for each anatomical structure.

1. The cerebrum and spinal cord _____

2. The meninges _____

3. Under the dura mater _____

4. The brain _____

5. A nerve _____

6. Within the skull _____

Pathology

Term	Word Parts	Definition
Medical Specialties		
anesthesiology (an-es-thee-zee-ALL-oh-jee)	an- = without esthesi/o = sensation, feeling -logy = study of	Branch of medicine specializing in all aspects of anesthesia, including for surgical procedures, resuscitation measures, and management of acute and chronic pain; physician is *anesthesiologist*
neurology (noo-RALL-oh-jee)	neur/o = nerve -logy = study of	Branch of medicine concerned with diagnosis and treatment of diseases and conditions of the nervous system; physician is *neurologist*
neurosurgery (noo-roh-SER-jer-ee)	neur/o = nerve	Branch of medicine concerned with treating conditions and diseases of the nervous system by surgical means; physician is *neurosurgeon*
Signs and Symptoms		
absence seizure		Type of epileptic seizure that lasts only a few seconds to half a minute, characterized by loss of awareness and absence of activity; also known as *petit mal seizure*
analgesia (an-al-JEE-zee-ah)	an- = without alges/o = sense of pain -ia = condition	Absence of pain
anesthesia (an-es-THEE-zha)	an- = without esthesi/o = feeling, sensation -ia = condition	Condition in which there is lack of feeling or sensation
aphasia (ah-FAY-zee-ah)	a- = without -phasia = speech	Inability to communicate verbally or in writing due to damage of speech or language centers in the brain
ataxia (ah-TAK-see-ah)	a- = without -taxia = muscle coordination	Lack of muscle coordination
aura (AW-ruh)		Sensations, such as seeing colors or smelling an unusual odor, that occur just prior to epileptic seizure or migraine headache

Pathology (continued)

Term	Word Parts	Definition
cephalalgia (seff-al-AL-jee-ah)	cephal/o = head -algia = pain	Headache (HA)
coma (KOH-mah)		Profound unconsciousness resulting from illness or injury
conscious (KON-shus)		Condition of being awake and aware of surroundings
convulsion (kon-VUL-shun)		Severe involuntary muscle contractions and relaxations; have a variety of causes, such as epilepsy, fever, and toxic conditions
delirium (deh-LEER-ee-um)	de- = without	Abnormal mental state characterized by confusion, disorientation, and agitation
dementia (deh-MEN-sha)	de- = without ment/o = mind -ia = condition	Progressive impairment of intellectual function that interferes with performing activities of daily living; patients have little awareness of their condition; found in disorders such as Alzheimer's
dysphasia (dis-FAY-zee-ah)	dys- = abnormal, difficult -phasia = speech	Difficulty communicating verbally or in writing due to damage of speech or language centers in the brain
focal seizure (FOH-kal)	-al = pertaining to	Localized seizure often affecting one limb
hemiparesis (hem-ee-pah-REE-sis)	hemi- = half -paresis = weakness	Weakness or loss of motion on one side of the body
hemiplegia (hem-ee-PLEE-jee-ah)	hemi- = half -plegia = paralysis	Paralysis on only one side of the body
hyperesthesia (high-per-es-THEE-zee-ah)	hyper- = excessive esthesi/o = feeling, sensation -ia = condition	Condition of abnormally heightened sense of feeling, sense of pain, or sensitivity to touch
monoparesis (mon-oh-pah-REE-sis)	mono- = one -paresis = weakness	Muscle weakness in one limb
monoplegia (mon-oh-PLEE-jee-ah)	mono- = one -plegia = paralysis	Paralysis of one limb
neuralgia (noo-RAL-jee-ah)	neur/o = nerve -algia = pain	Nerve pain
palsy (PAWL-zee)		Temporary or permanent loss of ability to control movement
paralysis (pah-RAL-ih-sis)		Temporary or permanent loss of function or voluntary movement
paraplegia (pair-ah-PLEE-jee-ah)	para- = two like parts of a pair -plegia = paralysis	Paralysis of lower portion of the body and both legs (the two like parts of a pair)
paresthesia (pair-es-THEE-zee-ah)	para- = abnormal esthesi/o = sensation, feeling -ia = condition	Abnormal sensation such as burning or tingling
quadriplegia (kwod-rih-PLEE-jee-ah)	quadri- = four -plegia = paralysis	Paralysis of all four limbs
seizure (SEE-zyoor)		Sudden, uncontrollable onset of symptoms, such as in epileptic seizure

Pathology (continued)

Term	Word Parts	Definition
semiconscious (sem-ee-KON-shus)	semi- = partial	State of being aware of surroundings and responding to stimuli only part of the time
syncope (SIN-koh-pee)		Fainting
tonic-clonic seizure	ton/o = tone clon/o = rapid contracting and relaxing -ic = pertaining to	Type of severe epileptic seizure characterized by loss of consciousness and convulsions; seizure alternates between strong continuous muscle spasms (tonic) and rhythmic muscle contraction and relaxation (clonic); also known as *grand mal seizure*
tremor (TREM-or)		Involuntary, repetitive, alternating movement of a part of the body
unconscious (un-KON-shus)	un- = not	State of being unaware of surroundings, with the inability to respond to stimuli
Brain		
Alzheimer's disease (AD) (ALTS-high-merz)		Chronic, organic mental disorder consisting of dementia, which is more prevalent in adults after age 65; involves progressive disorientation, apathy, speech and gait disturbances, and loss of memory; named for German neurologist Alois Alzheimer
anencephaly (an-en-SEFF-ah-lee)	an- = without encephal/o = brain	Congenital defect in which portions of the brain (usually the cerebrum) do not develop; child born with condition is missing a portion of the brain, cranium, and scalp; condition usually fatal within a few hours of birth
astrocytoma (ass-troh-sigh-TOH-mah)	astr/o = star cyt/o = cell -oma = tumor	Tumor of brain or spinal cord composed of astrocytes, one type of neuroglial cells that has arms projecting off it like a star
brain tumor		Intracranial mass, either benign or malignant; benign tumor of the brain can still be fatal since it will grow and cause pressure on normal brain tissue
cerebellitis (sair-eh-bell-EYE-tis)	cerebell/o = cerebellum -itis = inflammation	Inflammation of the cerebellum
cerebral aneurysm (AN-yoo-rizm)	cerebr/o = cerebrum -al = pertaining to	Localized abnormal dilation of blood vessel, usually artery; result of congenital defect or weakness in wall of vessel; ruptured aneurysm is common cause of hemorrhagic cerebrovascular accident (see Figure 12-9 ■)

■ **Figure 12-8** CT scan showing large malignant tumor in left hemisphere of the brain. *(Puwadol Jaturawutthichai/ Shutterstock)*

Pathology (continued)

Term	Word Parts	Definition

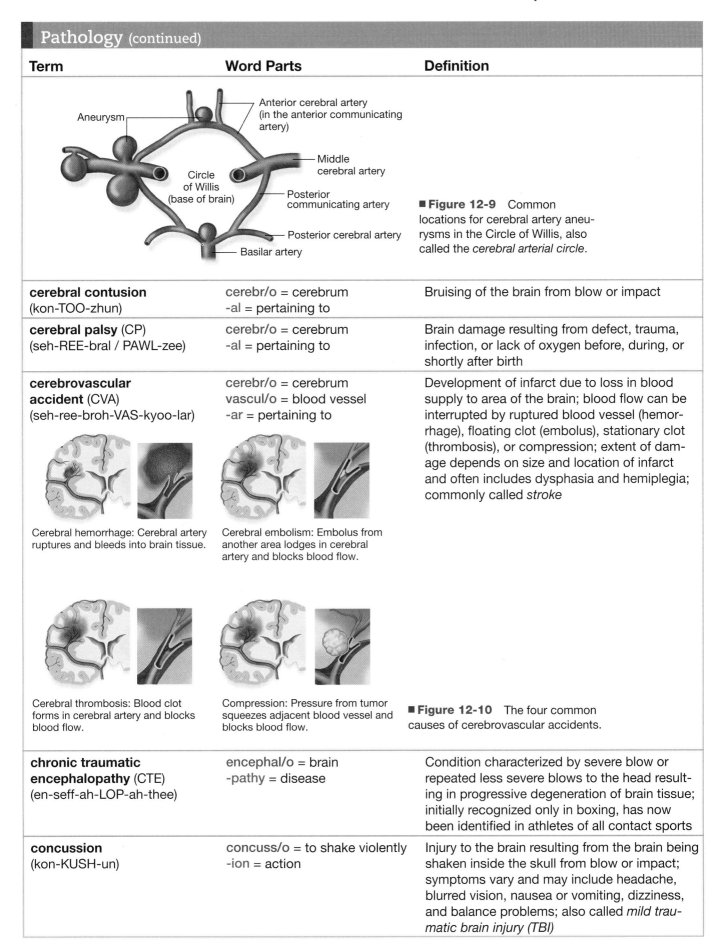

■ **Figure 12-9** Common locations for cerebral artery aneurysms in the Circle of Willis, also called the *cerebral arterial circle*.

cerebral contusion (kon-TOO-zhun)	cerebr/o = cerebrum -al = pertaining to	Bruising of the brain from blow or impact
cerebral palsy (CP) (seh-REE-bral / PAWL-zee)	cerebr/o = cerebrum -al = pertaining to	Brain damage resulting from defect, trauma, infection, or lack of oxygen before, during, or shortly after birth
cerebrovascular accident (CVA) (seh-ree-broh-VAS-kyoo-lar)	cerebr/o = cerebrum vascul/o = blood vessel -ar = pertaining to	Development of infarct due to loss in blood supply to area of the brain; blood flow can be interrupted by ruptured blood vessel (hemorrhage), floating clot (embolus), stationary clot (thrombosis), or compression; extent of damage depends on size and location of infarct and often includes dysphasia and hemiplegia; commonly called *stroke*

Cerebral hemorrhage: Cerebral artery ruptures and bleeds into brain tissue.

Cerebral embolism: Embolus from another area lodges in cerebral artery and blocks blood flow.

Cerebral thrombosis: Blood clot forms in cerebral artery and blocks blood flow.

Compression: Pressure from tumor squeezes adjacent blood vessel and blocks blood flow.

■ **Figure 12-10** The four common causes of cerebrovascular accidents.

| **chronic traumatic encephalopathy** (CTE) (en-seff-ah-LOP-ah-thee) | encephal/o = brain -pathy = disease | Condition characterized by severe blow or repeated less severe blows to the head resulting in progressive degeneration of brain tissue; initially recognized only in boxing, has now been identified in athletes of all contact sports |
| **concussion** (kon-KUSH-un) | concuss/o = to shake violently -ion = action | Injury to the brain resulting from the brain being shaken inside the skull from blow or impact; symptoms vary and may include headache, blurred vision, nausea or vomiting, dizziness, and balance problems; also called *mild traumatic brain injury (TBI)* |

Pathology (continued)

Term	Word Parts	Definition
encephalitis (en-seff-ah-LYE-tis)	encephal/o = brain -itis = inflammation	Inflammation of the brain
epilepsy (EP-ih-lep-see)		Recurrent disorder of the brain in which seizures and loss of consciousness occur as result of uncontrolled electrical activity of neurons in the brain
hydrocephalus (high-droh-SEFF-ah-lus)	hydr/o = water cephal/o = head	Accumulation of cerebrospinal fluid within ventricles of the brain, causing the head to be enlarged; treated by creating artificial shunt for fluid to leave the brain; if left untreated, may lead to seizures and mental retardation

Bulging fontanel

Enlarged ventricles

Catheter tip in ventricle

Valve

Blocked aqueduct

Shunt

■ **Figure 12-11**   Hydrocephalus. The figure on the left is a child with the enlarged ventricles of hydrocephalus. The figure on the right is the same child with a shunt to send the excess cerebrospinal fluid to the abdominal cavity.

Term	Word Parts	Definition
migraine (MY-grain)		Specific type of headache characterized by severe head pain, sensitivity to light, dizziness, and nausea
Parkinson's disease (PARK-in-sons)		Chronic disorder of the nervous system with fine tremors, muscular weakness, rigidity, and shuffling gait; named for British physician James Parkinson
Reye's syndrome (RISE / SIN-drohm)		Combination of symptoms first recognized by Australian pathologist R. D. K. Reye that includes acute encephalopathy and damage to various organs, especially the liver; occurs in children under age 15 who have had a viral infection; also associated with taking aspirin; for this reason, it's not recommended for children to use aspirin

Pathology (continued)

Term	Word Parts	Definition
shaken baby syndrome (SBS)		Caused by violent shaking of infant or toddler; symptoms may include subdural hematoma, brain swelling, and bleeding in retina of the eyes; usually no evidence of external trauma; also called *abusive head trauma (AHT)*
transient ischemic attack (TIA) (TRAN-zee-ent / iss-KEEM-ik)	isch/o = to hold back -emic = pertaining to a blood condition	Temporary interference with blood supply to the brain, causing neurological symptoms such as dizziness, numbness, and hemiparesis; may eventually lead to full-blown stroke (cerebrovascular accident)
traumatic brain injury (TBI)	-tic = pertaining to	Damage to the brain resulting from impact (such as car accident), blast waves (such as an explosion), or penetrating projectile (such as a bullet); symptoms may be mild, moderate, or severe and may include loss of consciousness, headache, vomiting, loss of motor coordination, and dizziness
Spinal Cord		
amyotrophic lateral sclerosis (ALS) (ay-my-oh-TROH-fik / LAT-er-al / skleh-ROH-sis)	a- = without my/o = muscle -trophic = pertaining to development later/o = side -al = pertaining to scler/o = hard -osis = abnormal condition	Condition with muscular weakness and atrophy due to degeneration of motor neurons of the spinal cord; also called *Lou Gehrig's disease*, after New York Yankees baseball player who died from this disease
meningocele (meh-NIN-goh-seel)	mening/o = meninges -cele = protrusion	Congenital condition in which the meninges protrude through opening in the vertebral column (see Figure 12-12A ■); see *spina bifida*
myelitis (my-eh-LYE-tis)	myel/o = spinal cord -itis = inflammation	Inflammation of the spinal cord
myelomeningocele (my-eh-loh-meh-NIN-goh-seel)	myel/o = spinal cord mening/o = meninges -cele = protrusion	Congenital condition in which meninges and spinal cord protrude through opening in the vertebral column (see Figure 12-12B ■); see *spina bifida*
poliomyelitis (poh-lee-oh-my-eh-LYE-tis)	poli/o = gray matter myel/o = spinal cord -itis = inflammation	Viral inflammation of gray matter of the spinal cord; results in varying degrees of paralysis; may be mild and reversible or may be severe and permanent; disease has been almost eliminated due to discovery of vaccine in the 1950s
spina bifida (SPY-nah / BIF-ih-dah)	spin/o = spine bi- = two	Congenital defect in walls of the spinal canal in which laminae of the vertebra do not meet or close (see Figure 12-12C ■); may result in meningocele or myelomeningocele— meninges or the spinal cord being pushed through opening

Pathology (continued)

Term	Word Parts	Definition

A. Meningocele

B. Myelomeningocele

C. Spina bifida

■ **Figure 12-12** A) Meningocele, the meninges sac protrudes through the opening in the vertebra. B) Myelomeningocele, the meninges sac and spinal cord protrude through the opening in the vertebra. C) Spina bifida occulta, the vertebra is not complete, but there is no protrusion of nervous system structures.

Term	Word Parts	Definition
spinal cord injury (SCI)	spin/o = spine -al = pertaining to	Damage to the spinal cord as result of trauma; spinal cord may be bruised or completely severed

Nerves

Term	Word Parts	Definition
Bell's palsy (BELLZ / PAWL-zee)		One-sided facial paralysis due to inflammation of facial nerve, probably viral in nature; patient cannot control salivation, tearing of the eyes, or expression, but most will eventually recover
Guillain-Barré syndrome (GHEE-yan / bah-RAY)		Disease of the nervous system in which nerves lose their myelin covering; may be caused by autoimmune reaction; characterized by loss of sensation and/or muscle control starting in the legs; symptoms then move toward trunk and may even result in paralysis of the diaphragm
multiple sclerosis (MS) (MULL-tih-pl / skleh-ROH-sis)	scler/o = hard -osis = abnormal condition	Inflammatory disease of the central nervous system in which there is extreme weakness and numbness due to loss of myelin insulation from around nerves that result in "hard" patches called plaques to appear
myasthenia gravis (my-as-THEE-nee-ah / GRAV-iss)	my/o = muscle -asthenia = weakness	Disease with severe muscular weakness and fatigue due to insufficient neurotransmitter at a synapse
neuroma (noo-ROH-mah)	neur/o = nerve -oma = tumor	Nerve tumor or tumor of connective tissue sheath around a nerve
neuropathy (noo-ROP-ah-thee)	neur/o = nerve -pathy = disease	General term for disease or damage to a nerve

Pathology (continued)

Term	Word Parts	Definition
polyneuritis (pol-ee-noo-RYE-tis)	poly- = many neur/o = nerve -itis = inflammation	Inflammation of two or more nerves
radiculitis (rah-dik-yoo-LYE-tis)	radicul/o = nerve root -itis = inflammation	Inflammation of a nerve root; may be caused by herniated nucleus pulposus
radiculopathy (rah-dik-yoo-LOP-ah-thee)	radicul/o = nerve root -pathy = disease	Refers to condition that occurs when a herniated nucleus pulposus puts pressure on a nerve root; symptoms include pain and numbness along path of affected nerve
shingles (SHING-lz)		Eruption of painful blisters on body along a nerve path caused by *Herpes zoster* virus infection of nerve root; virus initially introduced into body during chickenpox infection but becomes dormant in nerve cells; reactivation of virus later in life results in shingles

■ **Figure 12-13** Photograph of the skin eruptions associated with shingles. *(Stephen VanHorn/Shutterstock)*

Term	Word Parts	Definition
trigeminal neuralgia (trye-JEM-ih-nal / noo-RAL-jee-ah)	tri- = three -al = pertaining to neur/o = nerve -algia = pain	Chronic disorder characterized by sudden, sharp pain on one side of face in area served by the trigeminal cranial nerve; usually caused by pressure on and irritation of nerve or may be sign of multiple sclerosis; also called *tic douloureux*

Meninges

Term	Word Parts	Definition
epidural hematoma (ep-ih-DOO-ral / hee-mah-TOH-mah)	epi- = above dur/o = dura mater -al = pertaining to hemat/o = blood -oma = mass	Mass of blood in space outside the dura mater of the brain and spinal cord
meningioma (meh-nin-jee-OH-mah)	meningi/o = meninges -oma = tumor	Tumor in the meninges
meningitis (men-in-JYE-tis)	mening/o = meninges -itis = inflammation	Inflammation of the meninges around brain or spinal cord caused by bacterial or viral infection; symptoms include fever, headache, neck stiffness, lethargy, vomiting, irritability, and photophobia

Pathology (continued)

Term	Word Parts	Definition
subdural hematoma (sub-DOO-ral / hee-mah-TOH-mah)	sub- = under dur/o = dura mater -al = pertaining to hemat/o = blood -oma = mass	Mass of blood forming beneath the dura mater if the meninges are torn by trauma; may exert fatal pressure on the brain if hematoma not drained by surgery

■ **Figure 12-14** A subdural hematoma. A meningeal vein is ruptured and blood has accumulated in the subdural space, producing pressure on the brain.

PRACTICE AS YOU GO

D. Pathology Matching

Match each pathology term to its definition.

1. _____ aura
2. _____ meningitis
3. _____ coma
4. _____ shingles
5. _____ syncope
6. _____ palsy
7. _____ absence seizure
8. _____ tonic-clonic seizure
9. _____ meningocele
10. _____ concussion

a. mild traumatic brain injury
b. sensations before a seizure
c. seizure with convulsions
d. congenital hernia of meninges
e. seizure without convulsion
f. inflammation of meninges
g. profound unconsciousness
h. *Herpes zoster* infection
i. fainting
j. loss of ability to control movement

Diagnostic Procedures

Term	Word Parts	Definition
Clinical Laboratory Tests		
cerebrospinal fluid analysis (seh-ree-broh-SPY-nal / ah-NAL-ih-sis)	cerebr/o = cerebrum spin/o = spine -al = pertaining to	Laboratory examination of clear, watery, colorless fluid from within brain and spinal cord; infections and abnormal presence of blood can be detected in this test
Diagnostic Imaging		
brain scan		Image of the brain taken after injection of radioactive isotopes into circulation
cerebral angiography (seh-REE-bral / an-jee-OG-rah-fee)	cerebr/o = cerebrum -al = pertaining to angi/o = vessel -graphy = process of recording	X-ray of blood vessels of the brain after injection of radiopaque dye
echoencephalography (ek-oh-en-seff-ah-LOG-rah-fee)	encephal/o = brain -graphy = process of recording	Recording of ultrasonic echoes of the brain; useful in determining abnormal patterns of shifting in the brain
myelogram (MY-eh-loh-gram)	myel/o = spinal cord -gram = record	X-ray record of the spinal cord
myelography (my-eh-LOG-rah-fee)	myel/o = spinal cord -graphy = process of recording	Injection of radiopaque dye into the spinal canal; X-ray is then taken to examine normal and abnormal outlines made by dye
positron emission tomography (PET) (POZ-ih-tron / ee-MISH-un / toh-MOG-rah-fee)	tom/o = to cut -graphy = process of recording	Image of the brain cut along a plane produced by measuring gamma rays emitted from the brain after injecting glucose tagged with positively charged isotopes; measurement of glucose uptake by brain tissue indicates measurement of metabolic activity
Additional Diagnostic Tests		
Babinski's reflex (bah-BIN-skeez)		Reflex test developed by French neurologist Joseph Babinski to determine lesions and abnormalities in the nervous system; Babinski's reflex is present if great toe extends instead of flexes when lateral sole of the foot is stroked; normal response to this stimulation is flexion of the toe
electroencephalogram (EEG) (ee-lek-troh-en-SEFF-ah-loh-gram)	electr/o = electricity encephal/o = brain -gram = record	Record of the brain's electrical patterns
electroencephalography (EEG) (ee-lek-troh-en-seff-ah-LOG-rah-fee)	electr/o = electricity encephal/o = brain -graphy = process of recording	Recording electrical activity of the brain by placing electrodes at various positions on the scalp; also used in sleep studies to determine if there is a normal pattern of activity during sleep

Diagnostic Procedures (continued)

Term	Word Parts	Definition
lumbar puncture (LP) (LUM-bar / PUNK-chur)	lumb/o = low back -ar = pertaining to	Puncture with needle into lumbar area (usually fourth intervertebral space) to withdraw fluid for examination and for injection of anesthesia; also called *spinal puncture* or *spinal tap*

L1 vertebra
Lumbar puncture needle
Coccyx
Skin
Fat
Interspinous ligament
L4
L5
Extradural "space"
Tip end of spinal cord
CSF in lumbar cistern
Dura mater
Sacrum

■ **Figure 12-15**
A lumbar puncture. The needle is inserted between the lumbar vertebrae and into the spinal canal.

Term	Word Parts	Definition
nerve conduction velocity		Test to determine if nerves have been damaged by recording rate an electrical impulse is able to travel along a nerve; if nerve is damaged, velocity will be decreased

Therapeutic Procedures

Anesthesia

Term	Word Parts	Definition
anesthesia (an-es-THEE-zha)	an- = without esthesi/o = sensation, feeling -ia = condition	Administering medication to produce loss of feeling or sensation
general anesthesia (GA) (an-es-THEE-zha)		Produces loss of consciousness including absence of pain sensation; patient's vital signs (VS)—heart rate, breathing rate, pulse, and blood pressure—are carefully monitored when using general anesthetic
intravenous (IV) anesthesia (in-trah-VEE-nus / an-es-THEE-zha)	intra- = within ven/o = vein -ous = pertaining to	Route for administering general anesthesia via injection into vein
inhalation anesthesia (in-hah-LAY-shun / an-es-THEE-zha)	in- = inward hal/o = to breathe	Route for administering general anesthesia by breathing it in
local anesthesia (an-es-THEE-zha)	-al = pertaining to	Produces loss of sensation in one localized part of body; patient remains conscious
regional anesthesia (an-es-THEE-zha)	-al = pertaining to	Interrupts patient's pain sensation in region of body, such as the arm; anesthetic is injected near nerve that will be blocked from sensation; also called *nerve block*

Therapeutic Procedures (continued)

Term	Word Parts	Definition
subcutaneous anesthesia (sub-kyoo-TAY-nee-us / an-es-THEE-zha)	sub- = under cutane/o = skin -ous = pertaining to	Method of applying local anesthesia involving injecting anesthetic under the skin; for example, used to deaden skin prior to suturing a laceration
topical anesthesia (TOP-ih-kal / an-es-THEE-zha)	topic/o = a specific area -al = pertaining to	Method of applying local anesthesia involving placing liquid or gel directly onto specific area of skin; for example, used on the skin, cornea, or gums
Medical Procedures		
nerve block		Injection of regional anesthetic to stop passage of sensory or pain impulses along a nerve path
transcutaneous electrical nerve stimulation (TENS) (trans-kyoo-TAY-nee-us)	trans- = across cutane/o = skin -ous = pertaining to electr/o = electricity -ical = pertaining to	Application of mild electrical current by device with electrodes placed on skin over a painful area; relieves pain by interfering with nerve signal to the brain on pain nerve
Surgical Procedures		
carotid endarterectomy (kah-ROT-id / end-ar-teh-REK-toh-mee)	endo- = within arteri/o = artery -ectomy = surgical removal	Surgical procedure for removing obstruction within carotid artery, a major artery in the neck that carries oxygenated blood to the brain; developed to prevent strokes, but is found to be useful only in severe stenosis with transient ischemic attack
cerebrospinal fluid shunt (seh-ree-broh-SPY-nal)	cerebr/o = cerebrum spin/o = spine -al = pertaining to	Surgical procedure in which bypass is created to drain cerebrospinal fluid; used to treat hydrocephalus by draining excess cerebrospinal fluid from the brain and diverting it to abdominal cavity
laminectomy (lam-ih-NEK-toh-mee)	-ectomy = surgical removal	Removal of a portion of a vertebra, called the *lamina*, in order to relieve pressure on spinal nerve
neurectomy (noo-REK-toh-mee)	neur/o = nerve -ectomy = surgical removal	Surgical removal of a nerve
neuroplasty (NOOR-oh-plas-tee)	neur/o = nerve -plasty = surgical repair	Surgical repair of a nerve
neurorrhaphy (noo-ROR-ah-fee)	neur/o = nerve -rrhaphy = suture	To suture a nerve back together; actually refers to suturing connective tissue sheath around the nerve
tractotomy (trak-TOT-oh-mee)	-otomy = cutting into	Precision cutting of a nerve tract in the spinal cord; used to treat intractable pain or muscle spasms

PRACTICE AS YOU GO

E. Procedure Matching

Match each procedure term with its definition.

1. _____ brain scan
2. _____ lumbar puncture
3. _____ cerebral angiography
4. _____ EEG
5. _____ PET scan
6. _____ nerve block
7. _____ neurorrhaphy
8. _____ myelogram

a. image made by measuring gamma rays
b. record of brain's electrical activity
c. obtains CSF from around spinal cord
d. regional injection of anesthetic
e. diagnostic image made with radioactive isotopes
f. X-ray of spinal cord
g. X-ray of brain's blood vessels
h. suture together sheath around a nerve

Pharmacology

Classification	Word Parts	Action	Examples
analgesic (an-al-JEE-zik)	an- = without alges/o = sense of pain -ic = pertaining to	Treats minor to moderate pain without loss of consciousness	aspirin, Bayer, Ecotrin; acetaminophen, Tylenol; ibuprofen, Motrin
anesthetic (an-es-THET-ik)	an- = without esthesi/o = feeling, sensation -tic = pertaining to	Produces loss of sensation or loss of consciousness	lidocaine, Xylocaine; pentobarbital, Nembutal; propofol, Diprivan; procaine, Novocain
anticonvulsant (an-tye-kon-VUL-sant)	anti- = against	Reduces excitability of neurons and therefore prevents uncontrolled neuron activity associated with seizures	carbamazepine, Tegretol; phenobarbital, Nembutal
dopaminergic drugs (doh-pah-men-ER-jik)	-ic = pertaining to	Treat Parkinson's disease by either replacing dopamine that is lacking or increasing strength of dopamine that is present	levodopa; L-dopa, Larodopa; levodopa/carbidopa, Sinemet
hypnotic (hip-NOT-ik)	-ic = pertaining to	Promotes sleep	secobarbital, Seconal; temazepam, Restoril
narcotic analgesic (nar-KOT-ik)	-ic = pertaining to an- = without alges/o = sense of pain -ic = pertaining to	Treats severe pain; has potential to be habit forming if taken for prolonged time; also called *opiate*	morphine, MS Contin; oxycodone, OxyContin; meperidine, Demerol
sedative (SED-ah-tiv)		Has relaxing or calming effect	amobarbital, Amytal; butabarbital, Butisol

Abbreviations

AD	Alzheimer's disease	**ICP**	intracranial pressure
AHT	abusive head trauma	**IV**	intravenous
ALS	amyotrophic lateral sclerosis	**LP**	lumbar puncture
ANS	autonomic nervous system	**MS**	multiple sclerosis
CNS	central nervous system	**PET**	positron emission tomography
CP	cerebral palsy	**PNS**	peripheral nervous system
CSF	cerebrospinal fluid	**SBS**	shaken baby syndrome
CTE	chronic traumatic encephalopathy	**SCI**	spinal cord injury
CVA	cerebrovascular accident	**TBI**	traumatic brain injury
CVD	cerebrovascular disease	**TENS**	transcutaneous electrical nerve stimulation
EEG	electroencephalogram, electroencephalography	**TIA**	transient ischemic attack
GA	general anesthesia	**VS**	vital signs
HA	headache		

PRACTICE AS YOU GO

F. What's the Abbreviation?

1. cerebrospinal fluid _____
2. cerebrovascular disease _____
3. electroencephalogram _____
4. intracranial pressure _____
5. positron emission tomography _____
6. cerebrovascular accident _____
7. autonomic nervous system _____

AT A GLANCE

Word Parts

Presented here are the most common word parts (with their meanings) used to build mental health terms.

Combining Forms

amnes/o	forgetfulness	neur/o	nerve
anxi/o	fear, worry	obsess/o	besieged by thoughts
compuls/o	drive, compel	phob/o	irrational fear
delus/o	false belief	phren/o	mind
depress/o	to press down	psych/o	mind
hallucin/o	imagined perception	pyr/o	fire
klept/o	to steal	schiz/o	split
ment/o	mind	soci/o	society
narc/o	stupor, sleep		

Suffixes

-iatrist	physician	-mania	frenzy
-iatry	medical treatment	-phoria	condition to bear
-lepsy	seizure		

Mental Health Disciplines

Psychology

abnormal psychology

clinical psychologist (sigh-KALL-oh-jist)

normal psychology

psychology (sigh-KALL-oh-jee)

Psychology is the study of human behavior and thought processes. This behavioral science is primarily concerned with understanding how human beings interact with their physical environment and with each other. Behavior can be divided into two categories: normal and abnormal. The study of **normal psychology** includes how the personality develops, how people handle stress, and the stages of mental development. In contrast, **abnormal psychology** studies and treats behaviors that are outside of normal and that are detrimental to the person or society. These maladaptive behaviors range from occasional difficulty coping with stress, to bizarre actions and beliefs, to total withdrawal. A **clinical psychologist**, though not a physician, is a specialist in evaluating and treating persons with mental and emotional disorders.

> **Med Term Tip**
>
> All social interactions pose some problems for some people. These problems are not necessarily abnormal. One means of judging if behavior is abnormal is to compare one person's behavior with others in the community. Also, if a person's behavior interferes with the activities of daily living, it is often considered abnormal.

Psychiatry

psychiatric nurse (sigh-kee-AT-rik)

psychiatric social worker

psychiatrist (sigh-KIGH-ah-trist)

psychiatry (sigh-KIGH-ah-tree)

Psychiatry is the branch of medicine that deals with the diagnosis, treatment, and prevention of mental disorders. A **psychiatrist** is a medical physician specializing in the care of patients with mental, emotional, and behavioral disorders. Other health professions also have specialty areas in caring for clients with mental illness. Good examples are **psychiatric nurses** and **psychiatric social workers**.

> **What's In A Name?**
>
> Look for these word parts:
> **psych/o** = mind
> **-iatric** = pertaining to medical treatment
> **-iatrist** = physician
> **-iatry** = medical treatment
> **-logist** = one who studies
> **-logy** = study of

Pathology

The legal definition of mental disorder is "impaired judgment and lack of self-control." The guide for terminology and classifications relating to psychiatric disorders is the *Diagnostic and Statistical Manual of Mental Disorders, Fifth Edition* (DSM-5), which is published by the American Psychiatric Association (2013). The DSM organizes mental disorders into 19 major diagnostic categories of disorders. These categories and examples of conditions included in each are described below.

> **Med Term Tip**
>
> Mental disorders are sometimes more simply characterized by whether they are a *neurosis* or a *psychosis*. Neuroses are inappropriate coping mechanisms to handle stress, such as phobias and panic attacks. Psychoses involve extreme distortions of reality and disorganization of a person's thinking, including bizarre behaviors, hallucinations, and delusions. Schizophrenia is an example of a psychosis.

Term	Word Parts	Definition
Anxiety Disorders	anxi/o = fear, worry dis- = apart	Characterized by persistent worry and apprehension
general anxiety disorder (ang-ZYE-eh-tee)	anxi/o = fear, worry dis- = apart	Feeling of dread in absence of clearly identifiable stress trigger
panic disorder	-ic = pertaining to dis- = apart	Feeling of intense apprehension, terror, or sense of impending danger
phobias (FOH-bee-ahs)	phob/o = irrational fear -ia = condition	Irrational fear, such as *arachnophobia*, the fear of spiders

Pathology (continued)

Term	Word Parts	Definition
Bipolar and Related Disorders	bi- = two -ar = pertaining to dis- = apart	
bipolar disorder (BPD)	bi- = two -ar = pertaining to	Alternation between periods of deep depression and mania
	Med Term Tip The healthcare professional must take all threats of suicide from patients seriously. Psychologists tell us that there is no clear suicide type, which means that we cannot predict who will actually take his or her own life. Always tell the physician caring for the person about any discussion a patient has concerning suicide. If you believe a patient is in danger of suicide, do not be afraid to ask, "Are you thinking about suicide?"	
Depressive Disorders	depress/o = to press down dis- = apart	Characterized by instability in mood
major depressive disorder	depress/o = to press down dis- = apart	Feelings of hopelessness, helplessness, worthlessness; lack of pleasure in any activity; potential for suicide
mania (MAY-nee-ah)	-mania = frenzy	Displaying extreme elation, hyperactivity, excessive talkativeness, impaired judgment, distractibility, and grandiose delusions
Disruptive, Impulse Control, and Conduct Disorders	dis- = apart	Inability to resist impulse to perform some act that is harmful to individual or others
explosive disorder	ex- = outward dis- = apart	Violent rages
kleptomania (klep-toh-MAY-nee-ah)	klept/o = to steal -mania = frenzy	Uncontrollable impulse to steal
pyromania (pye-roh-MAY-nee-ah)	pyr/o = fire -mania = frenzy	Uncontrollable impulse to set fires
Dissociative Disorders	dis- = apart soci/o = society	Disorders in which severe emotional conflict is so repressed that a split in personality may occur or person may lose memory
dissociative amnesia (dih-SOH-see-ah-tiv / am-NEE-zee-ah)	dis- = apart soci/o = society amnes/o = forgetfulness -ia = condition	Loss of memory
dissociative identity disorder	dis- = apart soci/o = society	Having two or more distinct personalities
Elimination Disorders	dis- = apart	
encopresis		Act of voiding feces in inappropriate places after toilet training
enuresis (en-yoo-REE-sis)		Act of voiding urine in inappropriate places after toilet training
Feeding and Eating Disorders		Abnormal behaviors related to eating

Pathology (continued)

Term	Word Parts	Definition
anorexia nervosa (an-oh-REK-see-ah / ner-VOH-sah)	an- = without -orexia = appetite	Disorder characterized by distorted body image, pathological fear of becoming fat, and severe weight loss due to excessive dieting

■ **Figure 12-16**
Photograph of a young woman suffering from anorexia nervosa, posterior view. *(Den Rise/Shutterstock)*

Term	Word Parts	Definition
bulimia (boo-LEE-mee-ah)	-ia = condition	Condition of binge eating and intentional vomiting
Gender Dysphoria	dys- = abnormal -phoria = condition to bear	
gender dysphoria (dis-FOR-ee-ah)	dys- = abnormal -phoria = condition to bear	Occurs when birth gender is contrary to gender with which person identifies; includes both male to female (MTF) and female to male (FTM)
Neurocognitive Disorders	neur/o = nerve dis- = apart	Deterioration of mental functions due to temporary or permanent brain dysfunction
Alzheimer's disease (AD) (ALTS-high-merz)	dis- = apart	Degenerative brain disorder with gradual loss of cognitive abilities
dementia (deh-MEN-sha)	de- = without ment/o = mind -ia = condition	Progressive confusion and disorientation
Neurodevelopmental Disorders	neur/o = nerve -al = pertaining to dis- = apart	Impairment in growth or development of the central nervous system
attention-deficit/hyperactivity disorder (ADHD)	hyper- = excessive dis- = apart	Inattention and impulsive behavior
autism spectrum disorder (AW-tizm)	auto- = self -ism = state of dis- = apart	Range of conditions involving deficits in social interaction, communication skills, and restricted patterns of behavior
intellectual development disorder	-al = pertaining to dis- = apart	Below-average intellectual functioning
Obsessive–Compulsive and Related Disorders	dis- = apart	Characterized by obsessive preoccupations and repetitive behaviors
obsessive–compulsive disorder (OCD) (ob-SESS-iv / kom-PUHL-siv)	obsess/o = besieged by thoughts compuls/o = drive, compel dis- = apart	Performing repetitive rituals to reduce anxiety caused by persistent thoughts, ideas, or impulses

Pathology (continued)

Term	Word Parts	Definition
Paraphilic Disorders	para- = abnormal -philic = pertaining to being attracted to dis- = apart	Disorders include aberrant sexual activity and sexual dysfunction
pedophilic disorder (pee-doh-FILL-ik)	ped/o = child -philic = pertaining to being attracted to dis- = apart	Sexual interest in children
sexual masochism disorder (MAS-oh-kizm)	-al = pertaining to -ism = state of dis- = apart	Gratification derived from being hurt or abused
voyeuristic disorder (VOY-er-iss-tik)	-tic = pertaining to	Gratification derived from observing others engaged in sexual acts
Personality Disorders	dis- = apart	Inflexible or maladaptive behavior patterns that affect person's ability to function in society
antisocial personality disorder	anti- = against soci/o = society -al = pertaining to dis- = apart	Behaviors that are against legal or social norms
narcissistic personality disorder (nar-sih-SIS-tik)	dis- = apart	Abnormal sense of self-importance
paranoid personality disorder	dis- = apart	Exaggerated feelings of persecution
Schizophrenia Spectrum and Other Psychotic Disorders	schiz/o = split phren/o = mind -ia = condition	Mental disorders characterized by distortions of reality
delusional disorder (dee-LOO-zhun-al)	delus/o = false belief -al = pertaining to dis- = apart	False belief held even in face of contrary evidence
hallucination (hah-loo-sih-NAY-shun)	hallucin/o = imagined perception	Perceiving something that is not there
Sexual Dysfunctions	-al = pertaining to dys- = abnormal, difficult	Having difficulty during any stage of normal sexual activity that negatively impacts quality of life
erectile dysfunction	-ile = pertaining to dys- = difficult	Pertaining to difficulty achieving or maintaining erection
premature ejaculation	pre- = before	Ejaculation of semen before or shortly after penetration
Sleep–Wake Disorders	dis- = apart	Disorders relating to either sleeping or wakefulness
insomnia disorder (in-SOM-nee-ah)	in- = not somn/o = sleep -ia = condition	Condition of inability to sleep
narcolepsy (NAR-koh-lep-see)	narc/o = stupor, sleep -lepsy = seizure	Recurring episodes of sleeping during daytime and often difficulty sleeping at night
Somatic Symptom and Related Disorders	somat/o = body -ic = pertaining to dis- = apart	Patient has physical symptoms for which no physical disease can be determined
conversion disorder	vers/o = to turn dis- = apart	Anxiety is transformed into physical symptoms such as heart palpitations, paralysis, or blindness

Pathology (continued)

Term	Word Parts	Definition
somatic symptom disorder (SSD)	somat/o = body -ic = pertaining to dis- = apart	Having physical symptoms that cause distress and disrupt daily life; includes pre-occupation with symptoms and behaviors based on symptoms
Substance Use and Addictive Disorders	dis- = apart	
gambling disorder	dis- = apart	Inability to stop gambling
substance use disorder	dis- = apart	Overindulgence or dependence on chemical substances including alcohol, illegal drugs, and prescription drugs
Trauma- and Stressor-Related Disorders	dis- = apart	
posttraumatic stress disorder (PTSD)	post- = after -ic = pertaining to dis- = apart	Results from exposure to actual or implied death, serious injury, or sexual violence; condition impairs person's social interactions and capacity to work

PRACTICE AS YOU GO

G. Pathology Matching

Match each term to its description.

_____ **1.** panic disorder

_____ **2.** autism spectrum disorder

_____ **3.** dementia

_____ **4.** anorexia nervosa

_____ **5.** narcolepsy

_____ **6.** mania

_____ **7.** conversion disorder

_____ **8.** gambling disorder

_____ **9.** enuresis

_____ **10.** pyromania

a. type of feeding and eating disorder

b. type of disruptive, impulse control, and conduct disorder

c. type of sleep–wake disorder

d. type of anxiety disorder

e. type of substance use and addictive disorder

f. type of somatic symptom and related disorder

g. type of neurodevelopmental disorder

h. type of elimination disorder

i. type of depressive disorder

j. type of neurocognitive disorder

Therapeutic Procedures

Term	Word Parts	Definition
electroconvulsive therapy (ECT) (ee-lek-troh-kon-VUL-siv)	electr/o = electricity	Procedure occasionally used for cases of prolonged major depression; once-controversial treatment involves placement of electrode on one or both sides of patient's head and a current is turned on, briefly causing convulsive seizure; low level of voltage is used in modern electroconvulsive therapy, and patient is administered muscle relaxant and anesthesia; when first introduced in the 1940s, was very primitive and convulsions were not controlled in any manner; advocates of treatment today correctly state that it is a more effective way to treat severe depression than using drugs; not effective with disorders other than depression, such as schizophrenia and alcoholism

Therapeutic Procedures (continued)

Term	Word Parts	Definition
Psychopharmacology (sigh-koh-far-mah-KALL-oh-jee)	psych/o = mind pharmac/o = drug -logy = study of	Study of effects of drugs on the mind and particularly use of drugs in treating mental disorders; main classes of drugs for treatment of mental disorders are:
antidepressant drugs	anti- = against depress/o = to press down	Classified as stimulants; alter patient's mood by affecting levels of neurotransmitters in the brain; antidepressants, such as serotonin norepinephrine reuptake inhibitors, are nonaddictive but can produce unpleasant side effects such as dry mouth, weight gain, blurred vision, and nausea
antipsychotic drugs	anti- = against psych/o = mind -tic = pertaining to	These major tranquilizers include chlorpromazine (Thorazine), haloperidol (Haldol), clozapine (Clozaril), and risperidone; these drugs have transformed treatment of patients with psychoses and schizophrenia by reducing patient agitation and panic and shortening schizophrenic episodes; one side effect of these drugs is involuntary muscle movements, which approximately one-fourth of all adults who take the drugs develop
lithium		Special category of drug used successfully to calm patients who suffer from bipolar disorder (depression alternating with manic excitement)
minor tranquilizers		Include Valium and Xanax; also classified as central nervous system depressants and are prescribed for anxiety
Psychotherapy (sigh-koh-THAIR-ah-pee)	psych/o = mind -therapy = treatment	Method of treating mental disorders by mental rather than chemical or physical means; includes:
family and group psychotherapy	psych/o = mind -therapy = treatment	Often described as solution focused, therapist places minimal emphasis on patient past history and strong emphasis on having patient state and discuss goals and then find a way to achieve them
humanistic psychotherapy	-tic = pertaining to psych/o = mind -therapy = treatment	Therapist does not delve into patients' past when using these methods; instead, it is believed that patients can learn how to use their own internal resources to deal with their problems; therapist creates therapeutic atmosphere, which builds patient self-esteem and encourages discussion of problems, thereby gaining insight in how to handle them; also called *client-centered* or *nondirective psychotherapy*
psychoanalysis	psych/o = mind	Method of obtaining detailed account of past and present emotional and mental experiences from patient to determine source of problem and eliminate effects; system developed by Sigmund Freud that encourages patient to discuss repressed, painful, or hidden experiences with hope of eliminating or minimizing problem

Abbreviations

AD	Alzheimer's disease	**MA**	mental age
ADD	attention-deficit disorder	**MMPI**	Minnesota Multiphasic Personality Inventory
ADHD	attention-deficit/hyperactivity disorder	**MTF**	male to female
BPD	bipolar disorder	**OCD**	obsessive–compulsive disorder
CA	chronological age	**PTSD**	posttraumatic stress disorder
DSM	*Diagnostic and Statistical Manual of Mental Disorders*	**SAD**	seasonal affective disorder
ECT	electroconvulsive therapy	**SSD**	somatic symptom disorder
FTM	female to male		

Chapter Review

Real-World Applications

Medical Record Analysis

This Discharge Summary contains 12 medical terms. Underline each term and write it in the list below the report. Then explain each term as you would to a nonmedical person.

Discharge Summary

Admitting Diagnosis:	Paraplegia following motorcycle accident
Final Diagnosis:	Comminuted L2 fracture with epidural hematoma and spinal cord injury resulting in complete paraplegia at the L2 level.
History of Present Illness:	Patient is a 23-year-old male who was involved in a motorcycle accident. He was unconscious for 35 minutes but was fully aware of his surroundings upon regaining consciousness. He was immediately aware of total anesthesia and paralysis below the waist.
Summary of Hospital Course:	CT scan revealed extensive bone destruction at the fracture site and that the spinal cord was severed. Patient was unable to voluntarily contract any lower extremity muscles and was not able to feel touch or pinpricks. Lumbar laminectomy with spinal fusion was performed to stabilize the fracture and remove the epidural hematoma. The immediate postoperative recovery period proceeded normally. Patient began physical therapy and occupational therapy. After two months, X-rays indicated full healing of the spinal fusion and patient was transferred to a rehabilitation institute.
Discharge Plans:	Patient was transferred to a rehabilitation institute to continue intensive PT and OT.

Term	Explanation
1. _____	_____
2. _____	_____
3. _____	_____
4. _____	_____
5. _____	_____
6. _____	_____
7. _____	_____
8. _____	_____
9. _____	_____
10. _____	_____
11. _____	_____
12. _____	_____

Chart Note Transcription

The chart note below contains 11 phrases that can be reworded with a medical term presented in this chapter. Each phrase is identified with an underline. Determine the medical term and write your answers in the space provided.

Pearson General Hospital Consultation Report

Task   Edit   View   Time Scale   Options   Help   Download   Archive   Date: 17 May 2017

Current Complaint: Patient is a 38-year-old female referred to the <u>specialist in the treatment of diseases of the nervous system</u> **1** by her family physician with complaints of <u>difficulty with speech</u>, **2** <u>loss of motion on one side of the body</u>, **3** and <u>severe involuntary muscle contractions</u>. **4**

Past History: Patient is married and nulliparous. Has been healthy prior to current symptoms.

Signs and Symptoms: Her husband reports he first noted loss of motion on one side of the body when she began to drag her left foot. It has progressed to involve both left upper and lower extremities, with approximately a 50% loss in control of left lower extremity and a 25% loss of control in left upper extremity. Difficulty with speech is mild and mainly with recalling the names of common objects. Severe involuntary muscle contractions appear to be triggered by stress and last approximately two minutes. Results of a <u>recording of the electrical activity of the brain</u> **5** and a <u>puncture with a needle into the low back to withdraw fluid for examination</u> **6** were normal. However, an <u>injection with radioactive isotopes</u> **7** revealed the presence of a mass in the right <u>outer layer of the largest section of the brain</u>. **8**

Diagnosis: <u>Astrocyte tumor</u> **9** in the right <u>outer layer of the largest section of the brain</u> **8**

Treatment: A right <u>skull incision</u> **10** was performed to permit <u>the surgical use of extreme cold</u> **11** to destroy the tumor. Patient experienced moderate improvement in <u>loss of motion on one side of the body</u> **3** and <u>severe involuntary muscle contractions</u>, **4** but <u>difficulty with speech</u> **2** was unchanged.

1. _____

2. _____

3. _____

4. _____

5. _____

6. _____

7. _____

8. _____

9. _____

10. _____

11. _____

Case Study

Below is a case study presentation of a patient with a condition discussed in this chapter. Read the case study and answer the questions below. Some questions will ask for information not included within this chapter. Use your text, a medical dictionary, or any other reference material you choose to answer these questions.

Anna Moore, an 83-year-old female, is admitted to the ER with aphasia, hemiparesis on her left side, syncope, and delirium. Her daughter called the ambulance after discovering her mother in this condition at home. Mrs. Moore has a history of hypertension, atherosclerosis, and diabetes mellitus. She was admitted to the hospital after a brain scan revealed an infarct in the right cerebral hemisphere, leading to a diagnosis of CVA of the middle cerebral artery.

(lofoto/Shutterstock)

Questions

1. What pathological condition does Mrs. Moore have? Look this condition up in a reference source and include a short description of it.

   _____

   _____

2. List and define each of the patient's presenting symptoms in the ER.

   _____

   _____

3. The patient has a history of three significant conditions. Describe each in your own words.

   _____

   _____

4. What diagnostic test did the physician perform? Describe this test and the results in your own words.

   _____

   _____

5. What is an *infarct* and what causes it?

   _____

   _____

6. List and describe the four common causes of a CVA.

   _____

   _____

Practice Exercises

A. Terminology Matching

Match each cranial nerve to its function.

1. _____ olfactory		a. carries facial sensory impulses
2. _____ optic		b. turns eye to side
3. _____ oculomotor		c. controls tongue muscles
4. _____ trochlear		d. controls eye muscles and pupils
5. _____ trigeminal		e. swallowing
6. _____ abducens		f. controls facial muscles
7. _____ facial		g. controls oblique eye muscles
8. _____ vestibulocochlear		h. smell
9. _____ glossopharyngeal		i. controls neck and shoulder muscles
10. _____ vagus		j. hearing and equilibrium
11. _____ accessory		k. vision
12. _____ hypoglossal		l. supplies most organs in abdominal and thoracic cavities

B. Word Building Practice

The combining form **neur/o** refers to the *nerve*. Use it to write a term that means:

1. inflammation of the nerve _____

2. specialist in nerves _____

3. pain in the nerve _____

4. inflammation of many nerves _____

5. removal of a nerve _____

6. surgical repair of a nerve _____

7. nerve tumor _____

8. suture of a nerve _____

The combining form **mening/o** refers to the *meninges* or *membranes*. Use it to write a term that means:

9. inflammation of the meninges _____

10. protrusion of the meninges _____

11. protrusion of the spinal cord and the meninges _____

The combining form **encephal/o** refers to the *brain*. Use it to write a term that means:

12. X-ray record of the brain _____

13. disease of the brain _____

14. inflammation of the brain _____

15. protrusion of the brain _____

The combining form **cerebr/o** refers to the *cerebrum*. Use it to write a term that means:

16. pertaining to the cerebrum and spinal cord _____

17. pertaining to the cerebrum _____

C. Using Abbreviations

Fill in each blank with the appropriate abbreviation.

1. Joseph's inattention and impulsive behavior led to a diagnosis of _____.

2. Performing repetitive rituals to reduce anxiety is the hallmark of _____.

3. A(n) _____ is also called a *spinal tap*.

4. A(n) _____ measures the metabolic activity of tissue.

5. _____ is caused by the loss of the myelin sheath around nerves.

6. Juanita suffered a(n) _____ from an auto accident, but luckily the spinal cord was only bruised and not severed.

7. _____ is commonly called *Lou Gehrig's disease*.

8. In a(n) _____, the neurological symptoms are temporary.

9. The newborn has _____ resulting from lack of oxygen during a difficult delivery.

10. The brain damage from the _____ included hemiplegia and dysphasia.

D. Define the Procedures and Tests

1. myelography _____

2. cerebral angiography _____

3. Babinski's reflex _____

4. nerve conduction velocity _____

5. cerebrospinal fluid analysis _____

6. PET scan _____

7. echoencephalography _____

8. lumbar puncture _____

E. Complete the Term

For each definition given below, fill in the blank with the word part that completes the term.

Definition	Term
1. treatment of the mind	_____therapy
2. condition of being without a mind	de_____ia
3. pertaining to without sense of pain	an_____ic
4. record of the spinal cord	_____gram
5. process of recording electricity of the brain	electro_____graphy
6. pertaining to under the dura	sub_____al
7. inflammation of the meninges	_____itis
8. inflammation of many nerves	poly_____itis
9. abnormal hardened condition	_____osis
10. action of shaking violently	_____ion
11. nerve root disease	_____pathy
12. pertaining to without feeling/sensation	an_____tic
13. fire frenzy	pyro_____
14. condition of not sleeping	in_____ia

F. Define the Term

1. astrocytoma   _____

2. epilepsy   _____

3. anesthesia   _____

4. hemiparesis   _____

5. neurosurgeon   _____

6. analgesia   _____

7. focal seizure   _____

8. quadriplegia   _____

9. subdural hematoma   _____

10. intrathecal   _____

G. Terminology Matching

Match each term to its definition.

1. _____ neurologist

2. _____ cerebrovascular accident

3. _____ concussion

4. _____ aphasia

5. _____ migraine

a. sudden attack

b. type of severe headache

c. loss of intellectual ability

d. physician who treats nerve problems

e. stroke

6. _____ seizure

f. mild traumatic brain injury

7. _____ dementia

g. loss of ability to speak

8. _____ ataxia

h. congenital anomaly

9. _____ spina bifida

i. state of being unaware

10. _____ unconscious

j. lack of muscle coordination

H. Fill in the Blank

Parkinson's disease	transient ischemic attack	cerebral palsy	cerebrospinal fluid shunt
Bell's palsy	subdural hematoma	amyotrophic lateral sclerosis	nerve conduction velocity
delirium	cerebral aneurysm		

1. Dr. Martin noted that a 96-year-old patient suffered from _____ when she determined that he was confused, disoriented, and agitated.

2. Lucinda's _____ resulted in increasing muscle weakness as the motor neurons in her spinal cord degenerated.

3. The diagnosis of _____ was correct because the weakness affected only one side of Charles's face.

4. A cerebral angiogram was ordered because Dr. Larson suspected Mrs. Constantine had a(n) _____.

5. Roberta's symptoms included fine tremors, muscular weakness, rigidity, and a shuffling gait, leading to a diagnosis of _____.

6. Matthew's hydrocephalus required the placement of a(n) _____.

7. Because Mae's hemiparesis was temporary, the final diagnosis was _____.

8. Following a car accident, a CT scan showed a(n) _____ was putting pressure on the brain, necessitating immediate neurosurgery.

9. Birth trauma resulted in the newborn developing _____.

10. A(n) _____ test was performed in order to pinpoint the exact position of the nerve damage.

I. Pharmacology Challenge

Fill in the classification for each drug description, then match the brand name.

Drug Description	Classification	Brand Name
1. _____ produces loss of sensation	_____	a. L-dopa
2. _____ treats Parkinson's disease	_____	b. Amytal
3. _____ promotes sleep	_____	c. OxyContin
4. _____ medication for mild pain	_____	d. Seconal
5. _____ produces a calming effect	_____	e. Xylocaine
6. _____ treats severe pain	_____	f. Tegretol
7. _____ treats seizures	_____	g. Motrin

J. Terminology Matching

Match each term to its clue.

1. _____ neurocognitive disorder
2. _____ elimination disorder
3. _____ dissociative disorder
4. _____ eating disorder
5. _____ sleep–wake disorder
6. _____ depressive disorder
7. _____ impulse control disorder
8. _____ somatic symptom disorder
9. _____ personality disorder
10. _____ paraphilic disorder
11. _____ anxiety disorder

a. conversion disorder
b. kleptomania
c. pedophilic disorder
d. narcissistic personality
e. insomnia
f. mania
g. panic attacks
h. amnesia
i. dementia
j. anorexia nervosa
k. enuresis

K. Name the Treatment

Identify each mental health treatment from its description.

1. depressant drugs prescribed for anxiety _____
2. client-centered psychotherapy _____
3. drug used to calm patients with bipolar disorder _____
4. reduces patient agitation and panic and shortens schizophrenic episodes _____
5. obtains a detailed account of the past and present emotional and mental experiences _____
6. stimulants that alter the patient's mood by affecting neurotransmitter levels _____

L. Name the Anesthesia

Identify the type of anesthesia for each description.

1. produces loss of consciousness and absence of pain _____
2. produces loss of sensation in one localized part of the body _____
3. anesthetic applied directly onto a specific skin area _____
4. also referred to as a nerve block _____

M. Anatomical Adjectives

Fill in the blank with the missing noun or adjective.

Noun	Adjective
1. cerebellum	_____
2. _____	thalamic
3. _____	cerebral
4. _____	vertebral
5. within the skull	_____
6. _____	spinal
7. brain	_____
8. pons	_____
9. medulla oblongata	_____
10. _____	neural
11. meninges	_____
12. _____	ventricular

N. Spelling Practice

Some of the following terms are misspelled. Identify the incorrect terms and spell them correctly in the blank provided.

1. anesthesiology _____
2. cephalgia _____
3. voyeuristic _____
4. postraumatic _____
5. hallucination _____
6. hyperesthesia _____
7. quadraplegia _____
8. hydrocephalis _____
9. amyotropic _____
10. echoencephalography _____

O. Complete the Statement

1. _____ is a behavioral science that studies human behavior and thought processes.

   _____ is a branch of medicine that diagnoses and treats mental disorders.

2. _____ nerves serve the skin and skeletal muscles.

3. The _____ nervous system is involved with the control of involuntary bodily functions.

4. _____ neurons are afferent neurons and _____ neurons are efferent neurons.

5. Cerebrospinal fluid is found in the _____ space.

6. The midbrain, pons, and medulla oblongata make up the _____.

7. The occipital lobe of the cerebrum controls _____.

8. _____ is a fatty substance that insulates some axons.

Labeling Exercises

Image A

Write the labels for this figure on the numbered lines provided.

1. _____

2. _____

3. _____

Image B

Write the labels for this figure on the numbered lines provided.

1. _____

2. _____

3. _____

4. _____

5. _____

6. _____

7. _____

Image C

Write the labels for this figure on the numbered lines provided.

1. _____

2. _____

3. _____

4. _____

5. _____

6. _____

7. _____

8. _____

9. _____

MyLab Medical Terminology™

MyLab Medical Terminology is a premium online homework management system that includes a host of features to help you study. Registered users will find:

- A multitude of activities and assignments built within the MyLab platform

- Powerful tools that track and analyze your results—allowing you to create a personalized learning experience

- Videos and audio pronunciations to help enrich your progress

- Streaming lesson presentations (Guided Lectures) and self-paced learning modules

- A space where you and your instructors can check your progress and manage your assignments

Chapter 13

Special Senses: The Eye and Ear

Learning Objectives

Upon completion of this chapter, you will be able to

1. Identify and define the combining forms, suffixes, and prefixes introduced in this chapter.
2. Correctly spell and pronounce medical terms and major anatomical structures relating to the eye and ear.
3. Locate and describe the major structures of the eye and ear and their functions.
4. Describe the process of vision.
5. Describe the path of sound vibration.
6. Identify and define eye and ear anatomical terms.
7. Identify and define selected eye and ear pathology terms.
8. Identify and define selected eye and ear diagnostic procedures.
9. Identify and define selected eye and ear therapeutic procedures.
10. Identify and define selected medications relating to the eye and ear.
11. Define selected abbreviations associated with the eye and ear.

SECTION I: THE EYE

AT A GLANCE

Function

The eye contains the sensory receptor cells for vision.

Structures

The primary structures that comprise the eye:

eyeball	**eye muscles**
sclera	**eyelids**
choroid	**conjunctiva**
retina	**lacrimal apparatus**

Word Parts

Presented here are the most common word parts (with their meanings) used to build eye terms. For a more comprehensive list, refer to the Terminology section of this chapter.

Combining Forms

ambly/o	dull, dim	**mi/o**	lessening
aque/o	water	**mydr/i**	widening
blast/o	immature	**nyctal/o**	night
blephar/o	eyelid	**ocul/o**	eye
chromat/o	color	**ophthalm/o**	eye
conjunctiv/o	conjunctiva	**opt/o**	eye, vision
corne/o	cornea	**optic/o**	eye, vision
cycl/o	ciliary body	**papill/o**	optic disk
dacry/o	tears	**phac/o**	lens
dipl/o	double	**phot/o**	light
emmetr/o	correct, proper	**presby/o**	old age
glauc/o	gray	**pupill/o**	pupil
ir/o	iris	**retin/o**	retina
irid/o	iris	**scler/o**	sclera
kerat/o	cornea	**stigmat/o**	point
lacrim/o	tears	**uve/o**	choroid
macul/o	macula lutea	**vitre/o**	glassy

Suffixes

-ician	specialist	**-opsia**	vision condition
-metrist	specialist in measuring	**-phobia**	fear
-opia	vision condition	**-tropia**	turned condition

Prefixes

eso-	inward
exo-	outward
myo-	to shut

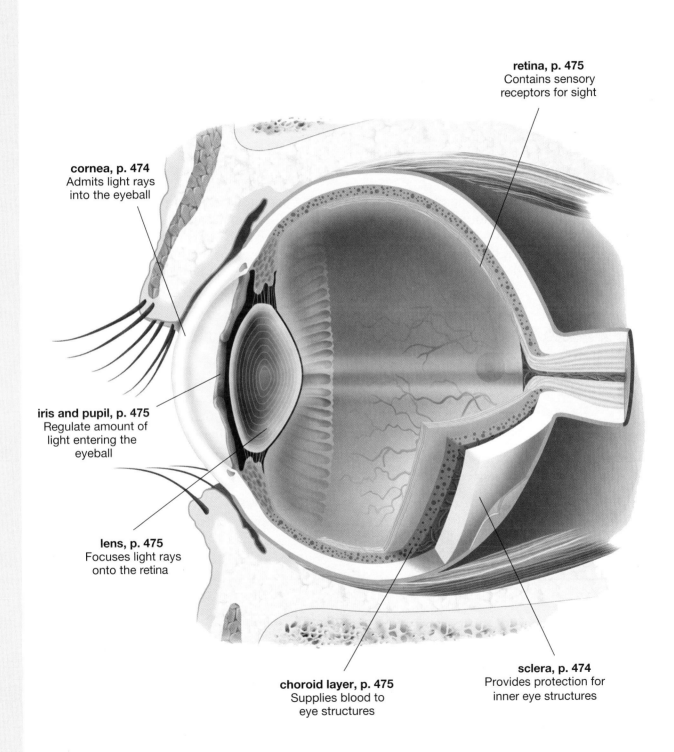

retina, p. 475
Contains sensory
receptors for sight

cornea, p. 474
Admits light rays
into the eyeball

iris and pupil, p. 475
Regulate amount of
light entering the
eyeball

lens, p. 475
Focuses light rays
onto the retina

choroid layer, p. 475
Supplies blood to
eye structures

sclera, p. 474
Provides protection for
inner eye structures

Anatomy and Physiology of the Eye

conjunctiva (kon-junk-TYE-vah)   lacrimal apparatus (LAK-rim-al)
eye muscles   ophthalmology (off-thal-MALL-oh-jee)
eyeball   optic nerve (OP-tik)
eyelids

The study of the eye is known as **ophthalmology** (Ophth). The **eyeball** is the incredible organ of sight that transmits an external image by way of the nervous system—the **optic nerve**—to the brain. The brain then translates these sensory impulses into an image with computer-like accuracy.

In addition to the eyeball, several external structures play a role in vision. These are the **eye muscles**, **eyelids**, **conjunctiva**, and **lacrimal apparatus**.

The Eyeball

choroid (KOR-oyd)   retina (RET-ih-nah)
orbit   sclera (SKLAIR-ah)

Each of the two eyeballs is housed in and protected by the **orbit**, an opening in the skull formed by a portion of the frontal, zygomatic, maxillary, ethmoid, sphenoid, lacrimal, and palatine bones. The actual eyeball is composed of three layers: the **sclera**, the **choroid**, and the **retina**. Light rays enter the eyeball through the anterior structures of the sclera and are focused onto the sensory receptor cells of the retina where they are converted to electrical signals that travel to the brain via the optic nerve.

Sclera

cornea (KOR-nee-ah)   refracts

The outer layer, the sclera, provides a tough protective coating for the inner structures of the eye. Another term for the sclera is the *white of the eye*.

The anterior portion of the sclera is called the **cornea** (see Figure 13-1 ■). This clear, transparent area of the sclera allows light to enter the interior of the eyeball. The cornea actually bends, or **refracts**, the light rays.

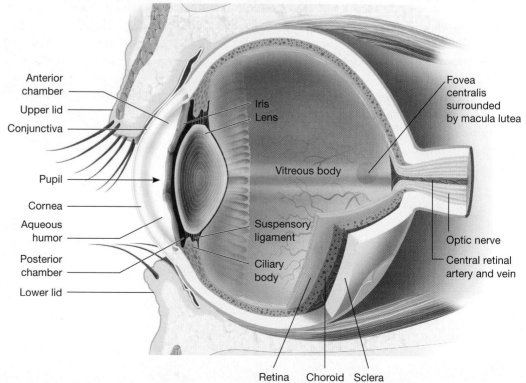

■ Figure 13-1 The internal structures of the eye.

Choroid

ciliary body (SIL-ee-air-ee)   lens
iris   pupil

The second or middle layer of the eyeball is called the *choroid*. This opaque layer distributes the blood supply for the eye.

The anterior portion of the choroid layer consists of the **iris**, **pupil**, and **ciliary body** (see again Figure 13-1). The iris is the colored portion of the eye and contains smooth muscle. The pupil is the opening in the center of the iris that allows light rays to enter the eyeball. The iris muscles contract or relax to change the size of the pupil, thereby controlling how much light enters the interior of the eyeball. Immediately posterior to the iris is a ring of smooth muscle called the ciliary body. Sitting in the center of the ring is the **lens**. The lens is not actually part of the choroid layer, but it is attached to the ciliary body by many thin ligaments called *suspensory ligaments*. The muscular ciliary body contracts or relaxes to pull on the edge of the lens, changing the shape of the lens so it can focus incoming light onto the retina.

Retina

aqueous humor (AY-kwee-us)   optic disk
cones   retinal blood vessels (RET-ih-nal)
fovea centralis (FOH-vee-ah / sen-TRAH-lis)   rods
macula lutea (MAK-yoo-lah / LOO-tee-ah)   vitreous humor (VIT-ree-us)

The third and innermost layer of the eyeball is the retina. It contains the sensory receptor cells (**rods** and **cones**) that respond to light rays. Rods are active in dim light and help the eye to see in gray tones. Cones are active only in bright light and are responsible for color vision. When someone looks directly at an object, the image falls on an area called the **macula lutea**, or "yellow spot" (see again Figure 13-1). In the center of the macula lutea is a depression called the **fovea centralis**, meaning *central pit*. This pit contains a high concentration of sensory receptor cells and, therefore, is the point of clearest vision. Also visible on the retina is the **optic disk**. This is the point where the **retinal blood vessels** enter and exit the eyeball and where the optic nerve leaves the eyeball (see Figure 13-2 ■). There are no sensory receptor cells in the optic disk and therefore it causes a blind spot in each eye's field of vision. Because the blind spot of each eye is set to the side, one eye is able to cover for the missing information from the other. For this reason, a person is not generally aware of their existence. The interior spaces of the eyeball are not empty. The spaces between the cornea and lens are filled with **aqueous humor**, a watery fluid, and the large open area between the lens and retina contains **vitreous humor**, a semisolid gel.

■ **Figure 13-2** Photograph of the retina of the eye. The optic disk appears yellow and the retinal arteries radiate out from it. The darker area in the center of the photo is the macula lutea. *(Left Handed Photography/Shutterstock)*

Muscles of the Eye

oblique muscles (oh-BLEEK)   **rectus muscles** (REK-tus)

Six muscles connect the actual eyeball to the skull (see Figure 13-3 ■). These muscles allow for change in the direction of each eye's sightline. In addition, they provide support for the eyeball in the eye socket. Children may be born with a weakness in some of these muscles and may require treatments such as eye exercises or even surgery to correct this problem, commonly referred to as crossed eyes or *strabismus* (see Figure 13-4 ■). The muscles involved are the four **rectus** and two **oblique muscles**. Rectus (meaning *straight*) muscles pull the eye up, down, left, or right in a straight line. Oblique muscles are on an angle and produce diagonal eye movement.

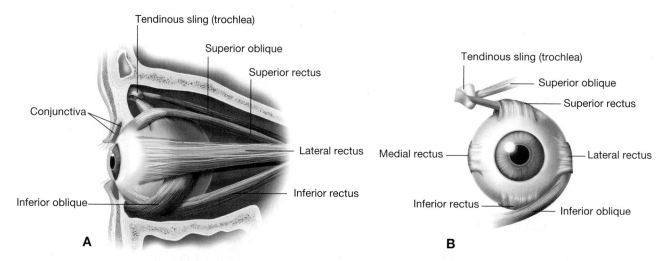

■ **Figure 13-3**   The arrangement of the external eye muscles, A) lateral and B) anterior views.

■ **Figure 13-4**   Examples of common forms of strabismus. A) Esotropia with the right eye turning inward. *(Biophoto Associates/Science Source)* B) Exotropia with the right eye turning outward. *(Gwen Shockey/Science Source)*

The Eyelids

cilia (SIL-ee-ah)   **sebaceous glands** (sih-BAY-shus)
eyelashes

A pair of eyelids over each eyeball provides protection from foreign particles, injury from the sun and intense light, and trauma (see again Figure 13-1). Both the upper and lower edges of the eyelids have **eyelashes**, or **cilia**, that protect the eye from foreign particles. In addition, **sebaceous glands** located in the eyelids secrete lubricating oil onto the eyeball.

Conjunctiva

mucous membrane (MYOO-kus)

The conjunctiva of the eye is a **mucous membrane** lining. It forms a continuous covering on the underside of each eyelid and across the anterior surface of each eyeball (see again Figure 13-1). This serves as protection for the eye by sealing off the eyeball in the socket.

> **What's In A Name?**
> Look for these word parts:
> **muc/o** = mucus
> **-ous** = pertaining to

Lacrimal Apparatus

lacrimal canals	**nasolacrimal duct** (nay-zoh-LAK-rim-al)
lacrimal gland	tears
nasal cavity	

The **lacrimal gland** is located under the outer upper corner of each eyelid. These glands produce **tears**. Tears serve the important function of washing and lubricating the anterior surface of the eyeball. **Lacrimal canals**, located in the inner corner of the eye socket, then collect the tears and drain them into the **nasolacrimal duct**. This duct ultimately drains the tears into the **nasal cavity** (see Figure 13-5 ■).

> **What's In A Name?**
> Look for these word parts:
> **lacrim/o** = tears
> **nas/o** = nose
> **-al** = pertaining to

- Superior lacrimal (tear) gland
- Inferior lacrimal (tear) gland
- Lacrimal sac
- Lacrimal canals
- Nasolacrimal duct (drains into the nasal cavity)

■ **Figure 13-5** The structure of the lacrimal apparatus.

How Vision Works

When light rays strike the eye, they first pass through the cornea, pupil, aqueous humor, lens, and vitreous humor (see Figure 13-6 ■). They then strike the retina and stimulate the rods and cones. When the light rays hit the retina, an upside-down image is sent along nerve impulses to the optic nerve (see Figure 13-7 ■). The optic nerve transmits these impulses to the brain, where the upside-down image is translated into the right-side-up image being looked at.

Vision requires proper functioning of four mechanisms:

1. Coordination of the external eye muscles so that both eyes move together.
2. The correct amount of light admitted by the pupil.
3. The correct focus of light on the retina by the lens.
4. The optic nerve transmitting sensory images to the brain.

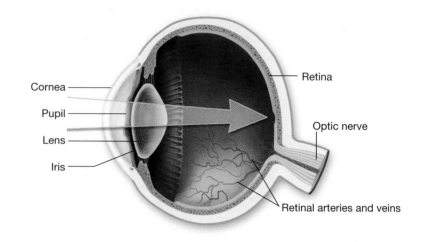

■ **Figure 13-6** The path of light through the cornea, iris, lens, and striking the retina.

Cornea — Pupil — Lens — Iris — Retina — Optic nerve — Retinal arteries and veins

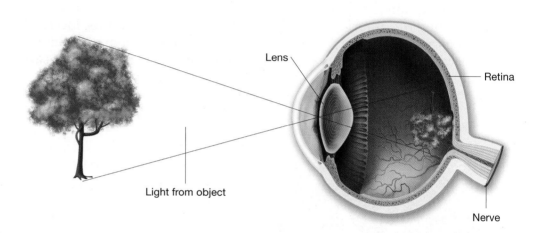

■ **Figure 13-7** The image formed on the retina is inverted. The brain rights the image as part of the interpretation process.

Lens — Retina — Light from object — Nerve

PRACTICE AS YOU GO

A. Complete the Statement

1. The study of the eye is _____.

2. Another term for eyelashes is _____.

3. The glands responsible for tears are called _____ glands.

4. The clear, transparent portion of the sclera is called the _____.

5. The innermost layer of the eye, which is composed of sensory receptors, is the _____.

6. The pupil of the eye is actually a hole in the _____.

7. The _____ layer of the eyeball distributes the blood supply to the eyeball.

8. _____ are active in bright light and perceive color. _____ are active in dim light and see in gray tones.

9. _____ muscles pull the eyeball in a straight line, whereas _____ muscles produce diagonal eye movement.

10. The _____ is a mucous membrane covering the anterior surface of the eyeball.

Terminology
Word Parts Used to Build Eye Terms

The following lists contain the combining forms, suffixes, and prefixes used to build terms in the remaining sections of this chapter.

Combining Forms

aden/o	gland	**emmetr/o**	correct, proper	**opt/o**	eye, vision
ambly/o	dull, dim	**esthesi/o**	sensation, feeling	**optic/o**	eye, vision
angi/o	vessel	**glauc/o**	gray	**papill/o**	optic disk
bi/o	life	**ir/o**	iris	**phac/o**	lens
blast/o	immature	**irid/o**	iris	**phot/o**	light
blephar/o	eyelid	**kerat/o**	cornea	**pneum/o**	air
chromat/o	color	**lacrim/o**	tears	**presby/o**	old age
conjunctiv/o	conjunctiva	**macul/o**	macula lutea	**pupill/o**	pupil
corne/o	cornea	**mi/o**	lessening	**retin/o**	retina
cry/o	cold	**myc/o**	fungus	**scler/o**	sclera
cycl/o	ciliary body	**mydr/i**	widening	**stigmat/o**	point
cyst/o	sac	**nyctal/o**	night	**ton/o**	tone
dacry/o	tears	**ocul/o**	eye	**uve/o**	choroid
dipl/o	double	**ophthalm/o**	eye	**xer/o**	dry

Suffixes

-al	pertaining to	**-logy**	study of	**-pexy**	surgical fixation
-algia	pain	**-malacia**	abnormal softening	**-phobia**	fear
-ar	pertaining to	**-meter**	instrument to measure	**-plasty**	surgical repair
-ary	pertaining to	**-metrist**	specialist in measuring	**-plegia**	paralysis
-atic	pertaining to			**-ptosis**	drooping
-ectomy	surgical removal	**-metry**	process of measuring	**-rrhagia**	abnormal flow condition
-edema	swelling	**-oma**	tumor; mass		
-graphy	process of recording	**-opia**	vision condition	**-scope**	instrument for viewing
-ia	condition	**-opsia**	vision condition	**-scopy**	process of visually examining
-ic	pertaining to	**-osis**	abnormal condition		
-ician	specialist	**-otomy**	cutting into	**-tic**	pertaining to
-ism	state of	**-pathy**	disease	**-tropia**	turned condition
-itis	inflammation				

Prefixes

a-	without	**exo-**	outward	**intra-**	within
an-	without	**extra-**	outside of	**micro-**	small
anti-	against	**hemi-**	half	**mono-**	one
de-	without	**hyper-**	excessive	**myo-**	to shut
eso-	inward				

Adjective Forms of Anatomical Terms

Term	Word Parts	Definition
conjunctival (kon-junk-TYE-val)	conjunctiv/o = conjunctiva -al = pertaining to	Pertaining to conjunctiva
corneal (KOR-nee-al)	corne/o = cornea -al = pertaining to	Pertaining to cornea
	Word Watch Be careful using the combining forms **core/o** meaning *pupil* and **corne/o** meaning *cornea*.	
extraocular (eks-trah-OK-yoo-lar)	extra- = outside of ocul/o = eye -ar = pertaining to	Pertaining to being outside the eyeball; for example, the extra-ocular eye muscles
intraocular (in-trah-OK-yoo-lar)	intra- = within ocul/o = eye -ar = pertaining to	Pertaining to within the eye
iridal (IR-id-al)	irid/o = iris -al = pertaining to	Pertaining to iris
lacrimal (LAK-rim-al)	lacrim/o = tears -al = pertaining to	Pertaining to tears
macular (MAK-yoo-lar)	macul/o = macula lutea -ar = pertaining to	Pertaining to macula lutea
ocular (OK-yoo-lar)	ocul/o = eye -ar = pertaining to	Pertaining to eye
ophthalmic (off-THAL-mik)	ophthalm/o = eye -ic = pertaining to	Pertaining to eye
optic (OP-tik)	opt/o = eye, vision -ic = pertaining to	Pertaining to eye or vision
optical (OP-tih-kal)	optic/o = eye, vision -al = pertaining to	Pertaining to eye or vision
pupillary (PYOO-pih-lair-ee)	pupill/o = pupil -ary = pertaining to	Pertaining to pupil
retinal (RET-ih-nal)	retin/o = retina -al = pertaining to	Pertaining to retina
scleral (SKLAIR-al)	scler/o = sclera -al = pertaining to	Pertaining to sclera
uveal (YOO-vee-al)	uve/o = choroid -al = pertaining to	Pertaining to choroid layer of eye

PRACTICE AS YOU GO

B. Give the adjective form for each term.

1. The pupil _____

2. The eye or vision _____ or _____

3. The retina _____

4. Tears   _____

5. Within the eye   _____

6. Outside of the eye _____

Pathology

Term	Word Parts	Definition
Medical Specialties		
ophthalmology (Ophth) (off-thal-MALL-oh-jee)	ophthalm/o = eye -logy = study of	Branch of medicine involving diagnosis and treatment of conditions and diseases of the eye and surrounding structures; physician is *ophthalmologist*
optician (op-TISH-an)	opt/o = vision -ician = specialist	Vision specialist trained in grinding and fitting corrective lenses
optometrist (op-TOM-eh-trist)	opt/o = vision -metrist = specialist in measuring	Doctor of optometry
optometry (op-TOM-eh-tree)	opt/o = vision -metry = process of measuring	Medical profession specializing in examining the eyes, testing visual acuity, and prescribing corrective lenses
Signs and Symptoms		
blepharoptosis (blef-ah-rop-TOH-sis)	blephar/o = eyelid -ptosis = drooping	Drooping eyelid
cycloplegia (sigh-kloh-PLEE-jee-ah)	cycl/o = ciliary body -plegia = paralysis	Paralysis of ciliary body that, in turn, changes shape of lens and makes it difficult to bring images into focus
diplopia (dip-LOH-pee-ah)	dipl/o = double -opia = vision condition	Condition of seeing double
emmetropia (EM) (em-eh-TROH-pee-ah)	emmetr/o = correct, proper -opia = vision condition	State of normal vision
iridoplegia (ir-id-oh-PLEE-jee-ah)	irid/o = iris -plegia = paralysis	Paralysis of the iris that, in turn, changes size of the pupil and makes it difficult to regulate amount of light entering the eye
nyctalopia (nik-tah-LOH-pee-ah)	nyctal/o = night -opia = vision condition	Difficulty seeing in dim light; also called *night blindness*; usually due to damaged rods
	Med Term Tip The simple translation of *nyctalopia* is *night vision*. However, it is used to mean *night blindness*.	
ophthalmalgia (off-thal-MAL-jee-ah)	ophthalm/o = eye -algia = pain	Eye pain
ophthalmoplegia (off-thal-moh-PLEE-jee-ah)	ophthalm/o = eye -plegia = paralysis	Paralysis of one or more of the extraocular eye muscles
ophthalmorrhagia (off-thal-moh-RAY-jee-ah)	ophthalm/o = eye -rrhagia = abnormal flow condition	Bleeding from the eye
papilledema (pap-il-eh-DEE-mah)	papill/o = optic disk -edema = swelling	Swelling of the optic disk; often as result of increased intraocular pressure; also called *choked disk*

Pathology (continued)

Term	Word Parts	Definition
photophobia (foh-toh-FOH-bee-ah)	phot/o = light -phobia = fear	Although term translates into *fear of light*, actually means strong sensitivity to bright light
presbyopia (prez-bee-OH-pee-ah)	presby/o = old age -opia = vision condition	Expected changes in vision due to normal aging process; resulting in difficulty in focusing for near vision (such as reading)
scleromalacia (sklair-oh-mah-LAY-shee-ah)	scler/o = sclera -malacia = abnormal softening	Softening of the sclera
xerophthalmia (zeer-off-THAL-mee-ah)	xer/o = dry ophthalm/o = eye -ia = condition	Condition of dry eyes

Eyeball

Term	Word Parts	Definition
achromatopsia (ah-kroh-mah-TOP-see-ah)	a- = without chromat/o = color -opsia = vision condition	Severe congenital deficiency in color vision; complete color blindness; more common in males
amblyopia (am-blee-OH-pee-ah)	ambly/o = dull, dim -opia = vision condition	Loss of vision not as result of eye pathology; usually occurs in patients who see two images; in order to see only one image, the brain will no longer recognize image being sent to it by one of the eyes; may occur if strabismus is not corrected; condition is not treatable with prescription lens; commonly referred to as *lazy eye*
astigmatism (Astigm) (ah-STIG-mah-tizm)	a- = without stigmat/o = point -ism = state of	Condition in which light rays are focused unevenly on the retina (no sharp point of focus), causing distorted image, due to abnormal curvature of the cornea
cataract (KAT-ah-rakt)		Development of an opaque or cloudy lens, resulting in diminished vision; most common causes are aging, eye trauma, or radiation (especially sunlight) exposure, but may be present at birth; treatment is usually surgical removal of lens with cataract and replacement with prosthetic lens

> **Med Term Tip**
>
> The term *cataract* comes from the Latin word meaning *waterfall*. This refers to how a person with a cataract sees the world—as if looking through a waterfall.

■ **Figure 13-8** Photograph of a person with a cataract in the right eye. *(ARZTSAMUI/Shutterstock)*

Term	Word Parts	Definition
corneal abrasion	corne/o = cornea -al = pertaining to	Scraping injury to the cornea; if it does not heal, may develop into ulcer
glaucoma (glaw-KOH-mah)	glauc/o = gray -oma = mass	Increase in intraocular pressure, which, if untreated, may result in atrophy (wasting-away) of optic nerve and blindness; treated with medication and surgery; there is increased risk of developing glaucoma in persons over age 60, those of African ancestry, people who have sustained serious eye injury, or anyone with family history of diabetes or glaucoma

> **Med Term Tip**
>
> The term *glaucoma* was first used by the ancient Greeks to describe the dull, glazed appearance of a blind eye, not an actual color change.

Pathology (continued)

Term	Word Parts	Definition
hyperopia (high-per-OH-pee-ah)	hyper- = excessive -opia = vision condition	With this condition person can see things in distance but has trouble reading material at close range; also known as *farsightedness;* condition is corrected with converging or biconvex lenses

■ **Figure 13-9** Hyperopia (farsightedness). In the uncorrected top figure, the image would come into focus behind the retina, making the image on the retina blurry. The bottom image shows how a biconvex lens corrects this condition.

iritis (eye-RYE-tis)	ir/o = iris -itis = inflammation	Inflammation of the iris
keratitis (kair-ah-TYE-tis)	kerat/o = cornea -itis = inflammation	Inflammation of the cornea

> **Word Watch**
> Be careful using the combining form **kerat/o**, which means both *cornea* and the hard protein *keratin.*

legally blind		Describes person who has severely impaired vision; usually defined as having visual acuity of 20/200 that cannot be improved with corrective lenses or having visual field of less than 20 degrees
macular degeneration (MAK-yoo-lar)	macul/o = macula lutea -ar = pertaining to	Deterioration of macular area of the retina of the eye; may be treated with laser surgery to destroy blood vessels beneath the macula
monochromatism (mon-oh-KROH-mah-tizm)	mono- = one chromat/o = color -ism = state of	Unable to perceive one color

Pathology (continued)

Term	Word Parts	Definition
myopia (MY) (my-OH-pee-ah)	myo- = to shut -opia = vision condition	With this condition person can see things close up but distance vision is blurred; also known as *nearsightedness*; condition is corrected with diverging or biconcave lenses; named because persons with myopia often partially shut their eyes, squint, in order to see more clearly

> **Med Term Tip**
>
> The term *myopia* appears to use the combining form **my/o**, which means *muscle*. This combining form comes from the Greek word *mys*. But in this case the term uses the prefix **myo-**, which comes from the Greek word *myo* or *myein*, meaning *to shut*.

Myopia (nearsightedness)

Corrected with biconcave lens

■ **Figure 13-10** Myopia (nearsightedness). In the uncorrected top figure, the image comes into focus in front of the retina, making the image on the retina blurry. The bottom image shows how a biconcave lens corrects this condition.

Term	Word Parts	Definition
oculomycosis (ok-yoo-loh-my-KOH-sis)	ocul/o = eye myc/o = fungus -osis = abnormal condition	Fungus infection of the eye
retinal detachment (RET-ih-nal)	retin/o = retina -al = pertaining to	Occurs when the retina becomes separated from the choroid layer; separation seriously damages blood vessels and nerves, resulting in blindness; may be treated with surgical or medical procedures to stabilize the retina and prevent separation
retinitis pigmentosa (ret-ih-NYE-tis / pig-men-TOH-sah)	retin/o = retina -itis = inflammation	Progressive disease of the eye resulting in the retina becoming sclerosed (hard), pigmented (colored), and atrophied (wasting-away); no known cure for this condition
retinoblastoma (ret-ih-noh-blas-TOH-mah)	retin/o = retina blast/o = immature -oma = tumor	Malignant eye tumor occurring in children, usually under age 3; requires enucleation
retinopathy (ret-in-OP-ah-thee)	retin/o = retina -pathy = disease	General term for disease affecting the retina
scleritis (skler-EYE-tis)	scler/o = sclera -itis = inflammation	Inflammation of the sclera

Pathology (continued)

Term	Word Parts	Definition
uveitis (yoo-vee-EYE-tis)	uve/o = choroid -itis = inflammation	Inflammation of the choroid layer

Conjunctiva

Term	Word Parts	Definition
conjunctivitis (kon-junk-tih-VYE-tis)	conjunctiv/o = conjunctiva -itis = inflammation	Inflammation of the conjunctiva usually as result of bacterial infection, but may also be caused by viruses and allergens; commonly called *pinkeye*
pterygium (teh-RIJ-ee-um)		Hypertrophied conjunctival tissue in inner corner of the eye

Eyelids

Term	Word Parts	Definition
blepharitis (blef-ah-RYE-tis)	blephar/o = eyelid -itis = inflammation	Inflammation of the eyelid
hordeolum (hor-DEE-oh-lum)		Refers to a *stye* (or *sty*), a small purulent inflammatory infection of a sebaceous gland of the eyelid; treated with hot compresses and/or surgical incision

Lacrimal Apparatus

Term	Word Parts	Definition
dacryoadenitis (dak-ree-oh-ad-eh-NYE-tis)	dacry/o = tears aden/o = gland -itis = inflammation	Inflammation of the lacrimal gland
dacryocystitis (dak-ree-oh-sis-TYE-tis)	dacry/o = tears cyst/o = sac -itis = inflammation	Inflammation of the lacrimal sac

Eye Muscles

Term	Word Parts	Definition
esotropia (ET) (ess-oh-TROH-pee-ah)	eso- = inward -tropia = turned condition	Inward turning of the eye; also called *cross-eyed*; example of a form of strabismus (muscle weakness of the eye)
exotropia (XT) (eks-oh-TROH-pee-ah)	exo- = outward -tropia = turned condition	Outward turning of the eye; also called *wall-eyed*; also an example of strabismus (muscle weakness of the eye)
strabismus (strah-BIZ-mus)		Eye muscle weakness commonly seen in children resulting in eyes looking in different directions at the same time; may be corrected with glasses, eye exercises, and/or surgery

Brain-Related Vision Pathologies

Term	Word Parts	Definition
hemianopia (hem-ee-ah-NOH-pee-ah)	hemi- = half an- = without -opia = vision condition	Loss of vision in half of visual field; a stroke patient may suffer from this disorder
nystagmus (niss-TAG-mus)		Jerky-appearing involuntary eye movements, usually left and right; often an indication of brain injury

PRACTICE AS YOU GO

C. Pathology Matching

Match each pathology term to its definition.

1. _____ emmetropia   a. opacity of the lens
2. _____ hyperopia   b. a form of strabismus
3. _____ cataract   c. nearsightedness
4. _____ astigmatism   d. due to abnormal curvature of cornea
5. _____ esotropia   e. lazy eye
6. _____ xerophthalmia   f. involuntary movements of the eye
7. _____ myopia   g. farsightedness
8. _____ nystagmus   h. normal vision
9. _____ amblyopia   i. dry eyes
10. _____ presbyopia   j. vision loss due to normal aging

Diagnostic Procedures

Term	Word Parts	Definition
Eye Examination Tests		
color vision tests		Use of polychromic (multicolored) charts to determine ability of patient to recognize color; most common is Ishihara test for red-green color blindness

■ **Figure 13-11** An example of color blindness test. A person with red-green color blindness would not be able to distinguish the green 27 from the surrounding red circles.

Term	Word Parts	Definition
fluorescein angiography (floor-ESS-see-in / an-jee-OG-rah-fee)	angi/o = vessel -graphy = process of recording	Process of injecting dye (fluorescein) to observe movement of blood and detect lesions in macular area of the retina; used to determine if there is detachment of the retina
fluorescein staining (floor-ESS-see-in)		Application of dye eyedrops of bright green fluorescent color used to look for corneal abrasions or ulcers
keratometer (kair-ah-TOM-eh-ter)	kerat/o = cornea -meter = instrument to measure	Instrument used to measure curvature of the cornea

Diagnostic Procedures (continued)

Term	Word Parts	Definition
keratometry (kair-ah-TOM-eh-tree)	kerat/o = cornea -metry = process of measuring	Measurement of curvature of the cornea using instrument called *keratometer*
ophthalmoscope (off-THAL-moh-skohp)	ophthalm/o – eye -scope = instrument for viewing	Instrument used to examine inside of the eye through the pupil
ophthalmoscopy (off-thal-MOSS-koh-pee)	ophthalm/o = eye -scopy = process of visually examining	Examination of interior of the eyes using instrument called *ophthalmoscope*; pupil is dilated in order to see cornea, lens, and retina; used to identify abnormalities in blood vessels of the eye and some systemic diseases

■ **Figure 13-12** Examination of the interior of the eye using an ophthalmoscope. *(Monkey Business Images/ Shutterstock)*

Term	Word Parts	Definition
optometer (op-TOM-eh-ter)	opt/o = vision -meter = instrument to measure	Instrument used to measure how well the eye is able to focus images clearly on the retina
refractive error test (ree-FRAK-tiv)		Vision test for defect in ability of the eye to accurately focus image that is hitting it; refractive errors result in myopia and hyperopia
slit lamp microscopy	micro- = small -scopy = process of visually examining	Process of visually examining conjunctiva, cornea, iris, and lens of the eye
Snellen chart (SNEL-en)		Chart used for testing distance vision named for Dutch ophthalmologist Herman Snellen; contains letters of varying sizes and is administered from a distance of 20 feet; person who can read at 20 feet what average person can read at this distance is said to have 20/20 vision
tonometry (tohn-OM-eh-tree)	ton/o = tone -metry = process of measuring	Measurement of intraocular pressure of the eye using *tonometer* to check for condition of glaucoma; generally part of normal eye exam for adults
visual acuity (VA) test (VIZH-oo-al / ah-KYOO-ih-tee)	-al = pertaining to	Measurement of sharpness of patient's vision; usually, Snellen chart is used for this test in which patient identifies letters from a distance of 20 feet

Therapeutic Procedures

Terms	Word Parts	Definition
Surgical Procedures		
blepharectomy (blef-ah-REK-toh-mee)	blephar/o = eyelid -ectomy = surgical removal	Surgical removal of all or part of the eyelid
blepharoplasty (BLEF-ah-roh-plas-tee)	blephar/o = eyelid -plasty = surgical repair	Surgical repair of the eyelid; common plastic surgery to correct blepharoptosis
conjunctivoplasty (kon-JUNK-tih-voh-plas-tee)	conjunctiv/o = conjunctiva -plasty = surgical repair	Surgical repair of the conjunctiva
cryopexy (KRY-oh-pek-see)	cry/o = cold -pexy = surgical fixation	Surgical fixation of the retina by using extreme cold
enucleation (ee-noo-klee-AY-shun)		Surgical removal of an eyeball
intraocular lens (IOL) **implant** (in-trah-OK-yoo-lar)	intra- = within ocul/o = eye -ar = pertaining to	Use of artificial lens to replace the lens removed during cataract surgery
iridectomy (ir-ih-DEK-toh-mee)	irid/o = iris -ectomy = surgical removal	Surgical removal of a small portion of the iris
iridosclerotomy (ir-ih-doh-skleh-ROT-oh-mee)	irid/o = iris scler/o = sclera -otomy = cutting into	To cut into iris and sclera
keratoplasty (KAIR-ah-toh-plas-tee)	kerat/o = cornea -plasty = surgical repair	Surgical repair of the cornea is simple translation of this term utilized to mean corneal transplant
laser-assisted in situ keratomileusis (LASIK) (in-SIGH-tyoo / kair-ah-toh-mih-LOO-sis)	kerat/o = cornea	Correction of myopia using laser surgery to remove corneal tissue
laser photocoagulation (LAY-zer / foh-toh-koh-ag-yoo-LAY-shun)	phot/o = light	Use of laser beam to destroy very small precise areas of the retina; may be used to treat retinal detachment or macular degeneration

■Figure 13-13   LASIK surgery uses a laser to reshape the cornea. *(Mehmetcan/Shutterstock)*

Therapeutic Procedures (continued)

Terms	Word Parts	Definition
phacoemulsification (fay-koh-ee-mull-sih-fih-KAY-shun)	phac/o = lens	Use of high-frequency sound waves to emulsify (liquefy) a lens with a cataract, which is then aspirated (removed by suction) with a needle
photorefractive keratectomy (PRK) (foh-toh-ree-FRAK-tiv / kair-ah-TEK-toh-mee)	phot/o = light kerat/o = cornea -ectomy = surgical removal	Surgical use of laser to reshape the cornea and correct errors of refraction
pneumatic retinopexy (noo-MAT-ik / ret-ih-noh-PEK-see)	pneum/o = air -atic = pertaining to retin/o = retina -pexy = surgical fixation	Surgical injection of gas bubble into the eye and positioning the head so that bubble presses against area of detached retina
radial keratotomy (RK) (RAY-dee-al / kair-ah-TOT-oh-mee)	-al = pertaining to kerat/o = cornea -otomy = cutting into	Spokelike incisions around the cornea that result in it becoming flatter; surgical treatment for myopia
retinopexy (ret-ih-noh-PEK-see)	retin/o = retina -pexy = surgical fixation	Surgical fixation of the retina; one treatment for a detaching retina
scleral buckling (SKLAIR-al)	scler/o = sclera -al = pertaining to	Placing a band of silicone around outside of the sclera that stabilizes a detaching retina
sclerotomy (skleh-ROT-oh-mee)	scler/o = sclera -otomy = cutting into	To cut into the sclera
strabotomy (strah-BOT-oh-mee)	-otomy = cutting into	Incision into the eye muscles in order to correct strabismus

PRACTICE AS YOU GO

D. Procedure Matching

Match each procedure term to its definition.

1. _____ fluorescein staining   **a.** examining the interior of the eyeball

2. _____ ophthalmoscopy   **b.** corneal transplant

3. _____ tonometry   **c.** liquefies a cataract

4. _____ enucleation   **d.** looks for corneal abrasions or ulcers

5. _____ keratoplasty   **e.** surgical removal of an eyeball

6. _____ phacoemulsification   **f.** measures intraocular pressure

Pharmacology

Classification	Word Parts	Action	Examples
anesthetic ophthalmic solution (off-THAL-mik)	an- = without esthesi/o = sensation, feeling -tic = pertaining to ophthalm/o = eye -ic = pertaining to	Eyedrops for pain relief associated with eye infections, corneal abrasions, or surgery	proparacain, Ak-Taine, Ocu-Caine; tetracaine, Opticaine, Pontocaine
antibiotic ophthalmic solution (off-THAL-mik)	anti- = against bi/o = life -tic = pertaining to ophthalm/o = eye -ic = pertaining to	Eyedrops for treatment of bacterial eye infections	erythromycin, Del-Mycin, Ilotycin Ophthalmic
antiglaucoma medications (an-tye-glaw-KOH-mah)	anti- = against glauc/o = gray -oma = mass	Reduce intraocular pressure by lowering amount of aqueous humor in the eyeball; may achieve this by either reducing production of aqueous humor or increasing its outflow	timolol, Betimol, Timoptic; acetazolamide, Ak-Zol, Dazamide; prostaglandin analogs, Lumigan, Xalatan
artificial tears		Medications, many of them over-the-counter, to treat dry eyes	buffered isotonic solutions, Akwa Tears, Refresh Plus, Moisture Eyes
miotic drops (my-OT-ik)	mi/o = lessening -tic = pertaining to	Any substance that causes the pupil to constrict (lessen); these medications may also be used to treat glaucoma	physostigmine, Eserine Sulfate, Isopto Eserine; carbachol, Carbastat, Miostat
mydriatic drops (mid-ree-AT-ik)	mydr/i = widening -atic = pertaining to	Any substance that causes the pupil to dilate (widen) by paralyzing iris and/or ciliary body muscles; particularly useful during eye examinations and eye surgery	atropine sulfate, Atropine-Care Ophthalmic, Atropisol Ophthalmic
ophthalmic decongestants	ophthalm/o = eye -ic = pertaining to de- = without	Over-the-counter medications that constrict the arterioles of the eye and reduce redness and itching of the conjunctiva	tetrahydrozoline, Visine, Murine

Abbreviations

ARMD	age-related macular degeneration	**LASIK**	laser-assisted in situ keratomileusis
Astigm	astigmatism	**MY**	myopia
c.gl.	correction with glasses	**Ophth**	ophthalmology
D	diopter (lens strength)	**PERRLA**	pupils equal, round, react to light and accommodation
DVA	distance visual acuity	**PRK**	photorefractive keratectomy
ECCE	extracapsular cataract extraction	**REM**	rapid eye movement
EENT	eyes, ears, nose, and throat	**RK**	radial keratotomy
EM	emmetropia	**s.gl.**	without correction or glasses
EOM	extraocular movement	**SMD**	senile macular degeneration
ET	esotropia	**VA**	visual acuity
ICCE	intracapsular cataract extraction	**VF**	visual field
IOL	intraocular lens	**XT**	exotropia
IOP	intraocular pressure		

PRACTICE AS YOU GO

E. What's the Abbreviation?

1. intraocular lens _____

2. emmetropia _____

3. exotropia _____

4. myopia _____

5. extraocular movement _____

6. visual acuity _____

AT A GLANCE

Function

The ear contains the sensory receptors for hearing and equilibrium (balance).

Structures

The primary structures that comprise the ear:

external ear   **middle ear**

auricle   **inner ear**

Word Parts

Presented here are the most common word parts (with their meanings) used to build ear terms. For a more comprehensive list, refer to the Terminology section of this chapter.

Combining Forms

acous/o	hearing	**labyrinth/o**	labyrinth (inner ear)
audi/o	hearing	**myring/o**	tympanic membrane
audit/o	hearing	**ot/o**	ear
aur/o	ear	**salping/o**	auditory tube (eustachian tube)
auricul/o	ear	**staped/o**	stapes
cerumin/o	cerumen	**tympan/o**	tympanic membrane
cochle/o	cochlea	**vestibul/o**	vestibule

Suffixes

-cusis	hearing
-otia	ear condition

The Ear Illustrated

auricle, p. 494
Directs sound
waves into the
ear canal

middle ear, p. 495
Transmits sound
waves to the
inner ear

inner ear, p. 495
Contains sensory
receptors for
hearing and
balance

external ear, p. 494
Transmits sound
waves to the
middle ear

Anatomy and Physiology of the Ear

audiology (aw-dee-ALL-oh-jee)

cochlear nerve (KOH-klee-ar)

equilibrium (ee-kwih-LIB-ree-um)

external ear

hearing

inner ear

middle ear

otology (oh-TALL-oh-jee)

vestibular nerve (ves-TIB-yoo-lar)

vestibulocochlear nerve
(ves-tib-yoo-loh-KOH-klee-ar)

The study of the ear is referred to as **otology** (Oto), and the study of hearing disorders is called **audiology**. While there is a large amount of overlap between these two areas, there are also examples of ear problems that do not affect hearing. The ear is responsible for two senses: **hearing** and **equilibrium**, or the body's sense of balance. Hearing and equilibrium sensory information is carried to the brain by cranial nerve VIII, the **vestibulocochlear nerve**. This nerve is divided into two major branches. The **cochlear nerve** carries hearing information, and the **vestibular nerve** carries equilibrium information.

The ear is subdivided into three areas: **external ear**, **middle ear**, and **inner ear**.

External Ear

auditory canal (AW-dih-tor-ee)

auricle (AW-rih-kl)

cerumen (seh-ROO-men)

external auditory meatus (AW-dih-tor-ee /
mee-AY-tus)

pinna (PIN-ah)

tympanic membrane (tim-PAN-ik)

The external ear consists of three parts: the **auricle**, the **auditory canal**, and the **tympanic membrane** (see Figure 13-14 ■). The auricle or **pinna** is what is commonly referred to as the *ear* because this is the only visible portion. The auricle with its earlobe has a unique shape in each person and functions like a funnel to capture sound waves as they go past the outer ear and channel them through the **external auditory meatus**. The sound then moves along the auditory canal and causes the

Labels: Pinna, Cartilage, External auditory meatus, Auditory canal, Mastoid process, Lobe, Temporal bone, Malleus (hammer), Incus (anvil), Semicircular canals (equilibrium), Vestibular nerve, Cochlear nerve, Cochlea (hearing), Oval window, Stapes (stirrup), Eustachian tube, Tympanic membrane (eardrum), Internal carotid artery, Internal jugular vein

■ **Figure 13-14** The internal structures of the outer, middle, and inner ear.

tympanic membrane (eardrum) to vibrate. The tympanic membrane actually separates the external ear from the middle ear. Earwax or **cerumen** is produced in oil glands in the auditory canal. This wax helps to protect and lubricate the ear. It is also just barely liquid at body temperature. This causes cerumen to slowly flow out of the auditory canal, carrying dirt and dust with it. Therefore, the auditory canal is self-cleaning.

> **Med Term Tip**
>
> The term *tympanic membrane* comes from the Greek word for *drumhead*. The tympanic membrane or eardrum vibrates to sound waves like a drum head.

Middle Ear

auditory tube (AW-dih-tor-ee)
eustachian tube (yoo-STAY-shee-en)
incus (ING-kus)
malleus (MAL-ee-us)

ossicles (OSS-ih-kls)
oval window
stapes (STAY-peez)

The middle ear is located in a small cavity in the temporal bone of the skull. This air-filled cavity contains three tiny bones called **ossicles** (see Figure 13-15 ■). These three bones—the **malleus**, **incus**, and **stapes**—are vital to the hearing process. They amplify the vibrations in the middle ear and transmit them to the inner ear from the malleus to the incus and finally to the stapes. The stapes, the last of the three ossicles, is attached to a very thin membrane that covers the opening to the inner ear called the **oval window**.

   The **eustachian tube** or **auditory tube** connects the nasopharynx with the middle ear (see again Figure 13-14). Each time a person swallows, the eustachian tube opens. This connection allows pressure to equalize between the middle ear cavity and the atmospheric pressure.

> **Med Term Tip**
>
> The three ossicles in the middle ear are the tiniest bones in the body and are sometimes referred to by terms that are similar to their shape. Thus, the malleus is called the hammer, the incus is the anvil, and the stapes is the stirrup (see again Figure 13-15).

Tympanic membrane —
— Malleus
— Incus
— Stapes
— Oval window

■ **Figure 13-15**   Close-up view of the ossicles within the middle ear. These three bones extend from the tympanic membrane to the oval window.

Inner Ear

cochlea (KOH-klee-ah)
labyrinth (LAB-ih-rinth)
organ of Corti (KOR-tee)
saccule (SAK-yool)

semicircular canals
utricle (YOO-trih-kl)
vestibule (VES-tih-byool)

The inner ear is also located in a cavity within the temporal bone (see again Figure 13-14). This fluid-filled cavity is referred to as the **labyrinth** because of its shape. The first structure of the inner ear is the **vestibule**. Each of the remaining inner ear structures—the **cochlea** (the sensory organ for hearing) and the **semicircular canals**, **utricle**, and **saccule** (the sensory organs for equilibrium)—open off the vestibule. Each of these organs contains hair cells, which are the actual sensory receptor cells. In the cochlea, the hair cells are referred to collectively as the **organ of Corti**.

> **What's In A Name?**
>
> Look for these word parts:
> -ar = pertaining to
> -ule = small
> semi- = partial

> **Med Term Tip**
>
> The term *vestibule* comes from the Latin word *vestibulum*, meaning *entrance*. It received this name because it is the entryway into the inner ear.

How Hearing Works

conductive hearing loss (kon-DUK-tiv)
sensorineural hearing loss (sen-soh-ree-NOO-ral)

Figure 13-16 ■ outlines the path of sound through the outer ear and middle ear and into the cochlea of the inner ear. Sound waves traveling down the external auditory canal strike the eardrum, causing it to vibrate. The ossicles conduct these vibrations across the middle ear from the eardrum to the oval window. Oval window movements initiate vibrations in the fluid that fills the cochlea. As the fluid vibrations strike a hair cell, they bend the small hairs and stimulate the nerve ending. The nerve ending then sends an electrical impulse to the brain on the cochlear portion of the vestibulocochlear nerve.

Hearing loss can be divided into two main categories: **conductive hearing loss** and **sensorineural hearing loss**. Conductive refers to disease or malformation of the outer or middle ear. All sound is weaker and muffled in conductive hearing loss since it is not conducted correctly to the inner ear. Sensorineural hearing loss is the result of damage or malformation of the inner ear (cochlea) or the cochlear nerve. In this hearing loss, some sounds are distorted and heard incorrectly. There can also be a combination of both conductive and sensorineural hearing loss.

Path of sound vibrations

| Outer ear | Middle ear | Inner ear |

Outer ear:
- Pinna
- External auditory canal
- Tympanic membrane

Middle ear:
- Malleus
- Incus
- Stapes
- Oval window

Inner ear:
- Cochlea
- Auditory fluids
- Organ of Corti
- Auditory nerve fibers
- Cerebral cortex

■ **Figure 13-16** The path of sound waves through the outer, middle, and inner ear.

PRACTICE AS YOU GO

F. Complete the Statement

1. The three bones in the middle ear are the _____, _____, and _____.

2. The study of the ear is called _____.

3. Another term for the eardrum is _____.

4. _____ is produced in the oil glands in the auditory canal.

5. The _____ tube connects the nasopharynx with the middle ear.

6. The _____ is responsible for conducting impulses from the ear to the brain.

7. The ear is responsible for the senses of _____ and _____.

8. _____ hearing loss refers to disease or malformation of the outer or middle ear.

Terminology

Word Parts Used to Build Ear Terms

The following lists contain the combining forms, suffixes, and prefixes used to build terms in the remaining sections of this chapter.

Combining Forms

acous/o	hearing	cochle/o	cochlea	presby/o	old age
audi/o	hearing	labyrinth/o	labyrinth	py/o	pus
audit/o	hearing	laryng/o	larynx	rhin/o	nose
aur/o	ear	myc/o	fungus	salping/o	auditory tube
auricul/o	ear	myring/o	tympanic membrane	staped/o	stapes
bi/o	life	neur/o	nerve	tympan/o	tympanic membrane
cerumin/o	cerumen	ot/o	ear	vestibul/o	vestibule

Suffixes

-al	pertaining to	-logy	study of	-rrhagia	abnormal flow
-algia	pain	-meter	instrument to measure	-rrhea	discharge
-ar	pertaining to	-metry	process of measuring	-rrhexis	rupture
-cusis	hearing	-oma	mass; tumor	-sclerosis	hardening
-ectomy	surgical removal	-ory	pertaining to	-scope	instrument to visually examine
-emetic	pertaining to vomiting	-osis	abnormal condition	-scopy	process of visually examining
-gram	record	-otia	ear condition		
-ic	pertaining to	-otomy	cutting into	-tic	pertaining to
-itis	inflammation	-plasty	surgical repair		

Prefixes

an-	without	bi-	two	micro-	small
anti-	against	macro-	large	mono-	one

Adjective Forms of Anatomical Terms

Term	Word Parts	Definition
acoustic (ah-KOOS-tik)	acous/o = hearing -tic = pertaining to	Pertaining to hearing
auditory (AW-dih-tor-ee)	audit/o = hearing -ory = pertaining to	Pertaining to hearing
aural (AW-ral)	aur/o = ear -al = pertaining to	Pertaining to the ear

> **Word Watch**
> Be careful when using two terms that sound very similar—*aural* meaning *pertaining to the ear* and *oral* meaning *pertaining to the mouth.*

Term	Word Parts	Definition
auricular (aw-RIK-yoo-lar)	auricul/o = ear -ar = pertaining to	Pertaining to the ear
binaural (bye-NOR-al)	bi- = two aur/o = ear -al = pertaining to	Pertaining to both ears
cochlear (KOH-klee-ar)	cochle/o = cochlea -ar = pertaining to	Pertaining to cochlea
monaural (mon-AW-ral)	mono- = one aur/o = ear -al = pertaining to	Pertaining to one ear
otic (OH-tik)	ot/o = ear -ic = pertaining to	Pertaining to the ear
tympanic (tim-PAN-ik)	tympan/o = tympanic membrane -ic = pertaining to	Pertaining to tympanic membrane
vestibular (ves-TIB-yoo-lar)	vestibul/o = vestibule -ar = pertaining to	Pertaining to vestibule

PRACTICE AS YOU GO

G. Give the adjective form for each term.

1. The cochlea _____

2. The ear _____, _____, or _____

3. The vestibule _____

4. Hearing _____ or _____

5. One ear _____

Pathology

Term	Word Parts	Definition
Medical Specialties		
audiology (aw-dee-ALL-oh-jee)	audi/o = hearing -logy = study of	Medical specialty involved with measuring hearing function and identifying hearing loss; specialist is an *audiologist*
otorhinolaryngology (ENT) (oh-toh-rye-noh-lair-in-GALL-oh-jee)	ot/o = ear rhin/o = nose laryng/o = larynx -logy = study of	Branch of medicine involving the diagnosis and treatment of conditions and diseases of the ear, nose, and throat; also referred to as *ENT*; physician is an *otorhinolaryngologist*
Signs and Symptoms		
macrotia (mah-KROH-shee-ah)	macro- = large -otia = ear condition	Condition of having abnormally large ears
microtia (my-KROH-shee-ah)	micro- = small -otia = ear condition	Condition of having abnormally small ears
otalgia (oh-TAL-jee-ah)	ot/o = ear -algia = pain	Ear pain
otopyorrhea (oh-toh-pye-oh-REE-ah)	ot/o = ear py/o = pus -rrhea = discharge	Discharge of pus from the ear
otorrhagia (oh-toh-RAY-jee-ah)	ot/o = ear -rrhagia = abnormal flow	Bleeding from the ear
presbycusis (prez-bih-KYOO-sis)	presby/o = old age -cusis = hearing condition	Normal loss of hearing that can accompany aging process
residual hearing (rih-ZID-joo-al)	-al = pertaining to	Amount of hearing still present after damage has occurred to auditory mechanism
tinnitus (tin-EYE-tus)		Ringing in the ears
tympanorrhexis (tim-pan-oh-REK-sis)	tympan/o = tympanic membrane -rrhexis = rupture	Rupture of the tympanic membrane
vertigo (VER-tih-goh)		Dizziness caused by sensation that room is spinning
Hearing Loss		
anacusis (an-ah-KYOO-sis)	an- = without -cusis = hearing	Total absence of hearing; inability to perceive sound; also called *deafness*
deafness		Inability to hear or having some degree of hearing impairment
External Ear		
ceruminosis (seh-roo-mih-NOH-sis)	cerumin/o = cerumen -osis = abnormal condition	Excessive accumulation of earwax resulting in hard wax plug; sound becomes muffled
otitis externa (OE) (oh-TYE-tis / eks-TER-nah)	ot/o = ear -itis = inflammation	External ear infection; may be caused by bacteria or fungus; also called *otomycosis* and commonly referred to as *swimmer's ear*

Pathology (continued)

Term	Word Parts	Definition
otomycosis (oh-toh-my-KOH-sis)	ot/o = ear myc/o = fungus -osis = abnormal condition	Fungal infection of the ear; one type of otitis externa
Middle Ear		
myringitis (mir-in-JYE-tis)	myring/o = tympanic membrane -itis = inflammation	Inflammation of the tympanic membrane
otitis media (OM) (oh-TYE-tis / MEE-dee-ah)	ot/o = ear -itis = inflammation	Seen frequently in children; commonly referred to as *middle ear infection*; often preceded by upper respiratory infection during which pathogens move from the pharynx to the middle ear via the eustachian tube; fluid accumulates in the middle ear cavity; fluid may be watery, *serous otitis media*, or full of pus, *purulent otitis media*
otosclerosis (oh-toh-sklair-OH-sis)	ot/o = ear -sclerosis = hardening	Loss of mobility of the stapes bone, leading to progressive hearing loss
salpingitis (sal-pin-JIGH-tis)	salping/o = auditory tube -itis = inflammation	Inflammation of the auditory tube

> **Word Watch**
> Be careful using the combining form **salping/o**, which can mean either *eustachian tube* or *fallopian tube*.

Term	Word Parts	Definition
tympanitis (tim-pan-EYE-tis)	tympan/o = tympanic membrane -itis = inflammation	Inflammation of the tympanic membrane
Inner Ear		
acoustic neuroma (ah-KOOS-tik / noo-ROH-mah)	acous/o = hearing -tic = pertaining to neur/o = nerve -oma = tumor	Benign tumor of eighth cranial nerve sheath; pressure causes symptoms such as tinnitus, headache, dizziness, and progressive hearing loss
labyrinthitis (lab-ih-rin-THIGH-tis)	labyrinth/o = labyrinth -itis = inflammation	May affect both hearing and equilibrium portions of inner ear; also referred to as *inner ear infection*
Ménière's disease (may-nee-AIRZ)		Abnormal condition within the labyrinth of inner ear that can lead to progressive loss of hearing; symptoms are vertigo, hearing loss, and tinnitus (ringing in the ears); named for French physician Prosper Ménière

PRACTICE AS YOU GO

H. Terminology Matching

Match each term to its definition.

1. _____ anacusis   **a.** small ears
2. _____ otitis externa   **b.** dizziness
3. _____ microtia   **c.** ringing in the ears

4. _____ otopyorrhea   **d.** a fungal infection

5. _____ labyrinthitis   **e.** absence of hearing

6. _____ tinnitus   **f.** ruptured eardrum

7. _____ otosclerosis   **g.** pus discharge from the ear

8. _____ vertigo   **h.** swimmer's ear

9. _____ otomycosis   **i.** loss of mobility of stapes

10. _____ tympanorrhexis   **j.** inner ear infection

Diagnostic Procedures

Term	Word Parts	Definition
Audiology Tests		
audiogram (AW-dee-oh-gram)	audi/o = hearing -gram = record	Graphic record that illustrates results of audiometry
audiometer (aw-dee-OM-eh-ter)	audi/o = hearing -meter = instrument to measure	Instrument to measure hearing
audiometry (aw-dee-OM-eh-tree)	audi/o = hearing -metry = process of measuring	Test of hearing ability by determining lowest and highest intensity (decibels) and frequencies (hertz) that person can distinguish; patient may sit in soundproof booth and receive sounds through earphones as technician decreases sound or lowers tones

■ **Figure 13-17** Audiometry exam being administered to a young child who is wearing the earphones through which sounds are given. *(Capifrutta/Shutterstock)*

decibel (dB) (DES-ih-bel)		Measures intensity or loudness of a sound; zero decibels is quietest sound measured and 120 dB is loudest sound commonly measured
hertz (Hz)		Measurement of frequency or pitch of sound; lowest pitch on audiogram is 250 Hz; measurement can go as high as 8000 Hz, which is highest pitch measured

Diagnostic Procedures (continued)

Term	Word Parts	Definition
Rinne and Weber tuning-fork tests (RIN-eh / VAY-ber)		Tests that assess both nerve and bone conduction of sound; physician holds a tuning fork, an instrument that produces a constant pitch when struck, against or near bones on side of the head
Otology Tests		
otoscope (OH-toh-skohp)	ot/o = ear -scope = instrument to visually examine	Instrument to view inside the ear canal
otoscopy (oh-TOSS-koh-pee)	ot/o = ear -scopy = process of visually examining	Examination of ear canal, eardrum, and outer ear using *otoscope*

Med Term Tip

Small children are prone to placing objects in their ears. In some cases, as with peas and beans, these become moist in the ear canal and swell, which makes removal difficult. *Otoscopy*, or the examination of the ear using an *otoscope*, can aid in identifying and removing the cause of hearing loss if it is due to foreign bodies.

■ **Figure 13-18** An otoscope, used to visually examine the external auditory ear canal and tympanic membrane. *(Patrick Watson/Pearson Education, Inc.)*

Term	Word Parts	Definition
tympanogram (TIM-pah-noh-gram)	tympan/o = tympanic membrane -gram = record	Graphic record that illustrates results of tympanometry
tympanometer (tim-pah-NOM-eh-ter)	tympan/o = tympanic membrane -meter = instrument to measure	Instrument used to measure the movement of the tympanic membrane
tympanometry (tim-pah-NOM-eh-tree)	tympan/o = tympanic membrane -metry = process of measuring	Measurement of the movement of the tympanic membrane; can indicate the presence of pressure in the middle ear
Balance Test		
falling test		Test used to observe balance and equilibrium; patient is observed balancing on one foot, then with one foot in front of the other, and then walking forward with eyes open; same test is conducted with patient's eyes closed; swaying and falling with the eyes closed can indicate ear and equilibrium malfunction

Therapeutic Procedures

Term	Word Parts	Definition

Audiology Procedures

American Sign Language (ASL)		Nonverbal method of communicating in which the hands and fingers are used to indicate words and concepts; used by both persons who are deaf and persons with speech impairments

■ **Figure 13-19**   Two women having a conversation using American Sign Language. *(Vladimir Mucibabic/Shutterstock)*

hearing aid		Apparatus or mechanical device used by persons with impaired hearing to amplify sound; also called *amplification device*

Surgical Procedures

cochlear implant (KOH-klee-ar)	cochle/o = cochlea -ar = pertaining to	Mechanical device surgically placed under the skin behind outer ear (pinna) that converts sound signals into magnetic impulses to stimulate the auditory nerve; can be beneficial for those with profound sensorineural hearing loss

■ **Figure 13-20**   Photograph of a child with a cochlear implant. This device sends electrical impulses directly to the brain. *(George Dodson/Pearson Education, Inc.)*

Term	Word Parts	Definition
labyrinthectomy (lab-ih-rin-THEK-toh-mee)	labyrinth/o = labyrinth -ectomy = surgical removal	Surgical removal of the labyrinth
labyrinthotomy (lab-ih-rin-THOT-oh-mee)	labyrinth/o = labyrinth -otomy = cutting into	To cut into the labyrinth
myringectomy (mir-in-JEK-toh-mee)	myring/o = tympanic membrane -ectomy = surgical removal	Surgical removal of the tympanic membrane
myringoplasty (mir-IN-goh-plas-tee)	myring/o = tympanic membrane -plasty = surgical repair	Surgical repair of the tympanic membrane

Therapeutic Procedures (continued)

Term	Word Parts	Definition
myringotomy (mir-in-GOT-oh-mee)	myring/o = tympanic membrane -otomy = cutting into	Surgical puncture of the eardrum with removal of fluid and pus from middle ear to eliminate persistent ear infection and excessive pressure on the tympanic membrane; pressure equalizing tube is placed in the tympanic membrane to allow for drainage of middle ear cavity; tube typically falls out on its own
otoplasty (OH-toh-plas-tee)	ot/o = ear -plasty = surgical repair	Surgical repair of the external ear
pressure equalizing tube (PE tube)		Small tube surgically placed in child's eardrum to assist in drainage of trapped fluid and to equalize pressure between middle ear cavity and atmosphere
salpingotomy (sal-pin-GOT-oh-mee)	salping/o = auditory tube -otomy = cutting into	To cut into the auditory tube
stapedectomy (stay-peh-DEK-toh-mee)	staped/o = stapes -ectomy = pertaining to	Removal of the stapes bone to treat otosclerosis (hardening of the bone); a prosthesis or artificial stapes may be implanted
tympanectomy (tim-pah-NEK-toh-mee)	tympan/o = tympanic membrane -ectomy = surgical removal	Surgical removal of the tympanic membrane
tympanoplasty (TIM-pah-noh-plas-tee)	tympan/o = tympanic membrane -plasty = surgical repair	Surgical repair of the tympanic membrane
tympanotomy (tim-pah-NOT-oh-mee)	tympan/o = tympanic membrane -otomy = cutting into	To cut into the tympanic membrane

PRACTICE AS YOU GO

I. Procedure Matching

Match each procedure term to its definition.

1. _____ myringotomy   **a.** removal of stapes bone

2. _____ tympanoplasty   **b.** reconstruction of eardrum

3. _____ otoplasty   **c.** surgical puncture of eardrum

4. _____ stapedectomy   **d.** repairs external ear

5. _____ Rinne and Weber   **e.** drains off fluid

6. _____ falling test   **f.** treats sensorineural hearing loss

7. _____ PE tube   **g.** tuning-fork tests

8. _____ cochlear implant   **h.** balance test

Pharmacology

Classification	Word Parts	Action	Examples
antibiotic otic solution (OH-tik)	anti- = against bi/o = life -tic = pertaining to ot/o = ear -ic = pertaining to	Eardrops to treat otitis externa	Neomycin, polymyxin B and hydrocortisone solution, Otocort, Cortisporin, Otic Care
antiemetic (an-tye-ee-MEH-tik)	anti- = against -emetic = pertaining to vomiting	Effective in treating nausea associated with vertigo	meclizine, Antivert, Meni-D; prochlorperazine, Compazine
wax emulsifiers		Substances used to soften earwax to prevent buildup within the external ear canal	carbamide peroxide, Debrox Drops, Murine Ear Wax Removal Drops

Abbreviations

ASL	American Sign Language	OE	otitis externa
BC	bone conduction	OM	otitis media
dB	decibel	Oto	otology
EENT	eyes, ears, nose, and throat	PE tube	pressure equalizing tube
ENT	ears, nose, and throat	PORP	partial ossicular replacement prosthesis
HEENT	head, eyes, ears, nose, and throat	SOM	serous otitis media
Hz	hertz	TORP	total ossicular replacement prosthesis

PRACTICE AS YOU GO

J. What's the Abbreviation?

1. otitis externa _____
2. eyes, ears, nose, and throat _____
3. bone conduction _____
4. pressure equalizing tube _____
5. otitis media _____

Chapter Review

Real-World Applications

Medical Record Analysis

This Ophthalmology Consultation Report contains 11 medical terms. Underline each term and write it in the list below the report. Then explain each term as you would to a nonmedical person.

Ophthalmology Consultation Report

Reason for Consultation:	Evaluation of progressive loss of vision in right eye
History of Present Illness:	Patient is a 79-year-old female who has noted gradual deterioration of vision and increasing photophobia during the past year, particularly in the right eye. She states that it feels like there is a film over her right eye. She denies any change in vision in her left eye. Patient has used corrective lenses her entire adult life for hyperopia.
Results of Physical Examination:	Visual acuity test showed no change in this patient's long-standing hyperopia. The pupils react properly to light. Intraocular pressure is normal. Ophthalmoscopy after application of mydriatic drops revealed presence of large opaque cataract in lens of right eye. There is a very small cataract forming in the left eye. There is no evidence of retinopathy, macular degeneration, or keratitis.
Assessment:	Diminished vision in right eye secondary to cataract
Recommendations:	Phacoemulsification of cataract followed by prosthetic lens implant.

Term	Explanation
1. _____	_____
2. _____	_____
3. _____	_____
4. _____	_____
5. _____	_____
6. _____	_____
7. _____	_____
8. _____	_____
9. _____	_____
10. _____	_____
11. _____	_____

Chart Note Transcription

The chart note below contains 10 phrases that can be reworded with a medical term presented in this chapter. Each phrase is identified with an underline. Determine the medical term and write your answers in the space provided.

Pearson General Hospital Consultation Report

Task   Edit   View   Time Scale   Options   Help   Download   Archive   Date: 17 May 2017

Current Complaint: An eight-year-old female was referred to the <u>specialist in the treatment of diseases of the ears, nose, and throat</u> **1** by her pediatrician for evaluation of chronic left <u>middle ear infection</u>. **2**

Past History: Patient's mother reports that her daughter began to experience recurrent ear infections at approximately six months of age. Frequency of the infections has increased during the past two years, and she is missing school. Mother also reports the child's teacher feels she is having difficulty hearing in the classroom.

Signs and Symptoms: <u>Both ears</u> **3** <u>visual examination of the external ear canal and eardrum</u> **4** revealed that the <u>membrane between the external ear canal and middle ear</u> **5** is normal on the right and bulging on the left. An excessive amount of <u>earwax</u> **6** was noted in both ears. <u>Measurement of the movement of the eardrum</u> **7** indicates that there is a buildup of fluid in the left middle ear. <u>Tests of hearing ability</u> **8** report normal hearing on the right and <u>loss of hearing as a result of the blocking of sound transmission in the middle ear</u> **9** on the left. Patient also noted to have acute pharyngitis with purulent drainage at time of evaluation.

Diagnosis: Hearing loss secondary to chronic left middle ear infection

Treatment: Left <u>eardrum incision</u> **10** with placement of pressure equalizing tube for drainage.

1. _____

2. _____

3. _____

4. _____

5. _____

6. _____

7. _____

8. _____

9. _____

10. _____

Case Study

Below is a case study presentation of a patient with a condition discussed in this chapter. Read the case study and answer the questions below. Some questions will ask for information not included within this chapter. Use your text, a medical dictionary, or any other reference material you choose to answer these questions.

This 35-year-old male musician was seen in the EENT clinic complaining of a progressive hearing loss over the past 15 years. He is now unable to hear what is being said if there is any environmental noise present. He states that he has played with a group of musicians using amplified instruments and no earplugs for the past 20 years. External ear structures appear normal bilaterally with otoscopy. Tympanometry is normal bilaterally. Audiometry reveals diminished hearing bilaterally. Rinne and Weber tuning-fork tests indicate that the patient has a moderate amount of conductive hearing loss but rule out sensorineural hearing loss. Diagnosis is moderate bilateral conductive hearing loss as a result of prolonged exposure to loud noise. Patient is referred for evaluation for a hearing aid.

(MY - Music/Alamy Stock Photo)

Questions

1. Which type of hearing loss does this patient appear to have? Look this condition up in a reference source and include a short description of it.

   _____

   _____

2. Explain how the other type of hearing loss (the type ruled out by the Rinne and Weber tuning-fork tests) is different from what this patient has.

   _____

   _____

3. What diagnostic tests did the physician perform? Describe them in your own words.

   _____

   _____

4. Explain the difference between a hearing aid and a cochlear implant.

   _____

   _____

5. How do you think this patient could have avoided this hearing loss?

   _____

   _____

Practice Exercises

A. Pharmacology Challenge

Fill in the classification for each drug description, then match the brand name.

	Drug Description	Classification	Brand Name
1.	_____ treats dry eyes	_____	a. Atropine-Care
2.	_____ reduces intraocular pressure	_____	b. Visine
3.	_____ eardrops for ear infection	_____	c. Timoptic
4.	_____ dilates pupil	_____	d. Opticaine
5.	_____ treats nausea from vertigo	_____	e. Debrox Drops
6.	_____ eyedrops for bacterial infection	_____	f. Eserine Sulfate
7.	_____ reduces eye redness	_____	g. Antivert
8.	_____ constricts pupil	_____	h. Refresh Plus
9.	_____ softens cerumen	_____	i. Otocort
10.	_____ eyedrops for pain	_____	j. Del-Mycin

B. Word Building Practice

The combining form **blephar/o** refers to the *eyelid*. Use it to write a term that means:

1. inflammation of the eyelid _____

2. surgical repair of the eyelid _____

3. drooping of the upper eyelid _____

The combining form **retin/o** refers to the *retina*. Use it to write a term that means:

4. a disease of the retina _____

5. surgical fixation of the retina _____

The combining form **ophthalm/o** refers to the *eye*. Use it to write a term that means:

6. the study of the eye _____

7. pertaining to the eye _____

8. an eye examination using a scope _____

The combining form **irid/o** refers to the *iris*. Use it to write a term that means:

9. iris paralysis _____

10. removal of the iris _____

The combining form **ot/o** refers to the *ear*. Write a word that means:

11. ear surgical repair _____

12. pus flow from the ear _____

13. pain in the ear _____

14. inflammation of the ear _____

The combining form **tympan/o** refers to the *eardrum*. Write a word that means:

15. eardrum rupture   _____

16. eardrum incision   _____

17. eardrum inflammation   _____

The combining form **audi/o** refers to *hearing*. Write a word that means:

18. record of hearing   _____

19. instrument to measure hearing _____

20. study of hearing   _____

C. Complete the Term

For each definition given below, fill in the blank with the word part that completes the term.

Definition	Term
1. instrument to visually examine the ear	_____scope
2. surgical fixation of the retina	_____pexy
3. without hearing	ana_____
4. drooping eyelid	_____ptosis
5. specialist in measuring vision	_____metrist
6. instrument to measure eardrum	_____meter
7. cutting into the cornea	_____otomy
8. old-age vision condition	presby_____
9. surgical removal of the iris	_____ectomy
10. process of measuring hearing	_____metry
11. eye pain	_____algia
12. hardening of the ear	_____sclerosis
13. inflammation of the conjunctiva	_____itis
14. large ear condition	macr_____
15. state of one color	mono_____ism

D. Using Abbreviations

Fill in each blank with the appropriate abbreviation.

1. _____ is a condition in which light rays focus unevenly on the retina because of an uneven cornea.

2. _____ is a branch of medicine that diagnoses and treats conditions of the ears, nose, and throat.

3. A _____ test measures the sharpness of vision.

4. _____ may be caused by bacteria or fungus in the external ear.

5. _____ is commonly called *cross-eyed* because the eye is turned inward.

6. _____ tubes equalize pressure between the middle ear and the external atmosphere.

7. _____ surgery uses a laser to correct myopia.

8. _____ is commonly called *nearsightedness*.

9. _____, a common infection in children, causes fluid to accumulate in the middle ear cavity.

10. Cataracts are commonly corrected by replacing the lens with a(n) _____ implant.

E. Fill in the Blank

emmetropia	tonometry	Ménière's disease
hyperopia	cataract	hordeolum
acoustic neuroma	strabismus	myopia
otorhinolaryngologist	presbycusis	
conjunctivitis	inner ear	

1. Cheri is having a regular eye checkup. The pressure-reading test that the physician will do to detect glaucoma is

   _____.

2. Carlos's ophthalmologist tells him that he has normal vision. This is called _____.

3. Ana has been given an antibiotic eye ointment for pinkeye. The medical term for this condition is _____.

4. Adrian is nearsighted and cannot read signs in the distance. This is called _____.

5. Ivan is scheduled to have surgery to have the opaque lens of his right eye removed. This condition is a(n)

   _____.

6. Roberto has developed a stye on the corner of his left eye. He has been told to treat it with hot compresses. This condition is called a(n) _____.

7. Judith has twin boys with crossed eyes that will require surgical correction. The medical term for this condition is

   _____.

8. Beth is farsighted and has difficulty reading textbooks. Her eyeglass correction will be for _____.

9. Grace was told by her physician that her hearing loss was a part of the aging process. The term for this is

   _____.

10. Stacey is having frequent middle ear infections and wishes to be treated by a specialist. She would go to a(n)

    _____.

11. Warren was told that his dizziness may be caused by a problem in the _____ area.

12. Shantel is suffering from an abnormal condition of the inner ear, vertigo, and tinnitus. She may have _____.

13. Keisha was told that her tumor of the eighth cranial nerve was benign, but she still experienced a hearing loss as a result of the tumor. This tumor is called a(n) _____.

F. Define the Term

1. amblyopia   _____

2. diplopia   _____

3. mydriatic   _____

4. miotic   _____

5. presbyopia   _____

6. tinnitus   _____

7. stapes _____

8. tympanometry _____

9. eustachian tube _____

10. labyrinth _____

11. audiogram _____

12. otitis media _____

G. Anatomical Adjectives

Fill in the blank with the missing noun or adjective.

Noun	Adjective
1. conjunctiva	_____
2. _____	auditory
3. cornea	_____
4. _____	auricular
5. within the eye	_____
6. _____	otic
7. tears	_____
8. _____	iridal
9. one ear	_____
10. sclera	_____
11. _____	ocular
12. retina	_____
13. eardrum	_____
14. _____	ophthalmic
15. cochlea	_____

H. Spelling Practice

Some of the following terms are misspelled. Identify the incorrect terms and spell them correctly in the blank provided.

1. opthalmology _____

2. otosclerosis _____

3. dacryoadenitis _____

4. emetropia _____

5. labyrinthtitis _____

6. presbyopia _____

7. stapedectomy _____

8. monochromism _____

9. otopyorhea _____

10. astigmatism _____

I. Complete the Statement

1. <u>In order</u>, the structures light rays pass through to strike the retina are: _____, _____, _____, _____, and _____.

2. Tears ultimately drain into the _____.

3. _____ eye muscles pull the eyeball left, right, up, or down in a straight line. _____ eye muscles move the eyeball diagonally.

4. The _____ is a mucous membrane that covers and protects the front of the eyeball.

5. Eyelashes are called _____.

6. The ciliary body is part of the _____ layer of the eyeball.

7. The three ossicles are _____, _____, and _____.

8. With _____ hearing loss, the problem is with the outer or middle ear and sound is muffled. In _____ hearing loss, the problem is with the inner ear or cochlear nerve and impulses are not successfully sent to the brain.

9. The blind spot in each eyeball is caused by the _____.

10. The _____ nerve carries hearing information and the _____ nerve carries equilibrium information.

MyLab Medical Terminology™

MyLab Medical Terminology is a premium online homework management system that includes a host of features to help you study. Registered users will find:

- A multitude of activities and assignments built within the MyLab platform
- Powerful tools that track and analyze your results—allowing you to create a personalized learning experience
- Videos and audio pronunciations to help enrich your progress
- Streaming lesson presentations (Guided Lectures) and self-paced learning modules
- A space where you and your instructors can check your progress and manage your assignments

Labeling Exercises

Image A

Write the labels for this figure on the numbered lines provided.

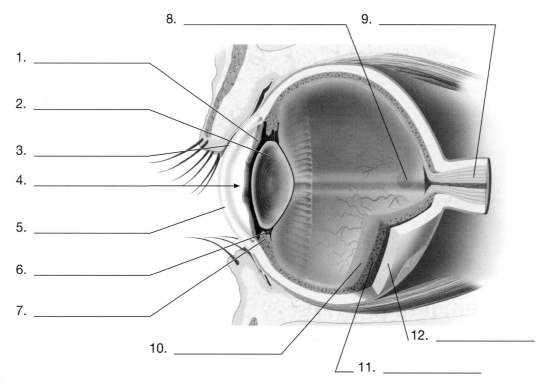

8. _____

9. _____

1. _____

2. _____

3. _____

4. _____

5. _____

6. _____

7. _____

10. _____

11. _____

12. _____

Image B

Write the labels for this figure on the numbered lines provided.

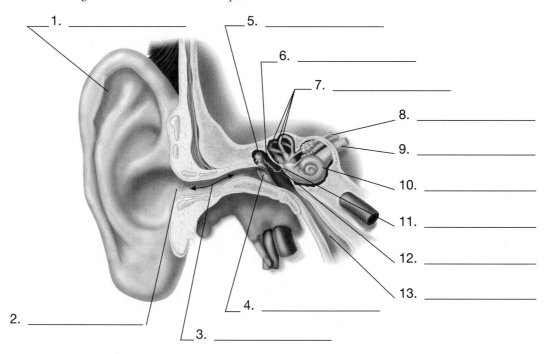

1. _____

5. _____

6. _____

7. _____

8. _____

9. _____

10. _____

11. _____

12. _____

13. _____

2. _____

3. _____

4. _____

Appendices

Appendix I
Word Parts Arranged Alphabetically and Defined

The word parts that have been presented in this textbook are summarized here with their definitions for quick reference. Prefixes are listed first, followed by combining forms and suffixes.

Prefix	Definition	Prefix	Definition
a-	without	macro-	large
ab-	away from	micro-	small
ad-	toward	mono-	one
allo-	other, different from usual	multi-	many
an-	without	myo-	to shut
ante-	before, in front of	neo-	new
anti-	against	non-	not
auto-	self	nulli-	none
bi-	two	pan-	all
brady-	slow	para-	beside; abnormal; two like
circum-	around		parts of a pair
contra-	against	per-	through
de-	without	peri-	around
di-	two	poly-	many
dis-	apart	post-	after
dys-	painful; difficult; abnormal	pre-	before
e-	outward	primi-	first
endo-	within; inner	pro-	before
epi-	above	pseudo-	false
eso-	inward	quadri-	four
eu-	normal	re-	again
ex-	outward	retro-	backward; behind
exo-	outward	semi-	partial
extra-	outside of	sub-	under
hemi-	half	tachy-	fast
hetero-	different	tetra-	four
homo-	same	trans-	across
hyper-	excessive	tri-	three
hypo-	below; insufficient	ultra-	beyond
in-	not; inward	un-	not
inter-	between	xeno-	foreign
intra-	within		

Combining Form	Definition	Combining Form	Definition
abdomin/o	abdomen	adip/o	fat
acous/o	hearing	adren/o	adrenal glands
acr/o	extremities	adrenal/o	adrenal glands
aden/o	gland	aer/o	air
adenoid/o	adenoids	agglutin/o	clumping

515

Combining Form	Definition	Combining Form	Definition
albin/o	white	cerebr/o	cerebrum
alges/o	sense of pain	cerumin/o	cerumen
alveol/o	alveolus	cervic/o	neck, cervix
ambly/o	dull, dim	chem/o	chemical, drug
amnes/o	forgetfulness	chol/e	bile, gall
amni/o	amnion	cholangi/o	bile duct
an/o	anus	cholecyst/o	gallbladder
andr/o	male	choledoch/o	common bile duct
angi/o	vessel	chondr/o	cartilage
ankyl/o	stiff joint	chori/o	chorion
anter/o	front	chrom/o	color
anthrac/o	coal	chromat/o	color
anxi/o	fear, worry	cirrh/o	yellow
aort/o	aorta	cis/o	to cut
append/o	appendix	clavicul/o	clavicle
appendic/o	appendix	cleid/o	clavicle
aque/o	water	clon/o	rapid contracting and relaxing
arteri/o	artery	coagul/o	clotting
arteriol/o	arteriole	coccyg/o	coccyx
arthr/o	joint	cochle/o	cochlea
articul/o	joint	col/o	colon
astr/o	star	colon/o	colon
atel/o	incomplete	colp/o	vagina
ather/o	fatty substance	compuls/o	drive, compel
atri/o	atrium	concuss/o	to shake violently
audi/o	hearing	coni/o	dust
audit/o	hearing	conjunctiv/o	conjunctiva
aur/o	ear	corne/o	cornea
auricul/o	ear	coron/o	heart
axill/o	axilla	corpor/o	body
azot/o	nitrogenous waste	cortic/o	outer layer
bacteri/o	bacteria	cost/o	rib
balan/o	glans penis	crani/o	skull
bar/o	weight	crin/o	to secrete
bas/o	base	crur/o	leg
bi/o	life	cry/o	cold
blast/o	immature	crypt/o	hidden
blephar/o	eyelid	culd/o	cul-de-sac
brachi/o	arm	cutane/o	skin
bronch/o	bronchus	cyan/o	blue
bronchi/o	bronchus	cycl/o	ciliary body
bronchiol/o	bronchiole	cyst/o	sac, urinary bladder
bucc/o	cheek	cyt/o	cell
burs/o	sac	dacry/o	tears
calc/o	calcium	delus/o	false belief
carcin/o	cancer	dent/o	tooth
cardi/o	heart	depress/o	to press down
carp/o	carpus	derm/o	skin
caud/o	tail	dermat/o	skin
cauter/o	to burn	diaphor/o	profuse sweating
cec/o	cecum	diaphragmat/o	diaphragm
centr/o	center	dilat/o	to widen
cephal/o	head	dipl/o	double
cerebell/o	cerebellum	dist/o	away from

Combining Form	Definition	Combining Form	Definition
diverticul/o	pouch	hymen/o	hymen
dors/o	back	hyster/o	uterus
duct/o	to bring	iatr/o	physician, medicine, treatment
duoden/o	duodenum		
dur/o	dura mater	ichthy/o	scaly, dry
electr/o	electricity	idi/o	distinctive
embol/o	plug	ile/o	ileum
embry/o	embryo	ili/o	ilium
emmetr/o	correct, proper	immun/o	protection
encephal/o	brain	infer/o	below
enter/o	small intestine	inguin/o	groin
eosin/o	rosy red	iod/o	iodine
epididym/o	epididymis	ir/o	iris
epiglott/o	epiglottis	irid/o	iris
episi/o	vulva	isch/o	to hold back
epitheli/o	epithelium	ischi/o	ischium
erythr/o	red	jejun/o	jejunum
esophag/o	esophagus	kal/i	potassium
esthesi/o	sensation, feeling	kerat/o	hard, horny, cornea
estr/o	female	ket/o	ketones
extens/o	to stretch out	keton/o	ketones
fasci/o	fibrous band	kinesi/o	movement
femor/o	femur	klept/o	to steal
fet/o	fetus	kyph/o	hump
fibr/o	fibers	labi/o	lip
fibrin/o	fibers	labyrinth/o	labyrinth (inner ear)
fibul/o	fibula	lacrim/o	tears
flex/o	to bend	lact/o	milk
fus/o	pouring	lamin/o	lamina (part of vertebra)
gastr/o	stomach	lapar/o	abdomen
genit/o	genital	laryng/o	larynx
gingiv/o	gums	later/o	side
glauc/o	gray	leuk/o	white
gli/o	glue	lingu/o	tongue
glomerul/o	glomerulus	lip/o	fat
gloss/o	tongue	lith/o	stone
gluc/o	glucose	lob/o	lobe
glute/o	buttock	lord/o	bent backward
glyc/o	sugar	lumb/o	loin (low back)
glycos/o	sugar, glucose	lymph/o	lymph
gonad/o	sex glands	lymphaden/o	lymph node
granul/o	granules	lymphangi/o	lymph vessel
gynec/o	female	macul/o	macula lutea
habilitat/o	ability	mamm/o	breast
hal/o	to breathe	mandibul/o	mandible
hallucin/o	imagined perception	mast/o	breast
hem/o	blood	maxill/o	maxilla
hemat/o	blood	meat/o	meatus
hepat/o	liver	medi/o	middle
hidr/o	sweat	medull/o	inner region, medulla oblongata
hist/o	tissue		
home/o	sameness	melan/o	black
humer/o	humerus	men/o	menses, menstruation
hydr/o	water	mening/o	meninges

Combining Form	Definition	Combining Form	Definition
meningi/o	meninges	pareun/o	sexual intercourse
ment/o	mind	pariet/o	cavity wall
metacarp/o	metacarpus	patell/o	patella
metatars/o	metatarsus	path/o	disease
metr/o	uterus	pector/o	chest
mi/o	lessening	ped/o	child; foot
mineral/o	minerals, electrolytes	pedicul/o	lice
morph/o	shape	pelv/o	pelvis
muc/o	mucus	pen/o	penis
muscul/o	muscle	perine/o	perineum
my/o	muscle	peripher/o	away from center
myc/o	fungus	peritone/o	peritoneum
mydr/i	widening	phac/o	lens
myel/o	bone marrow, spinal cord	phag/o	eat, swallow
myocardi/o	heart muscle	phalang/o	phalanges
myos/o	muscle	pharmac/o	drug
myring/o	tympanic membrane	pharyng/o	pharynx
narc/o	stupor, sleep	phleb/o	vein
nas/o	nose	phob/o	irrational fear
nat/o	birth	phon/o	sound
natr/o	sodium	phot/o	light
necr/o	death	phren/o	mind
nephr/o	kidney	physic/o	body
neur/o	nerve	pineal/o	pineal gland
neutr/o	neutral	pituit/o	pituitary gland
noct/i	night	pituitar/o	pituitary gland
nucle/o	nucleus	plant/o	sole of foot
nyctal/o	night	pleur/o	pleura
o/o	egg	pneum/o	lung, air
obsess/o	besieged by thoughts	pneumon/o	lung, air
ocul/o	eye	pod/o	foot
odont/o	tooth	poli/o	gray matter
olig/o	scanty	polyp/o	polyp
onych/o	nail	pont/o	pons
oophor/o	ovary	poster/o	back
ophthalm/o	eye	presby/o	old age
opt/o	eye, vision	proct/o	rectum and anus
optic/o	eye, vision	prostat/o	prostate gland
or/o	mouth	prosthet/o	addition
orch/o	testes	protein/o	protein
orchi/o	testes	proxim/o	near to
orchid/o	testes	psych/o	mind
orth/o	straight	pub/o	genital region, pubis
oste/o	bone	pulmon/o	lung
ot/o	ear	pupill/o	pupil
ov/i	ovum	py/o	pus
ov/o	ovum	pyel/o	renal pelvis
ovari/o	ovary	pylor/o	pylorus
ox/i	oxygen	pyr/o	fire
ox/o	oxygen	radi/o	radius; ray (X-ray)
palat/o	palate	radic/o	root
pancreat/o	pancreas	radicul/o	nerve root
papill/o	optic disk	rect/o	rectum
parathyroid/o	parathyroid gland	ren/o	kidney

Combining Form	Definition	Combining Form	Definition
retin/o	retina	therm/o	heat
rhin/o	nose	thorac/o	chest
rhytid/o	wrinkle	thromb/o	clot
rotat/o	to revolve	thym/o	thymus gland
sacr/o	sacrum	thyr/o	thyroid gland
salping/o	uterine (fallopian) tubes, auditory tube (eustachian tube)	thyroid/o	thyroid gland
		tibi/o	tibia
sanguin/o	blood	tom/o	to cut
sarc/o	flesh	ton/o	tone
scapul/o	scapula	tonsill/o	tonsils
schiz/o	split	topic/o	a specific area
scler/o	hard, sclera	tox/o	poison
scoli/o	crooked	toxic/o	poison
seb/o	oil	trache/o	trachea
sept/o	wall	trich/o	hair
septic/o	infection	tuss/o	cough
sialaden/o	salivary gland	tympan/o	tympanic membrane
sigmoid/o	sigmoid colon	uln/o	ulna
sinus/o	sinus	ungu/o	nail
soci/o	society	ur/o	urine
somat/o	body	ureter/o	ureter
somn/o	sleep	urethr/o	urethra
son/o	sound	urin/o	urine
spermat/o	sperm	uter/o	uterus
sphygm/o	pulse	uve/o	choroid
spin/o	spine	vagin/o	vagina
spir/o	breathing	valv/o	valve
splen/o	spleen	valvul/o	valve
spondyl/o	vertebrae	varic/o	dilated vein
staped/o	stapes	vas/o	vessel, vas deferens
stern/o	sternum	vascul/o	blood vessel
steth/o	chest	ven/o	vein
stigmat/o	point	ventr/o	belly
super/o	above	ventricul/o	ventricle
synov/o	synovial membrane	venul/o	venule
synovi/o	synovial membrane	vers/o	to turn
system/o	system	vertebr/o	vertebra
tars/o	tarsus	vesic/o	sac, bladder
ten/o	tendon	vesicul/o	seminal vesicle
tend/o	tendon	vestibul/o	vestibule
tendin/o	tendon	viscer/o	internal organ
testicul/o	testes	vitre/o	glassy
thalam/o	thalamus	vulv/o	vulva
thec/o	sheath (meninges)	xer/o	dry

Suffix	Definition	Suffix	Definition
-ac	pertaining to	-asthenia	weakness
-al	pertaining to	-atic	pertaining to
-algia	pain	-blast	immature
-an	pertaining to	-capnia	carbon dioxide
-apheresis	removal, carry away	-cardia	heart condition
-ar	pertaining to	-cele	protrusion
-arche	beginning	-centesis	puncture to withdraw fluid
-ary	pertaining to	-cide	to kill

Suffix	Definition	Suffix	Definition
-clasia	to surgically break	-lysis	to destroy (to break down)
-crit	separation of	-lytic	destruction
-cusis	hearing	-malacia	abnormal softening
-cyesis	state of pregnancy	-mania	frenzy
-cyte	cell	-manometer	instrument to measure pressure
-cytic	pertaining to cells	-megaly	enlarged
-cytosis	more than the normal number of cells	-meter	instrument for measuring
-derma	skin condition	-metrist	specialist in measuring
-desis	to fuse	-metry	process of measuring
-dipsia	thirst	-nic	pertaining to
-dynia	pain	-oid	resembling
-eal	pertaining to	-ole	small
-ectasis	dilation	-oma	tumor, mass
-ectomy	surgical removal	-opia	vision condition
-edema	swelling	-opsia	vision condition
-emesis	vomiting	-opsy	view of
-emetic	pertaining to vomiting	-orexia	appetite
-emia	blood condition	-ory	pertaining to
-emic	pertaining to a blood condition	-ose	pertaining to
-gen	that which produces	-osis	abnormal condition
-genesis	produces	-osmia	smell
-genic	producing	-ostomy	surgically create an opening
-globin	protein	-otia	ear condition
-globulin	protein	-otomy	cutting into
-gram	record	-ous	pertaining to
-graph	to record	-para	to bear (offspring)
-graphy	process of recording	-paresis	weakness
-gravida	pregnant woman	-partum	childbirth
-ia	condition	-pathy	disease
-iac	pertaining to	-penia	abnormal decrease, too few
-iasis	abnormal condition	-pepsia	digestion
-iatric	pertaining to medical treatment	-pexy	surgical fixation
-iatrist	physician	-phage	to eat
-iatry	medical treatment	-phagia	eat, swallow
-ic	pertaining to	-phasia	speech
-ical	pertaining to	-phil	attracted to
-ician	specialist	-philia	condition of being attracted to
-ile	pertaining to	-philic	pertaining to being attracted to
-ine	pertaining to	-phobia	fear
-ion	action	-phonia	voice
-ior	pertaining to	-phoresis	carrying
-ism	state of	-phoria	condition to bear
-ist	specialist	-phylaxis	protection
-istry	specialty of	-plasia	formation of cells
-itis	inflammation	-plasm	formation
-kinesia	movement	-plastic	pertaining to formation
-lepsy	seizure	-plastin	formation
-listhesis	slipping	-plasty	surgical repair
-lith	stone	-plegia	paralysis
-lithiasis	condition of stones	-pnea	breathing
-logic	pertaining to study of	-poiesis	formation
-logist	one who studies	-porosis	porous
-logy	study of	-prandial	pertaining to a meal

Suffix	Definition	Suffix	Definition
-pressor	to press down	-taxia	muscle coordination
-ptosis	drooping	-tension	pressure
-ptysis	spitting	-therapy	treatment
-rrhage	abnormal flow	-thorax	chest
-rrhagia	abnormal flow condition	-tic	pertaining to
-rrhagic	pertaining to abnormal flow	-tocia	labor, childbirth
-rrhaphy	to suture	-tome	instrument to cut
-rrhea	discharge	-tonia	tone
-rrhexis	rupture	-tonic	pertaining to tone
-salpinx	uterine tube	-toxic	pertaining to poison
-sclerosis	hardening	-tripsy	surgical crushing
-scope	instrument for viewing	-trophic	pertaining to development
-scopic	pertaining to visually examining	-trophy	development
-scopy	process of visually examining	-tropia	turned condition
-spasm	involuntary muscle contraction	-tropic	pertaining to stimulating
-spermia	condition of sperm	-tropin	to stimulate
-stasis	standing still	-ule	small
-stenosis	narrowing	-uria	condition of the urine

Appendix II
Word Parts Arranged Alphabetically by Definition

The definitions of the word parts that have been presented in this textbook are presented here and are arranged alphabetically. Prefixes are listed first, followed by combining forms and suffixes.

Definition	Prefix
abnormal	dys-, para-
above	epi-
across	trans-
after	post-
again	re-
against	anti-, contra-
all	pan-
apart	dis-
around	circum-, peri-
away from	ab-
backward	retro-
before	ante-, pre-, pro-
behind	retro-
below	hypo-
beside	para-
between	inter-
beyond	ultra-
different	hetero-
different from usual	allo-
difficult	dys-
excessive	hyper-
false	pseudo-
fast	tachy-
first	primi-
foreign	xeno-
four	quadri-, tetra-
half	hemi-
in front of	ante-
inner	endo-

Definition	Prefix
insufficient	hypo-
inward	eso-, in-
large	macro-
many	multi-, poly-
new	neo-
none	nulli-
normal	eu-
not	in-, non-, un-
one	mono-
other	allo-
outside of	extra-
outward	e-, ex-, exo-
painful	dys-
partial	semi-
same	homo-
self	auto-
slow	brady-
small	micro-
three	tri-
through	per-
to shut	myo-
toward	ad-
two	bi-, di-
two like parts of a pair	para-
under	sub-
within	endo-, intra-
without	a-, an-, de-

Definition	Combining Form
ability	habilitat/o
above	super/o
addition	prosthet/o
adenoids	adenoid/o
adrenal glands	adren/o, adrenal/o
air	aer/o, pneum/o
alveolus	alveol/o
amnion	amni/o
anus	an/o
aorta	aort/o
appendix	append/o, appendic/o
arm	brachi/o
arteriole	arteriol/o
artery	arteri/o
atrium	atri/o
auditory tube (eustachian tube)	salping/o

Definition	Combining Form
away from	dist/o
away from center	peripher/o
axilla	axill/o
back	dors/o, poster/o
bacteria	bacteri/o
base	bas/o
belly	ventr/o
below	infer/o
to bend	flex/o
bent backward	lord/o
besieged by thoughts	obsess/o
bile	chol/e
bile duct	cholangi/o
birth	nat/o
black	melan/o
bladder	vesic/o

Definition	Combining Form	Definition	Combining Form
blood	hem/o, hemat/o, sanguin/o	cul-de-sac	culd/o
		to cut	cis/o, tom/o
blood vessel	vascul/o	death	necr/o
blue	cyan/o	diaphragm	diaphragmat/o
body	corpor/o, physic/o, somat/o	dilated vein	varic/o
		dim	ambly/o
bone	oste/o	disease	path/o
bone marrow	myel/o	distinctive	idi/o
brain	encephal/o	double	dipl/o
breast	mamm/o, mast/o	drive	compuls/o
to breathe	hal/o	drug	chem/o, pharmac/o
breathing	spir/o	dry	ichthy/o, xer/o
to bring	duct/o	dull	ambly/o
bronchiole	bronchiol/o	duodenum	duoden/o
bronchus	bronch/o, bronchi/o	dura mater	dur/o
to burn	cauter/o	dust	coni/o
buttock	glute/o	ear	aur/o, auricul/o, ot/o
calcium	calc/o		
cancer	carcin/o	eat	phag/o
carpus	carp/o	egg	o/o
cartilage	chondr/o	electricity	electr/o
cavity wall	pariet/o	electrolytes	mineral/o
cecum	cec/o	embryo	embry/o
cell	cyt/o	epididymis	epididym/o
center	centr/o	epiglottis	epiglott/o
cerebellum	cerebell/o	epithelium	epitheli/o
cerebrum	cerebr/o	esophagus	esophag/o
cerumen	cerumin/o	extremities	acr/o
cervix	cervic/o	eye	ocul/o, ophthalm/o, opt/o, optic/o
cheek	bucc/o		
chemical	chem/o	eyelid	blephar/o
chest	pector/o, steth/o, thorac/o	false belief	delus/o
		fat	adip/o, lip/o
child	ped/o	fatty substance	ather/o
chorion	chori/o	fear	anxi/o
choroid	uve/o	feeling	esthesi/o
ciliary body	cycl/o	female	estr/o, gynec/o
clavicle	clavicul/o, cleid/o	femur	femor/o
clot	thromb/o	fetus	fet/o
clotting	coagul/o	fibers	fibr/o, fibrin/o
clumping	agglutin/o	fibrous band	fasci/o
coal	anthrac/o	fibula	fibul/o
coccyx	coccyg/o	fire	pyr/o
cochlea	cochle/o	flesh	sarc/o
cold	cry/o	foot	ped/o, pod/o
colon	col/o, colon/o	forgetfulness	amnes/o
color	chrom/o, chromat/o	front	anter/o
common bile duct	choledoch/o	fungus	myc/o
compel	compuls/o	gall	chol/e
conjunctiva	conjunctiv/o	gallbladder	cholecyst/o
cornea	corne/o, kerat/o	genital	genit/o
correct	emmetr/o	genital region	pub/o
cough	tuss/o	gland	aden/o
crooked	scoli/o	glans penis	balan/o

Definition	Combining Form	Definition	Combining Form
glassy	vitre/o	lymph node	lymphaden/o
glomerulus	glomerul/o	lymph vessel	lymphangi/o
glucose	gluc/o, glycos/o	macula lutea	macul/o
glue	gli/o	male	andr/o
granules	granul/o	mandible	mandibul/o
gray	glauc/o	maxilla	maxill/o
gray matter	poli/o	meatus	meat/o
groin	inguin/o	medicine	iatr/o
gums	gingiv/o	medulla oblongata	medull/o
hair	trich/o	meninges	mening/o,
hard	kerat/o, scler/o		meningi/o
horny	kerat/o	menses, menstruation	men/o
head	cephal/o	metacarpus	metacarp/o
hearing	acous/o, audi/o, audit/o	metatarsus	metatars/o
heart	cardi/o, coron/o	middle	medi/o
heart muscle	myocardi/o	milk	lact/o
heat	therm/o	mind	ment/o, phren/o,
hidden	crypt/o		psych/o
to hold back	isch/o	minerals	mineral/o
humerus	humer/o	mouth	or/o
hump	kyph/o	movement	kinesi/o
hymen	hymen/o	mucus	muc/o
ileum	ile/o	muscle	muscul/o, my/o,
ilium	ili/o		myos/o
imagined perception	hallucin/o	nail	onych/o, ungu/o
immature	blast/o	near to	proxim/o
incomplete	atel/o	neck	cervic/o
infection	septic/o	nerve	neur/o
inner region	medull/o	nerve root	radicul/o
internal organ	viscer/o	neutral	neutr/o
iodine	iod/o	night	noct/i, nyctal/o
iris	ir/o, irid/o	nitrogenous waste	azot/o
irrational fear	phob/o	nose	nas/o, rhin/o
ischium	ischi/o	nucleus	nucle/o
jejunum	jejun/o	oil	seb/o
joint	arthr/o, articul/o	old age	presby/o
ketones	ket/o, keton/o	optic disk	papill/o
kidney	nephr/o, ren/o	outer layer	cortic/o
labyrinth (inner ear)	labyrinth/o	ovary	oophor/o, ovari/o
lamina (part of vertebra)	lamin/o	ovum	ov/o, ov/i
larynx	laryng/o	oxygen	ox/o, ox/i
leg	crur/o	pain	alges/o
lens	phac/o	palate	palat/o
lessening	mi/o	pancreas	pancreat/o
lice	pedicul/o	parathyroid gland	parathyroid/o
life	bi/o	patella	patell/o
light	phot/o	pelvis	pelv/o
lip	labi/o	penis	pen/o
liver	hepat/o	perineum	perine/o
lobe	lob/o	peritoneum	peritone/o
loin (low back)	lumb/o	phalanges	phalang/o
lung	pneum/o, pneumon/o, pulmon/o	pharynx	pharyng/o
		physician	iatr/o
lymph	lymph/o	pineal gland	pineal/o

Definition	Combining Form	Definition	Combining Form
pituitary gland	pituitar/o	side	later/o
pleura	pleur/o	sigmoid colon	sigmoid/o
plug	embol/o	sinus	sinus/o
point	stigmat/o	skin	cutane/o, derm/o, dermat/o
poison	tox/o, toxic/o		
polyp	polyp/o	skull	crani/o
pons	pont/o	sleep	narc/o, somn/o
potassium	kal/i	small intestine	enter/o
pouch	diverticul/o	society	soci/o
pouring	fus/o	sodium	natr/o
to press down	depress/o	sole of foot	plant/o
profuse sweating	diaphor/o	sound	phon/o, son/o
proper	emmetr/o	specific area	topic/o
prostate gland	prostat/o	sperm	spermat/o
protection	immun/o	spinal cord	myel/o
protein	protein/o	spine	spin/o
pubis	pub/o	spleen	splen/o
pulse	sphygm/o	split	schiz/o
pupil	pupill/o	stapes	staped/o
pus	py/o	star	astr/o
pylorus	pylor/o	to steal	klept/o
radius	radi/o	sternum	stern/o
radiation	radi/o	stiff joint	ankyl/o
rapid contracting and relaxing	clon/o	stomach	gastr/o
		stone	lith/o
rectum	rect/o	straight	orth/o
ray (X-ray)	radi/o	to stretch out	extens/o
rectum and anus	proct/o	stupor	narc/o
red	erythr/o	sugar	glyc/o, glycos/o
renal pelvis	pyel/o	swallow	phag/o
retina	retin/o	sweat	hidr/o
to revolve	rotat/o	synovial membrane	synov/o, synovi/o
rib	cost/o	system	system/o
root	radic/o	tail	caud/o
rosy red	eosin/o	tarsus	tars/o
sac	burs/o, cyst/o, vesic/o	tears	dacry/o, lacrim/o
sacrum	sacr/o	tendon	ten/o, tend/o, tendin/o
salivary gland	sialaden/o		
sameness	home/o	testes	orch/o, orchi/o, orchid/o, testicul/o
scaly	ichthy/o		
scanty	olig/o	thalamus	thalam/o
scapula	scapul/o	thymus gland	thym/o
sclera	scler/o	thyroid gland	thyr/o, thyroid/o
to secrete	crin/o	tibia	tibi/o
seminal vesicle	vesicul/o	tissue	hist/o
sensation	esthesi/o	tone	ton/o
sense of pain	alges/o	tongue	gloss/o, lingu/o
sex glands	gonad/o	tonsils	tonsill/o
sexual intercourse	pareun/o	tooth	dent/o, odont/o
to shake violently	concuss/o	trachea	trache/o
shape	morph/o	treatment	iatr/o
sheath (meninges)	thec/o	to turn	vers/o

Definition	Combining Form	Definition	Combining Form
tympanic membrane	**tympan/o, myring/o**	venule	**venul/o**
ulna	**uln/o**	vision	**opt/o, optic/o**
ureter	**ureter/o**	water	**hydr/o**
urethra	**urethr/o**	worry	**anxi/o**
urinary bladder	**cyst/o**	to widen	**dilat/o**
urine	**ur/o, urin/o**	yellow	**cirrh/o**
uterine (fallopian) tubes	**salping/o**		

Definition	Suffix	Definition	Suffix
abnormal condition	**-iasis, -osis**	drooping	**-ptosis**
abnormal decrease	**-penia**	ear condition	**-otia**
abnormal flow	**-rrhage**	to eat	**-phage**
abnormal flow (pertaining to)	**-rrhagic**	eat	**-phagia**
abnormal flow condition	**-rrhagia**	enlarged	**-megaly**
abnormal softening	**-malacia**	fear	**-phobia**
action	**-ion**	fixation (surgical)	**-pexy**
appetite	**-orexia**	flow condition (abnormal)	**-rrhagia**
attracted to	**-phil**	formation	**-plasm, -plastin,**
to bear (offspring)	**-para**		**-poiesis**
beginning	**-arche**	formation (pertaining to)	**-plastic**
being attracted to (condition of)	**-philia**	formation of cells	**-plasia**
being attracted to (pertaining to)	**-philic**	frenzy	**-mania**
		to fuse	**-desis**
blood condition	**-emia**	hardening	**-sclerosis**
blood condition (pertaining to a)	**-emic**	hearing	**-cusis**
breathing	**-pnea**	heart condition	**-cardia**
carbon dioxide	**-capnia**	immature	**-blast**
carry away	**-apheresis**	inflammation	**-itis**
carrying	**-phoresis**	instrument for measuring	**-meter**
cell	**-cyte**	instrument for viewing	**-scope**
cells (pertaining to)	**-cytic**	instrument to cut	**-tome**
chest	**-thorax**	instrument to measure pressure	**-manometer**
childbirth	**-partum, -tocia**		
condition	**-ia**	involuntary muscle contraction	**-spasm**
condition (abnormal)	**-iasis, -osis**	to kill	**-cide**
condition of being attracted to	**-philia**	labor	**-tocia**
condition of sperm	**-spermia**	laws (pertaining to)	**-nomics**
condition of stones	**-lithiasis**	mass	**-oma**
condition of the urine	**-uria**	meal (pertaining to a)	**-prandial**
condition to bear	**-phoria**	measure pressure (instrument to)	**-manometer**
crushing (surgical)	**-tripsy**		
cut (instrument to)	**-tome**	measuring (instrument for)	**-meter**
cutting into	**-otomy**	measuring (process of)	**-metry**
decrease, too few (abnormal)	**-penia**	medical treatment	**-iatry**
to destroy (to break down)	**-lysis**	medical treatment (pertaining to)	**-iatric**
destruction	**-lytic**		
development	**-trophy**	more than the normal number of cells	**-cytosis**
development (pertaining to)	**-trophic**		
digestion	**-pepsia**	movement	**-kinesia**
dilation	**-ectasis**	muscle coordination	**-taxia**
discharge	**-rrhea**	narrowing	**-stenosis**
disease	**-pathy**	one who studies	**-logist**

Definition	Suffix	Definition	Suffix
opening (surgically create an)	-ostomy	speech	-phasia
pain	-algia, -dynia	sperm (condition of)	-spermia
paralysis	-plegia	spitting	-ptysis
pertaining to	-ac, -al, -an, -ar,	standing still	-stasis
	-ary, -atic, -eal, -ia,	state of	-ism
	-iac, -ic, -ical, -ile,	state of pregnancy	-cyesis
	-ine, -ior, -nic, -ory,	to stimulate	-tropin
	-ose, -ous, -tic	stimulating (pertaining to)	-tropic
pertaining to a blood condition	-emic	stone	-lith
pertaining to a meal	-prandial	stones (condition of)	-lithiasis
pertaining to abnormal flow	-rrhagic	study of	-logy
pertaining to being attracted to	-philic	study of (pertaining to)	-logic
pertaining to cells	-cytic	surgical crushing	-tripsy
pertaining to development	-trophic	surgical fixation	-pexy
pertaining to formation	-plastic	surgical removal	-ectomy
pertaining to medical treatment	-iatric	surgical repair	-plasty
pertaining to poison	-toxic	surgically create an opening	-ostomy
pertaining to stimulating	-tropic	to suture	-rrhaphy
pertaining to study of	-logic	swallow	-phagia
pertaining to tone	-tonic	swelling	-edema
pertaining to visually examining	-scopic	that which produces	-gen
pertaining to vomiting	-emetic	thirst	-dipsia
physician	-iatrist	to bear (offspring)	-para
poison (pertaining to)	-toxic	to destroy (to break down)	-lysis
porous	-porosis	to eat	-phage
pregnant woman	-gravida	to fuse	-desis
pressure	-tension	to kill	-cide
process of measuring	-metry	to press down	-pressin,
process of recording	-graphy		-pressor
process of visually examining	-scopy	to record	-graph
produces	-genesis	to shine through	-lucent
producing	-genic	to stimulate	-tropin
protection	-phylaxis	to suture	-rrhaphy
protein	-globin, -globulin	tone	-tonia
protrusion	-cele	tone (pertaining to)	-tonic
puncture to withdraw fluid	-centesis	too few	-penia
recording (process of)	-graphy	treatment	-therapy
record	-gram	tumor	-oma
removal	-apheresis	turned condition	-tropia
removal (surgical)	-ectomy	the urine (condition of)	-uria
repair (surgical)	-plasty	uterine tube	-salpinx
resembling	-oid	view of	-opsy
rupture	-rrhexis	viewing (instrument for)	-scope
seizure	-lepsy	vision condition	-opia, -opsia
separation of	-crit	visually examining	-scopic
to shine through	-lucent	(pertaining to)	
skin condition	-derma	visually examining (process of)	-scopy
slipping	-listhesis	voice	-phonia
small	-ole, -ule, -osmia	vomiting	-emesis
softening (abnormal)	-malacia	vomiting (pertaining to)	-emetic
specialist	-ician, -ist	weakness	-asthenia,
specialist in measuring	-metrist		-paresis
specialty of	-istry		

Appendix III
Abbreviations

Abbreviation	Meaning
i̇	one
i̇ i̇	two
i̇ i̇ i̇	three
#	number
α	alpha
ā	before
AB	abortion
ABGs	arterial blood gases
ac	before meals
ACR	albumin/creatinine ratio
ACTH	adrenocorticotropic hormone
AD	Alzheimer's disease
ad lib	as desired
ADD	attention-deficit disorder
ADH	antidiuretic hormone
ADHD	attention-deficit/hyperactivity disorder
ADLs	activities of daily living
AE	above elbow
AED	automated external defibrillator
AF	atrial fibrillation
AGN	acute glomerulonephritis
AHT	abusive head trauma
AI	artificial insemination
AIDS	acquired immunodeficiency syndrome
AK	above knee
AKI	acute kidney injury
ALL	acute lymphocytic leukemia
ALS	amyotrophic lateral sclerosis
ALT	alanine transaminase
AMI	acute myocardial infarction
AML	acute myeloid leukemia
ANA	antinuclear antibody
Angio	angiography
ANS	autonomic nervous system
ante	before
AP	anteroposterior
APAP	acetaminophen (Tylenol)
aq	aqueous (water)
ARC	AIDS-related complex
ARDS	adult (or acute) respiratory distress syndrome
ARF	acute renal failure
ARMD	age-related macular degeneration
AROM	active range of motion
AS	arteriosclerosis
ASD	atrial septal defect
ASHD	arteriosclerotic heart disease

Abbreviation	Meaning
ASL	American Sign Language
AST	aspartate transaminase
Astigm	astigmatism
ATN	acute tubular necrosis
AV, A-V	atrioventricular
β	beta
Ba	barium
basos	basophils
BBB	bundle branch block (L for left; R for right)
BC	bone conduction
BCC	basal cell carcinoma
BDT	bone density testing
BE	barium enema, below elbow
bid	twice a day
BK	below knee
BM	bowel movement
BMI	body mass index
BMR	basal metabolic rate
BMT	bone marrow transplant
BNO	bladder neck obstruction
BP	blood pressure
BPD	bipolar disorder
BPH	benign prostatic hyperplasia
bpm	beats per minute
Bronch	bronchoscopy
BS	bowel sounds
BSE	breast self-examination
BUN	blood urea nitrogen
bx, BX	biopsy
c̄	with
C&S	culture and sensitivity
c.gl.	correction with glasses
C1, C2, etc.	first cervical vertebra, second cervical vertebra, etc.
Ca	calcium
CA	chronological age
CABG	coronary artery bypass graft
CAD	coronary artery disease
cap(s)	capsule(s)
CAPD	continuous ambulatory peritoneal dialysis
CAT	computerized axial tomography
cath	catheterization
CBC	complete blood count
CBD	common bile duct
CC	cardiac catheterization, chief complaint, clean catch urine specimen
CCU	coronary care unit

Abbreviation	Meaning
C. diff	*Clostridium difficile*
CF	cystic fibrosis
CHF	congestive heart failure
Cl⁻	chloride
CK	creatine kinase
CLL	chronic lymphocytic leukemia
CML	chronic myeloid leukemia
CNS	central nervous system
CO_2	carbon dioxide
CoA	coarctation of the aorta
COPD	chronic obstructive pulmonary disease
CPAP	continuous positive airway pressure
CP	cerebral palsy, chest pain
CPK	creatine phosphokinase
CPR	cardiopulmonary resuscitation
CRE	carbapenem-resistant Enterobacteriaceae
CRF	chronic renal failure
crit	hematocrit
CS, C-section	cesarean section
CSD	congenital septal defect
CSF	cerebrospinal fluid
CT	calcitonin, computerized tomography
CTA	clear to auscultation
CTE	chronic traumatic encephalopathy
CTS	carpal tunnel syndrome
CV	cardiovascular
CVA	cerebrovascular accident
CVD	cerebrovascular disease
CVS	chorionic villus sampling
Cx	cervix
CXR	chest X-ray
cysto	cystoscopy
D	diopter (lens strength)
d	day
D&C	dilation and curettage
dB	decibel
d/c, DC	discontinue
DEA	Drug Enforcement Administration
decub	decubitus ulcer, lying down
Derm, derm	dermatology
DEXA	dual-energy X-ray absorptiometry
DI	diabetes insipidus, diagnostic imaging
diff	differential
dil	dilute
DISC, disc	discontinue
disp	dispense
DJD	degenerative joint disease
DM	diabetes mellitus
DOE	dyspnea on exertion

Abbreviation	Meaning
DPT	diphtheria, pertussis, tetanus injection
DRE	digital rectal exam
DSA	digital subtraction angiography
DSM	*Diagnostic and Statistical Manual of Mental Disorders*
DTR	deep tendon reflex
DVA	distance visual acuity
DVT	deep vein thrombosis
DXA	dual-energy X-ray absorptiometry
ECC	extracorporeal circulation
ECCE	extracapsular cataract extraction
ECG	electrocardiogram
ECHO	echocardiography
ECT	electroconvulsive therapy
ED	erectile dysfunction
EDD	estimated date of delivery
EEG	electroencephalogram, electroencephalography
EENT	eyes, ears, nose, and throat
EGD	esophagogastroduodenoscopy
eGFR	estimated glomerular filtration rate
EKG	electrocardiogram
EM	emmetropia
EMB	endometrial biopsy
EMG	electromyogram
ENT	ears, nose, and throat
EOM	extraocular movement
eos	eosinophils
eosins	eosinophils
ERCP	endoscopic retrograde cholangiopancreatography
ERT	estrogen replacement therapy
ERV	expiratory reserve volume
ESR	erythrocyte sedimentation rate
ESRD	end-stage renal disease
ESWL	extracorporeal shockwave lithotripsy
et	and
ET	esotropia
EU	excretory urography
FBS	fasting blood sugar
FDA	Food and Drug Administration
FEKG	fetal electrocardiogram
FHR	fetal heart rate
FHT	fetal heart tone
fib	fibrillation
flu	influenza
FOBT	fecal occult blood test
FRC	functional residual capacity
FS	frozen section
FSH	follicle-stimulating hormone
FTM	female to male
FTND	full-term normal delivery
Fx, FX	fracture

Abbreviation	Meaning
GI	gastrointestinal
GI	first pregnancy
GA	general anesthesia
GB	gallbladder X-ray
GC	gonorrhea
GERD	gastroesophageal reflux disease
GH	growth hormone
gm	gram
gr	grain
grav I	first pregnancy
gt	drop
GTT	glucose tolerance test
gtt	drops
GU	genitourinary
GVHD	graft versus host disease
GYN	gynecology
H_2O	water
HA	headache
HAI	healthcare-associated infection
HAV	hepatitis A virus
Hb	hemoglobin
HBV	hepatitis B virus
HCG, hCG	human chorionic gonadotropin
HCl	hydrochloric acid
HCO_3^-	bicarbonate
HCT, Hct	hematocrit
HCV	hepatitis C virus
HD	Hodgkin's disease, hemodialysis
HDN	hemolytic disease of the newborn
HDV	hepatitis D virus
HEENT	head, ears, eyes, nose, and throat
HEV	hepatitis E virus
Hgb	hemoglobin
HIV	human immunodeficiency virus
HMD	hyaline membrane disease
HNP	herniated nucleus pulposus
HPV	human papillomavirus
H. pylori	*Helicobacter pylori*
HRT	hormone replacement therapy
HSG	hysterosalpingography
HSV-1	herpes simplex virus type 1
HTN	hypertension
Hz	hertz
I&D	incision and drainage
I&O	intake and output
IBD	inflammatory bowel disease
IBS	irritable bowel syndrome
IC	inspiratory capacity
ICCE	intracapsular cataract extraction
ICD	implantable cardioverter-defibrillator
ICP	intracranial pressure
ICU	intensive care unit
ID	intradermal
IDDM	insulin-dependent diabetes mellitus

Abbreviation	Meaning
Ig	immunoglobulins (IgA, IgD, IgE, IgG, IgM)
IM	intramuscular
inj	injection
IOL	intraocular lens
IOP	intraocular pressure
IPD	intermittent peritoneal dialysis
IPPB	intermittent positive pressure breathing
IRDS	infant respiratory distress syndrome
IRV	inspiratory reserve volume
IUD	intrauterine device
IV	intravenous
IVC	intravenous cholangiography
IVF	*in vitro* fertilization
IVP	intravenous pyelogram
JRA	juvenile rheumatoid arthritis
K^+	potassium
kg	kilogram
KS	Kaposi's sarcoma
KUB	kidneys, ureters, bladder
L	liter
L1, L2, etc.	first lumbar vertebra, second lumbar vertebra, etc.
LASIK	laser-assisted in situ keratomileusis
lat	lateral
LBW	low birth weight
LE	lower extremity
LH	luteinizing hormone
LLE	left lower extremity
LLL	left lower lobe
LLQ	left lower quadrant
LMP	last menstrual period
LP	lumbar puncture
LUE	left upper extremity
LUL	left upper lobe
LUQ	left upper quadrant
LVH	left-ventricular hypertrophy
lymphs	lymphocytes
MA	mental age
mcg	microgram
MD	muscular dystrophy
MDI	metered-dose inhaler
mEq	milliequivalent
MERS	Middle East respiratory syndrome
mg	milligram
MI	myocardial infarction, mitral insufficiency
mL	milliliter
MM	malignant melanoma
mm Hg	millimeters of mercury
MMPI	Minnesota Multiphasic Personality Inventory
mono	mononucleosis

Abbreviation	Meaning
monos	monocytes
MR	mitral regurgitation
MRSA	methicillin-resistant *Staphylococcus aureus*
MS	musculoskeletal, mitral stenosis, multiple sclerosis
MSH	melanocyte-stimulating hormone
MTF	male to female
MTX	methotrexate
MUA	manipulation under anesthesia
MVP	mitral valve prolapse
N&V	nausea and vomiting
Na$^+$	sodium
NB	newborn
NF	necrotizing fasciitis
NG	nasogastric (tube)
NHL	non-Hodgkin's lymphoma
NIDDM	non-insulin-dependent diabetes mellitus
NK	natural killer cells
noc	night
NPH	neutral protamine Hagedorn (insulin)
NPO	nothing by mouth
NS	nephrotic syndrome, normal saline
NSAID	nonsteroidal anti-inflammatory drug
O&P	ova and parasites
O$_2$	oxygen
OA	osteoarthritis
OB	obstetrics
OCD	obsessive–compulsive disorder
OCPs	oral contraceptive pills
od	overdose
OE	otitis externa
oint	ointment
OM	otitis media
Ophth	ophthalmology
OR	operating room
ORIF	open reduction–internal fixation
Orth, ortho	orthopedics
OT	occupational therapy
OTC	over the counter
Oto	otology
oz	ounce
p̄	after
P	phosphorus, pulse
PI	first delivery
PA	posteroanterior, pernicious anemia
PAC	premature atrial contraction
Pap	Papanicolaou test
para I	first delivery
PBI	protein-bound iodine
pc	after meals
PCP	pneumocystis pneumonia
PCV	packed cell volume

Abbreviation	Meaning
PDA	patent ductus arteriosus
PDR	*Physician's Desk Reference*
PE	pulmonary embolism
PE tube	pressure equalizing tube
per	through, with
PERRLA	pupils equal, round, react to light and accommodation
PET	positron emission tomography
PFT	pulmonary function test
pH	acidity or alkalinity of a solution
PharmD	registered pharmacist
PID	pelvic inflammatory disease
PIH	pregnancy-induced hypertension
PMN	polymorphonuclear neutrophil
PMS	premenstrual syndrome
PNS	peripheral nervous system
po	by mouth
PO	phone order
polys	polymorphonuclear neutrophil
PORP	partial ossicular replacement prosthesis
pp	postprandial
PPD	purified protein derivative
PRK	photorefractive keratectomy
PRL	prolactin
prn	as needed
pro-time	prothrombin time
PROM	passive range of motion
prot	protocol
PSA	prostate-specific antigen
pt	patient
PT	physical therapy, prothrombin time
PTC	percutaneous transhepatic cholangiography
PTCA	percutaneous transluminal coronary angioplasty
PTH	parathyroid hormone
PTSD	posttraumatic stress disorder
PUD	peptic ulcer disease
PVC	premature ventricular contraction
PVD	peripheral vascular disease
q	every
qam	every morning
qh	every hour
qid	four times a day
R	respiration, roentgen
RA	rheumatoid arthritis, room air
RAI	radioactive iodine
RBC	red blood cell
RDS	respiratory distress syndrome
REM	rapid eye movement
Rh+	Rh-positive
Rh-	Rh-negative
RIA	radioimmunoassay
RK	radial keratotomy

Abbreviation	Meaning	Abbreviation	Meaning
RLE	right lower extremity	T_4	thyroxine
RLL	right lower lobe	tab(s)	tablet(s)
RLQ	right lower quadrant	TAH-BSO	total abdominal hysterectomy–bilateral salpingo-oophorectomy
RML	right middle lobe		
ROM	range of motion	TB	tuberculosis
RP	retrograde pyelogram	TBI	traumatic brain injury
RPh	registered pharmacist	tbsp	tablespoon
RPR	rapid plasma reagin (test for syphilis)	TENS	transcutaneous electrical nerve stimulation
RUE	right upper extremity		
RUL	right upper lobe	TFT	thyroid function test
RUQ	right upper quadrant	THA	total hip arthroplasty
RV	reserve volume	THR	total hip replacement
Rx	take	TIA	transient ischemic attack
s̄	without	tid	three times a day
s.gl.	without correction or glasses	TKA	total knee arthroplasty
S1	first heart sound	TKR	total knee replacement
S2	second heart sound	TLC	total lung capacity
SA, S-A	sinoatrial	TO	telephone order
SAD	seasonal affective disorder	top	apply topically
SARS	severe acute respiratory syndrome	TORP	total ossicular replacement prosthesis
SBS	shaken baby syndrome		
SCC	squamous cell carcinoma	tPA	tissue plasminogen activator
SCI	spinal cord injury	TPN	total parenteral nutrition
SCIDS	severe combined immunodeficiency syndrome	TPR	temperature, pulse, and respiration
		TSH	thyroid-stimulating hormone
sed rate	erythrocyte sedimentation rate	tsp	teaspoon
segs	segmented neutrophils	TSS	toxic shock syndrome
SG	skin graft, specific gravity	tTG	tissue transglutaminase
SIDS	sudden infant death syndrome	TUR	transurethral resection
Sig	label as follows/directions	TURP	transurethral resection of the prostate
SK	streptokinase		
sl	sublingual	TV	tidal volume
SLE	systemic lupus erythematosus	U/A, UA	urinalysis
SMD	senile macular degeneration	UC	urine culture, uterine contractions
SOB	shortness of breath	UE	upper extremity
sol	solution	UGI	upper gastrointestinal series
SOM	serous otitis media	URI	upper respiratory infection
sp. gr.	specific gravity	US	ultrasound
SPP	suprapubic prostatectomy	UTI	urinary tract infection
SSD	somatic symptom disorder	UV	ultraviolet
stat	at once/immediately	V fib	ventricular fibrillation
STD	sexually transmitted disease	VA	visual acuity
STI	sexually transmitted infection	VC	vital capacity
STSG	split-thickness skin graft	VCUG	voiding cystourethrography
Subc, Subq	subcutaneous	VD	venereal disease
suppos, supp	suppository	VF	visual field
susp	suspension	VO	verbal order
syr	syrup	VS	vital signs
T & A	tonsillectomy and adenoidectomy	VSD	ventricular septal defect
T	tablespoon	VT	ventricular tachycardia
t	teaspoon	WBC	white blood cell
T1, T2, etc.	first thoracic vertebra, second thoracic vertebra, etc.	wt	weight
		x	times
T_3	triiodothyronine	XT	exotropia

Abbreviations to Be Avoided

Abbreviations make writing notes faster, but they also create the possibility of being misunderstood. For this reason, the Joint Commission on Accreditation of Healthcare Organizations (JCAHO) and the Institute for Safe Medication Practices (ISMP) publishes lists of error-prone abbreviations that are not to be used. The following table presents these abbreviations and what should be used instead. The Joint Commission (TJC) has determined that the first seven abbreviations (marked with an *) must appear on an accredited institution's "Do Not Use" list of abbreviations.

Abbreviation	Intended Meaning	Potential Problem	Recommendation
IU*	International Unit	Mistaken for "IV" or "10"	Write "international unit"
MS, MSO$_4$, and MgSO$_4$*	morphine sulfate, magnesium sulfate	Mistaken for each other	Write "morphine sulfate" or "magnesium sulfate"
Not using a zero before a decimal point (0.X)*	.X mg	Decimal point is missed	Always write a zero before a decimal point (0.X mg)
q.d. or QD*	every day	Mistaken for "qid"	Write "daily"
q.o.d. or QOD*	every other day	Mistaken for "qd" or for "qid"	Write "every other day"
U or u*	unit	Mistaken for "0," "4," or "cc"	Write "unit"
Using a zero after a decimal point*	X.0 mg	Decimal point is missed	Never write a zero by itself after a decimal point (X mg is correct)
@	at	Mistaken for "2"	Write "at"
&	and	Mistaken for "2"	Write "and"
< and >	lesser than and greater than	Mistakenly read as the opposite symbol	Write "lesser than" and "greater than"
+	and	Mistaken for "4"	Write "and"
°	hour	Mistaken for "0"	Write "hr," "h," or "hour"
i/d	one daily	Mistaken for "tid"	Write "one daily"
μg	microgram	Mistaken for "mg"	Write "mcg"
3	dram	Mistaken for "3"	Write "dram"
AS, AD, AU and OS, OD, OU	left ear, right ear, both ears and left eye, right eye, both eyes	Mistaken for each other (for example, "AS" and "OS")	Write "left ear," "right ear," "both ears," "left eye," "right eye," and "both eyes"
BT	bedtime	Mistaken for "bid"	Write "bedtime"
cc	cubic centimeter	Mistaken for "U" (units)	Since a cubic centimeter is equal to a milliliter, write "mL"
D/C	discharge	Mistaken to mean "discontinue"	Write "discharge"
Dose and unit of measure run together (such as 10mg or 100mL)	10 mg or 100 mL	Mistaken for "100 mg" or "1000 mL"	Use adequate space between dose and unit of measure
Drug name and dose run together (such as Inderal40 mg)	Inderal 40 mg	Mistaken for "Inderal 140 mg"	Use adequate space between drug name and dose
hs or HS	half-strength or at bedtime	Meanings can be mistaken for each other	Write "half-strength" or "at bedtime"
IJ	injection	Mistaken for "IV"	Write "injection"
IN	intranasal	Mistaken for "IM" or "IV"	Write "intranasal" or "NAS"

Abbreviation	Intended Meaning	Potential Problem	Recommendation
Large numbers without proper comma (such as 100000)	100,000	Mistaken for "1,000,000"	Always use commas in large numbers
o.d. or OD	once daily	Mistaken for "right eye (OD)" or "overdose"	write "daily"
OJ	orange juice	Mistaken for "right eye (OD)"	write "orange juice"
Per os	by mouth	"os" can be mistaken to mean "left eye"	write "PO," "orally," or "by mouth"
Period following abbreviation such as mg. or mL.	mg or mL	Period mistaken for "1"	Write "mg" or "mL"
qhs	every bedtime	Mistaken for "qhr"	Write "bedtime"
qn	every night	Mistaken for "qh"	Write "nightly"
q1d	every day	Mistaken for "qid"	Write "daily"
q6PM	every day at 6:00 p.m.	Mistaken to mean "every 6 hours"	Write "daily at 6 p.m."
SC, SQ, sub q	subcutaneous	SC mistaken for "SL," SQ mistaken for "5 every," the separate q mistaken for "every"	Write "Subq," "Subc," or "subcutaneous"
ss	sliding scale or one-half	Mistaken for each other and for "55"	Write "sliding scale," "one-half," or "1/2"
SSRI and SSI	sliding scale regular insulin and sliding scale insulin	Mistaken for "selective-serotonin reuptake inhibitor" and "strong solution of iodine"	Write "sliding scale (insulin)"
tiw or TIW	three times a week	Mistaken for "three times a day" or "twice weekly"	Write "3 times weekly"
UD	as directed (*ut dictum*)	Mistaken for unit dose	Write "as directed"
x3d	for three days	Mistaken to mean "for 3 doses"	Write "for three days"

Answer Keys

Chapter 1 Answers
Practice As You Go

A. 1. word root, combining vowel, prefix, suffix
2. combining form 3. o 4. suffix 5. prefix
B. 1. cardiology 2. gastrology 3. dermatology
4. ophthalmology 5. immunology 6. nephrology
7. hematology 8. gynecology 9. neurology
10. pathology
C. 1. tachy-, fast 2. pseudo-, false 3. hypo-,
insufficient 4. inter-, between 5. eu-, normal
6. post-, after 7. mono-, one 8. sub-, under
D. 1. pulmonology 2. rhinorrhea 3. nephromalacia
4. cardiomegaly 5. gastrotomy 6. dermatitis
7. laryngectomy 8. arthroplasty
E. 1. metastases 2. ova 3. nuclei 4. phalanges
5. appendices 6. vertebrae
F. 1. c 2. a 3. e 4. d 5. b
G. 1. c 2. a 3. b
H. 1. true 2. false 3. true 4. false 5. true
I. 1. e 2. d 3. f 4. a 5. c 6. b

Practice Exercises

A. 1. l 2. e 3. j 4. f 5. d 6. k 7. m 8. o 9. g 10. n 11. b
12. h 13. a 14. c 15. i
B. 1. without 2. slow 3. without 4. normal 5. excessive
6. between 7. before 8. under 9. not 10. many
11. within 12. outside 13. two 14. all 15. above
16. against 17. fast 18. insufficient 19. through
20. around
C. 1. study of 2. paralysis 3. discharge 4. narrowing 5. treatment 6. pertaining to 7. that which
produces 8. destruction 9. view of 10. surgical
removal 11. hardening 12. pertaining to 13. pain
14. surgical fixation 15. process of measuring
16. pertaining to 17. surgical repair 18. cutting into
19. instrument for viewing 20. pertaining to
D. 1. cardiomalacia 2. gastrostomy 3. rhinoplasty
4. hypertrophy 5. pathology 6. neuroma
7. gastroenterology 8. otitis 9. chemotherapy
10. carcinogen
E. 1. life 2. cancer 3. heart 4. chemical 5. to cut
6. skin 7. small intestine 8. stomach 9. female
10. blood 11. protection 12. voice box 13. kidney
14. nerve 15. eye 16. ear 17. disease 18. lung
19. nose
F. 1. diagnoses 2. diverticula 3. bursae 4. bronchi
5. arteries

G. 1. *Physician's Desk Reference* (PDR) 2. pharmacist
3. generic or nonproprietary 4. brand or
proprietary 5. the chemical formula 6. Drug
Enforcement Administration
H. 1. Pravachol, 20 milligrams each, label instructions, take one every night, supply with 30, refill
three times with no substitutions 2. Lanoxin,
0.125 milligrams each, label instructions, take
3 now and then 2 every morning, supply with
100 and may refill as needed 3. Synthroid,
0.075 milligrams each, label instructions, take
1 every day, supply with 100 and may refill four
times 4. Norvasc, 5 milligrams each, label instructions, take 1 every morning, supply with 60 and
no refills

Chapter 2 Answers
Practice As You Go

A. 1. cells, tissues, organs, systems, body 2. cytoplasm, nucleus, cell membrane 3. epithelial
4. cardiac, skeletal, smooth 5. connective
6. neurons
B. 1. integumentary, d 2. cardiovascular, i 3. digestive, g 4. female reproductive, b 5. musculoskeletal (skeletal), a 6. respiratory, j 7. urinary, c 8. male
reproductive, f 9. nervous, h 10. musculoskeletal
(muscular), e
C. 1. c 2. a 3. b
D. 1. cephalic 2. pubic 3. crural 4. gluteal 5. cervical
6. brachial 7. dorsum 8. thoracic
E. 1. anatomical 2. right lower 3. cranial, spinal
4. nine 5. right inguinal 6. pleural, pericardial
F. 1. inferior or caudal 2. supine 3. lateral 4. ventral
or anterior 5. deep 6. apex 7. distal 8. posterior or
dorsal 9. cephalic or superior
G. 1. d 2. f 3. a 4. b 5. c 6. e

Practice Exercises

A. 1. epi-, above 2. peri-, around 3. hypo-, insufficient or below 4. retro-, behind or backward
B. 1. j 2. i 3. f 4. g 5. a 6. c 7. d 8. b 9. h 10. l 11. e
12. m 13. f 14. m 15. k
C. 1. MS 2. lat 3. RUQ 4. CV 5. GI 6. AP 7. OB
8. LLQ
D. 1. thoracic 2. head 3. neck 4. brachial 5. gluteal
6. leg 7. spine 8. dorsum 9. abdominal 10. skull

E. **1.** proxim/o, proximal **2.** super/o, superior
3. medi/o, medial **4.** ventr/o, ventral **5.** caud/o, caudal **6.** anter/o, anterior **7.** later/o, lateral **8.** dors/o, dorsal **9.** infer/o, inferior **10.** poster/o, posterior
F. **1.** a **2.** c **3.** f **4.** e **5.** a **6.** d **7.** b **8.** e **9.** c **10.** b
G. **1.** sublingual **2.** rectal **3.** topical **4.** intradermal
5. intramuscular **6.** intravenous **7.** oral
H. **1.** spelled correctly **2.** hypochondriac **3.** integumentary **4.** spelled correctly **5.** spelled correctly
6. spelled correctly **7.** intravenous **8.** sagittal
9. spelled correctly **10.** epithelium
I. **1.** otorhinolaryngology **2.** cardiology **3.** gynecology **4.** orthopedics **5.** ophthalmology **6.** urology
7. dermatology **8.** gastroenterology

Labeling Exercises

A. **1.** cephalic **2.** cervical **3.** thoracic **4.** brachial
5. abdominal **6.** pelvic **7.** pubic **8.** crural **9.** trunk
10. vertebral **11.** dorsum **12.** gluteal
B. **1.** frontal or coronal plane **2.** sagittal or median plane **3.** transverse or horizontal plane

Chapter 3 Answers
Practice As You Go

A. **1.** epidermis, dermis **2.** hypodermis or subcutaneous layer **3.** basal cell **4.** fat cells or lipocytes
5. dermis **6.** keratin **7.** melanin **8.** corium **9.** nail bed **10.** sebaceous, sweat
B. **1.** ungual **2.** dermal, cutaneous, or dermic **3.** epidermal **4.** hypodermic, subcutaneous **5.** intradermal
C. **1.** e **2.** f **3.** i **4.** j **5.** a **6.** c **7.** l **8.** g **9.** k **10.** h **11.** d **12.** b
D. **1.** h **2.** i **3.** j **4.** e **5.** c **6.** a **7.** f **8.** g **9.** b **10.** d
E. **1.** FS **2.** I&D **3.** ID **4.** Subq or Subc **5.** UV **6.** BX or bx **7.** C&S **8.** BCC **9.** decub **10.** Derm or derm

Real-World Applications
Medical Record Analysis

1. basal cell carcinoma—Cancerous tumor of the basal cell layer of the epidermis. A frequent type of skin cancer that rarely metastasizes or spreads. These cancers can arise on sun-exposed skin.
2. lesions—A general term for a wound, injury, or abnormality.
3. biopsies—A piece of tissue is removed by syringe and needle, knife, punch, or brush to examine under a microscope. Used to aid in diagnosis.
4. excised—To surgically cut out.
5. pruritus—Severe itching.
6. anterior—Pertaining to the front side of the body.
7. erythema—Redness or flushing of the skin.

8. depigmentation—Loss of normal skin color or pigment.
9. epidermis—The superficial layer of the skin.
10. dermis—The deeper layer of the skin.
11. dermatoplasty—Skin grafting; transplantation of skin.

Chart Note Transcription

1. ulcer 2. dermatologist 3. pruritus 4. erythema
5. pustules 6. dermis 7. necrosis 8. culture and sensitivity 9. cellulitis 10. debridement

Case Study

1. Systemic lupus erythematosus; another example is rheumatoid arthritis.
2. Erythema—Skin redness; photosensitivity—Intolerance to strong light; alopecia—Baldness; stiffness in joints.
3. Exfoliative cytology and fungal scrapings—in both tests cells are scraped away from the skin and examined under a microscope in order to make a diagnosis; in order to make sure the rash was not caused by something else like a fungal infection.
4. Internist—oral anti-inflammatory medication to reduce pain, swelling, and stiffness in joints; dermatologist—anti-inflammatory corticosteroid cream to reduce the red rash.
5. Completing examinations and various diagnostic tests in order to collect information necessary for a diagnosis.

Practice Exercises

A. **1.** cryosurgery **2.** onychomalacia **3.** allograft
4. necrosis **5.** diaphoresis **6.** xenograft
7. anhidrosis **8.** seborrhea **9.** pediculosis
10. liposuction **11.** dermatology **12.** trichomycosis **13.** ichthyosis **14.** rhytidectomy
15. xeroderma
B. **1.** redness involving superficial layer of skin
2. burn damage through epidermis and into dermis causing vesicles **3.** burn damage to full thickness of epidermis and dermis
C. **1.** flat, discolored area **2.** small, solid raised spot less than 0.5 cm **3.** fluid-filled sac **4.** cracklike lesion **5.** raised spot containing pus **6.** small, round swollen area **7.** fluid-filled blister **8.** open sore **9.** firm, solid mass larger than 0.5 cm **10.** torn or jagged wound
D. **1.** dermatitis **2.** dermatosis **3.** dermatome
4. dermatologist **5.** dermatoplasty **6.** dermatology
7. melanoma **8.** melanocyte **9.** scleroderma
10. leukoderma **11.** erythroderma **12.** onychomalacia
13. paronychia **14.** onychophagia **15.** onychectomy
E. **1.** decub **2.** SLE **3.** C&S **4.** MM **5.** SG **6.** I&D
7. SCC, BCC **8.** Derm or derm

F. **1.** xeroderma **2.** petechiae **3.** tinea **4.** scabies
5. paronychia **6.** Kaposi's sarcoma **7.** impetigo
8. keloid **9.** exfoliative cytology **10.** frozen section
G. **1.** antifungal, e **2.** antipruritic, c **3.** antiparasit-
ic, a **4.** corticosteroid cream, b **5.** anesthetic, f
6. antibiotic, d
H. **1.** spelled correctly **2.** chemabrasion **3.** rhytidectomy
4. spelled correctly **5.** hyperhidrosis **6.** paronychia
7. spelled correctly **8.** spelled correctly **9.** decubitus **10.** spelled correctly
I. **1.** sweat glands, sebaceous glands, hair, nails
2. basal layer **3.** melanin **4.** collagen **5.** fat
6. keratin **7.** sebum **8.** sudoriferous

Labeling Exercises

A. **1.** epidermis **2.** dermis **3.** subcutaneous layer
4. sweat gland **5.** sweat duct **6.** hair shaft
7. sebaceous gland **8.** arrector pili muscle
9. sensory receptors
B. **1.** epidermis **2.** dermis **3.** subcutaneous layer
4. sebaceous gland **5.** arrector pili muscle **6.** hair
shaft **7.** hair follicle **8.** hair root **9.** papilla
C. **1.** free edge **2.** lateral nail groove **3.** lunula **4.** nail
bed **5.** nail body **6.** cuticle **7.** nail root

Chapter 4 Answers
Practice As You Go

A. **1.** osseous **2.** joint, ligaments **3.** diaphysis, epiphysis **4.** head, condyle, epicondyle, trochanter,
tubercle, tuberosity **5.** sinus, foramen, fossa, fissure
B. **1.** patella **2.** tarsus **3.** clavicle **4.** femur **5.** phalanges **6.** carpus **7.** tibia **8.** scapula **9.** phalanges
C. **1.** femoral **2.** sternal **3.** clavicular **4.** coccygeal
5. maxillary **6.** tibial **7.** patellar **8.** phalangeal **9.** hu-
meral **10.** pubic
D. **1.** e **2.** d **3.** j **4.** b **5.** g **6.** i **7.** a **8.** c **9.** f **10.** h
E. **1.** e **2.** c **3.** f **4.** a **5.** d **6.** b
F. **1.** TKR **2.** HNP **3.** UE **4.** L5 **5.** AK **6.** Fx or FX
7. NSAID
G. **1.** smooth **2.** myoneural or neuromuscular **3.** skel-
etal, smooth, cardiac
H. **1.** e **2.** d **3.** b **4.** c **5.** a **6.** h **7.** g **8.** f
I. **1.** d **2.** g **3.** a **4.** h **5.** e **6.** c **7.** f **8.** b
J. **1.** IM **2.** DTR **3.** MD **4.** EMG **5.** CTS

Real-World Applications
Medical Record Analysis

1. osteoarthritis—Joint inflammation resulting in
degeneration of the bones and joints, especially
those bearing weight. Results in bone rubbing
against bone.
2. bilateral—Pertaining to both sides.

3. TKA—Surgical reconstruction of a knee joint by
implanting a prosthetic knee joint. Also called *total
knee replacement (TKR)*.
4. orthopedic surgeon—Physician that specializes in
the diagnosis and treatment of conditions of the
musculoskeletal system using surgical means.
5. Radiographs — An X-ray image.
6. physical therapy—Treats disorders using physical
means and methods; includes joint motion and
muscle strength.
7. therapeutic exercise — Specific exercises planned
to improve range of motion and muscle strength
8. gait training—Learning how to walk.
9. occupational therapy—Assists patients to regain,
develop, and improve skills that are important for
independent functioning.
10. ADLs—Activities of daily living.

Chart Note Transcription

1. Colles' fracture (fx) **2.** cast **3.** fracture **4.** orthopedist
5. osteoporosis **6.** dual-energy X-ray absorptiometry
(DXA, DEXA) **7.** flexion **8.** extension **9.** comminuted
fracture (FX, Fx) **10.** femur **11.** total hip arthroplasty
(THA)

Case Study

1. Rheumatoid arthritis.
2. Cartilage damage and crippling deformities.
3. Osteoarthritis.
4. Bone scan—Radioactive dye is used to visualize
the body; erythrocyte sedimentation rate—
A blood test that can determine if a person has an
inflammatory disease.
5. Anti-inflammatory medication to reduce inflammation and provide some pain relief; physical therapy—
Treatment using warm water and exercises to
maintain the flexibility of the joints.
6. Acute—Brief disease, also used to mean sudden
and severe disease; chronic—Disease of a long
duration.

Practice Exercises

A. **1.** osteocyte **2.** osteoblast **3.** osteoporosis
4. osteopathy **5.** osteotomy **6.** osteotome
7. osteomyelitis **8.** osteomalacia **9.** osteochondroma
10. myopathy **11.** myoplasty **12.** myorrhaphy
13. electromyogram **14.** myasthenia **15.** tenodynia
16. tenorrhaphy **17.** arthrodesis **18.** arthroplasty
19. arthrotomy **20.** arthritis **21.** arthrocentesis
22. arthralgia **23.** chondrectomy **24.** chondroma
25. chondromalacia
B. **1.** cervical, 7 **2.** thoracic, 12 **3.** lumbar, 5
4. sacrum, 1 (5 fused) **5.** coccyx, 1 (3–5 fused)

C. 1. osteoporosis 2. myorrhexis 3. scoliosis 4. dystonia 5. kinesiology 6. lordosis 7. spondylolisthesis 8. arthrocentesis 9. abduction 10. osteoarthritis 11. osteoclasia 12. chondromalacia 13. muscular 14. myasthenia 15. tendinitis 16. bursitis 17. myeloma 18. arthrodesis

D. 1. osteoporosis 2. rickets 3. lateral epicondylitis 4. herniated nucleus pulposus 5. osteogenic sarcoma 6. scoliosis 7. pseudohypertrophic muscular dystrophy 8. systemic lupus erythematosus 9. spondylolisthesis 10. carpal tunnel syndrome

E. 1. axial, 1, upper jaw 2. appendicular, 16, wrist bones 3. appendicular, 2, shoulder blade 4. appendicular, 2, kneecap 5. axial, 1, breast bone 6. appendicular, 2, thigh bone 7. appendicular, 10, forefoot bone 8. appendicular, 2, shin bone 9. appendicular, 2, collar bone 10. axial, 2, cheek bone

F. 1. CTS 2. DEXA or DXA 3. MD 4. THA or THR 5. EMG 6. RA 7. Fx or FX 8. NSAID

G. 1. surgical repair of cartilage 2. slow movement 3. porous bone 4. abnormal increase in lumbar spine curve (swayback) 5. lack of development 6. bone marrow tumor 7. artificial substitute for a body part 8. cutting into skull 9. puncture of a joint to withdraw fluid 10. bursa inflammation

H. 1. nonsteroidal anti-inflammatory drugs, b 2. corticosteroids, e 3. skeletal muscle relaxants, a 4. bone reabsorption inhibitors, c 5. calcium supplements, d

I. 1. massage 2. mobilization 3. hydrotherapy 4. ultrasound 5. thermotherapy 6. phonophoresis 7. cryotherapy 8. gait training

J. 1. c 2. h 3. f 4. g 5. d 6. e 7. a 8. b

K. 1. spelled correctly 2. pseudohypertrophic 3. polymyositis 4. spelled correctly 5. spelled correctly 6. osteochondroma 7. spondylosis 8. spelled correctly 9. spelled correctly 10. exostosis

Labeling Exercises

A. 1. skull 2. cervical vertebrae 3. sternum 4. ribs 5. thoracic vertebrae 6. lumbar vertebrae 7. ilium 8. pubis 9. ischium 10. femur 11. patella 12. tibia 13. fibula 14. tarsus 15. metatarsus 16. phalanges 17. maxilla 18. mandible 19. scapula 20. humerus 21. ulna 22. radius 23. sacrum 24. coccyx 25. carpus 26. metacarpus 27. phalanges

B. 1. proximal epiphysis 2. diaphysis 3. distal epiphysis 4. articular cartilage 5. epiphyseal line 6. spongy or cancellous bone 7. compact or cortical bone 8. medullary cavity

C. 1. periosteum 2. synovial membrane 3. articular cartilage 4. joint cavity 5. joint capsule

Chapter 5 Answers
Practice As You Go

A. 1. cardiology 2. endocardium, myocardium, epicardium 3. sinoatrial node 4. away from 5. tricuspid, pulmonary, mitral (bicuspid), aortic 6. atria, ventricles 7. pulmonary 8. apex 9. septum 10. systole, diastole

B. 1. arteries, veins, capillaries 2. veins 3. arteries 4. capillaries 5. systolic, diastolic

C. 1. cardiac or coronary 2. interventricular 3. arterial 4. venular 5. myocardial 6. atrial

D. 1. f 2. h 3. d 4. g 5. b 6. i 7. a 8. c 9. e 10. j

E. 1. c 2. g 3. j 4. a 5. d 6. b 7. i 8. e 9. f 10. h

F. 1. MVP 2. VSD 3. PTCA 4. V fib 5. DVT 6. ASHD 7. CoA 8. tPA 9. CV 10. ECC

Real-World Applications
Medical Record Analysis

1. hypertension—Blood pressure above the normal range.

2. tachycardia—The condition of having a fast heart rate, typically more than 100 beats/minute while at rest.

3. congestive heart failure (CHF)—Pathological condition of the heart in which there is a reduced outflow of blood from the left side of the heart because the left ventricle myocardium has become too weak to efficiently pump blood. Results in weakness, breathlessness, and edema.

4. mitral valve prolapse—Condition in which the cusps or flaps of the heart valve are too loose and fail to shut tightly, allowing blood to flow backward through the valve when the heart chamber contracts. Most commonly occurs in the mitral valve, but may affect any of the heart valves.

5. palpitations—Pounding, racing heartbeats.

6. electrocardiography (EKG)—Process of recording the electrical activity of the heart. Useful in the diagnosis of abnormal cardiac rhythm and heart muscle (myocardium) damage.

7. cardiac biomarkers—Blood test to determine the level of proteins specific to heart muscles in the blood. An increase in these proteins may indicate heart muscle damage such as a myocardial infarction. These proteins include creatine kinase (CK) and troponin.

8. echocardiography—Noninvasive diagnostic method using ultrasound to visualize internal cardiac structures. Cardiac valve activity can be evaluated using this method.

9. stress test—Method for evaluating cardiovascular fitness. The patient is placed on a treadmill or a bicycle and then subjected to steadily increasing levels of work. An EKG and oxygen levels are taken while the patient exercises. The test is stopped if abnormalities occur on the EKG. Also called an *exercise test* or a *treadmill test*.

10. angiocardiography—X-rays taken after the injection of an opaque material into a blood vessel. Can be performed on the aorta as an aortic angiogram, on the heart as an angiocardiogram, and on the brain as a cerebral angiogram.

11. coronary artery disease (CAD)—Insufficient blood supply to the heart muscle due to an obstruction of one or more coronary arteries. May be caused by atherosclerosis and may cause angina pectoris and myocardial infarction.

12. myocardial infarction—Condition caused by the partial or complete occlusion or closing of one or more of the coronary arteries. Symptoms include a squeezing pain or heavy pressure in the middle of the chest (angina pectoris). A delay in treatment could result in death. Also referred to as a *heart attack*.

13. mitral valvoplasty—Removal of a diseased heart valve and replacement with an artificial valve.

Chart Note Transcription

1. angina pectoris 2. bradycardia 3. hypertension 4. myocardial infarction (MI) 5. electrocardiogram (EKG, ECG) 6. cardiac biomarkers 7. coronary artery disease (CAD) 8. cardiac catheterization 9. stress test (treadmill test) 10. percutaneous transluminal coronary angioplasty (PTCA) 11. coronary artery bypass graft (CABG)

Case Study

1. Heart attack; condition caused by the partial or complete occlusion or closing of one or more of the coronary arteries. Symptoms include a squeezing pain or heavy pressure in the middle of the chest (angina pectoris). A delay in treatment could result in death.

2. The main complaint, the one the patient is most aware of or most anxious about.

3. Angina pectoris—Condition in which there is severe pain with a sensation of constriction around the heart; caused by a deficiency of oxygen to the heart muscle.

4. Nausea—Feeling of need to vomit; dyspnea—Difficulty breathing; diaphoresis—Profuse sweating.

5. Cardiac biomarkers; angiocardiography; cardiac scan; electrocardiography; stress testing; cardiac catheterization; Holter monitor.

6. Smokes; overweight; family history; sedentary lifestyle. He can stop smoking, lose weight, and become more active.

Practice Exercises

A. 1. cardiac 2. cardiomyopathy 3. cardiomegaly 4. tachycardia 5. bradycardia 6. electrocardiogram 7. angiostenosis 8. angiitis 9. angiospasm 10. arterial 11. arteriosclerosis 12. arteriole 13. endocarditis 14. epicarditis 15. myocarditis

B. 1. aortic 2. atrial 3. heart 4. venous 5. arteriole 6. ventricle 7. valvular 8. myocardial 9. venular 10. heart 11. blood vessel 12. artery

C. 1. angiogram 2. tachycardia 3. cardiomyopathy 4. endocarditis 5. arteriosclerosis 6. hypertension 7. atheroma 8. phlebitis 9. thrombolytic 10. embolectomy 11. intracoronary 12. valvoplasty

D. 1. pulmonary, systemic 2. myocardium 3. septum 4. tricuspid, mitral or bicuspid, pulmonary, aortic 5. sinoatrial node 6. coronary 7. Blood pressure 8. capillary bed

E. 1. BBB 2. MI 3. PAC 4. EKG or ECG 5. ECHO 6. PTCA 7. ECC 8. DVT 9. CHF 10. CSD

F. 1. thin flexible tube 2. an area of dead tissue 3. a blood clot 4. pounding heartbeat 5. backflow 6. weakened and ballooning arterial wall 7. complete stoppage of heart activity 8. serious cardiac arrhythmia 9. heart attack 10. varicose veins in anal region

G. 1. murmur 2. defibrillation 3. hypertension 4. pacemaker 5. varicose veins 6. angina pectoris 7. CCU 8. MI 9. angiography 10. echocardiogram 11. Holter monitor 12. CHF

H. 1. antiarrhythmic, e 2. antilipidemic, g 3. cardiotonic, f 4. diuretic, h 5. anticoagulant, b 6. fibrinolytic, a 7. vasodilator, d 8. calcium channel blocker, c

I. 1. cardiomyopathy 2. tachycardia 3. spelled correctly 4. spelled correctly 5. spelled correctly 6. spelled correctly 7. spelled correctly 8. infarction 9. arrhythmia 10. angiitis

Labeling Exercises

A. 1. pulmonary arteries 2. vena cavae 3. right atrium 4. right ventricle 5. systemic veins 6. capillary bed of lungs 7. pulmonary veins 8. aorta 9. left atrium 10. left ventricle 11. systemic arteries 12. systemic capillary beds

B. 1. superior vena cava 2. aorta 3. pulmonary trunk 4. pulmonary valve 5. right atrium 6. tricuspid valve 7. right ventricle 8. inferior vena cava 9. pulmonary artery 10. pulmonary vein 11. left atrium 12. aortic valve 13. mitral or bicuspid valve 14. left ventricle 15. endocardium 16. myocardium 17. pericardium

Chapter 6 Answers
Practice As You Go

A. **1.** phagocytosis **2.** erythrocytes (red blood cells), leukocytes (white blood cells), platelets (thrombocytes) **3.** plasma **4.** hemostasis **5.** ABO system, Rh factor
B. **1.** hematic or sanguineous **2.** leukocytic **3.** thrombocytic **4.** fibrinous **5.** erythrocytic
C. **1.** d **2.** e **3.** c **4.** b **5.** a
D. **1.** c **2.** e **3.** a **4.** b **5.** d
E. **1.** ALL **2.** BMT **3.** eosins or eos **4.** HCT or Hct or crit **5.** PA **6.** CBC **7.** diff **8.** WBC **9.** noc **10.** pc
F. **1.** spleen, tonsils, thymus **2.** thoracic duct, right lymphatic duct **3.** axillary, cervical, mediastinal, inguinal **4.** active acquired **5.** antibody-mediated
G. **1.** splenic **2.** lymphatic **3.** tonsillar **4.** thymic **5.** lymphangial
H. **1.** c **2.** a **3.** d **4.** e **5.** b
I. **1.** e **2.** c **3.** d **4.** a **5.** b
J. **1.** AIDS **2.** ARC **3.** HIV **4.** mono **5.** KS **6.** Ig **7.** SCIDS **8.** PCP

Real-World Applications
Medical Record Analysis

1. splenomegaly—An enlarged spleen.
2. non-Hodgkin's lymphoma—Cancer of the lymphatic tissues other than Hodgkin's lymphoma.
3. spleen—An organ located in the upper left quadrant of the abdomen. Consists of lymphatic tissue that is highly infiltrated with blood vessels. It filters out and destroys old red blood cells.
4. splenectomy—The surgical removal of the spleen.
5. Monospot—A blood test for infectious mononucleosis.
6. HIV antigen/antibody immunoassay —A blood test for HIV infection. HIV antigen (foreign viral proteins) can be detected shortly after exposure and antibodies produced by the body in response to an HIV infection can be detected 2–8 weeks after exposure.
7. Magnetic resonance imaging (MRI)—Medical imaging that uses radio-frequency radiation as its source of energy. It does not require the injection of contrast medium or exposure to ionizing radiation. The technique is useful for visualizing large blood vessels, the heart, the brain, and soft tissues.
8. tumor—Abnormal growth of tissue that may be benign or malignant.
9. biopsy—A piece of tissue is removed by syringe and needle, knife, punch, or brush to examine under a microscope. Used to aid in diagnosis.
10. chemotherapy—Treating diseases, especially cancer, with chemicals that are toxic to cells of the body.

Chart Note Transcription

1. hematologist **2.** HIV antigen/antibody immunoassay **3.** prothrombin time **4.** complete blood count (CBC) **5.** erythropenia **6.** thrombopenia **7.** leukocytosis **8.** bone marrow aspiration **9.** leukemia **10.** homologous transfusion

Case Study

1. Acute lymphocytic leukemia.
2. High fever; thrombopenia—Too few platelets; epistaxis—Nosebleed; gingival bleeding—Gums bleeding; petechiae—Pinpoint bruises; ecchymoses—Large black and blue bruises.
3. Bone marrow aspiration—Sample of bone marrow is removed by aspiration with a needle and examined for diseases.
4. A diagnosis based on the results of the physician's direct examination rather than based on other tests like X-rays and labwork.
5. Chemotherapy—Treating disease by using chemicals that have a toxic effect on the body, especially cancerous tissue.
6. Remission—A period during which the symptoms of a disease or disorder leave. Can be temporary.

Practice Exercises

A. **1.** splenomegaly **2.** splenectomy **3.** splenotomy **4.** lymphocytes **5.** lymphoma **6.** lymphadenopathy **7.** lymphadenoma **8.** lymphadenitis **9.** immunologist **10.** immunoglobulin **11.** immunology **12.** hematic **13.** hematoma **14.** hematopoiesis **15.** hemolytic **16.** hemoglobin **17.** leukopenia **18.** erythropenia **19.** pancytopenia **20.** leukocytosis **21.** erythrocytosis **22.** thrombocytosis **23.** erythrocyte **24.** leukocyte **25.** lymphocyte
B. **1.** HCT or Hct or crit **2.** HIV, AIDS **3.** ESR or sed rate **4.** GVHD **5.** C&S **6.** PCP **7.** Pro-time or PT **8.** AML, ALL **9.** RBC, WBC **10.** PA
C. **1.** erythrocytosis **2.** hyperlipidemia **3.** leukopenia **4.** hemoglobin **5.** phlebotomy **6.** fibrinolytic **7.** morphology **8.** hematocrit **9.** pathology **10.** lymphedema **11.** lymphangioma **12.** immunotherapy **13.** tonsillectomy **14.** myeloma **15.** splenomegaly
D. **1.** polycythemia vera **2.** mononucleosis **3.** anaphylactic shock **4.** HIV **5.** Kaposi's sarcoma **6.** autoimmune diseases **7.** Hodgkin's disease **8.** pneumocystis **9.** aplastic **10.** pernicious
E. **1.** reverse transcriptase inhibitor, e **2.** anticoagulant, a **3.** antihemorrhagic, d **4.** antihistamine, h **5.** immunosuppressant, f **6.** fibrinolytic, b **7.** hematinic, g **8.** corticosteroid, c **9.** antiplatelet agent, i

F. **1.** d **2.** f **3.** b **4.** g **5.** a **6.** e **7.** c
G. **1.** treatment with an antibody injection **2.** blood test for mononucleosis **3.** infections seen in immunocompromised patients **4.** intense itching **5.** tissue's response to injury **6.** blood transfusion from another person **7.** caused by vitamin B_{12} deficiency **8.** cancer of blood-forming bone marrow **9.** rapid flow of blood, bleeding **10.** blood poisoning
H. **1.** axillary **2.** sanguineous or hematic **3.** lymph vessel **4.** fibers **5.** spleen **6.** thymus gland **7.** thrombocytic **8.** leukocytic **9.** erythrocytic **10.** tonsils
I. **1.** tonsillitis **2.** spelled correctly **3.** spelled correctly **4.** spelled correctly **5.** inflammation **6.** spelled correctly **7.** autologous **8.** spelled correctly **9.** pancytopenia **10.** dyscrasia
J. **1.** hemoglobin **2.** eosinophils, basophils, neutrophils, monocytes, lymphocytes **3.** Platelet **4.** donor, recipient **5.** lacteals **6.** Lymph nodes **7.** spleen **8.** cellular

Labeling Exercises

A. **1.** plasma **2.** red blood cells or erythrocytes **3.** platelets or thrombocytes **4.** white blood cells or leukocytes
B. **1.** cervical nodes **2.** mediastinal nodes **3.** axillary nodes **4.** inguinal nodes
C. **1.** thymus gland **2.** lymph node **3.** tonsil **4.** spleen **5.** lymphatic vessels

Chapter 7 Answers
Practice As You Go

A. **1.** nasal cavity, pharynx, larynx, trachea, bronchial tubes, lungs **2.** pharynx **3.** epiglottis **4.** 3, 2 **5.** alveoli **6.** pleura **7.** bronchioles, alveoli
B. **1.** c **2.** f **3.** a **4.** h **5.** g **6.** b **7.** e **8.** d
C. **1.** laryngeal **2.** pulmonary **3.** paranasal **4.** alveolar **5.** nasal **6.** diaphragmatic
D. **1.** e **2.** i **3.** h **4.** a **5.** j **6.** d **7.** b **8.** g **9.** f **10.** c
E. **1.** f **2.** c **3.** e **4.** a **5.** d **6.** b
F. **1.** URI **2.** PFT **3.** O_2 **4.** CO_2 **5.** COPD **6.** Bronch **7.** TB **8.** IRDS

Real-World Applications
Medical Record Analysis

1. asthma—Disease caused by various conditions, such as allergens, and resulting in constriction of the bronchial airways, dyspnea, coughing, and wheezing. Can cause violent spasms of the bronchi (bronchospasms) but is generally not a life-threatening condition. Medication can be very effective.
2. dyspnea—Term describing difficult or labored breathing.
3. cyanosis—Refers to the bluish tint of skin that is receiving an insufficient amount of oxygen or circulation.
4. expiration—To breathe out; exhale.
5. phlegm—Thick mucus secreted by the membranes that line the respiratory tract. When phlegm is coughed through the mouth, it is called *sputum*. Phlegm is examined for color, odor, and consistency.
6. auscultation—To listen to body sounds, usually using a stethoscope.
7. rhonchi—Somewhat musical sound during expiration, often found in asthma or infection. Caused by spasms of the bronchial tubes. Also called *wheezing*.
8. arterial blood gases (ABGs)—Testing for the gases present in the blood. Generally used to assist in determining the levels of oxygen (O_2) and carbon dioxide (CO_2) in the blood.
9. hypoxemia—The condition of having an insufficient amount of oxygen in the bloodstream.
10. spirometry—Procedure to measure lung capacity using a *spirometer*.
11. Proventil—Medication that relaxes muscle spasms in bronchial tubes. Used to treat asthma.
12. bronchospasms—An involuntary muscle spasm of the smooth muscle in the wall of the bronchus.

Chart Note Transcription

1. dyspnea **2.** tachypnea **3.** arterial blood gases (ABGs) **4.** hypoxemia **5.** auscultation **6.** crackles **7.** purulent **8.** sputum **9.** CXR **10.** pneumonia **11.** endotracheal intubation

Case Study

1. Pneumonia.
2. Dyspnea—Difficulty breathing; dizziness; orthopnea—Comfortable breathing only while sitting up; elevated temperature, cough.
3. Auscultation (listening to the body sounds) revealed crackles (abnormal sound); chest X-ray revealed fluid in the upper lobe of the right lung.
4. A method of determining a patient's general health and heart and lung function by measuring pulse (100 BPM and rapid), respiratory rate (24 breaths/min and labored), temperature (102°F), and blood pressure (180/110).
5. IV antibiotics—Medicine to kill bacteria given into a vein; intermittent positive pressure breathing—Method of assisting patients in breathing by using a machine that produces an increased pressure.

6. The IV antibiotics were changed to oral antibiotics—she started taking pills.

Practice Exercises

A. **1.** exchange of O_2 and CO_2 **2.** ventilation **3.** exchange of O_2 and CO_2 in the lungs **4.** exchange of O_2 and CO_2 at cellular level **5.** diaphragm **6.** volume of air in the lungs after a maximal inhalation or inspiration **7.** amount of air entering lungs in a single inspiration or leaving lungs in single expiration of quiet breathing **8.** air remaining in the lungs after a forced expiration **9.** nasal cavity, pharynx, larynx, trachea, bronchial tubes, lungs **10.** respiratory rate, temperature, heart rate, blood pressure

B. **1.** rhinitis **2.** rhinorrhea **3.** rhinoplasty **4.** laryngitis **5.** laryngospasm **6.** laryngoscopy **7.** laryngeal **8.** laryngectomy **9.** laryngoplasty **10.** laryngoplegia **11.** bronchial **12.** bronchitis **13.** bronchoscopy **14.** bronchogenic **15.** bronchospasm **16.** thoracotomy **17.** thoracalgia **18.** thoracic **19.** tracheotomy **20.** tracheostenosis **21.** endotracheal **22.** dyspnea **23.** tachypnea **24.** orthopnea **25.** apnea

C. **1.** anosmia **2.** bradypnea **3.** laryngoplegia **4.** hemoptysis **5.** rhinorrhagia **6.** dysphonia **7.** pharyngitis **8.** bronchiectasis **9.** anthracosis **10.** pneumothorax **11.** oximeter **12.** laryngoscopy **13.** pleurocentesis **14.** cardiopulmonary **15.** tracheostenosis

D. **1.** inhalation or inspiration **2.** hemoptysis **3.** pulmonary emboli **4.** sinusitis **5.** pharyngitis **6.** pneumothorax **7.** pertussis **8.** pleurotomy **9.** pleurodynia **10.** nasopharyngitis

E. **1.** ENT **2.** COPD **3.** CF **4.** IRDS **5.** PE **6.** SIDS **7.** ABGs **8.** CXR **9.** PFT **10.** CPAP

F. **1.** cardiopulmonary resuscitation **2.** thoracentesis **3.** respirator **4.** supplemental oxygen **5.** patent **6.** ventilation-perfusion scan **7.** sputum cytology **8.** hyperventilation **9.** rhonchi **10.** anthracosis

G. **1.** decongestant, f **2.** antitussive, a **3.** antibiotic, c **4.** expectorant, g **5.** mucolytic, h **6.** bronchodilator, d **7.** antihistamine, e **8.** corticosteroid, b

H. **1.** alveolar **2.** lung **3.** thoracic **4.** bronchus **5.** tracheal **6.** epiglottis **7.** mucous **8.** pharyngeal **9.** bronchiole **10.** septum

I. **1.** nasopharyngeal **2.** spelled correctly **3.** cannula **4.** hemoptysis **5.** bronchodilator **6.** spelled correctly **7.** spelled correctly **8.** spelled correctly **9.** spelled correctly **10.** pneumoconiosis

Labeling Exercises

A. **1.** pharynx and larynx **2.** trachea **3.** nasal cavity **4.** bronchial tubes **5.** lungs

B. **1.** nares **2.** paranasal sinuses **3.** nasal cavity **4.** hard palate **5.** soft palate **6.** palatine tonsil **7.** epiglottis **8.** vocal cords **9.** esophagus **10.** trachea

C. **1.** trachea **2.** right upper lobe **3.** right middle lobe **4.** right lower lobe **5.** apex of lung **6.** left upper lobe **7.** left lower lobe **8.** diaphragm

Chapter 8 Answers
Practice As You Go

A. **1.** gastrointestinal (GI) **2.** gut, alimentary canal, gastrointestinal tract, mouth, anus **3.** digesting food, absorbing nutrients, eliminating waste **4.** incisors, cuspids or canines **5.** bicuspids or premolars, molars **6.** crown, root **7.** enamel **8.** deciduous, permanent

B. **1.** oropharynx **2.** peristalsis **3.** hydrochloric acid, chyme **4.** duodenum, jejunum, ileum **5.** villi **6.** ileocecal valve, anus, cecum, colon, rectum **7.** sigmoid **8.** defecation

C. **1.** salivary glands, liver, gallbladder, pancreas **2.** amylase, carbohydrates **3.** bile, emulsification, gallbladder **4.** duodenum, buffers, pancreatic enzymes

D. **1.** duodenal **2.** nasogastric **3.** hepatic **4.** pancreatic **5.** cholecystic or cystic **6.** sublingual **7.** esophageal **8.** sigmoidal

E. **1.** i **2.** f **3.** c **4.** a **5.** j **6.** l **7.** e **8.** b **9.** k **10.** d **11.** g **12.** o **13.** h **14.** n **15.** m

F. **1.** f **2.** g **3.** e **4.** h **5.** b **6.** a **7.** d **8.** c

G. **1.** NG **2.** GI **3.** HBV **4.** FOBT **5.** IBD **6.** HSV-1 **7.** AST **8.** pc **9.** PUD **10.** GERD

Real-World Applications
Medical Record Analysis

1. epigastric—Pertaining to the area above the stomach.
2. anemia—A large group of conditions characterized by a reduction in the number of red blood cells or the amount of hemoglobin in the blood; results in less oxygen reaching the tissues.
3. melena—Passage of dark tarry stool. Color is the result of digestive enzymes working on blood in the gastrointestinal tract.
4. dyspepsia—An "upset stomach."
5. antacids—Medication to neutralize stomach acid.
6. complete blood count (CBC)—A combination of blood tests including red blood cell count, white blood cell count, hemoglobin, hematocrit, white blood cell differential, and platelet count.

7. fecal occult blood—Laboratory test on the feces to determine if microscopic amounts of blood are present. Also called *hemoccult* or *stool guaiac*.

8. *Helicobacter pylori*—A bacteria that may damage the lining of the stomach setting up the conditions for peptic ulcer disease to develop.

9. gastroscopy—Procedure in which a flexible *gastroscope* is passed through the mouth and down the esophagus in order to visualize inside the stomach. Used to diagnose peptic ulcers and gastric carcinoma.

10. ulcer—An open sore or lesion in the skin or mucous membrane.

11. peptic ulcer disease—Ulcer occurring in the lower portion of the esophagus, stomach, and/or duodenum; thought to be caused by the acid of gastric juices. Initial damage to the protective lining of the stomach may be caused by a *Helicobacter pylori* (*H. pylori*) bacterial infection. If the ulcer extends all the way through the wall of the stomach, it is called a *perforated ulcer*, which requires immediate surgery to repair.

12. gastrectomy—Surgical removal of the stomach.

Chart Note Transcription

1. gastroenterologist 2. constipation 3. cholelithiasis 4. cholecystectomy 5. gastroesophageal reflux disease 6. ascites 7. lower gastrointestinal series 8. polyposis 9. colonoscopy 10. sigmoid colon 11. colectomy 12. colostomy

Case Study

1. Severe RUQ pain—Severe pain is located in the upper right corner of the abdomen; nausea—Feeling the urge to vomit; scleral jaundice—The whites of the eye have a yellowish cast to them.

2. Gallbladder, right kidney, majority of the liver, a small portion of the pancreas, portion of colon and small intestine.

3. Gallstones blocking the common bile duct so bile can't drain into the small intestine.

4. Abdominal ultrasound—The use of high-frequency sound waves to produce an image of an organ, such as the gallbladder; percutaneous transhepatic cholangiography (PTC)—Procedure in which contrast medium is injected directly into the liver to visualize the bile ducts; used to detect obstructions such as gallstones in the common bile duct.

5. Cholelithiasis is the condition of having gallstones present in the gallbladder, they may not be causing any symptoms; cholecystitis is the inflammation of the gallbladder that occurs when gallstones block the flow of bile out of the gallbladder.

6. Laparoscopic cholecystectomy—The gallbladder was removed through a very small abdominal incision with the assistance of a laparoscope.

Practice Exercises

A. 1. gastritis 2. gastroenterology 3. gastrectomy 4. gastroscopy 5. gastralgia 6. gastromegaly 7. gastrotomy 8. esophagitis 9. esophagoscopy 10. esophagoplasty 11. esophageal 12. esophagectomy 13. proctopexy 14. proctoptosis 15. proctitis 16. proctologist 17. cholecystectomy 18. cholecystolithiasis 19. cholecystolithotripsy 20. cholecystitis 21. laparoscope 22. laparotomy 23. laparoscopy 24. hepatoma 25. hepatomegaly 26. hepatic 27. hepatitis 28. pancreatitis 29. pancreatic 30. colostomy 31. colitis

B. 1. pharyngoplasty 2. hepatoma 3. gastrectomy 4. polyposis 5. sigmoidoscope 6. postprandial 7. cholecystogram 8. pancreatitis 9. sialadenitis 10. anorexia 11. hematemesis 12. bradypepsia 13. gastroenterology 14. dysphagia 15. periodontal

C. 1. TPN, NG 2. UGI 3. O&P 4. IBS 5. PUD 6. GERD 7. N&V 8. AST, ALT 9. FOBT 10. BM

D. 1. visual exam of the colon 2. tooth X-ray 3. bright red blood in the stool 4. blood test to determine amount of waste product bilirubin in the bloodstream 5. weight loss and wasting from a chronic illness 6. use of NG tube to wash out stomach 7. surgical repair of hernia 8. pulling teeth 9. surgical crushing of common bile duct stone 10. surgically create a connection between two organs or vessels

E. 1. liver biopsy 2. colostomy 3. barium swallow 4. lower GI series 5. colectomy 6. fecal occult blood test 7. choledocholithotripsy 8. total parenteral nutrition 9. gastric stapling 10. intravenous cholecystography 11. colonoscopy 12. ileostomy

F. 1. d 2. g 3. h 4. e 5. f 6. b 7. c 8. a

G. 1. antidiarrheal, f 2. proton pump inhibitor, h 3. antiemetic, d 4. H₂-receptor antagonist, a 5. anorexiant, b 6. laxative, c 7. antacid, e 8. antiviral, g

H. 1. spelled correctly 2. salivary 3. ileocecal 4. submandibular 5. spelled correctly 6. spelled correctly 7. spelled correctly 8. proctoptosis 9. spelled correctly 10. antidiarrheal

I. 1. buccal 2. cholecystic 3. jejunum 4. colon and rectum 5. hypoglossal or sublingual 6. small intestine 7. pancreas 8. dental 9. lip 10. sigmoid colon 11. pharyngeal 12. gastric 13. duodenum 14. hepatic 15. oral

J. **1.** buffers, pancreatic enzymes **2.** bile, liver **3.** amylase **4.** ileocecal valve, anus **5.** small intestine **6.** pyloric sphincter **7.** peristalsis **8.** epiglottis **9.** cuspids or canines, incisors, bicuspids or premolars, molars **10.** gingiva

Labeling Exercises

A. **1.** salivary glands **2.** esophagus **3.** pancreas **4.** small intestine **5.** oral cavity **6.** stomach **7.** liver and gallbladder **8.** colon

B. **1.** esophagus **2.** cardiac or lower esophageal sphincter **3.** pyloric sphincter **4.** duodenum **5.** antrum **6.** fundus of stomach **7.** rugae **8.** body of stomach

C. **1.** cystic duct **2.** common bile duct **3.** gallbladder **4.** duodenum **5.** liver **6.** hepatic duct **7.** pancreas **8.** pancreatic duct

Chapter 9 Answers
Practice As You Go

A. **1.** nephrons **2.** Bowman's capsule, loop of Henle **3.** smooth muscle **4.** retroperitoneal **5.** glomerulus **6.** calyx **7.** two, one **8.** micturition, voiding

B. **1.** homeostasis **2.** filtration, reabsorption, secretion **3.** electrolytes **4.** peritubular **5.** Specific gravity **6.** muscle

C. **1.** ureteral **2.** renal **3.** glomerular **4.** urinary **5.** urethral

D. **1.** c **2.** g **3.** h **4.** i **5.** f **6.** e **7.** d **8.** b **9.** a **10.** j

E. **1.** f **2.** e **3.** h **4.** a **5.** g **6.** c **7.** d **8.** b

F. **1.** kidneys, ureters, bladder **2.** catheterization **3.** cystoscopy **4.** genitourinary **5.** extracorporeal shockwave lithotripsy **6.** urinary tract infection **7.** urine culture **8.** retrograde pyelogram **9.** acute renal failure **10.** blood urea nitrogen **11.** chronic renal failure **12.** water

Real-World Applications
Medical Record Analysis

1. hematuria—The presence of blood in the urine.
2. pyelonephritis—Inflammation of the renal pelvis and the kidney. One of the most common types of kidney disease. It may be the result of a lower urinary tract infection that moved up to the kidney by way of the ureters. There may be large quantities of white blood cells and bacteria in the urine. Blood (hematuria) may even be present in the urine in this condition. Can occur with any untreated or persistent case of cystitis.
3. chronic cystitis—Urinary bladder inflammation.
4. dysuria—Difficult or painful urination.

5. clean catch urinalysis—Laboratory test that consists of the physical, chemical, and microscopic examination of urine.
6. pyuria—The presence of pus in the urine.
7. culture and sensitivity—Laboratory test of urine for bacterial infection. Attempt to grow bacteria on a culture medium in order to identify it and determine which antibiotics it is sensitive to.
8. pathogen—Anything, such as bacteria, viruses, fungi, or toxins, that may cause disease.
9. antibiotic—Medication used to treat bacterial infections of the urinary tract.
10. cystoscopy—Visual examination of the urinary bladder using an instrument called a *cystoscope*.
11. bladder neck obstruction—Blockage of the bladder outlet. Often caused by an enlarged prostate gland in males.
12. congenital—Present from birth.
13. catheterized—Insertion of a tube through the urethra and into the urinary bladder for the purpose of withdrawing urine or inserting dye.

Chart Note Transcription

1. urologist **2.** hematuria **3.** cystitis **4.** clean-catch specimen **5.** urinalysis (U/A, UA) **6.** pyuria **7.** retrograde pyelogram **8.** ureter **9.** ureterolith **10.** extracorporeal shockwave lithotripsy (ESWL) **11.** calculi

Case Study

1. Cystitis—Inflammation of the urinary bladder; pyelonephritis—Inflammation of the renal pelvis and the kidney. One of the most common types of kidney disease. It may be the result of a lower urinary tract infection that moved up to the kidney by way of the ureters. There may be large quantities of white blood cells and bacteria in the urine. Blood (hematuria) may even be present in the urine in this condition. Can occur with any untreated or persistent case of cystitis.
2. Fever; chills; fatigue; urgency—Feeling the need to urinate immediately; frequency—Urge to urinate more often than normal; dysuria—Difficult or painful urination; hematuria—Blood in the urine; cloudy urine with a fishy smell—Urine was not clear and smelled bad.
3. Clean catch specimen—Urine sample obtained after cleaning off the urinary opening and catching or collecting a urine sample in midstream (halfway through the urination process) to minimize contamination from the genitalia; U/A (urinalysis)—A physical, chemical, and microscopic examination of the urine; urine C&S (culture & sensitivity)—Test for the presence and identification of bacteria in

the urine; KUB (kidneys, ureters, and bladder)—An X-ray of the urinary organs.

4. Pyuria—Pus in the urine; bacteriuria—Bacteria in the urine; acidic pH—Indicates a urinary tract infection; culture and sensitivity—Revealed a common type of bacteria; KUB—Pyelonephritis.

5. Antibiotic—To kill the bacteria; push fluids—To flush out the bladder.

6. Clear, pale yellow to deep gold color, aromatic odor, specific gravity between 1.010–1.030, pH between 5.0–8.0, very little protein, no glucose, ketones, or blood.

Practice Exercises

A. 1. nephropexy 2. nephrogram 3. nephrolithiasis 4. nephrectomy 5. nephritis 6. nephropathy 7. nephrosclerosis 8. cystitis 9. cystorrhagia 10. cystoplasty 11. cystoscope 12. cystalgia 13. pyeloplasty 14. pyelitis 15. pyelogram 16. ureterolith 17. ureterectasis 18. ureterostenosis 19. urethritis 20. urethroscope 21. oliguria 22. hematuria 23. proteinuria 24. glycosuria 25. pyuria

B. 1. cystopexy 2. lithotripsy 3. pyeloplasty 4. urinalysis 5. nephroptosis 6. pyuria 7. ureterectasis 8. glomerulonephritis 9. meatotomy 10. urethralgia

C. 1. antispasmodic, b 2. antibiotic, c 3. diuretic, a

D. 1. urination or voiding urine 2. increases urine production 3. pain associated with kidney stone 4. inserting a tube through urethra into the bladder 5. inflammation of renal pelvis 6. inflammation of glomeruli in the kidney 7. cutting into an organ to remove stone 8. bedwetting 9. enlargement of urethral opening 10. damage to glomerulus secondary to diabetes mellitus 11. lab test of chemical composition of urine 12. decrease in force of urine stream

E. 1. anuria 2. hematuria 3. calculus or nephrolith 4. lithotripsy 5. urethritis 6. pyuria 7. bacteriuria 8. dysuria 9. ketonuria 10. proteinuria 11. polyuria

F. 1. HD 2. ESWL 3. cysto 4. IVP 5. KUB 6. C&S 7. BNO 8. UTI

G. 1. renal transplant 2. nephropexy 3. urinary tract infection 4. pyelolithectomy 5. renal biopsy 6. ureterectomy 7. cystostomy 8. cystoscopy 9. IVP

H. 1. bladder 2. ureteral 3. urine 4. renal 5. glomerulus 6. renal pelvis 7. meatal 8. urethral

I. 1. spelled correctly 2. nephrosclerosis 3. spelled correctly 4. spelled correctly 5. incontinence 6. spelled correctly 7. cystocele 8. catheterization 9. spelled correctly 10. lithotripsy

J. 1. nitrogenous wastes 2. renal corpuscle 3. electrolytes 4. rugae 5. loop of Henle 6. urethra, ureters 7. hilum 8. cortex, medulla

Labeling Exercises

A. 1. kidney 2. urinary bladder 3. ureter 4. male urethra 5. female urethra

B. 1. cortex 2. medulla 3. calyx 4. renal pelvis 5. renal papilla 6. renal pyramid 7. ureter

C. 1. efferent arteriole 2. glomerular (Bowman's) capsule 3. glomerulus 4. afferent arteriole 5. proximal convoluted tubule 6. descending nephron loop 7. distal convoluted tubule 8. collecting tubule 9. ascending nephron loop 10. peritubular capillaries

Chapter 10 Answers
Practice As You Go

A. 1. uterine tubes 2. vulva 3. estrogen, progesterone 4. menopause 5. ovum 6. endometrium 7. hymen 8. lactation

B. 1. placenta, umbilical cord 2. gestation 3. dilation, expulsion, placental 4. crowning 5. breech 6. amnion, chorion

C. 1. embryonic 2. fetal 3. uterine 4. ovarian 5. mammary 6. vaginal

D. 1. b 2. h 3. g 4. c 5. a 6. i 7. j 8. d 9. e 10. f

E. 1. e 2. g 3. d 4. a 5. h 6. c 7. b 8. f

F. 1. GI or grav I 2. AI 3. UC 4. FTND 5. IUD 6. D&C 7. HRT 8. gyn or GYN 9. AB 10. OCPs

G. 1. urinary, reproductive 2. testes, epididymis, penis 3. foreskin 4. testes 5. bulbourethral glands 6. testosterone 7. perineum

H. 1. testicular 2. spermatic 3. vesicular 4. penile 5. prostatic

I. 1. b 2. e 3. a 4. c 5. f 6. d

J. 1. c 2. a 3. d 4. b 5. e

K. 1. ED 2. GC 3. DRE 4. TURP 5. STI

Real-World Applications
Medical Record Analysis

1. gestation—The length of time of pregnancy, normally about 40 weeks.

2. amniocentesis—Puncturing of the amniotic sac using a needle and syringe for the purpose of withdrawing amniotic fluid for testing. Can assist in determining fetal maturity, development, and genetic disorders.

3. fetus—The unborn infant from approximately week 9 until birth.

4. obstetrician—Branch of medicine specializing in the diagnosis and treatment of women during pregnancy and childbirth, and immediately after childbirth. Physician is called an *obstetrician*.

5. multigravida—A woman who has been pregnant two or more times.

6. nullipara—A woman who has not given birth to a live infant.
7. miscarriage—Unplanned loss of a pregnancy due to the death of the embryo or fetus before the time it is viable, also referred to as a *spontaneous abortion*.
8. pelvic ultrasound—Use of high-frequency sound waves to produce an image or photograph of an organ, such as the uterus, ovaries, or fetus.
9. placenta previa—A placenta that is implanted in the lower portion of the uterus and, in turn, blocks the birth canal.
10. abruptio placentae—Emergency condition in which the placenta tears away from the uterine wall prior to delivery of the infant. Requires immediate delivery of the baby.
11. placenta—The organ that connects the fetus to the mother's uterus, supplies fetus with oxygen and nutrients.
12. C-section—Surgical delivery of a baby through an incision into the abdominal and uterine walls.

Chart Note Transcription

1. ejaculation 2. cryptorchidism 3. orchidopexy 4. vasectomy 5. ejaculation 6. digital rectal exam (DRE) 7. prostate cancer 8. prostate-specific antigen (PSA) 9. benign prostatic hyperplasia (BPH) 10. transurethral resection of the prostate (TUR, TURP)

Case Study

1. Genital herpes.
2. Fever—She has a temperature; malaise—A feeling of general discomfort; dysuria—Painful urination; vaginal leukorrhea—A white discharge or flow from the vagina.
3. Vesicles—Small fluid-filled blisters; ulcers—Craterlike erosions of the skin; erythema—Redness; edema—Swelling.
4. An abnormality located on the body in some area outside of the genital region.
5. To feel with your hands.
6. There is a risk of passing the virus to the baby as it passes through the birth canal.

Practice Exercises

A. 1. GYN, OB 2. PMS 3. HDN 4. CVS 5. OCPs, IUD 6. HPV 7. STI 8. PSA 9. TUR or TURP 10. TSS
B. 1. the formation of mature sperm 2. accumulation of fluid within the testes 3. surgical removal of the prostate gland by inserting a device through the urethra and removing prostate tissue 4. inability to father children due to a problem with spermatogenesis 5. surgical removal of the testes 6. surgical removal of part or all of the vas deferens

7. removal of the testicles in the male or the ovaries in the female 8. the normal length of time of pregnancy, about 40 weeks 9. first bowel movement of newborn 10. a woman who has never been pregnant 11. difficult labor and childbirth 12. discharge from the uterus other than the menstrual flow 13. a benign fibrous growth 14. benign cysts forming in the breast 15. placenta implants in lower uterus and blocks birth canal
C. 1. colposcopy 2. colposcope 3. cervicectomy 4. cervicitis 5. hysteropexy 6. hysterectomy 7. hysterorrhexis 8. oophoritis 9. oophorectomy 10. mammogram 11. mammoplasty 12. amniotomy 13. amniorrhea 14. prostatectomy 15. prostatitis 16. orchiectomy 17. orchioplasty 18. orchiotomy 19. aspermia 20. oligospermia 21. spermatogenesis 22. spermatolysis
D. 1. balanoplasty 2. hyperplasia 3. cryptorchidism 4. varicocele 5. oligospermia 6. oophorectomy 7. colposcope 8. salpingocyesis 9. lactorrhea 10. endometriosis 11. pyosalpinx 12. neonatology 13. menorrhagia 14. primigravida 15. hysterorrhexis
E. 1. conization 2. stillbirth 3. puberty 4. premenstrual syndrome 5. laparoscopy 6. fibroid tumor 7. D&C 8. eclampsia 9. endometriosis 10. cesarean section
F. 1. e 2. i 3. h 4. c 5. a 6. d 7. g 8. b 9. f
G. 1. androgen therapy, f 2. oxytocin, a 3. antiprostatic agent, b 4. birth control pills, g 5. spermatocide, d 6. erectile dysfunction agent, h 7. hormone replacement therapy, i 8. abortifacient, e 9. fertility drug, c
H. 1. amniotic 2. cervical 3. embryonic 4. endometrium 5. mammary 6. ovary 7. uterus 8. fetus 9. vesicular 10. sperm 11. testicular 12. glans penis 13. epididymal 14. prostate gland 15. penile
I. 1. spelled correctly 2. epispadias 3. spelled correctly 4. circumcision 5. spelled correctly 6. spelled correctly 7. mammogram 8. preeclampsia 9. spelled correctly 10. premenstrual
J. 1. follicle-stimulating hormone, luteinizing hormone, estrogen, progesterone 2. ovulation 3. uterine tube or fallopian tube 4. lactation 5. embryo 6. expulsion 7. spermatogenesis 8. prostate gland

Labeling Exercises

A. 1. uterine tube or fallopian tube 2. ovary 3. fundus of uterus 4. corpus (body) of uterus 5. cervix 6. vagina 7. clitoris 8. labium majora 9. labium minora
B. 1. seminal vesicle 2. vas deferens 3. prostate gland 4. bulbourethral gland 5. urethra 6. epididymis 7. glans penis 8. testis
C. 1. areola 2. nipple 3. lactiferous gland 4. lactiferous duct 5. fat

Chapter 11 Answers

Practice As You Go

A. 1. d 2. g 3. i 4. a 5. j 6. b 7. e 8. f 9. h 10. c
B. 1. endocrinology 2. pituitary 3. gonads 4. cortico-
    steroids 5. circadian rhythm 6. iodine 7. Insulin,
    glucagon 8. thymus gland
C. 1. thymic 2. pancreatic 3. thyroidal 4. ovarian
    5. testicular
D. 1. b 2. a 3. e 4. h 5. j 6. i 7. f 8. g 9. c 10. d
E. 1. e 2. d 3. a 4. f 5. c 6. b 7. h 8. g
F. 1. NIDDM 2. IDDM 3. ACTH 4. PTH 5. T_3 6. TSH
    7. FBS 8. PRL

Real-World Applications

Medical Record Analysis

1. hyperglycemia—The condition of having a high
    level of sugar in the blood; associated with diabe-
    tes mellitus.
2. ketoacidosis—Acidosis due to an excess of acidic
    ketone bodies (waste products). A serious condi-
    tion requiring immediate treatment that can result
    in death for the diabetic patient if not reversed.
    Also called *diabetic acidosis.*
3. glycosuria—Having a high level of sugar excreted
    in the urine.
4. type 1 diabetes mellitus—Also called *insulin-
    dependent diabetes mellitus.* It develops early in
    life when the pancreas stops insulin production.
    Patient must take daily insulin injections.
5. polyuria—The condition of producing an exces-
    sive amount of urine.
6. polydipsia—Excessive feeling of thirst.
7. fasting blood sugar—Blood test to measure the
    amount of sugar circulating throughout the body
    after a 12-hour fast.
8. insulin—Medication administered to replace in-
    sulin for type 1 diabetics or to treat severe type 2
    diabetics.
9. glucose tolerance test—Test to determine the
    blood sugar level. A measured dose of glucose
    is given to a patient either orally or intravenously.
    Blood samples are then drawn at certain intervals
    to determine the ability of the patient to use glu-
    cose. Used for diabetic patients to determine their
    insulin response to glucose.
10. glucometer—A device designed for a diabetic to
    use at home to measure the level of glucose in the
    bloodstream.

Chart Note Transcription

1. endocrinologist 2. obesity 3. hirsutism 4. radioimmunoassay (RIA) 5. cortisol 6. adenoma 7. adrenal
cortex 8. Cushing's syndrome 9. adenoma 10. adrenal
cortex 11. adrenalectomy

Case Study

1. Diabetes mellitus.
2. Diaphoresis—Profuse sweating; rapid respirations—Breathing fast; rapid pulse—Fast heart
   rate; disorientation—Confused about his surroundings.
3. Blood serum test—Lab test to measure the levels
   of different substances in the blood, used to determine the function of endocrine glands.
4. Hyperglycemia—Blood level of glucose is too
   high; ketoacidosis—An excessive amount of acidic ketone bodies in the body.
5. Type 1, insulin-dependent, or juvenile diabetes
   mellitus because he has had it since childhood
   and he is taking insulin shots.
6. Type 2, non-insulin-dependent diabetes mellitus typically develops later in life. The pancreas
   produces normal to high levels of insulin, but the
   cells fail to respond to it. Patients may take oral
   hypoglycemic agents to improve insulin function,
   or may eventually have to take insulin.

Practice Exercises

A. 1. thyroidectomy 2. thyroidal 3. hyperthyroidism
    4. pancreatic 5. pancreatitis 6. pancreatectomy
    7. pancreatotomy 8. adrenal 9. adrenomegaly
    10. adrenopathy 11. thymoma 12. thymectomy
    13. thymic 14. thymitis
B. 1. thyroidectomy 2. glucometer 3. postpran-
    dial 4. hypothyroidism 5. hyperpituitarism
    6. acromegaly 7. hyponatremia 8. polydipsia
    9. adrenalitis 10. hypercalcemia 11. glycosuria
    12. thymoma
C. 1. HRT 2. RIA 3. FBS 4. DM 5. FSH, LH 6. PTH
    7. ACTH 8. TSH 9. ADH 10. T_3, T_4
D. 1. hormone obtained from cortex of adrenal
    gland 2. having excessive hair 3. a nerve condi-
    tion characterized with spasms of extremities;
    can occur from imbalance of pH and calcium or
    disorder of parathyroid gland 4. disorder of the
    retina occurring with diabetes mellitus 5. increase
    in blood sugar level 6. decrease in blood sugar
    level 7. another term for epinephrine; produced by
    inner portion of adrenal gland 8. hormone pro-
    duced by pancreas; essential for metabolism of
    blood sugar 9. toxic condition due to hyperactivity
    of thyroid gland 10. a condition resulting when the
    endocrine gland secretes more hormone than is
    needed by the body
E. 1. insulinoma 2. ketoacidosis 3. panhypopituitarism
    4. pheochromocytoma 5. Hashimoto's thyroiditis
    6. gynecomastia

F. 1. corticosteroids, e 2. human growth hormone therapy, a 3. oral hypoglycemic agent, d 4. anti-thyroid agent, c 5. insulin, f 6. thyroid replacement hormone, b

G. 1. f 2. i 3. a 4. c 5. j 6. e 7. b 8. g 9. d 10. h

H. 1. spelled correctly 2. glycosuria 3. spelled correctly 4. adrenalitis 5. spelled correctly 6. spelled correctly 7. Recklinghausen 8. hyperpituitarism 9. spelled correctly 10. radioimmunoassay

I. 1. ovarian 2. pancreatic 3. testicular 4. thymic 5. thyroidal 6. parathyroidal

J. 1. homeostasis 2. exocrine, endocrine 3. adrenal 4. islet, glucagon, insulin 5. calcium 6. pituitary 7. thymosin 8. basal metabolic rate (BMR)

Labeling Exercises

A. 1. pineal gland 2. thyroid and parathyroid glands 3. adrenal glands 4. pancreas 5. pituitary gland 6. thymus gland 7. ovary 8. testis

B. 1. pituitary gland 2. bone and soft tissue 3. GH 4. testes 5. FSH, LH 6. ovary 7. FSH, LH 8. thyroid gland 9. TSH 10. adrenal cortex 11. ACTH 12. breast 13. PRL

C. 1. liver 2. stomach 3. pancreas 4. beta cell 5. alpha cell 6. islets of Langerhans

Chapter 12 Answers
Practice As You Go

A. 1. brain, spinal cord 2. cranial, spinal 3. dendrites, nerve cell body, axon 4. myelin 5. cerebrum 6. cerebellum 7. eyesight 8. hearing, smell

B. 1. ascending, descending 2. efferent or motor, afferent or sensory 3. dura mater, arachnoid layer, pia mater 4. parasympathetic, sympathetic 5. somatic

C. 1. cerebrospinal 2. meningeal 3. subdural 4. encephalic 5. neural 6. intracranial

D. 1. b 2. f 3. g 4. h 5. i 6. j 7. e 8. c 9. d 10. a

E. 1. e 2. c 3. g 4. b 5. a 6. d 7. h 8. f

F. 1. CSF 2. CVD 3. EEG 4. ICP 5. PET 6. CVA 7. ANS

G. 1. d 2. g 3. j 4. a 5. c 6. i 7. f 8. e 9. h 10. b

Real-World Applications

Medical Record Analysis

1. paraplegia—Paralysis of the lower portion of the body and both legs.
2. comminuted fracture—Fracture in which the bone is shattered, splintered, or crushed into many small pieces or fragments.
3. epidural hematoma—Mass of blood in the space outside the dura mater of the brain and spinal cord.
4. spinal cord injury—Damage to the spinal cord as a result of trauma. Spinal cord may be bruised or completely severed.
5. unconscious—State of being unaware of surroundings, with the inability to respond to stimuli.
6. anesthesia—The lack of feeling or sensation.
7. paralysis—Temporary or permanent loss of function or voluntary movement.
8. computed tomography scan (CT scan)—An imaging technique that is able to produce a cross-sectional view of the body.
9. laminectomy—Removal of a portion of a vertebra, called the *lamina*, in order to relieve pressure on the spinal nerve.
10. spinal fusion—Surgical immobilization of adjacent vertebrae. This may be done for several reasons, including correction for a herniated disk.
11. physical therapy (PT)—Treats disorders using physical means and methods; includes joint motion and muscle strength.
12. occupational therapy (OT)—Assists patients to regain, develop, and improve skills that are important for independent functioning.

Chart Note Transcription

1. neurologist 2. dysphasia 3. hemiplegia 4. convulsions 5. electroencephalography (EEG) 6. lumbar puncture (LP) 7. brain scan 8. cerebral cortex 9. astrocytoma 10. craniotomy 11. cryosurgery

Case Study

1. Cerebrovascular accident (CVA or stroke).
2. aphasia—Inability to speak; hemiparesis—Weakness on one side of the body; syncope—Fainting; delirium—Abnormal mental state with confusion, disorientation, and agitation.
3. hypertension—High blood pressure; atherosclerosis—Hardening of arteries due to buildup of yellow fatty substances; diabetes mellitus—Inability to make or use insulin properly to control blood sugar levels.
4. brain scan—An image of the brain after injection of radioactive isotopes into the circulation; revealed an infarct in the right cerebral hemisphere.
5. infarct—An area of tissue within an organ that undergoes necrosis (death) following the loss of its blood supply.
6. hemorrhage—Ruptured blood vessel; thrombus—Stationary clot; embolus—Floating clot; compression—Pinching off a blood vessel.

Practice Exercises

A. **1.** h **2.** k **3.** d **4.** g **5.** a **6.** b **7.** f **8.** j **9.** e **10.** l **11.** i **12.** c

B. **1.** neuritis **2.** neurologist **3.** neuralgia **4.** polyneuritis **5.** neurectomy **6.** neuroplasty **7.** neuroma **8.** neurorrhaphy **9.** meningitis **10.** meningocele **11.** myelomeningocele **12.** encephalogram **13.** encephalopathy **14.** encephalitis **15.** encephalocele **16.** cerebrospinal **17.** cerebral

C. **1.** ADHD **2.** OCD **3.** LP **4.** PET **5.** MS **6.** SCI **7.** ALS **8.** TIA **9.** CP **10.** CVA

D. **1.** injecting radiopaque dye into spinal canal to examine under X-ray the outlines made by the dye **2.** X-ray of the blood vessels of the brain after the injection of radiopaque dye **3.** reflex test on bottom of foot to detect lesion and abnormalities of nervous system **4.** test that measures how fast an impulse travels along a nerve to pinpoint an area of nerve damage **5.** laboratory examination of fluid taken from the brain and spinal cord **6.** positron emission tomography to measure cerebral blood flow, blood volume, oxygen, and glucose uptake **7.** recording the ultrasonic echoes of the brain **8.** needle puncture into the spinal cavity to withdraw fluid

E. **1.** psychotherapy **2.** dementia **3.** analgesic **4.** myelogram **5.** electroencephalography **6.** subdural **7.** meningitis **8.** polyneuritis **9.** sclerosis **10.** concussion **11.** radiculopathy **12.** anesthetic **13.** pyromania **14.** insomnia

F. **1.** tumor of astrocyte cells **2.** seizure **3.** without sensation **4.** weakness of one-half of body **5.** physician that treats nervous system with surgery **6.** without sense of pain **7.** localized seizure of one limb **8.** paralysis of all four limbs **9.** accumulation of blood in the subdural space **10.** within the meninges

G. **1.** d **2.** e **3.** f **4.** g **5.** b **6.** a **7.** c **8.** j **9.** h **10.** i

H. **1.** delirium **2.** amyotrophic lateral sclerosis **3.** Bell's palsy **4.** cerebral aneurysm **5.** Parkinson's disease **6.** cerebrospinal fluid shunt **7.** transient ischemic attack **8.** subdural hematoma **9.** cerebral palsy **10.** nerve conduction velocity

I. **1.** anesthetic, e **2.** dopaminergic drugs, a **3.** hypnotic, d **4.** analgesic, g **5.** sedative, b **6.** narcotic analgesic, c **7.** anticonvulsant, f

J. **1.** i **2.** k **3.** h **4.** j **5.** e **6.** f **7.** b **8.** a **9.** d **10.** c **11.** g

K. **1.** minor tranquilizers **2.** humanistic psychotherapy **3.** lithium **4.** antipsychotic drugs **5.** psychoanalysis **6.** antidepressant drugs

L. **1.** general anesthesia **2.** local anesthesia **3.** topical anesthesia **4.** regional anesthesia

M. **1.** cerebellar **2.** thalamus **3.** cerebrum **4.** vertebra **5.** intracranial **6.** spine **7.** encephalic **8.** pontine **9.** medullary **10.** nerve **11.** meningeal **12.** ventricle

N. **1.** spelled correctly **2.** cephalalgia **3.** spelled correctly **4.** posttraumatic **5.** spelled correctly **6.** spelled correctly **7.** quadriplegia **8.** hydrocephalus **9.** amyotrophic **10.** spelled correctly

O. **1.** psychology, psychiatry **2.** somatic **3.** autonomic **4.** sensory, motor **5.** subarachnoid **6.** brainstem **7.** vision **8.** myelin

Labeling Exercises

A. **1.** brain **2.** spinal nerves **3.** spinal cord

B. **1.** dendrites **2.** nerve cell body **3.** unmyelinated region **4.** myelinated axon **5.** nucleus **6.** axon **7.** terminal end fibers

C. **1.** cerebrum **2.** diencephalon **3.** thalamus **4.** hypothalamus **5.** brainstem **6.** midbrain **7.** cerebellum **8.** pons **9.** medulla oblongata

Chapter 13 Answers
Practice As You Go

A. **1.** ophthalmology **2.** cilia **3.** lacrimal **4.** cornea **5.** retina **6.** iris **7.** choroid **8.** cones, rods **9.** rectus, oblique **10.** conjunctiva

B. **1.** pupillary **2.** optic or optical **3.** retinal **4.** lacrimal **5.** intraocular **6.** extraocular

C. **1.** h **2.** g **3.** a **4.** d **5.** b **6.** i **7.** c **8.** f **9.** e **10.** j

D. **1.** d **2.** a **3.** f **4.** e **5.** b **6.** c

E. **1.** IOL **2.** EM **3.** XT **4.** MY **5.** EOM **6.** VA

F. **1.** malleus, incus, stapes **2.** otology **3.** tympanic membrane **4.** cerumen **5.** eustachian or auditory **6.** vestibulocochlear nerve **7.** hearing, equilibrium **8.** conductive

G. **1.** cochlear **2.** otic or aural or auricular **3.** vestibular **4.** acoustic or auditory **5.** monaural

H. **1.** e **2.** h **3.** a **4.** g **5.** j **6.** c **7.** i **8.** b **9.** d **10.** f

I. **1.** c **2.** b **3.** d **4.** a **5.** g **6.** h **7.** e **8.** f

J. **1.** OE **2.** EENT **3.** BC **4.** PE tube **5.** OM

Real-World Applications
Medical Record Analysis

1. photophobia—Although the term translates into *fear of light*, it actually means a strong sensitivity to bright light.
2. hyperopia—With this condition a person can see things in the distance but has trouble reading material at close range. Also known as *farsightedness.* This condition is corrected with converging or biconvex lenses.
3. visual acuity test—Measurement of the sharpness of a patient's vision. Usually, a Snellen chart is used for this test in which the patient identifies letters from a distance of 20 feet.
4. intraocular—Pertaining to inside the eye.
5. ophthalmoscopy—Examination of the interior of the eyes using an instrument called an

ophthalmoscope. The physician dilates the pupil in order to see the cornea, lens, and retina. Used to identify abnormalities in the blood vessels of the eye and some systemic diseases.

6. mydriatic drops—Any substance that causes the pupil to dilate by paralyzing the iris and/or ciliary body muscles. Particularly useful during eye examinations and eye surgery.

7. cataract—Damage to the lens causing it to become opaque or cloudy, resulting in diminished vision. Treatment is usually surgical removal of the lens with the cataract and replacement with a prosthetic lens.

8. retinopathy—A general term for disease affecting the retina.

9. macular degeneration—Deterioration of the macular area of the retina of the eye. May be treated with laser surgery to destroy the blood vessels beneath the macula.

10. phacoemulsification—Use of high-frequency sound waves to emulsify (liquefy) a lens with a cataract, which is then aspirated (removed by suction) with a needle.

11. prosthetic lens implant—The use of an artificial lens to replace the lens removed during cataract surgery.

Chart Note Transcription

1. otorhinolaryngologist (ENT) 2. otitis media (OM)
3. binaural 4. otoscopy 5. tympanic membrane
6. cerumen 7. tympanometry 8. audiometry test
9. conductive hearing loss 10. myringotomy or tympanotomy

Case Study

1. Conductive hearing loss results from disease or malformation of the outer or middle ear; all sound is weaker because it is not conducted correctly to the inner ear.

2. Sensorineural hearing loss as a result of damage or malformation of the inner ear or the cochlear nerve.

3. Otoscopy examination of the auditory canal and middle ear; tympanometry measurement of the movement of the tympanic membrane; audiometry test for hearing ability; Rinne and Weber tuning-fork tests assess both the nerve and bone conduction of sound.

4. Hearing aids or amplification devices amplify sound and will work best for conductive hearing loss; cochlear implant is a device that converts sound signals into magnetic impulses to stimulate the auditory nerve and is used to treat profound sensorineural hearing loss.

6. Protect his ears better during playing music by wearing earplugs.

Practice Exercises

A. 1. artificial tears, h 2. antiglaucoma medication, c 3. antibiotic otic solution, i 4. mydriatic, a 5. antiemetic, g 6. antibiotic ophthalmic solution, j 7. ophthalmic decongestant, b 8. miotic, f 9. wax emulsifier, e 10. anesthetic ophthalmic solution, d

B. 1. blepharitis 2. blepharoplasty 3. blepharoptosis 4. retinopathy 5. retinopexy 6. ophthalmology 7. ophthalmic 8. ophthalmoscopy 9. iridoplegia 10. iridectomy 11. otoplasty 12. otopyorrhea 13. otalgia 14. otitis 15. tympanorrhexis 16. tympanotomy 17. tympanitis 18. audiogram 19. audiometer 20. audiology

C. 1. otoscope 2. retinopexy 3. anacusis 4. blepharoptosis 5. optometrist 6. tympanometer 7. keratotomy 8. presbyopia 9. iridectomy 10. audiometry 11. ophthalmalgia 12. otosclerosis 13. conjunctivitis 14. macrotia 15. monochromatism

D. 1. Astigm 2. ENT 3. VA 4. OE 5. ET 6. PE 7. LASIK 8. MY 9. OM 10. IOL

E. 1. tonometry 2. emmetropia 3. conjunctivitis 4. myopia 5. cataract 6. hordeolum 7. strabismus 8. hyperopia 9. presbycusis 10. otorhinolaryngologist 11. inner ear 12. Ménière's disease 13. acoustic neuroma

F. 1. dull/dim vision 2. double vision 3. enlarge or widen pupil 4. constrict pupil 5. vision changes due to normal aging 6. ringing in the ears 7. middle-ear bone 8. measures movement in eardrum 9. auditory tube 10. inner ear 11. results of hearing test 12. middle ear infection

G. 1. conjunctival 2. hearing 3. corneal 4. ear 5. intraocular 6. ear 7. lacrimal 8. iris 9. monaural 10. scleral 11. eye 12. retinal 13. tympanic 14. eye 15. cochlear

H. 1. ophthalmology 2. spelled correctly 3. spelled correctly 4. emmetropia 5. labyrinthitis 6. spelled correctly 7. spelled correctly 8. monochromatism 9. otopyorrhea 10. spelled correctly

I. 1. cornea, pupil; aqueous humor, lens, vitreous humor 2. nasal cavity 3. rectus, oblique 4. conjunctiva 5. cilia 6. choroid 7. incus, malleus, stapes 8. conductive, sensorineural 9. optic disk 10. auditory, vestibular

Labeling Exercises

A. 1. iris 2. lens 3. conjunctiva 4. pupil 5. cornea 6. suspensory ligaments 7. ciliary body 8. fovea centralis 9. optic nerve 10. retina 11. choroid 12. sclera

B. 1. pinna 2. external auditory meatus 3. auditory canal 4. tympanic membrane 5. malleus 6. incus 7. semicircular canals 8. vestibular nerve 9. cochlear nerve 10. cochlea 11. oval window 12. stapes 13. Eustachian tube

Glossary/Index

Note: Headings in **bold** indicate definitions. Page numbers with *t* indicate tables; those with *f* indicate figures.

A

Abbreviations, 13. *See also individual subject headings*

Abdominal aorta, 157*f*, 398*f*

Abdominal cavity, superior portion of abdominopelvic cavity, 40, 40*f*, 41*t*

Abdominal region, the abdomen, 38*t*, 39*f*

Abdominopelvic cavity, ventral cavity consisting of abdominal and pelvic cavities; contains digestive, urinary, and reproductive organs, 40–41, 41*t*–42*t*, 276*f*

Abducens nerve, 434*t*

Abduction, directional term meaning to move away from midline of body, 125*f*, 125*t*

Abnormal psychology, study and treatment of behaviors outside of normal and detrimental to person or society; these maladaptive behaviors range from occasional difficulty coping with stress, to bizarre actions and beliefs, to total withdrawal, 453

ABO system, major system of blood typing, 190

Abortifacient, medication that terminates a pregnancy, 369

Abortion (AB). *See* Elective abortion; Spontaneous abortion; Therapeutic abortion

Abrasion, scraping away a portion of skin surface, 65

Abruptio placentae, emergency condition in which placenta tears away from uterine wall prior to delivery of infant; requires immediate delivery of baby, 362

Abscess, a collection of pus in skin, 69

Absence seizure, type of epileptic seizure that lasts only a few seconds to half a minute, characterized by loss of awareness and absence of activity; also called *petit mal seizure,* 438

Accessory nerve, 434*t*

Abusive head trauma (AHT). *See* Shaken baby syndrome

Accessory organs of the skin, organs that are located within the dermis; includes hair, nails, sebaceous glands, and sweat glands, 60–62, 61*f*

Accessory organs of digestive system, organs that assist in digestion, but are not part of continuous tube from mouth to anus; includes liver, pancreas, gallbladder, and salivary glands, 270, 278–280, 279*f*, 291

ACE inhibitor drugs, medication that produces vasodilation and decreases blood pressure, 173

Achromatopsia, condition of color blindness; more common in males, 482

Acne, inflammatory disease of sebaceous glands and hair follicles resulting in papules and pustules, 69

Acne rosacea, chronic form of acne seen in adults involving redness, tiny pimples, and broken blood vessels, primarily on the nose and cheeks, 70

Acne vulgaris, common form of acne occurring in adolescence from oversecretion of oil glands; characterized by comedos, papules, and pustules, 70

Acoustic, pertaining to hearing, 498

Acoustic neuroma, benign tumor of eighth cranial nerve sheath; can cause symptoms from pressure being exerted on tissues, 500

Acquired immunity, protective response of body to a specific pathogen, 205

Acquired immunodeficiency syndrome (AIDS), disease involving a defect in cell-mediated immunity system; syndrome of opportunistic infections occurring in final stages of infection with human immunodeficiency virus (HIV); virus attacks T4 lymphocytes and destroys them, reducing person's ability to fight infection, 212

Acromegaly, chronic disease of adults resulting in elongation and enlargement of bones of head and extremities, 410, 410*f*

Action, type of movement a muscle produces, 124, 125*f*

Active acquired immunity, immunity developing after direct exposure to a pathogen, 205–206

Activities of daily living (ADLs), activities usually performed during a normal day, such as eating, dressing, and washing, 132

Acute care hospitals, hospitals that typically provide services to diagnose (laboratory, diagnostic imaging) and treat (surgery, medications, therapy) diseases for a short period of time; in addition, they usually provide emergency and obstetrical care; also called *general hospital,* 15*t*

Acute respiratory distress syndrome. *See* Adult respiratory distress syndrome

Acute tubular necrosis (ATN), damage to renal tubules due to presence of toxins in urine or to ischemia; results in oliguria, 325

Addison's disease, results from a deficiency in adrenocortical hormones; there may be increased pigmentation of skin, generalized weakness, and weight loss, 408

Additive, sum of action of two (or more) drugs given; in this case, total strength of medications is equal to sum of strength of each individual drug, 197

Adduction, directional term meaning to move toward midline of body, 125*f*, 125*t*

Adenocarcinoma, malignant adenoma in a glandular organ, 411

Adenoidectomy, surgical removal of adenoids, 215

Adenoiditis, inflammation of adenoids, 211

Adenoids, another term for pharyngeal tonsils; tonsils are a collection of lymphatic tissue found in nasopharynx to combat microorganisms entering body through nose or mouth, 205, 231–232

Azotemia, accumulation of nitrogenous waste in bloodstream; occurs when kidney fails to filter these wastes from blood, 323

B

B cells, common name for B lymphocytes, respond to foreign antigens by producing protective antibodies, 206

B lymphocytes, humoral immunity cells, which respond to foreign antigens by producing protective antibodies; simply referred to as *B cells*, 206

Babinski's reflex, reflex test to determine lesions and abnormalities in nervous system; Babinski's reflex is present if great toe extends instead of flexes when lateral sole of foot is stroked; normal response to this stimulation would be flexion, or upward movement, of toe, 447

Baby teeth. *See* Deciduous teeth

Bacteria, primitive, single-celled microorganisms that are present everywhere; some are capable of causing disease in humans, 205

Bacteriuria, bacteria in urine, 323

Balanic, pertaining to glans penis, 376

Balanitis, inflammation of skin covering glans penis, 378

Balanoplasty, surgical repair of glans penis, 380

Balanorrhea, discharge from glans penis, 377

Balloon angioplasty. *See* Percutaneous transluminal coronary angioplasty

Bariatric surgery, group of surgical procedures designed to treat morbid (extreme) obesity by reducing size of stomach or diverting food from portion of alimentary canal, 296

Barium enema (BE). *See* Lower gastrointestinal series

Barium swallow. *See* Upper gastrointestinal series

Barrier contraception, prevention of pregnancy using a device to prevent sperm from meeting ovum; includes condoms, diaphragms, and cervical caps, 367

Bartholin's glands, glands located on either side of vaginal opening that secrete mucus for vaginal lubrication, 351, 351*f*

Basal cell carcinoma (BCC), tumor of basal cell layer of epidermis; frequent type of skin cancer that rarely metastasizes or spreads; these cancers can arise on sun-exposed skin, 70, 70*f*

Basal layer, deepest layer of epidermis; this living layer constantly multiplies and divides to supply cells to replace cells that are sloughed off skin surface,58, 60

Basal metabolic rate (BMR), minimum rate of metabolism necessary to support functions of body at rest, 403–404

Base, directional term meaning bottom or lower part, 44*t*, 234

Basilic vein, 158*f*

Basophil (basos), granulocyte white blood cell that releases histamine and heparin in damaged tissues, 189*f*, 189*t*

Basophilic, pertaining to a leukocyte that attracts a basic pH stain, 192

Bell jar apparatus, 236*f*

Bell's palsy, one-sided facial paralysis due to inflammation of facial nerve, 444

Benign prostatic hyperplasia (BPH), enlargement of prostate gland commonly seen in males over age, 50, 378

Beta-blocker drugs, medications that treat hypertension and angina pectoris by lowering heart rate, 173

Biceps, arm muscle named for number of attachment points; *bi-* means *two* and biceps have two heads attached to bone, 119*f*, 124, 125*f*

Bicuspid valve, valve between left atrium and ventricle; prevents blood from flowing backward into atrium; has two cusps or flaps; also called *mitral valve*, 151–152, 153*f*

Bicuspids, premolar permanent teeth having two cusps or projections that assist in grinding food; humans have eight bicuspids, 271*f*, 272, 273*f*

Bilateral, pertaining to two sides, 5, 7

Bile, substance produced by liver and stored in gallbladder; added to chyme in duodenum and functions to emulsify fats so they can be digested and absorbed, 279

Bile duct, 279, 279*f*, 280

Bilirubin, waste product produced from destruction of worn-out red blood cells; disposed of by liver, 188

Binaural, referring to both ears, 498

Biopsy (BX, bx), piece of tissue is removed by syringe and needle, knife, punch, or brush to examine under a microscope; used to aid in diagnosis, 77

Bipolar disorder (BPD), mental disorder in which patient has alternating periods of depression and mania, 454

Bipolar and related disorders, a classification of psychiatric disorders in the DSM-5 characterized by alternation between periods of deep depression and mania; includes bipolar disorder (BPD),

Bitewing X-ray, X-ray taken with part of film holder held between teeth, and film held parallel to teeth, 293

Black lung. *See* Anthracosis

Bladder, 316*f*

Bladder cancer, cancerous tumor that arises from cells lining bladder; major symptom is hematuria, 327

Bladder neck obstruction (BNO), blockage of bladder outlet into urethra, 327

Blepharectomy, surgical removal of eyelid, 488

Blepharitis, inflammatory condition of eyelash follicles and glands of eyelids that results in swelling, redness, and crusts of dried mucus on lids; can be result of allergy or infection, 485

Blepharoplasty, surgical repair of eyelid, 488

Blepharoptosis, drooping eyelid, 481

Blind spot. *See* Optic disk

Blood, major component of hematic system; consists of watery plasma, red blood cells, and white blood cells, 33*t*, 186–199

abbreviations, 198–199

ABO system, 190

adjective forms of anatomical terms, 192

anatomy and physiology, 187*f*, 188–190, 189*f*, 189*t*, 190*f*

diagnostic procedures, 196, 196*f*

Bradypnea, slow breathing, 241

Brain, one of the largest organs in body and coordinates most body activities; center for all thought, memory, judgment, and emotion; each part of brain is responsible for controlling different body functions, such as temperature regulation and breathing; four sections include cerebrum, cerebellum, diencephalon, and brainstem, 30*f*, 31, 428, 429–431, 430*f*, 431*f*, 440–443, 440*f*, 441*f*, 442*f*

Brain scan, injection of radioactive isotopes into circulation to determine function and abnormality of brain, 447

Brainstem, area of brain with three components: medulla oblongata, pons, and midbrain; pathway for impulses to be conducted between brain and spinal cord; also contains centers that control respiration, heart rate, and blood pressure; in addition, 12 pairs of cranial nerves begin in brainstem, 429, 431

Brain tumor, intracranial mass, either benign or malignant; benign tumor of brain can be fatal since it will grow and cause pressure on normal brain tissue, 440, 440*f*

Brand name, name a pharmaceutical company chooses as trademark or market name for its drug; also called *proprietary* or *trade name*, 16

Breaking the water. *See* Amniotomy

Breast cancer, malignant tumor of breast; usually forms in milk-producing gland tissue or lining of milk ducts, 362, 362*f*

Breasts, milk-producing glands to provide nutrition for newborn; also called *mammary glands*, 348, 352, 352*f*, 362

Breech birth, placement of fetus in which buttocks or feet are presented first for delivery rather than head, 354, 355*f*

Bridge, dental appliance attached to adjacent teeth for support to replace missing teeth, 295

Broad spectrum, ability of drug to be effective against a wide range of microorganisms, 79

Bronchial, pertaining to the bronchi, 239

Bronchial tree, 233*f*

Bronchial tube, organ of respiratory system that carries air into each lung, 230, 233–234, 233*f*

Bronchiectasis, results from dilation of bronchus or bronchi that can result from infection; this abnormal stretching can be irreversible and result in destruction of bronchial walls; major symptom is large amount of purulent (pus-filled) sputum; rales (bubbling chest sound) and hemoptysis may be present, 241, 245

Bronchiolar, pertaining to a bronchiole, 239

Bronchioles, narrowest air tubes in lungs; each bronchiole terminates in tiny air sacs called *alveoli*, 233, 233*f*

Bronchitis, acute or chronic inflammation of lower respiratory tract that often occurs after other childhood infections such as measles, 245

Bronchodilator, medication that dilates or opens bronchi (airways in lungs) to improve breathing, 254

Bronchogenic carcinoma, malignant lung tumor that originates in bronchi; usually associated with history of cigarette smoking, 245, 245*f*

Bronchogram, X-ray record of lungs and bronchial tubes, 249

Bronchography, process of taking X-ray of lung after radiopaque substance has been placed into trachea or bronchial tube, 249

Bronchoplasty, surgical repair of a bronchial defect, 251

Bronchoscope, instrument to view inside a bronchus, 249

Bronchoscopy (Bronch), using bronchoscope to visualize bronchi; instrument can also be used to obtain tissue for biopsy and to remove foreign objects, 249, 250*f*

Bronchospasm, involuntary muscle spasm in bronchi, 241

Bronchus, distal end of trachea splits into left and right main bronchi as it enters each lung; each main bronchus is subdivided into smaller branches; smallest bronchi are bronchioles; each bronchiole ends in tiny air sacs called *alveoli*, 233

Bruise. *See* Hematoma

Buccal, (1) pertaining to cheeks; (2) drugs that are placed under lip or between cheek and gum, 45, 47*f*, 282

Buccolabial, pertaining to cheeks and lips, 282

Buffers, chemicals that neutralize acid, particularly stomach acid, 280

Bulbourethral gland, also called *Cowper's gland*; these two small male reproductive system glands are located on either side of urethra just distal to prostate; secretion from these glands neutralizes acidity in urethra and vagina, 373, 373*f*, 375

Bulimia, eating disorder characterized by recurrent binge eating and then purging of food with laxatives and vomiting, 455

Bulla, large blister; larger than a vesicle, 65

Bundle branch block (BBB), occurs when electrical impulse is blocked from travelling down atrioventricular bundle or bundle branches; results in ventricles beating at a different rate than atria; also called a *heart block*, 165

Bundle branches, part of conduction system of heart; electrical signal travels down interventricular septum, 153, 154*f*

Bundle of His. *See* Atrioventricular bundle

Bunion, inflammation of bursa of the great toe, 113

Bunionectomy, removal of bursa at joint of great toe, 116

Burn, damage to skin caused by heat, electricity, ultraviolet light, or caustic chemicals; full-thickness burn exists when all layers are burned, called *third-degree burn*; partial-thickness burn exists when first layer of skin, epidermis, is burned, and second layer of skin, dermis, is damaged, called *second-degree burn*; first-degree burn damages only epidermis, 70–72, 71*f*, 72*f*

Bursa, saclike connective tissue structure found in some joints; protects moving parts from friction; some common bursa locations are elbow, knee, and shoulder joints, 101, 102

Bursectomy, surgical removal of a bursa, 116

Bursitis, inflammation of bursa between bony prominences and muscles or tendons; common in shoulder and knee, 107

C

Cachexia, loss of weight and generalized wasting that occurs during a chronic disease, 284

Calcitonin (CT), hormone secreted by thyroid gland; stimulates deposition of calcium into bone, 397t, 403–404

Calcium (Ca⁺), inorganic substance found in plasma; important for bones, muscles, and nerves, 188, 400

Calcium channel blocker drugs, medications that treat hypertension, angina pectoris, and congestive heart failure by causing heart to beat less forcefully and less often, 173

Calcium supplements, maintaining high blood levels of calcium in association with vitamin D helps maintain bone density and treats osteomalacia, osteoporosis, and rickets, 118

Calculus, stone formed within organ by accumulation of mineral salts; found in kidney, renal pelvis, ureters, bladder, or urethra; plural is *calculi*, 323, 323f

Callus, mass of bone tissue that forms at fracture site during its healing, 107

Calyx, duct that connects renal papilla to renal pelvis; urine flows from collecting tubule through calyx and into renal pelvis, 314, 315f

Cancellous bone, bony tissue found inside a bone; contains cavities that hold red bone marrow; also called *spongy bone*, 92–93, 93f

Cancerous tumors, malignant growths in the body, 205

Candidiasis, yeastlike infection of skin and mucous membranes that can result in white plaques on tongue and vagina, 361

Canines, also called *cuspid teeth* or *eyeteeth*; permanent teeth located between incisors and bicuspids that assist in biting and cutting food; humans have four canine teeth, 272

Canker sores. *See* Aphthous ulcers

Capillaries, smallest blood or lymphatic vessels; blood capillaries are very thin to allow gas, nutrient, and waste exchange between blood and tissues; lymph capillaries collect lymph fluid from tissues and carry it to larger lymph vessels, 148, 148f, 155f, 156

Capillary bed, network of capillaries found in a given tissue or organ, 156

Carbapenem-resistant Enterobacteriaceae (CRE) **infection,** infection by group of bacteria resistant to powerful antibiotics, frequently occurs in healthcare settings, 213

Carbon dioxide (CO₂), waste product of cellular energy production; removed from cells by blood and eliminated from body by lungs, 148–149, 148f, 230

Carbuncle, inflammation and infection of skin and hair follicle that may result from several untreated boils; most commonly found on neck, upper back, or head, 75

Cardiac, pertaining to the heart, 161

Cardiac arrest, when heart stops beating and circulation ceases, 163

Cardiac biomarkers, blood test to determine level of proteins specific to heart muscles in blood; increase in these proteins may indicate heart muscle damage such as myocardial infarction; proteins include creatine kinase (CK) and troponin, 169

Cardiac catheterization (CC), passage of thin tube (catheter) through arm vein and blood vessel leading into heart; used to detect abnormalities, to collect cardiac blood samples, and to determine pressure within cardiac area, 169

Cardiac muscle, involuntary muscle found in heart, 122–123, 122f, 123f, 149

Cardiac scan, patient is given radioactive thallium intravenously and then scanning equipment is used to visualize heart; especially useful in determining myocardial damage, 169

Cardiac sphincter, also called *lower esophageal sphincter* or *gastroesophageal sphincter*; prevents food and gastric juices from backing up into esophagus, 275, 275f

Cardiac tamponade, pressure on heart resulting from fluid buildup inside pericardial sac, 163

Cardiologist, physician specializing in treating diseases and conditions of cardiovascular system, 162

Cardiology, branch of medicine specializing in conditions of cardiovascular system, 32t, 162

Cardiomegaly, abnormally enlarged heart, 163

Cardiomyopathy, general term for disease of myocardium that may be caused by alcohol abuse, parasites, viral infection, and congestive heart failure, 163

Cardiopulmonary resuscitation (CPR), emergency treatment provided by trained persons and given to patients when their respirations and heart stop; provides oxygen to brain, heart, and other vital organs until medical treatment can restore normal heart and pulmonary function, 170, 253

Cardiotonic, substance that strengthens the heart muscle, 173

Cardiovascular, pertaining to the heart and blood vessels, 32

Cardiovascular system (CV), system that transports blood to all areas of body; organs include heart and blood vessels (arteries, veins, and capillaries); also called *circulatory system*, 145–175

abbreviations, 174–175

adjective forms of anatomical terms, 160–161

anatomy and physiology, 147f, 148–159

diagnostic procedures, 168–170

functions, 32t, 146

medical specialties, 32t

pathology, 162–167

pharmacology, 173

terminology, 146, 159–160

therapeutic procedures, 170–172

Cardiovascular technologist/technician, healthcare professional trained to perform a variety of diagnostic and therapeutic procedures including electrocardiography, echocardiography, and exercise stress tests, 162

Cardioversion. *See* Defibrillation

Carotid artery, 157f

Carotid endarterectomy, surgical procedure for removing obstruction within carotid artery, major artery in neck that carries oxygenated blood to brain; developed to prevent strokes but found to be useful only in severe stenosis with TIA, 449

Carpal, pertaining to the carpus or wrist, 104

Carpal tunnel release, surgical cutting of ligament in wrist to relieve nerve pressure caused by carpal tunnel syndrome, which can be caused by repetitive motion such as typing, 133

Carpal tunnel syndrome (CTS), painful disorder of wrist and hand, induced by compression of median nerve as it passes under ligaments on palm side of wrist; symptoms include weakness, pain, burning, tingling, and aching in forearm, wrist, and hand, 130

Carpals, wrist bones in upper extremity, 92, 104

Carpus, collective name for the eight wrist bones in each upper extremity, 91f, 98, 99f, 100, 100f, 100t

Cartilage, strong, flexible connective tissue found in several locations in body, such as covering ends of bones in synovial joint, nasal septum, external ear, eustachian tube, larynx, trachea, bronchi, and intervertebral disks, 30f, 31, 92

Cartilaginous joints, joints that allow slight movement but hold bones firmly in place by solid piece of cartilage; example is pubic symphysis; fetal skeleton is composed of cartilaginous tissue, 101, 102f

Cast, application of solid material to immobilize extremity or portion of body as a result of fracture, dislocation, or severe injury; most often made of plaster of Paris or fiberglass, 117

Castration, surgical removal of testicles in male or ovaries in female, 380

Cataract, diminished vision resulting from lens of eye becoming opaque or cloudy; treatment is usually surgical removal of lens with cataract and replacement with prosthetic lens, 482, 482f

Catheter (cath), flexible tube inserted into body for purpose of moving fluids into or out of body; used in cardiovascular system to place dye into blood vessels so they may be visualized on X-rays; used in urinary system to drain urine from bladder, 169, 330

Catheterization, insertion of a tube through urethra and into urinary bladder for purpose of withdrawing urine or inserting dye, 330

Caudal, directional term meaning toward feet or tail, or below; akin to inferior, 43f, 43t

Cauterization, destruction of tissue by using caustic chemicals, electric currents, or by heating or freezing, 78

Cecal, pertaining to the cecum, 282

Cecum, first portion of colon; a blind pouch off beginning of large intestine; appendix originates at end, 276f, 277, 277f

Celiac disease, autoimmune condition affecting small intestine; caused by reaction to gluten; symptoms may include abdominal bloating and pain, diarrhea, and nutritional deficiencies, 288

Cell, basic unit of all living things; composes all tissues and organs in body; performs survival functions such as reproduction, respiration, metabolism, and excretion; some also able to carry on specialized functions, such as contraction by muscle cells and electrical impulse transmission by nerve cells, 27f, 28, 30f

Cell-mediated immunity, immunity resulting from activation of sensitized T lymphocytes; immune response causes antigens to be destroyed by direct action of cells; also called cellular immunity, 206

Cell membrane, outermost boundary of the cell, 28, 29f

Cellular immunity, also called cell-mediated immunity; process results in production of T cells and natural killer (NK) cells that directly attach to foreign cells; immune response fights invasion by viruses, bacteria, fungi, and cancer, 206–207

Cellulitis, inflammation of cellular or connective tissues, 72

Cementum, anchors root of a tooth into socket of jaw, 272, 273f

Central canal, canal that extends down length of spinal cord; contains cerebrospinal fluid, 432

Central nervous system (CNS), portion of nervous system consisting of brain and spinal cord; receives impulses from all over body, processes information, and then responds with action; consists of both gray and white matter, 428–429
 brain, 30f, 31, 428, 429–431, 430f, 431f, 440–443, 440f, 441f, 442f
 meninges, 428–429, 433, 433f, 445–446, 446f
 spinal cord, 30f, 31, 428, 431f, 432–433, 432f, 435f, 443–444, 444f

Cephalalgia, a headache, 439

Cephalic, 1) pertaining to the head; 2) directional term meaning toward the head, or above, 39f, 43f, 43t, 437

Cephalic region, head region of the body, 38t, 39f

Cephalic vein, 158f

Cerebellar, pertaining to cerebellum, 437

Cerebellitis, inflammation of cerebellum, 440

Cerebellum, second largest portion of brain, located beneath posterior portion of cerebrum; part of brain that aids in coordinating voluntary body movements and maintaining balance and equilibrium; attached to brainstem by pons; refined muscular movement is initiated in cerebrum, 429, 431f

Cerebral, pertaining to the cerebrum, 437

Cerebral aneurysm, localized abnormal dilatation of blood vessel, usually artery; result of congenital defect or weakness in wall of vessel; ruptured aneurysm is a common cause for hemorrhagic CVA, 440, 441f

Cerebral angiography, X-ray of blood vessels of brain after injection of radiopaque dye, 447

Cerebral contusion, bruising of brain from blow or impact; symptoms last longer than 24 hours and include unconsciousness, dizziness, vomiting, unequal pupil size, and shock, 441

Cerebral cortex, outer layer of cerebrum; composed of folds of gray matter called gyri, which are separated by sulci, 429

Cerebral hemispheres, divisions of cerebrum into right and left halves, 429–430

Cerebral palsy (CP), brain damage resulting from a defect, trauma, infection, or lack of oxygen before, during, or shortly after birth, 441

Comedo, medical term for blackhead; an accumulation of sebum in sebaceous gland that has become blackened; also called a *blackhead*, 65

Comminuted fracture, fracture in which bone is shattered, splintered, or crushed into many pieces or fragments; fracture is completely through bone, 108

Common bile duct (CBD), duct that carries bile from gallbladder to duodenum, 279–280, 279f

Common cold. *See* Nasopharyngitis

Common iliac artery, 157f

Common iliac vein, 158f

Common peroneal nerve, 435f

Compact bone, hard exterior surface bone; also called *cortical bone*, 92–93, 93f, 102f

Complemental air. *See* Inspiratory reserve volume

Complete blood count (CBC), a combination of blood tests; includes red blood cell count, white blood cell count, hemoglobin, hematocrit, white blood cell differential, and platelet count, 196

Compound fracture, open fracture in which skin has been broken through by fracture; also called an *open fracture*, 108, 108f

Compression fracture, fracture involving loss of height of vertebral body, 109

Computed tomography scan (CT scan), imaging technique able to produce cross-sectional view of body; X-ray pictures are taken at multiple angles through body and computer constructs composite cross-section from images.

Conception, fertilization of ovum by a sperm, 349–350

Concussion, injury to brain resulting from blow or impact; symptoms may include headache, blurred vision, nausea or vomiting, dizziness, and balance problems; also called *mild traumatic brain injury*, 441

Conductive hearing loss, loss of hearing as a result of blocking of sound transmission in middle ear and outer ear, 496

Condyle, refers to rounded portion at end of a bone, 94, 95f

Cones, sensory receptors of retina that are active in bright light and see in color, 475, 477

Confidentiality, 16

Congenital anomalies, birth defects, 112, 165, 286, 354

Congenital hypothyroidism, congenital condition due to lack of thyroid secretion that may result in arrested physical and mental development; formerly called *cretinism*, 411

Congenital septal defect (CSD), defect, present at birth, in wall separating two chambers of heart; results in a mixture of oxygenated and deoxygenated blood being carried to surrounding tissues; there can be atrial septal defect (ASD) and ventricular septal defect (VSD), 163

Congestive heart failure (CHF), pathological condition of heart in which there is reduced outflow of blood from left side of heart; results in weakness, breathlessness, and edema, 163

Conization, surgical removal of core of cervical tissue; also refers to partial removal of cervix, 367

Conjunctiva, protective mucous membrane lining on underside of each eyelid and across anterior surface of each eyeball, 474, 474f, 477, 485

Conjunctival, pertaining to conjunctiva, 480

Conjunctivitis, inflammation of conjunctiva; commonly called *pinkeye*, 485

Conjunctivoplasty, surgical repair of conjunctiva, 488

Connective tissue, supporting and protecting tissue in body structures; examples are fat or adipose tissue, cartilage, and bone, 28, 30f, 31

Conscious, condition of being awake and aware of surroundings, 439

Constipation, experiencing difficulty in defecation or infrequent defecation, 284

Consultation reports, document in patient's medical record; reports given by specialists whom physician has requested to evaluate patient, 14t

Contact dermatitis, skin irritation due to direct contact of skin with an allergen, 211

Continuous positive airway pressure (CPAP), machine that supplies constant and steady air pressure to keep airways open; treatment for sleep apnea, 251

Contracture, abnormal shortening of muscle, making it difficult to stretch muscle, 129

Contraindication, condition in which particular drug should not be used, 197

Controlled substances, drugs that have potential for being addictive (habit forming) or can be abused, 17, 18t

Contusion, injury caused by blow to body; causes swelling, pain, and bruising; skin is not broken, 65

Conversion disorder, disorder in which patient unconsciously substitutes physical signs or symptoms for anxiety; most common physical signs or symptoms are blindness, heart palpitations, and paralysis, 456

Convulsion, severe involuntary muscle contractions and relaxations; caused by a variety of things, such as epilepsy, fever, and toxic conditions, 439

Corium, living layer of skin located between epidermis and subcutaneous layer; also referred to as *dermis*, contains hair follicles, sweat glands, sebaceous glands, blood vessels, lymph vessels, sensory receptors, nerve fibers, and muscle fibers, 60

Cornea, portion of sclera that is clear and transparent and allows light to enter interior of eye; also plays role in bending light rays, 474, 474f, 477, 478f

Corneal, pertaining to cornea, 480

Corneal abrasion, scraping injury to cornea; if not allowed to heal, may develop into ulcer, 482

Coronal plane, vertical plane that divides body into front (anterior or ventral) and back (posterior or dorsal) sections; also called *frontal plane*, 37–38, 37f

Coronal section, sectional view of body produced by cut along frontal plane; also called *frontal section*, 37–38, 37f

Coronary, pertaining to heart, 161

Coronary arteries, group of three arteries that branch off aorta and carry blood to myocardium, 155, 156f, 171

Coronary artery bypass graft (CABG), open-heart surgery in which blood vessel is grafted to route blood around point of constriction in diseased coronary artery, 171

chronic lung disease to congenital and chronic heart problems, 242, 242f

Cycloplegia, paralysis of ciliary body which, in turn, changes shape of lens and makes it difficult to bring images into focus, 481

Cyst, fluid-filled sac under skin, 65, 65f

Cystalgia, bladder pain, 323

Cystectomy, surgical removal of bladder, 331

Cystic, (1) pertaining to urinary bladder; (2) pertaining to gallbladder, 282

Cystic duct, duct leading from gallbladder to common bile duct; carries bile, 279–280, 279f

Cystic fibrosis (CF), hereditary condition causing exocrine glands to malfunction; patient produces very thick mucus that causes severe congestion within lungs and digestive system; through more advanced treatment, many children are now living into adulthood with this disease, 246

Cystitis, inflammation of bladder, 318, 327

Cystocele, protrusion (or herniation) of urinary bladder into wall of vagina; may cause urinary frequency and urgency, 327, 361

Cystogram, record of bladder, 328

Cystography, process of instilling contrast material or dye into bladder by catheter to visualize urinary bladder on X-ray, 328

Cystolith, bladder stone, 323

Cystopexy, surgical fixation of bladder, 331

Cystoplasty, surgical repair of bladder, 331

Cystorrhagia, abnormal bleeding from bladder, 323

Cystoscope, instrument used to visually examine bladder, 329

Cystoscopy (cysto), visual examination of urinary bladder using instrument called *cystoscope*, 329

Cystostomy, creation of opening through abdominal wall and into bladder, 331

Cystotomy, incision into bladder, 331

Cytology, study of cells, 28

Cytoplasm, watery internal environment of a cell, 28, 29f

Cytotoxic, pertaining to poisoning cells, 206–207

D

Dacryoadenitis, inflammation of lacrimal gland, 485

Dacryocystitis, inflammation of tear sac, 485

Deafness, inability to hear or having some degree of hearing impairment, 499

Debridement, removal of foreign material and dead or damaged tissue from wound, 78

Decibel (dB), measures intensity or loudness of sound; zero decibels is quietest sound measured and 120 dB is loudest sound commonly measured, 501

Deciduous teeth, 20 teeth that begin to erupt around six months of age; eventually pushed out by permanent teeth; also called *baby teeth*, 272

Decongestant, substance that reduces nasal congestion and swelling, 254

Decubitus ulcer (decub), bedsore or pressure sore formed from pressure over bony prominences on body; caused by lack of blood flow, 72

Deep, directional term meaning away from surface of body, 44t

Deep tendon reflex (DTR), muscle contraction in response to stretch caused by striking muscle tendon with reflex hammer; test used to determine if muscles are responding properly, 132

Deep vein thrombosis (DVT), formation of blood clots in a vein deep in the body, usually in the legs, 167

Defecation, evacuation of feces from rectum, 277

Defibrillation, procedure that converts serious irregular heartbeats, such as fibrillation, by giving electric shocks to heart; also called *cardioversion*, 170, 170f

Degenerative joint disease (DJD). *See* Osteoarthritis

Deglutition, swallowing, 270–271

Delirium, state of mental confusion with lack of orientation to time and place, 439

Delivery, emergence of baby from birth canal, 354, 355f

Delusional disorder, false belief held with conviction even in face of strong evidence to contrary, 456

Dementia, progressive impairment of intellectual function that interferes with performing activities of daily living; patients have little awareness of their condition; found in disorders such as Alzheimer's, 439, 455

Dendrite, branched process off a neuron that receives impulses and carries them to cell body, 428, 429f

Dental, pertaining to teeth, 282

Dental caries, gradual decay and disintegration of teeth caused by bacteria that can result in inflamed tissue and abscessed teeth; commonly called a *tooth cavity*, 286

Dentalgia, tooth pain, 284

Dentin, main bulk of tooth; covered by enamel, 272, 273f

Dentist, practitioner of dentistry, 268

Dentistry, branch of healthcare involved with prevention, diagnosis, and treatment of conditions involving teeth, jaw, and mouth; practitioner is *dentist* or *oral surgeon*, 284

Denture, partial or complete set of artificial teeth that are set in plastic materials; substitute for natural teeth and related structures, 295

Deoxygenated, blood in veins that is low in oxygen content, 148, 148f

Depigmentation, loss of normal skin color or pigment, 65

Depression, downward movement, as in dropping shoulders, 126t

Depressive disorders, a classification of psychiatric disorders in the DSM-5 characterized by instability in mood; includes major depressive disorder and mania, 454

Dermabrasion, abrasion or rubbing using wire brushes or sandpaper, 78

Dermal, pertaining to skin, 64

Dermatitis, inflammation of skin, 72

Dermatologist, physician specialized in diagnosis and treatment of diseases of integumentary system, 65

Dermatology (Derm, derm), branch of medicine specializing in conditions of integumentary system, 32t, 65

Dermatome, instrument for cutting skin or thin transplants of skin, 78

Dermatoplasty, surgical repair of skin, 78

Dermatosis, abnormal condition of skin, 72

Dermic, pertaining to the skin, 64

Dermis, living layer of skin located between epidermis and subcutaneous layer; also referred to as *corium*; contains hair follicles, sweat glands, sebaceous glands, blood vessels, lymph vessels, sensory receptors, nerve fibers, and muscle fibers, 58, 59*f*, 60, 61*f*

Descending aorta, 153*f*

Descending colon, section of colon that descends left side of abdomen, 276*f*, 277, 277*f*

Descending nephron loop, 316*f*

Descending tracts, nerve tracts carrying motor signals down spinal cord to muscles, 432

Diabetes insipidus (DI), disorder caused by inadequate secretion of hormone by posterior lobe of pituitary gland; there may be polyuria and polydipsia, 410*f*

Diabetes mellitus (DM), serious disease in which pancreas fails to produce insulin or insulin does not work properly; consequently, patient has very high blood sugar; kidney will attempt to lower high blood sugar level by excreting excess sugar in urine, 409

Diabetic acidosis. *See* Ketoacidosis

Diabetic nephropathy, accumulation of damage to glomerulus capillaries due to chronic high blood sugars of diabetes mellitus, 325

Diabetic retinopathy, secondary complication of diabetes affecting blood vessels of retina, resulting in visual changes and even blindness, 409

Diagnostic and Statistical Manual of Mental Disorders, Fifth Edition (DSM-5), 453

Diagnostic reports, found in patient's medical record; consists of results of all diagnostic tests performed on patient, principally from clinical lab and medical imaging (e.g., X-ray and ultrasound), 14*t*

Diaphoresis, excessive or profuse sweating, 65

Diaphragm, major muscle of inspiration; separates thoracic from abdominal cavity, 40, 40*f*, 235–236, 236*f*

Diaphragmatic, pertaining to diaphragm, 239

Diaphragmatocele. *See* Hiatal hernia

Diaphysis, shaft portion of long bone, 92, 93*f*

Diarrhea, passing of frequent, watery bowel movements; usually accompanies gastrointestinal (GI) disorders, 284

Diastole, period of time during which heart chamber is relaxed, 152

Diastolic pressure, lower pressure within blood vessels during relaxation phase of heartbeat, 159

Diencephalon, portion of brain that contains two most critical areas of brain, thalamus and hypothalamus, 429, 430*f*

Digestive system, system that digests food and absorbs nutrients; organs include mouth, pharynx, esophagus, stomach, small and large intestines, liver, gallbladder, pancreas, and salivary glands; also called *gastrointestinal system*, 34*t*, 263–299, 268–299

abbreviations, 299

accessory organs of, 278–280, 279*f*

adjective forms of anatomical terms, 282–283

anatomy and physiology, 269*f*, 270–280

colon, 275–277, 276*f*, 277*f*

diagnostic procedures, 292–295

esophagus, 270, 271*f*, 272*f*, 274, 275*f*, 286

function, 268

gallbladder, 270, 279–279, 279*f*

liver, 270, 279, 279*f*

medical specialties, 34*t*

oral cavity, 270–271, 271*f*, 272*f*, 286

pancreas, 270, 279*f*, 280, 396, 397*t*, 399–400, 400*f*, 409

pathology, 284–291

pharmacology, 298–299

pharynx, 121, 205, 231–232, 231*f*, 272*f*, 274, 286

salivary glands, 270, 278, 279*f*

small intestine, 270, 275–277, 276*f*, 288–290

stomach, 270, 275, 275*f*, 286

teeth, 270–271, 271*f*, 272*f*, 273*f*

terminology, 268, 270, 280–281

therapeutic procedures, 295–298

Digital rectal exam (DRE), manual examination for enlarged prostate gland performed by palpating (feeling) prostate gland through wall of rectum, 380

Digital veins, 158*f*

Dilation and curettage (D&C), surgical procedure in which opening of cervix is dilated and uterus is scraped or suctioned of its lining or tissue; often performed after spontaneous abortion and to stop excessive bleeding from other causes, 367

Dilation stage, first stage of labor; begins with uterine contractions that press fetus against cervix causing it to dilate to 10 cm and become thin; thinning of cervix is called *effacement*, 354, 355*f*

Diphtheria, bacterial infection characterized by severe inflammation that can form membrane coating in upper respiratory tract that can cause marked difficulty breathing, 244

Diplopia, double vision, 481

Directional terms, 42–43, 43*t*–44*t*

Discharge summary, part of patient's medical record; comprehensive outline of patient's entire hospital stay; includes condition at time of admission, admitting diagnosis, test results, treatments and patient's response, final diagnosis, and follow-up plans, 14*t*

Dislocation, occurs when bones in joint are displaced from their normal alignment, 113

Disruptive, impulse control, and conduct disorders, a classification of psychiatric disorders in the DSM-5 characterized by the inability to resist impulses to perform some act harmful to individual or others; includes kleptomania, pyromania, and explosive disorder, 454

Dissociative amnesia, loss of memory, 454

Dissociative disorders, a classification of psychiatric disorders in the DSM-5 in which severe emotional conflict is so repressed that split in personality or memory loss occurs; includes dissociative amnesia and dissociative identity disorder, 454

Efferent, moving away from, 311

Efferent arteriole, arteriole that carries blood away from glomerulus, 315, 316*f*

Efferent neurons, carry impulses away from brain and spinal cord to muscles and glands; also called *motor neurons*, 433–434, 435*f*

Egg cell, 349*f*, 350*f*

Ejaculation, impulse of forcing seminal fluid from male urethra, 374

Elastin fibers, 229*f*

Elective abortion, legal termination of pregnancy for nonmedical reasons, 367

Electrocardiogram (ECG, EKG), record of electrical activity of heart; useful in diagnosis of abnormal cardiac rhythm and heart muscle (myocardium) damage, 154*f*, 169

Electrocardiography, process of recording electrical activity of heart, 169

Electrocautery, to destroy tissue with electric current, 78

Electroconvulsive therapy (ECT), procedure occasionally used for cases of prolonged major depression in which electrode is placed on one or both sides of patient's head and current is turned on briefly causing convulsive seizure; low level of voltage used in modern ECT, and patient is administered muscle relaxant and anesthesia; advocates today correctly state it is a more effective way to treat severe depression than using drugs; not effective with disorders other than depression, such as schizophrenia and alcoholism, 457

Electroencephalogram (EEG), record of brain's electrical activity, 447

Electroencephalography (EEG), recording electrical activity of brain by placing electrodes at various positions on scalp; also used in sleep studies to determine if there is a normal pattern of activity during sleep, 447

Electrolyte, chemical compound that separates into charged particles, or ionizes, in solution; sodium (Na⁺), potassium (K⁺), and chloride (Cl⁻) are examples of electrolytes, 318

Electromyogram (EMG), record of muscle electricity, 132

Electromyography, recording of electrical patterns of muscle in order to diagnose diseases, 132

Electronic Medical Record (EMR), digital version of patient's medical record created by using software program to enter patient information into computer or tablet, 14, 14*t*

Elephantiasis, inflammation, obstruction, and destruction of lymph vessels that results in enlarged tissues due to edema, 211

Elevation, muscle action that raises body part, as in shrugging the shoulders, 126*t*

Elimination disorders, classification of psychiatric disorders in DSM-5 involving inappropriate voiding of urine or feces; includes enuresis and encopresis, 454

Embolectomy, surgical removal of embolus or clot from a blood vessel, 171

Embolus, obstruction of blood vessel by blood clot that moves from another area, 162, 162*f*

Embryo, term to describe developing infant from fertilization until end of eighth week, 353–354, 354*f*

Embryonic, pertaining to embryo, 357

Emesis, vomiting; expulsion of stomach contents through mouth, 285

Emmetropia (EM), state of normal vision, 481

Emphysema, pulmonary condition that can occur as result of long-term heavy smoking; air pollution also worsens this disease; patient may not be able to breathe except in sitting or standing position, 246

Empyema, pus within pleural space, usually result of infection, 247

Emulsification, to make fats and lipids more soluble in water, 279

Enamel, hardest substance in body; covers outer surface of teeth, 272, 273*f*

Encephalic, pertaining to brain, 437

Encephalitis, inflammation of brain due to disease factors such as rabies, influenza, measles, or smallpox, 442

Encopresis, elimination disorder characterized by voiding feces in inappropriate places after toilet training, 454

Endarterectomy, removal of inside layer of an artery, 171

Endings
plural, 12
singular, 12

Endocarditis, inflammation of inner lining layer of heart; may be due to microorganisms or to abnormal immunological response, 164

Endocardium, inner layer of heart, which is very smooth and lines chambers of heart, 150, 150*f*

Endocervicitis, inflammation of inner aspect of cervix, 360

Endocrine glands, glandular system that secretes hormones directly into bloodstream rather than into duct; endocrine glands are frequently referred to as ductless glands; endocrine system includes thyroid gland, adrenal glands, parathyroid glands, pituitary gland, pancreas (islets of Langerhans), testes, ovaries, and thymus gland, 396, 396*t*–397*t*

Endocrine system, body system consisting of glands that secrete hormones directly into bloodstream; endocrine glands include adrenal glands, parathyroid glands, pancreas, pituitary gland, testes, ovaries, thymus gland, and thyroid gland, 35*t*, 393–415, 395*f*
abbreviations, 415
adjective forms of anatomical terms, 406
adrenal glands, 396, 398–399, 408–409
anatomy and physiology, 396–404, 396*t*–397*t*
diagnostic procedures, 412–413
medical specialties, 35*t*, 407
ovaries, 348–349, 348*f*, 349*f*, 360, 396, 396*t*–397*t*, 399, 399*f*
pancreas, 270, 279*f*, 280, 396, 397*t*, 399–400, 400*f*, 409
parathyroid glands, 396, 397*t*, 400, 401*f*, 409–410
pathology, 407–411
pharmacology, 414–415
pineal gland, 396, 397*t*, 400, 401*f*
pituitary gland, 396, 401–402, 401*f*, 402*f*, 410

Endocrinologist, physician who specializes in treatment of endocrine glands, 407

Endocrinology, branch of medicine specializing in conditions of endocrine system, 35t, 407

Endocrinopathy, disease of endocrine system, 407

Endometrial, pertaining to the endometrium, 357

Endometrial biopsy (EMB), taking sample of tissue from lining of uterus to test for abnormalities, 366

Endometrial cancer, cancer of endometrial lining of uterus, 360

Endometriosis, abnormal condition of endometrium tissue appearing throughout pelvis or on abdominal wall; this tissue is usually found within uterus, 362

Endometritis, inflammation of endometrial lining of uterus, 360

Endometrium, inner lining of uterus; contains rich blood supply and reacts to hormonal changes every month, which results in menstruation; during pregnancy, lining of uterus does not leave body but remains to nourish unborn child, 350, 350f

Endoscopic retrograde cholangiopancreatography (ERCP), using endoscope to X-ray bile and pancreatic ducts, 294

Endothelium, 153f

Endotracheal intubation, placing tube through mouth to create airway, 251, 251f

Enema, injection of fluid through rectum and into large intestine for purpose of cleansing bowel for testing, treating constipation, or administering drugs, 295

Enteric, pertaining to small intestine, 282

Enteritis, inflammation of only small intestine, 288

Enucleated, loss of cell's nucleus, 188

Enucleation, surgical removal of an eyeball, 488

Enuresis, elimination disorder characterized by the involuntary discharge of urine after age by which bladder control should have been established; usually occurs by age 5; *nocturnal enuresis* refers to bed-wetting at night, 324, 454

Eosinophil (eosins, eos), granulocyte white blood cells that destroy parasites and increase during allergic reactions, 189f, 189t

Eosinophilic, pertaining to [a leukocyte] that attracts a rosy red stain, 192

Epicardium, outer layer of heart; forms part of pericardium, 150, 150f

Epicondyle, projection located above or on condyle, 94, 95f

Epidermal, pertaining to above [upon] the skin, 64

Epidermis, superficial layer of skin; is composed of squamous epithelium cells; these are flat scalelike cells that are arranged in layers, called *stratified squamous epithelium*; many layers of epidermis create a barrier to infection; epidermis does not have a blood supply, so is dependent on deeper layers of skin for nourishment; however, deepest epidermis layer is called *basal layer*; these cells are alive and constantly dividing; older cells are pushed out toward surface by new cells forming beneath; during this process, they shrink and die, becoming filled with a protein called *keratin*; keratin-filled cells are sloughed off as dead cells, 58–60, 59f, 61f

Epididymal, pertaining to epididymis, 376

Epididymectomy, surgical removal of epididymis, 380

Epididymis, coiled tubule that lies on top of testes within scrotum; stores sperm as they are produced and turns into vas deferens, 373, 373f, 374, 378, 403f

Epididymitis, inflammation of epididymis causing pain and swelling in inguinal area, 378

Epidural hematoma, mass of blood in space outside dura mater of brain and spinal cord, 445

Epidural space, 433f

Epigastric, anatomical division of abdomen, middle section of upper row, 41f, 41t

Epiglottic, pertaining to epiglottis, 239

Epiglottis, flap of cartilage that covers larynx when swallowing; prevents food and drink from entering larynx and trachea, 231f, 232, 272f, 274

Epilepsy, recurrent disorder of brain in which convulsive seizures and loss of consciousness occur, 442

Epinephrine, hormone produced by adrenal medulla; also known as *adrenaline*; actions include increased heart rate and force of contraction, bronchodilation, and relaxation of intestinal muscles, 396t, 398–399

Epiphyseal line, 93f

Epiphysis, wide ends of a long bone, 92, 93f

Episiorrhaphy, to suture perineum after birth, 367

Episiotomy, surgical incision of perineum to facilitate delivery process; can prevent irregular tearing of tissue during birth, 367

Epispadias, congenital opening of urethra on dorsal surface of penis, 378

Epistaxis, nosebleed, 242

Epithelial tissue, tissue found throughout body as skin, outer covering of organs, and inner lining for tubular or hollow structures, 28, 30f

Epithelium, epithelial tissue composed of close-packed cells that form covering for and lining of body structures, 29, 30f

Equilibrium, sense of balance, 494

Erectile dysfunction (ED), inability to copulate due to inability to maintain erection; also called *impotence*, 378, 456

Erectile dysfunction agents, medications that temporarily produce erection in patients with erectile dysfunction, 382

Erectile tissue, tissue with numerous blood vessels and nerve endings; becomes filled with blood and enlarges in size in response to sexual stimulation, 351, 374

Eructation, burping of gas or stomach acid into mouth; belching, 285

Erythema, redness or flushing of skin, 66

Erythroblastosis fetalis. *See* Hemolytic disease of the newborn

Erythrocyte, also called *red blood cells* (RBCs); cells that contain hemoglobin, an iron-containing pigment that binds oxygen in order to transport it to cells of body, 188, 189*f*, 194–195, 194*f*

Erythrocyte sedimentation rate (ESR, sed rate), blood test to determine rate at which mature red blood cells settle out of blood after addition of anticoagulant; indicates of presence of inflammatory disease, 196

Erythrocytic, pertaining to red blood cells, 192

Erythrocytosis, too many red cells, 194

Erythroderma, red skin, 66

Erythropenia, too few red cells, 194

Eschar, thick layer of dead tissue and tissue fluid that develops over deep burn area, 66

Esophageal, pertaining to esophagus, 282

Esophageal varices, enlarged and swollen varicose veins in lower end of esophagus; they can rupture and result in serious hemorrhage, 286

Esophagogastroduodenoscopy (EGD), use of flexible fiber-optic scope to visually examine esophagus, stomach, and beginning of duodenum, 294

Esophagus, tube that carries food from pharynx to stomach, 270, 271*f*, 272*f*, 274, 275*f*, 286

Esotropia (ET), inward turning of eye; example of a form of strabismus (muscle weakness of eye), 476*f*, 485

Estimated glomerular filtration rate (eGFR), urine test to measure kidney function, 328

Estrogen, one of hormones produced by ovaries; works with progesterone to control menstrual cycle and is responsible for producing secondary sexual characteristics, 348–349, 396*t*, 399

Ethmoid bone, cranial bone, 95, 97, 97*f*, 97*t*

Eupnea, normal breathing, 242

Eustachian tube, tube or canal that connects middle ear with nasopharynx and allows for balance of pressure between outer and middle ear; infection can travel via mucous membranes of eustachian tube, resulting in middle ear infections; also called *auditory tube*, 231–232, 272*f*, 494*f*, 495

Eversion, directional term meaning turning outward, 126*t*, 127*f*

Ewing's sarcoma, malignant growth found in shaft of long bones that spreads through periosteum; removal is treatment of choice, as tumor will metastasize or spread to other organs, 110

Excisional biopsy, entire suspicious area of tissue removed for examination, 77

Excretory urography (EU), injection of dye into bloodstream followed by taking X-ray to trace action of kidney as it excretes dye in the urine, 329

Exfoliative cytology, scraping cells from tissue and then examining them under microscope, 77

Exhalation, to breathe air out of lungs; also called *expiration*, 230

Exocrine, 396

Exocrine glands, secrete substances into a duct; examples include tears and tear ducts, 396

Exophthalmos, condition in which eyeballs protrude, such as in Graves' disease; generally caused by overproduction of thyroid hormone, 407

Exostosis, bone spur, 110

Exotropia (XT), outward turning of eye; an example of strabismus (muscle weakness of eye), 476*f*, 485

Expectorant, substance that assists in removal of secretions from bronchopulmonary membranes, 254

Expiration. *See* Exhalation

Expiratory reserve volume (ERV), amount of air that can be forcibly exhaled after normal quiet respiration; also called *supplemental air*, 235*t*

Exploratory laparotomy, abdominal operation for purpose of examining abdominal organs and tissues for signs of disease or other abnormalities, 297

Explosive disorder, impulse control disorder in which patient is unable to control violent rages, 454

Expulsion stage, stage of labor and delivery during which baby is delivered, 354, 355*f*

Extension, movement that brings limb into or toward a straight condition, 125*f*, 126*t*

Extensor carpi, muscle named for its action, extension, 124

External auditory meatus, opening into external ear canal, 494, 494*f*

External ear, outermost portion of ear; consists of auricle, auditory canal, and eardrum, 494–495, 494*f*, 499

External fixation. *See* Fixation

External iliac artery, 157*f*

External iliac vein, 158*f*

External oblique, muscle named for direction of its fibers, on an oblique angle, 119*f*, 124

External respiration, exchange of oxygen and carbon dioxide that takes place in lungs, 230

External sphincter, ring of voluntary muscle that controls emptying of urine from bladder, 316–317

Extracorporeal circulation (ECC), during open heart surgery, routing of blood to heart-lung machine so it can be oxygenated and pumped to rest of body, 171

Extracorporeal shockwave lithotripsy (ESWL), use of ultrasound waves from outside the body to break up stones; process does not require surgery, 330, 330*f*

Extraction, removing or pulling teeth, 295

Extraocular, pertaining to being outside eyeball, for example, extraocular eye muscles, 480

Eye, 472–491

  abbreviations, 491

  adjective forms of anatomical terms, 480

  anatomy and physiology, 473*f*, 474–478

  conjunctiva, 474, 474*f*, 477, 485

  diagnostic procedures, 486–487

  eyeball, 474, 474*f*, 482–485

  eyelids, 474, 474*f*, 482–485

  lacrimal apparatus, 474, 474*f*, 482–485

  medical specialties, 481

  muscles, 476, 476*f*

  pathology, 481–485

  pharmacology, 490

  retina, 474–475, 474*f*, 475*f*, 477, 478*f*

  terminology, 472, 479–480

  therapeutic procedures, 488–489

  vision, 477, 478*f*

Eyeball, eye by itself, without any appendages such as eye muscles or tear ducts, 474, 474*f*, 482–485

it becomes more permeable and will allow protein and blood cells to enter filtrate; results in protein in urine (proteinuria) and hematuria, 325

Glomerulus, ball of capillaries encased by Bowman's capsule; within filtration stage of urine production, wastes filtered from blood leave glomerulus capillaries and enter Bowman's capsule, 315, 316*f*

Glossal, pertaining to tongue, 282

Glossopharyngeal nerve, 434*t*

Glottis, opening between vocal cords; air passes through glottis as it moves through larynx; changing tension of vocal cords changes size of opening, 232

Glucagon, hormone secreted by pancreas; stimulates liver to release glucose into blood, 280, 397*t* 399–400, 400*f*

Glucocorticoids, group of hormones secreted by adrenal cortex; regulate carbohydrate levels in body; cortisol is an example, 396*t*, 398

Glucometer, device for measuring level of glucose in bloodstream, 413

Glucose, form of sugar used by cells of body to make energy; transported to cells in blood, 188

Glucose tolerance test (GTT), determines blood sugar level; a measured dose of glucose is given to patient either orally or intravenously; blood samples are then drawn at certain intervals to determine ability of patient to utilize glucose; used for diabetic patients to determine their insulin response to glucose, 412

Gluteal, pertaining to buttocks, 39*f*

Gluteal region, refers to buttock region of body, 38*t*, 39*f*

Gluteus maximus, muscle named for its size and location; gluteus means "rump area" and maximus means "large," 124

Glycosuria, presence of sugar in the urine, 324, 407

Goiter, enlargement of thyroid gland, 411, 411*f*

Gonadotropins, general name for two anterior pituitary hormones, follicle-stimulating hormone and luteinizing hormone, 397*t*, 401–402, 402*f*

Gonads, organs responsible for producing sex cells; female gonads are ovaries, and they produce ova; male gonads are testes, and they produce sperm, 399

Gonorrhea, sexually transmitted inflammation of mucous membranes of either sex; can be passed on to infant during birth process, 379

Gout, type of arthritis; usually in first metatarsophalangeal joint; caused by high uric acid blood level, 113

Graft versus host disease (GVHD), serious complication of bone marrow transplant; immune cells from donor bone marrow (graft) attack recipient's (host's) tissues, 212

Grand mal seizure. *See* Tonic-clonic seizure

Granulocytes, granular polymorphonuclear leukocytes; three types: neutrophil, eosinophil, and basophil, 189, 189*t*

Graves' disease, condition resulting in overactivity of thyroid gland and can result in crisis situation; a type of *hyperthyroidism*, 411

Gray matter, tissue within central nervous system; consists of unsheathed or uncovered nerve cell bodies and dendrites, 428–429

Great saphenous vein, 158*f*

Greenstick fracture, fracture in which there is incomplete break; one side of bone is broken and other side is bent; commonly found in children due to their softer and more pliable bone structure, 109

Growth hormone (GH), hormone secreted by anterior pituitary that stimulates growth of body, 397*t*, 401–402, 402*f*

Guillain-Barré syndrome, disease of nervous system in which nerves lose their myelin covering; may be caused by autoimmune reaction; characterized by loss of sensation and/or muscle control in arms and legs; symptoms then move toward trunk and may even result in paralysis of diaphragm, 444

Gums, tissue around teeth; also called *gingiva*, 270–271, 271*f*

Gut, name for continuous muscular tube that stretches between mouth and anus; also called *alimentary canal*, 270

Gynecologist, physician specialized in treating conditions and diseases of female reproductive system, 359

Gynecology (GYN, gyn), branch of medicine specializing in conditions of female reproductive system, 34*t*, 359

Gynecomastia, development of breast tissue in males; may be symptom of adrenal feminization, 407

Gyri, convoluted, elevated portions of cerebral cortex; separated by fissures or sulci; singular is *gyrus*, 429–430, 431*f*

H

H. pylori **antibody test,** used to diagnose *H. pylori* infection causing peptic ulcer disease; may be performed on stool, breath, or tissue sample, 292

H₂-receptor antagonist, blocks production of stomach acids, 299

Hair, structure in integumentary system, 58, 59*f*, 60, 61*f*, 75

Hair follicle, cavities in dermis that contain hair root; hair grows longer from root, 60, 61*f*

Hair root, deeper cells that divide to grow hair longer, 60, 61*f*

Hair shaft, older keratinized cells that form most of length of a hair, 60, 61*f*

Hallucination, perception of something that is not there; may be visual, auditory, gustatory, or tactile, 456

Hammer. *See* Malleus

Hard palate, 95*t*, 231*f*, 267*f*, 272*f*

Hashimoto's thyroiditis, chronic form of thyroiditis, 411

Head, large ball-shaped end of a bone; may be separated from shaft of bone by area called *neck*, 94

Healthcare-associated infection (HAI), infection acquired from patients or healthcare workers; also called *nosocomial infection*, 207

Healthcare settings, 15, 15*t*

Health Insurance Portability and Accountability Act (HIPAA), 16

Health Maintenance Organization (HMO), organization that contracts with group of physicians and other healthcare workers to provide care exclusively for its members, 15*t*

Iliac, pertaining to ilium; one of pelvic bones, 105

Ilium, one of three bones that form the os coxae or innominate bone of the pelvis, 91*f*, 98, 100, 101*f*, 101*t*

Immune response, ability of lymphocytes to respond to specific antigens, 205–207, 206*f*

Immunity, body's ability to defend itself against pathogens, 205–207
  immune response, 205–207, 206*f*
  standard precautions, 207

Immunization, providing protection against communicable diseases by stimulating immune system to produce antibodies against that disease; also called *vaccination*, 205–206

Immunocompromised, having immune system unable to respond properly to pathogens, 212

Immunodeficiency disorder. *See* Immunocompromised

Immunoglobulin (Ig), antibodies secreted by B cells; all antibodies are immunoglobulins; assist in protecting body and its surfaces from invasion of bacteria; for example, immunoglobulin IgA in colostrum, first milk from mother, helps to protect newborn from infection, 206

Immunologist, physician who specializes in treating infectious diseases and other disorders of immune system, 209

Immunology, branch of medicine specializing in conditions of lymphatic and immune systems, 33*t*, 209

Immunosuppressants, substances that block certain actions of immune system; required to prevent rejection of transplanted organ, 215

Immunotherapy, boosting or strengthening of patient's immune system in order to treat disease, 215

Impacted fracture, fracture in which bone fragments are pushed into each other, 109

Impetigo, highly contagious staphylococcal skin infection, most commonly occurring on faces of children; begins as blisters that then rupture and dry into thick, yellow crust, 73, 73*f*

Implant, prosthetic device placed in jaw to which a tooth or denture may be anchored, 295

Implantable cardioverter-defibrillator (ICD), device implanted in heart that delivers electrical shock to restore normal heart rhythm; particularly useful for persons who experience ventricular fibrillation, 171

Incision and drainage (I&D), making incision to create opening for drainage of material such as pus, 78

Incisors, biting teeth in very front of mouth that function to cut food into smaller pieces; humans have eight incisors, 271*f*, 272, 273*f*

Incus, one of three ossicles of middle ear; also called *anvil*, 495, 495*f*

Infant respiratory distress syndrome (IRDS), lung condition most commonly found in premature infants characterized by tachypnea and respiratory grunting; also called *hyaline membrane disease* (HMD) and *respiratory distress syndrome of the newborn*, 246

Infarct, area of tissue within organ that undergoes necrosis (death) following loss of blood supply, 162

Inferior, directional term meaning toward feet or tail, or below; akin to *caudal*, 43*f*, 43*t*

Inferior vena cava, branch of vena cava that drains blood from abdomen and lower body, 152, 153*f*, 158*f*, 398*f*

Infertility, inability to produce children; generally defined as no pregnancy after properly timed intercourse for one year, 363

Inflammation, tissue response to injury from pathogens or physical agents; characterized by redness, pain, swelling, and feeling hot to touch, 210, 210*f*

Inflammatory bowel disease (IBD). *See* Ulcerative colitis

Influenza (flu), viral infection of respiratory system characterized by chills, fever, body aches, and fatigue; commonly called the *flu*, 246

Informed consent, medical record document, voluntarily signed by patient, or responsible party, that clearly describes purpose, methods, procedures, benefits, and risks of diagnostic or treatment procedure, 14*t*

Inguinal, pertaining to groin area; there is a collection of lymph nodes in this region that drain each leg, 209

Inguinal hernia, hernia or protrusion of intestine into inguinal region of body, 289, 289*f*

Inguinal nodes, 203*t*, 204*f*

Inhalation, (1) to breathe air into lungs; also called *inspiration*; (2) to introduce drugs into body by breathing them in, 45, 46*t*, 230

Inhalation anesthesia, general anesthesia administered by breathing it in, 448

Innate immunity. *See* Natural immunity

Inner ear, innermost section of ear; contains cochlea, semicircular canals, saccule, and utricle, 494, 494*f*, 495, 496*f*, 500

Inner ear infection. *See* Labyrinthitis

Innominate bone, also called *os coxae* or *hipbone*; pelvis portion of lower extremity; consists of ilium, ischium, and pubis and unites with sacrum and coccyx to form pelvis, 98, 100

Insertion, attachment of skeletal muscle to more movable bone in joint, 124, 125*f*

Insomnia disorder, sleeping disorder characterized by marked inability to fall asleep, 456

Inspiration. *See* Inhalation

Inspiratory capacity (IC), volume of air inhaled after normal exhale, 235*t*

Inspiratory reserve volume (IRV), air that can be forcibly inhaled after normal respiration has taken place; also called *complemental air*, 235*t*

Insulin, hormone secreted by pancreas; regulates level of sugar in bloodstream; the more insulin present in blood, the lower blood sugar will be, 280, 397*t*, 399–400, 400*f*, 414

Insulin-dependent diabetes mellitus (IDDM), also called *type 1 diabetes mellitus*; develops early in life when pancreas stops insulin production; people with IDDM must take daily insulin injections, 409

Insulinoma, tumor of islets of Langerhans cells of pancreas that secretes excessive amount of insulin, 409

Integument, another term for skin, 58

Integumentary system, skin and its appendages including sweat glands, oil glands, hair, and nails;

Ischemia, localized and temporary deficiency of blood supply due to obstruction of circulation, 162

Ischial, pertaining to ischium, one of pelvic bones, 105

Ischium, one of three bones forming os coxae or innominate bone of pelvis, 91*f*, 98, 100, 101*f*, 101*t*

Islets of Langerhans, regions within pancreas that secrete insulin and glucagon; also called *pancreatic islets*, 399–400, 400*f*

Isthmus, 404*f*

J

Jaundice, yellow cast to skin, mucous membranes, and whites of eyes caused by deposit of bile pigment from too much bilirubin in blood; bilirubin is a waste product produced when worn-out red blood cells are broken down; may be symptom of disorders such as gallstones blocking common bile duct or carcinoma of liver, 285

Jejunal, pertaining to jejunum, 282

Jejunostomy, 277

Jejunum, middle portion of small intestine; site of nutrient absorption, 275–276, 276*f*

Joint, point at which two bones meet; provides flexibility, 92, 101–102, 102*f*, 113–114, 114*f*

Joint capsule, elastic capsule that encloses synovial joints, 101, 102, 102*f*

Jugular vein, 158*f*

K

Kaposi's sarcoma (KS), form of skin cancer frequently seen in acquired immunodeficiency syndrome (AIDS) patients; consists of brownish-purple papules that spread from skin and metastasize to internal organs, 73, 212

Keloid, formation of scar after injury or surgery resulting in raised, thickened red area, 73, 73*f*

Keratin, hard protein substance produced by body; found in hair and nails, and filling inside of epidermal cells, 58, 60

Keratitis, inflammation of cornea, 483

Keratometer, instrument to measure cornea, 486

Keratometry, measurement of curvature of cornea using instrument called a *keratometer*, 487

Keratoplasty, surgical repair of cornea (corneal transplant), 488

Keratosis, overgrowth and thickening of epithelium, 73

Ketoacidosis, acidosis due to excess of ketone bodies (waste products); serious condition requiring immediate treatment as it may result in death for diabetic patient if not reversed, 409

Ketones, waste products in the bloodstream, 315, 320*t*

Ketonuria, ketones in urine, 324

Kidneys, two organs located in lumbar region of back behind parietal peritoneum; under muscles of back, just a little above waist; have concave or depressed area that gives them bean-shaped appearance; center of this concavity is called *hilum*, 313*f*, 314–315, 315*f*, 318

Kidneys, ureters, bladder (KUB), X-ray taken of abdomen demonstrating kidneys, ureters, and bladder without using any contrast dye; also called *flat-plate abdomen*, 329

Kinesiology, study of movement, 129

Kissing disease. *See* Mononucleosis

Kleptomania, impulse control disorder in which patient ls unable to refrain from stealing, 454

Kyphosis, abnormal increase in outward curvature of thoracic spine; also known as *hunchback* or *humpback*, 111, 112*f*

L

Labial, pertaining to the lips, 283

Labia majora, outer folds of skin that serves as protection for female external genitalia and urethral meatus, 348*f*, 351, 351*f*

Labia minora, inner folds of skin that serve as protection for female external genitalia and urethral meatus, 348*f*, 351, 351*f*

Labor, period of time beginning with uterine contractions and ending with birth of baby; there are three stages: dilation, expulsion, and placental stage, 354, 355*f*

Labyrinth, refers to inner ear; several fluid-filled cavities within temporal bone; labyrinth consists of cochlea, vestibule, and three semicircular canals; hair cells called *organ of Corti* line inner ear; hair cells change sound vibrations to electrical impulses and send impulses to brain via vestibulocochlear nerve, 494*f*, 495

Labyrinthectomy, surgical removal of labyrinth, 503

Labyrinthitis, labyrinth inflammation, 500

Labyrinthotomy, incision in labyrinth, 503

Laceration, torn or jagged wound; incorrectly used to describe a cut, 73

Lacrimal, pertaining to tears, 480

Lacrimal apparatus, consists of lacrimal gland, lacrimal canals, and nasolacrimal duct, 474, 474*f*, 477, 477*f*, 485

Lacrimal bone, facial bone, 95, 97, 97*f*, 97*t*

Lacrimal canals, located in inner corner of eye socket; collect tears and drain them into lacrimal sac, 477, 477*f*

Lacrimal gland, located in outer corner of each eyelid; washes anterior surface of eye with fluid called *tears*, 477, 477*f*

Lactation, function of secreting milk after childbirth from breasts or mammary glands, 352

Lacteals, lymphatic vessels in intestines that serve to absorb fats from diet, 202

Lactic, pertaining to milk, 358

Lactiferous ducts, carry milk from milk-producing glands to nipple, 352, 352*f*

Lactiferous glands, milk-producing glands in breast, 352, 352*f*

Lactorrhea, discharge of milk, 362

Laminectomy, removal of portion of a vertebra in order to relieve pressure on spinal nerve, 117, 449

Lymphocytic leukemia, type of leukemia in which abnormal white blood cells are lymphocytes; may be acute (rapid onset and progression) or chronic (slow onset and progression), 195

Lymphoma, tumor of lymphatic tissue, 211

M

Macrophage, phagocytic cells found in large quantities in lymph nodes; engulf foreign particles,205–206, 206*f*

Macrotia, abnormally large ears, 499

Macula lutea, area of retina onto which straight-ahead images are projected, 474*f*, 475, 475*f*

Macular, pertaining to macula lutea, 480

Macular degeneration, deterioration of macular area of retina of eye; may be treated with laser surgery to destroy blood vessels beneath macula, 483

Macule, flat, discolored area flush with skin surface; example would be freckle or birthmark, 66, 66*f*

Magnetic resonance imaging (MRI), use of electromagnetic energy to produce image of soft tissues in any plane of body; atoms behave differently when placed in strong magnetic field, when body is exposed to this magnetic field nuclei of body's atoms emit radio-frequency signals that can be used to create an image, 214, 214*f*

Major depressive disorder, mood disorder characterized by marked loss of interest in usually enjoyable activities, disturbances in sleep and eating patterns, fatigue, suicidal thoughts, and feelings of hopelessness, helplessness, and worthlessness, 454

Male reproductive system, responsible for producing sperm for reproduction; organs include testes, vas deferens, urethra, prostate gland, and penis, 35*t*, 371–382

abbreviations, 382
adjective forms of anatomical terms, 376
anatomy and physiology, 372*f*, 373–375
bulbourethral glands, 382
diagnostic procedures, 380
epididymis, 373, 373*f*, 374, 378
external organs of, 373–374, 373*f*
internal organs of, 374–375
medical specialties, 35*t*, 377
pathology, 377–379
penis, 373, 373*f*, 374, 378
pharmacology, 382
prostate gland, 373, 373*f*, 374, 378
seminal vesicles, 373, 373*f*, 374, 378
terminology, 371, 375–376
testes, 373–374, 373*f*, 377–378
therapeutic procedures, 380–381
vas deferens, 373–374, 373*f*, 377–378

Male urethra, 313*f*

Malignant melanoma (MM), cancerous, darkly pigmented tumor or mole on skin, 73, 73*f*

Malleus, one of three ossicles of middle ear; also called *hammer,* 495, 495*f*

Mammary, pertaining to breast, 358

Mammary glands, breasts; milk-producing glands to provide nutrition for newborn, 352, 352*f*

Mammogram, X-ray record of breast, 365

Mammography, process of X-raying breast, 365

Mammoplasty, surgical repair of breast, 368

Mandible, lower jawbone, 95, 97, 97*f*, 97*t*

Mandibular, pertaining to mandible or lower jaw, 105

Mania, depressive disorder characterized by extreme elation, hyperactivity, excessive talkativeness, impaired judgment, distractibility, and grandiose delusions, 454

Mantoux test. *See* Tuberculin skin test

Massage, kneading or applying pressure by hands to a part of patient's body to promote muscle relaxation and reduce tension, 132

Mastalgia, breast pain, 360

Mastectomy, surgical removal of breast, 368

Mastication, chewing, 270–271

Mastitis, inflammation of breast, common during lactation but can occur at any age, 362

Mastoid process, 124, 494*f*

Maxilla, upper jawbone, 95, 97, 97*f*, 97*t*

Maxillary, pertaining to maxilla or upper jaw, 105

Meatal, pertaining to meatus, 322

Meatotomy, surgical enlargement of urinary opening (meatus), 331

Meconium, substance that collects in intestines of fetus and becomes first stool of newborn, 358

Medial, directional term meaning to middle or near middle of body or structure, 43*f*, 44*t*

Median cubital vein, 158*f*

Median nerve, 435*f*

Median plane, when sagittal plane passes through middle of body, dividing it into equal right and left halves; also called *midsagittal plane,* 37–38, 37*f*

Mediastinal nodes, collection of lymph nodes located in mediastinum (central chest area) that drain chest, 203*t*, 204*f*

Mediastinum, central region of chest cavity; contains organs between lungs, including heart, aorta, esophagus, and trachea, 40, 40*f*, 149*f*, 234, 234*f*, 404*f*

Medical record, documents details of patient's hospital stay; each healthcare professional that has contact with patient in any capacity completes appropriate report of that contact and adds it to medical chart; permanent physical record of patient's day-to-day condition, when and what services received, and response to treatment; also called a *chart,* 13–14, 14*t*

Medical terms
interpreting, 11
pronouncing, 11
spelling, 11–12

Medulla, middle area of an organ; in endocrine system refers to adrenal medulla; in urinary system, refers to inner portion of kidney, 314, 315*f*

Medulla oblongata, portion of brainstem that connects spinal cord with brain; contains respiratory, cardiac, and blood pressure control centers, 429, 430*f*, 431, 431*f*, 434

Medullary, 1) pertaining to medulla or inner region; 2) pertaining to medulla oblongata, 105, 437

Mononucleosis (mono), acute infectious disease with large number of atypical lymphocytes; caused by Epstein-Barr virus; there may be abnormal liver function; commonly called *kissing disease*, 211

Monoparesis, weakness of one extremity, 439

Monoplegia, paralysis of one extremity, 439

Monospot, blood test to diagnose mononucleosis, 214

Morbid obesity. *See* Obesity

Motor neurons, nerves that carry activity instruction from CNS to muscles or glands out in body; also called *efferent neurons*, 123, 433, 435f

Mouth, external opening of alimentary canal; receives food; also called *oral cavity*, 270–271, 271f, 272f

Mucolytic, substance that liquefies mucus so it is easier to cough and clear it from respiratory tract, 254

Mucous, pertaining to mucus, 239

Mucous membrane, membrane that lines body passages that open directly to exterior of body, such as mouth and reproductive tract; secretes thick substance, or mucus; conjunctiva of eye is also a mucous membrane, 230, 477

Mucus, sticky fluid secreted by mucous membrane lining of respiratory tract; assists in cleansing air by trapping dust and bacteria, 230

Multigravida, woman with many (two or more) pregnancies, 359

Multipara, woman who has given birth to live infant many (two or more) times, 359

Multiple myeloma, cancer of lymphocytes that collect in bone marrow, resulting in bone marrow tumor, 212

Multiple sclerosis (MS), inflammatory disease of central nervous system in which there is extreme weakness and numbness due to loss of myelin insulation from around nerves that result in "hard" patches called plaques to appear, 444f

Murmur, extra heart sound as soft blowing sound or harsh click; may be soft and heard only with a stethoscope, or so loud it can be heard several feet away, 162

Muscle actions, 124, 125f, 125t, 126t, 127t

Muscle biopsy, removal of muscle tissue for pathological examination, 132

Muscle cells, 30f

Muscle fibers, bundles of muscle cells that form muscle, 122

Muscle wasting. *See* Atrophy

Muscles, bundles of parallel muscle tissue fibers; as fibers contract (shorten in length) they pull whatever they are attached to closer together; may move two bones closer together or make opening narrower; muscle contraction occurs when message is transmitted from brain through nervous system to muscles, 122, 428

Muscular, pertaining to muscles, 128

Muscular dystrophy (MD), inherited disease causing progressive muscle weakness and atrophy, 130

Muscular system, 120–134, 121f
abbreviations, 134
adjective forms of anatomical terms, 128
anatomy and physiology, 121f, 122–127, 122f, 123f, 125f, 126f, 127f
combining forms, 120, 128

diagnostic procedures, 131–132
functions, 32t
medical specialties, 32t
muscle types, 122–123, 122f, 123f
pathology, 129–131
pharmacology, 133
suffixes and prefixes, 128
terminology, 121, 124, 128
terminology for muscle actions, 124, 125f–127f
therapeutic procedures, 132–133

Muscular tissue, able to contract and shorten its length, thereby producing movement; may be under voluntary control (attached to bones) or involuntary control (heart and digestive organs), 28, 29, 30f

Musculoskeletal, pertaining to muscles and the skeleton, 128

Musculoskeletal system (MS), system providing support for body and produces movement; organs include muscles, tendons, bones, joints, and cartilage, 89–134. *See also* Muscular system; Skeletal system

Myalgia, muscle pain, 130

Myasthenia, lack of muscle strength, 130

Myasthenia gravis, disorder causing loss of muscle strength and paralysis; autoimmune disease, 444

Mycobacterium tuberculosis, bacteria responsible for causing tuberculosis, 247

Mycoplasma pneumonia, less severe but longer-lasting form of pneumonia caused by *Mycoplasma pneumoniae* bacteria; also called *walking pneumonia*, 246

Mydriatic drops, substance that causes pupil to dilate, 490

Myelin, tissue that wraps around many nerve fibers; composed of fatty material and functions as insulator, 428, 429f

Myelinated, nerve fibers covered with layer of myelin, 428–429

Myelitis, inflammation of spinal cord, 443

Myelogram, X-ray record of spinal cord after injection of meninges with radiopaque dye, 115, 447

Myelography, injection of radiopaque dye into spinal canal; X-ray is taken to examine normal and abnormal outlines made by dye, 115, 447

Myeloid leukemia, type of leukemia in which abnormal leukocytes are granulocytes, usually neutrophils, 195

Myeloma, tumor that forms in bone marrow tissue, 110

Myelomeningocele, congenital condition in which meninges and spinal cord protrude through spinal cord, 443, 444f

Myelonic, pertaining to spinal cord, 437

Myocardial, pertaining to heart muscle, 161

Myocardial infarction (MI), condition caused by partial or complete occlusion or closing of one or more of coronary arteries; symptoms include severe chest pain or heavy pressure in middle of chest; delay in treatment could result in death; also referred to as *MI* or *heart attack*, 164, 165f

Myocarditis, inflammation of heart muscle, 165

Myocardium, middle layer of muscle; thick and composed of cardiac muscle; layer produces heart contraction, 123, 150, 150f, 153f

Myometrium, middle muscle layer of uterus, 350, 350f

Myoneural junction, point at which nerve contacts muscle fiber; also called *neuromuscular junction*, 123

Myopathy, any disease of muscles, 130

Myopia, condition in which person can see things that are close up but distance vision is blurred; also known as *nearsightedness*, 484, 484f

Myoplasty, surgical repair of muscle, 133

Myorrhaphy, suture a muscle, 133

Myorrhexis, tearing a muscle, 130

Myotonia, muscle tone, 130

Myringectomy, surgical removal of eardrum, 503

Myringitis, eardrum inflammation, 500

Myringoplasty, surgical reconstruction of eardrum; also called *tympanoplasty*, 503

Myringotomy, surgical puncture of eardrum with removal of fluid and pus from middle ear, to eliminate persistent ear infection and excessive pressure on tympanic membrane; polyethylene tube is placed in tympanic membrane to allow for drainage of middle ear cavity, 504

Myxedema, condition resulting from hypofunction of thyroid gland; symptoms can include anemia, slow speech, enlarged tongue and facial features, edematous skin, drowsiness, and mental apathy, 411

N

Nail bed, connects nail body to connective tissue underneath, 61, 61f

Nail body, flat plate of keratin that forms most of nails, 61, 61f

Nail root, base of nail; nails grow longer from root, 61, 61f

Nails, structure in integumentary system, 58, 61, 61f, 76

Narcissistic personality disorder, personality disorder characterized by abnormal sense of self-importance, 456

Narcolepsy, sleep-wake disorder with recurring episodes of sleeping during the daytime, 456

Narcotic analgesic, drug used to treat severe pain; has potential to be habit forming if taken for prolonged time; also called *opiates*, 450

Nares, external openings of nose that open into nasal cavity, 230, 231f

Nasal, pertaining to nose, 239

Nasal bone, facial bone, 95, 97, 97f, 97t

Nasal cannula, two-pronged plastic device for delivering oxygen into nose; one prong is inserted into each naris, 251

Nasal cavity, large cavity just behind external nose that receives outside air; covered with mucous membrane to cleanse air; nasal septum divides nasal cavity into left and right halves, 33t, 230–231, 231f, 272f, 477

Nasal septum, flexible cartilage wall that divides nasal cavity into left and right halves; covered by mucous membrane, 230

Nasal steroids, nose spray to reduce inflammation and treat symptoms of nasal rhinitis, 215

Nasogastric (NG), pertaining to nose and stomach, 283

Nasogastric intubation (NG tube), flexible catheter is inserted into nose and down esophagus to stomach; may be used for feeding or to suction out stomach fluids, 296

Nasolacrimal duct, collects tears from inner corner of eye socket and drains them into nasal cavity, 477, 477f

Nasopharyngeal, pertaining to the nasopharynx, 239

Nasopharyngitis, inflammation of nasal cavity and throat; commonly called the *common cold*, 244

Nasopharynx, superior section of pharynx that receives air from nose, 231–232, 231f, 272f

Natural immunity, immunity not specific to particular disease and does not require prior exposure to pathogen; also called *innate immunity*, 205–206

Natural killer (NK) **cells,** T cells that can kill by entrapping foreign cells, tumor cells, and bacteria; also called *T8 cells*, 206–207

Nausea, urge to vomit, 285

Nearsightedness. *See* Myopia

Nebulizer. *See* Aerosol therapy

Neck, 1) the cervical region of the body; 2) narrow length of bone that connects ball of ball and-socket joint to diaphysis of long bone, 38t, 94, 95f

Necrosis, dead tissue, 67

Necrotizing fasciitis (NF), typically a bacterial infection resulting in death of body's soft tissue (skin, fat, and fascia); commonly called *flesh-eating disease*, 130

Neonate, term to describe newborn infant during first four weeks of life, 359

Neonatologist, specialist in treatment of newborn, 359

Neonatology, study of newborn, 359

Nephrectomy, surgical removal of a kidney, 331

Nephritis, inflammation of kidney, 326

Nephroblastoma. *See* Wilms' tumor

Nephrogram, X-ray of kidney, 329

Nephrolith, kidney stone, 324

Nephrolithiasis, presence of calculi in kidney, 326

Nephrolithotomy, incision into kidney to remove a stone, 332

Nephrologist, specialist in treatment of kidney disorders, 319

Nephrology, branch of medicine specializing in conditions of urinary system, 34t, 323

Nephroma, kidney tumor, 326

Nephromalacia, softening of kidney, 324

Nephromegaly, enlarged kidney, 324

Nephron, functional or working unit of kidney that filters blood and produces urine; more than 1 million in adult kidney; each consists of renal corpuscle and renal tubules, 314, 315, 316f

Nephron loop, portion of renal tubule; also called *loop of Henle*, 315, 316f

Nephropathy, kidney disease, 326

Nephropexy, surgical fixation of kidney, 332

Nephroptosis, drooping kidney, 326

Nephrosclerosis, hardening of kidney, 324

Nephrosis. *See* Nephrotic syndrome

Nephrostomy, creating new opening across body wall into kidney, 332

Nephrotic syndrome (NS), damage to glomerulus resulting in protein appearing in urine, proteinuria, and corresponding decrease in protein in bloodstream; also called *nephrosis*, 326

Nephrotomy, incision into kidney, 332

Nerve block, also referred to as *regional anesthesia*; anesthetic interrupts patient's pain sensation in particular region of body; anesthetic injected near nerve that will be blocked from sensation; patient usually remains conscious, 449

Nerve cell body, portion of nerve cell that includes nucleus, 428, 429f

Nerve cells. *See* Neuron

Nerve conduction velocity, test to determine if nerves have been damaged by recording rate an electrical impulse is able to travel along a nerve; if nerve is damaged, velocity will be decreased, 448

Nerve root, point where spinal or cranial nerve is attached to CNS, 433–434

Nerves, structures in nervous system that conduct electrical impulses from brain and spinal cord to muscles and other organs, 30f, 31, 428, 433–434, 444–445, 445f

Nervous system, coordinates all conscious and subconscious activities of body; organs include brain, spinal cord, and nerves, 35t, 426–451
  abbreviations, 451
  adjective forms of anatomical terms, 437
  anatomy and physiology, 427f, 428–435
  central, 451
  diagnostic procedures, 447–448
  medical specialties, 35t, 438
  nervous tissue, 28, 30f, 31, 428
  pathology, 438–446
  peripheral, 428, 433–435, 434t, 435f
  pharmacology, 450
  terminology, 426, 436–437
  therapeutic procedures, 448–449

Nervous tissue, conducts electrical impulses to and from brain and rest of body, 28, 30f, 31, 428

Neural, pertaining to nerves, 437

Neuralgia, nerve pain, 439

Neurectomy, surgical removal of a nerve, 449

Neurocognitive disorders, classification of psychiatric disorders in DSM-5 characterized by deterioration of mental functions due to temporary brain or permanent brain dysfunction; includes dementia and Alzheimer's disease, 455

Neurodevelopmental disorders, classification of psychiatric disorders in DSM-5 associated with impairment in growth or development of CNS; includes intellectual development disorder, attention-deficit/hyperactivity disorder, and autism spectrum disorder, 455

Neurogenic bladder, loss of nervous control that leads to retention; may be caused by spinal cord injury or multiple sclerosis, 327

Neuroglial, pertaining to glial cells that surround and support neurons, 437

Neuroglial cells, nervous tissue cells that perform support functions for neurons, 428

Neurologist, physician who specializes in disorders of nervous system, 438

Neurology, branch of medicine specializing in conditions of nervous system, 35t, 438

Neuroma, nerve tumor, 444

Neuromuscular junction, point at which motor neuron contacts muscle fiber; also called *myoneural junction*, 123

Neuron, name for individual nerve cell; neurons group together to form nerves and other nervous tissue, 29f, 30f, 31, 428

Neuropathy, disease of nerves, 444

Neuroplasty, surgical repair of nerves, 449

Neurorrhaphy, suture a nerve, 449

Neurosurgeon, physician who specializes in treating conditions and diseases of the nervous system by surgical means, 438

Neurosurgery, branch of medicine specializing in surgery on nervous system, 35t, 438

Neurotransmitter, chemical messenger that carries electrical impulse across gap between two neurons, 428

Neutrophil, granulocyte white blood cells that are important for phagocytosis; also most numerous of leukocytes, 189f, 189t

Neutrophilic, pertaining to [a leukocyte] that attracts a neutral pH stain, 192

Nevus, pigmented (colored) congenital skin blemish, birthmark, or mole; usually benign but may become cancerous, 67

Night blindness. *See* Nyctalopia

Nipple, point at which milk is released from breast, 352, 352f

Nitrogenous wastes, waste products that contain nitrogen; products, such as ammonia and urea, are produced during protein metabolism, 319

Nocturia, excessive urination during night; may or may not be abnormal, 324

Nodule, solid, raised group of cells, 67, 67f

Non-Hodgkin's lymphoma (NHL), cancer of lymphatic tissues other than Hodgkin's lymphoma, 211, 211f

Non-insulin-dependent diabetes mellitus (NIDDM), also called *type 2 diabetes mellitus*; develops later in life when pancreas produces insufficient insulin; persons may take oral hypoglycemics to stimulate insulin secretion, or may eventually have to take insulin, 409

Nonproprietary name, recognized and accepted official name for drug; each drug has only one generic name, which is not subject to trademark, so any pharmaceutical manufacturer may use it; also called *generic name*, 16

Nonsteroidal anti-inflammatory drugs (NSAIDs), large group of drugs including aspirin and ibuprofen that provide mild pain relief and anti-inflammatory benefits for conditions such as arthritis, 118

Norepinephrine, hormone secreted by adrenal medulla; a strong vasoconstrictor, 396t, 398–399

Normal psychology, behaviors that include how personality develops, how people handle stress, and stages of mental development, 453

Nosocomial infection, infection acquired as a result of hospital exposure; also called *healthcare-associated infection*, 207, 213

Nucleus, structure within a cell that contains DNA, 28, 29f

Nulligravida, woman who has never been pregnant, 359

Nullipara, woman who has never produced a viable baby, 359

Number prefixes, 7

Nurse, to breastfeed a baby, 352

Nurse's notes, medical record document that records patient's care throughout day; includes vital signs, treatment specifics, patient's response to treatment, and patient's condition, 14t

Nursing home, facility that provides long-term care for patients who need extra time to recover from illness or accident before they return home or for persons who can no longer care for themselves; also called *long-term care facility*, 15t

Nyctalopia, difficulty seeing in dim light; usually due to damaged rods; also called *night blindness*, 481

Nystagmus, jerky-appearing involuntary eye movement, 485

O

Obesity, having too much body fat leading to body weight that is above a healthy level; person whose weight interferes with normal activity and body function has *morbid obesity*, 285, 408

Oblique fracture, fracture at angle to bone, 109, 109f

Oblique muscles, oblique means "slanted"; two eye muscles are oblique muscles, 476, 476f

Obsessive-compulsive and related disorders, classification of psychiatric disorders in DSM-5 characterized by obsessive preoccupations and repetitive behaviors; caused by persistent thoughts, ideas, or impulses, 455

Obsessive-compulsive disorder (OCD), mental disorder in which person performs repetitive rituals in order to reduce anxiety, 455

Obstetrician, physician specializing in pregnancy and childbirth, 359

Obstetrics (OB), branch of medicine that treats women during pregnancy and childbirth, and immediately after childbirth, 34t, 359

Occipital bone, cranial bone, 95, 97, 97f, 97t

Occipital lobe, one of four cerebral hemisphere lobes; controls eyesight, 429–430, 431f

Occupational Safety and Health Administration (OSHA), federal agency that issued mandatory guidelines to ensure that all employees at risk of exposure to body fluids are provided with personal protective equipment, 207

Occupational therapist, healthcare professional that specializes in assisting persons to regain, develop, and improve skills important for independent functioning (activities of daily living), 129, 132f

Occupational therapy (OT), assists persons to regain, develop, and improve skills important for independent functioning (activities of daily living), specialist is *occupational therapist*, 129

Ocular, pertaining to eye, 480

Oculomotor nerve, 434t

Oculomycosis, condition of eye fungus, 484

Olfactory nerve, 434t

Oligomenorrhea, scanty menstrual flow, 360

Oligospermia, condition of having few sperm, 377

Oliguria, condition of scanty amount of urine, 324

Onychectomy, surgical removal of a nail, 78

Onychia, infected nailbed, 76

Onychomalacia, softening of nails, 67

Onychomycosis, abnormal condition of nail fungus, 76

Onychophagia, nail biting, 76

Oocyte, female sex cells or gametes produced in ovary; oocyte fuses with sperm to produce embryo; also called *ovum*, 348–349

Oogenesis, process of producing ova by the ovaries, 348

Oophorectomy, removal of an ovary, 368

Oophoritis, inflammation of an ovary, 360

Open fracture. *See* Compound fracture

Open reduction. *See* Reduction

Operative report, medical record report from surgeon detailing operation; includes pre- and postoperative diagnosis, specific details of surgical procedure itself, and how patient tolerated procedure, 14t

Ophthalmalgia, eye pain, 481

Ophthalmic, pertaining to eyes, 480

Ophthalmic decongestants, over-the-counter medications that constrict arterioles of eye, reduce redness and itching of conjunctiva, 490

Ophthalmologist, physician specialized in treating conditions and diseases of eye, 481

Ophthalmology (Ophth), branch of medicine specializing in condition of eye; physician is *ophthalmologist*, 36t, 474, 481

Ophthalmoplegia, paralysis of eye, 481

Ophthalmorrhagia, bleeding from the eye, 481

Ophthalmoscope, instrument to view inside eye, 487

Ophthalmoscopy, examination of interior of eyes using instrument called *ophthalmoscope*; pupil is dilated in order to see cornea, lens, and retina; identifies abnormalities in blood vessels of eye and some systemic diseases, 487, 487f

Opiates. *See* Narcotic analgesic

Opportunistic infections, infectious diseases associated with patients who have compromised immune systems and lowered resistance to infections and parasites, 212

Opposition, moves thumb away from palm; ability to move thumb into contact with other fingers, 126t

Optic, pertaining to eye, 480

Optical, pertaining to eye or vision, 480

Optic disk, area of retina associated with optic nerve; also called *blind spot*, 474f, 475, 475f

Optic nerve, second cranial nerve that carries impulses from retina to brain, 434t, 474, 474f, 477, 478f

Optician, grinds and fits corrective lenses and contacts as prescribed by physician or optometrist, 481

Optometer, instrument to measure vision, 487

Optometrist, doctor of optometry; provides care for eyes including examining eyes for diseases, assessing visual acuity, prescribing corrective lenses and eye treatments, and educating patients, 481

Optometry, process of measuring vision, 481

Otorrhagia, bleeding from ear, 499

Otosclerosis, progressive hearing loss caused by immobility of stapes bone, 500

Otoscope, instrument to view inside ear, 502

Otoscopy, examination of ear canal, eardrum, and outer ear using otoscope; foreign material can be removed from ear canal with this procedure, 502, 502f

Outer ear, 404f, 496f

Outpatient clinic, facility that provides services not requiring overnight hospitalization; services range from simple surgeries to diagnostic testing to therapy; also called *ambulatory care center* or *surgical center*, 15t

Ova, female sex cells or gametes produced in ovary; ovum fuses with sperm to produce embryo; singular is ovum; also called *oocyte*, 348–349, 399, 399f

Ova and parasites (O&P), laboratory examination of feces with microscope for presence of parasites or their eggs, 293

Oval window, division between middle and inner ear, 495, 495f

Ovarian, pertaining to ovaries, 358, 406

Ovarian carcinoma, cancer of ovary, 360

Ovarian cyst, sac that develops within ovary, 360

Ovaries, female gonads; two glands located on either side of lower abdominopelvic region of female; responsible for production of sex cells, ova, and hormones estrogen and progesterone, 348–349, 348f, 349f, 360, 396, 396t–397t, 399, 399f

Over-the-counter (OTC), drugs accessible in drugstores without prescription; also called *nonprescription drugs*, 17

Oviducts, tubes that carry ovum from ovary to uterus; also called *fallopian tubes* or *uterine tubes*, 349–350, 349f, 350f

Ovulation, release of an ovum from ovary, 348–349, 349f

Ovulation stimulant. *See* Fertility drug

Oximeter, instrument to measure oxygen, 250

Oximetry, process of measuring oxygen, 250

Oxygen (O_2), gaseous element absorbed by blood from air sacs in lungs; necessary for cells to make energy, 148–149, 148f, 230

Oxygenated, term for blood with a high oxygen level, 148, 148f

Oxytocin, hormone secreted by posterior pituitary; stimulates uterine contractions during labor and delivery, 369, 397t, 401–402, 402f

P

Pacemaker, another name for sinoatrial node of heart, 153, 154f

Pacemaker implantation, electrical device that substitutes for natural pacemaker of heart; controls beating of heart by series of rhythmic electrical impulses; external pacemaker has electrodes on outside of body; internal pacemaker has electrodes surgically implanted within chest wall, 171, 171f

Packed red cells, transfusion of only formed elements and without plasma, 197

Paget's disease, fairly common metabolic disease of bone from unknown causes; usually attacks middle-aged and older adults and is characterized by bone destruction and deformity, 111

Palate, roof of mouth; anterior portion is hard or bony, posterior portion is soft or flexible, 230, 270–271, 271f, 272f

Palatine bone, facial bone, 95, 97, 97f, 97t

Palatine tonsils, tonsils located in lateral wall of pharynx close to mouth, 205, 231–232, 271f, 272f

Palatoplasty, surgical repair of palate, 297

Pallor, abnormal paleness of skin, 67

Palpitations, pounding, racing heartbeat, 162

Palsy, temporary or permanent loss of ability to control movement, 439

Pancreas, digestive system organ that produces digestive enzymes; within endocrine system produces two hormones, insulin and glucagon, 270, 279f, 280, 396, 397t, 399–400, 400f, 409

Pancreatic, pertaining to pancreas, 283, 407

Pancreatic duct, carries pancreatic juices from pancreas to duodenum, 279f, 280

Pancreatic enzymes, digestive enzymes produced by pancreas and added to chyme in duodenum, 280

Pancreatic islets, regions within pancreas that secrete insulin and glucagon; also called *islets of Langerhans*, 399–400, 400f

Pancreatitis, inflammation of pancreas, 291

Pancytopenia, too few of all types of blood cells, 193

Panhypopituitarism, deficiency in all hormones secreted by pituitary gland; often recognized because of problems with glands regulated by pituitary—adrenal cortex, thyroid, ovaries, and testes, 410

Panic disorder, feeling of intense apprehension, terror, or sense of impending danger, 453

Pansinusitis, inflammation of all sinuses, 243

Pap (Papanicolaou) smear, test for early detection of cancer of cervix named after developer of test, George Papanicolaou, a Greek physician; a scraping of cells is removed from cervix for examination under a microscope, 365

Papilla, 61f

Papilledema, swelling of optic disk, often a result of increased intraocular pressure; also called *choked disk*, 481

Papule, small, solid, circular raised spot on surface of skin, often result of inflammation in oil gland, 67, 67f

Paracentesis, insertion of needle into abdominal cavity to withdraw fluid; tests to diagnose disease may be conducted on fluid, 295

Paralysis, temporary or permanent loss of function or voluntary movement, 439

Paranasal, pertaining to the sinuses beside the nose, 239

Paranasal sinuses, air-filled cavities within facial bones that open into nasal cavity; act as echo chamber during sound production, 230–231, 231f

Paranoid personality disorder, characterized by exaggerated feelings of persecution, 456

Paraphilic disorders, classification of psychiatric disorders in DSM-5 involving aberrant sexual activity;

Prefix, word part added in front of word root; frequently gives information about location of organ, number of parts or time (frequency); not all medical terms have prefix, 2–3, 5–7

Pregnancy, time from fertilization of ovum to birth of newborn, 348, 353–354, 353f, 354f, 355f, 358–359, 362–364

Pregnancy-induced hypertension (PIH). See Preeclampsia

Pregnancy test, chemical test that can determine pregnancy during first few weeks; can be performed in physician's office or with home-testing kit, 365

Premature, infant born prior to 37 weeks of gestation, 353

Premature atrial contraction (PAC), cardiac arrhythmia in which atria contract earlier than they should, 166

Premature ejaculation, release of semen before or shortly after penetration, 456

Premature ventricular contraction (PVC), cardiac arrhythmia in which ventricles contract earlier than they should, 166

Premenstrual syndrome (PMS), symptoms that develop just prior to onset of menstrual period; can include irritability, headache, tender breasts, and anxiety, 361

Premolar, another term for bicuspid teeth, 272

Prepatellar bursitis, pain and swelling in bursa between patella and skin; commonly called housemaid's knee, 113

Prepuce, also called foreskin; protective covering over glans penis; this covering of skin is removed during circumcision, 374

Presbycusis, loss of hearing that can accompany aging process, 499

Presbyopia, expected changes in vision due to normal aging process, resulting in difficulty in focusing for near vision (such as reading), 482

Prescription, written explanation to pharmacist regarding name of medication, dosage, and times of administration, 17, 18, 19f

Prescription drug, can only be ordered by licensed physician, dentist, or veterinarian, 17

Pressure equalizing tube (PE tube), small tube surgically placed in child's ear to assist in drainage of infection, 504

Priapism, persistent and painful erection due to pathological causes, not sexual arousal, 378

Primigravida, woman who has been pregnant once, 359

Primipara, woman who has given birth once, 359

Procedural suffixes, 10

Process, projection from surface of a bone, 94

Proctologist, specialist in anus and rectum, 284

Proctology, branch of medicine involved in diagnosis and treatment of diseases and disorders of anus and rectum, 34t, 284

Proctopexy, surgical fixation of rectum, 298

Proctoptosis, drooping rectum and anus, 290

Progesterone, one of hormones produced by ovaries; works with estrogen to control menstrual cycle, 348–349, 397t, 399

Prolactin (PRL), hormone secreted by anterior pituitary; stimulates milk production, 397t, 401–402, 402f

Prolapsed umbilical cord, when umbilical cord of baby is expelled first during delivery and is squeezed between baby's head and vaginal wall; presents emergency situation since baby's circulation is compromised, 363

Prolapsed uterus, fallen uterus that can cause cervix to protrude through vaginal opening; generally caused by weakened muscles from vaginal delivery or as a result of pelvic tumors pressing down, 361

Pronation, to turn downward or backward, as with hand or foot, 126t, 127f

Prone, directional term meaning lying horizontally facing downward, 44t

Pronunciation, of medical terms, 11

Prophylaxis, prevention of disease; for example, antibiotic can be used to prevent occurrence of bacterial infection, 254

Proprietary name, name a pharmaceutical company chooses as trademark or market name for its drug; also called brand or trade name, 16

Prostate cancer, slow-growing cancer that affects large number of males after age 50; PSA (prostate-specific antigen) test is used to assist in early detection of this disease, 378

Prostatectomy, surgical removal of prostate gland, 380

Prostate gland, within male reproductive system produces fluids that nourish sperm, 316f, 317f, 373, 373f, 375, 378

Prostate-specific antigen (PSA), blood test to screen for prostate cancer; elevated blood levels associated with prostate cancer, 380

Prostatic, pertaining to prostate gland, 376

Prostatitis, inflamed condition of prostate gland that may be result of infection, 378

Prosthesis, artificial device used as substitute for body part either congenitally missing or absent as result of accident or disease; for instance, artificial leg or hip prosthesis, 116

Prosthetic hip joint, 117, 117f

Prosthetics, healthcare profession specializing in making artificial body parts; person skilled in making and adjusting prostheses is a prosthetist; prosthesis is a manufactured substitute for any missing body part, such as an artificial leg, 107

Prosthetist, 107

Protease inhibitor drugs, medications that inhibit protease, enzyme viruses need to reproduce, 215

Protein-bound iodine (PBI) **test,** blood test to measure concentration of thyroxine (T4) circulating in bloodstream; iodine becomes bound to protein in blood and can be measured; useful in establishing thyroid function, 412

Proteinuria, protein in urine, 324

Prothrombin, protein element within blood that interacts with calcium salts to form thrombin, 189–190

Prothrombin time (pro-time, PT), measurement of time it takes for sample of blood to coagulate, 196

Proton pump inhibitor, blocks stomach's ability to secrete acid; used to treat peptic ulcers and gastroesophageal reflux disease, 299

Protozoans, single-celled organisms that can infect body, 205

Proximal, directional term meaning located closest to point of attachment to body, 43*f*, 44*t*

Proximal convoluted tubule, portion of renal tubule, 315, 316*f*

Pruritus, severe itching, 68

Pseudocyesis, false pregnancy, 363

Pseudohypertrophic muscular dystrophy, one type of inherited muscular dystrophy in which muscle tissue is gradually replaced by fatty tissue, giving the appearance of a strong and healthy muscle; also called *Duchenne's muscular dystrophy*, 130

Psoriasis, chronic inflammatory condition consisting of crusty papules forming patches with circular borders, 74, 74*f*

Psychiatric nurse, nurse with additional training in care of patients with mental, emotional, and behavioral disorders, 453

Psychiatric social worker, social worker with additional training in care of patients with mental, emotional, or behavioral disorders, 453

Psychiatrist, physician with specialized training in diagnosing and treating mental disorders; prescribes medication and conducts counseling, 453

Psychiatry, branch of medicine that deals with the diagnosis, treatment, and prevention of mental disorders, 453

Psychoanalysis, method of obtaining a detailed account of past and present emotional and mental experiences from patient to determine source of problem and eliminate effects, 458

Psychology, study of human behavior and thought process; behavioral science is primarily concerned with understanding how human beings interact with their physical environment and with each other, 453

Psychopharmacology, study of effects of drugs on mind and particularly use of drugs in treating mental disorders; main classes of drugs for treatment of mental disorders are antipsychotic drugs, antidepressant drugs, minor tranquilizers, and lithium, 458

Psychotherapy, method of treating mental disorders by mental rather than chemical or physical means; includes psychoanalysis, humanistic therapies, and family and group therapy, 458

Pterygium, hypertrophied conjunctival tissue in inner corner of eye, 485

Puberty, series of events leading up to a child becoming capable of reproduction, 350–351

Pubic, pertaining to pubis; one of pelvic bones, 39*f*, 105

Pubic region, genital region of body, 38*t*, 39*f*

Pubis, one of three bones that form os coxae or innominate bone, 91*f*, 98, 100, 101*f*, 101*t*

Pulmonary, pertaining to lung, 239

Pulmonary angiography, injecting dye into blood vessel for purpose of taking X-ray of arteries and veins of lungs, 249

Pulmonary artery, large artery that carries deoxygenated blood from right ventricle to lung, 152, 153*f*

Pulmonary capillaries, network of capillaries in lungs that tightly encase each alveolus; site of gas exchange, 233

Pulmonary circulation, transports deoxygenated blood from right side of heart to lungs where oxygen and carbon dioxide are exchanged; then carries oxygenated blood back to left side of heart, 148, 148*f*

Pulmonary edema, condition in which lung tissue retains excessive amount of fluid; results in labored breathing, 247

Pulmonary embolism (PE), blood clot or air bubble in pulmonary artery or one of its branches, 247

Pulmonary fibrosis, formation of fibrous scar tissue in lungs, which leads to decreased ability to expand lungs; may be caused by infections, pneumoconiosis, autoimmune diseases, and toxin exposure, 247

Pulmonary function test (PFT), group of diagnostic tests that give information regarding airflow in and out of the lungs, lung volumes, and gas exchange between the lungs and bloodstream, 235, 250

Pulmonary trunk, 149*f*, 150*f*

Pulmonary valve, semilunar valve between right ventricle and pulmonary artery in heart; prevents blood from flowing backward into ventricle, 151–152, 151*f*

Pulmonary veins, large veins that return oxygenated blood from lungs to left atrium, 152, 153*f*

Pulmonologist, physician specialized in treating diseases and disorders of respiratory system, 240

Pulmonology, branch of medicine specializing in conditions of respiratory system, 33*t*, 240

Pulp cavity, hollow interior of tooth; contains soft tissue made up of blood vessels, nerves, and lymph vessels, 272, 273*f*

Pulse (P), expansion and contraction produced by blood as it moves through artery; can be taken at several pulse points throughout body where artery is close to surface, 159

Punch biopsy, small cylinder of tissue is removed by an instrument that pierces through tissue like a hole punch, 77

Pupil, hole in center of iris; size is changed by iris dilating or constricting, 474*f*, 475, 477, 478*f*

Pupillary, pertaining to pupil, 480

Purified protein derivative (PPD). *See* Tuberculin skin tests

Purkinje fibers, part of conduction system of heart; found in ventricular myocardium, 153, 154*f*

Purpura, hemorrhages into skin and mucous membranes, 68, 68*f*

Purulent, pus-filled sputum, which can be result of infection, 68

Pustule, raised spot on skin containing pus, 68, 68*f*

Pyelitic, pertaining to renal pelvis, 322

Pyelitis, inflammation of renal pelvis, 326

Pyelogram, X-ray record of the renal pelvis, 329

Pyelonephritis, inflammation of renal pelvis and kidney; one of most common types of kidney disease; may be result of lower urinary tract infection that moved up to kidney by way of ureters; may be large quantities of white blood cells and bacteria in urine, and blood (hematuria) may even be present in urine in this condition; can occur with any untreated or persistent case of cystitis, 326

Pyeloplasty, surgical repair of renal pelvis, 332

Pyloric, pertaining to pylorus, 283

Pyloric sphincter, located at distal end of stomach; controls passage of food into duodenum, 275, 275f, 279f

Pyoderma, pus-producing skin infection, 68

Pyosalpinx, condition of having pus in fallopian tubes, 360

Pyothorax, condition of having pus in chest cavity, 243

Pyromania, impulse control disorder in which patient is unable to control impulse to start fires, 454

Pyrosis, pain and burning sensation usually caused by stomach acid splashing up into the esophagus; commonly called *heartburn*, 286

Pyuria, presence of pus in urine, 324

Q

Quadriplegia, paralysis of all four extremities; same as tetraplegia, 439

R

Radial, pertaining to radius; lower arm bone, 105

Radial artery, 157f

Radial keratotomy, spokelike incisions around cornea that result in it becoming flatter; surgical treatment for myopia, 489

Radial nerve, 435f

Radial vein, 158f

Radical mastectomy, surgical removal of breast tissue plus chest muscles and axillary lymph nodes; term radical is used to describe extensive surgical procedures designed to remove root cause of disease, 368

Radiculitis, nerve root inflammation, 445

Radiculopathy, disease of nerve root, 445

Radiograph, image produced by radiography (i.e., an X-ray), 115

Radiography, making of X-ray pictures, 115

Radioimmunoassay (RIA), test used to measure levels of hormones in plasma of blood, 412

Radius, one of forearm bones in upper extremity, 91f, 98, 99f, 100, 100f, 100t

Rales. *See* Crackles

Range of motion (ROM), maximum amount of movement allowed at a joint, from maximum flexion through maximum extension; measured as degrees of a circle, 101–102

Raynaud's phenomenon, periodic ischemic attacks affecting extremities of body, especially fingers, toes, ears, and nose; affected extremities become cyanotic and very painful; attacks are brought on by arterial constriction due to extreme cold or emotional stress, 167

Reabsorption, second phase of urine production; substances needed by body are reabsorbed as filtrate passes through kidney tubules, 318–319, 318f

Recklinghausen disease, excessive production of parathyroid hormone, which results in degeneration of bones, 410

Rectal, (1) pertaining to rectum; (2) substances introduced directly into rectal cavity in form of suppositories or solution; drugs may have to be administered by this route if patient is unable to take them by mouth due to nausea, vomiting, and surgery, 45, 47t, 283

Rectocele, protrusion or herniation of rectum into vagina, 361

Rectum, area at end of large intestine for storage of feces that leads to anal canal, 277, 277f, 348f

Rectus abdominis, muscle named for its location and direction of its fibers: rectus means *straight* and abdominis means *abdominal*, 119f, 124

Rectus muscles, rectus means *straight*; four of the eye muscles are rectus muscles, 476, 476f

Red blood cell count (RBC), blood test to determine number of erythrocytes in volume of blood; decrease in red blood cells may indicate anemia; increase may indicate polycythemia, 196

Red blood cell morphology, determines diseases such as sickle cell anemia through examination of blood for abnormalities in shape (morphology) of erythrocytes, 196

Red blood cells (RBCs), also called *erythrocytes*; contain hemoglobin and iron-containing pigment that binds oxygen in order to transport it to cells of body, 188, 189f

Red bone marrow, tissue that manufactures most of blood cells; found in cancellous bone cavities, 92–93

Reduction, correcting a fracture by realigning bone fragments; closed reduction is doing manipulation without entering body; open reduction is process of making surgical incision at site of fracture to do reduction, necessary when bony fragments need to be removed, or *internal fixation*, such as plates or pins, is required, 118

Refract, bending of light rays as they enter eye, 474

Refractive error test, eye examination performed by physician to determine and correct refractive errors in eye, 487

Regional anesthesia, anesthetic interrupts patient's pain sensation in a particular region of body; injected near nerve that will be blocked from sensation; patient usually remains conscious; also referred to as *nerve block*, 448

Regional ileitis. *See* Crohn's disease

Regurgitation, to flow backward; within cardiovascular system refers to blood flowing backward through valve; within digestive system refers to food flowing backward from stomach to mouth, 163, 286

Rehabilitation, process of treatment and exercise that can help person with disability attain maximum function and well-being, 133

Rehabilitation centers, facilities that provide intensive physical and occupational therapy; include inpatient and outpatient treatment, 15t

Sarcoidosis, autoimmune disease of unknown cause in which lesions may appear in liver, skin, lungs, lymph nodes, spleen, eyes, and small bones of hands and feet, 213

Scabies, contagious skin disease caused by egg-laying mite that causes intense itching; often seen in children, 74

Scapula, also called *shoulder blade*; upper extremity bone, 91*f*, 93*f*, 98, 99*f*, 100, 100*f*, 100*t*

Scapular, pertaining to scapula or shoulder blade, 105

Schedule I, drugs with highest potential for addiction and abuse; not accepted for medical use; examples are heroin and LSD, 17, 18*t*

Schedule II, drugs with high potential for addiction and abuse; accepted for medical use in United States; examples are codeine, cocaine, morphine, opium, and secobarbital, 17, 18*t*

Schedule III, drugs with moderate-to-low potential for addiction and abuse; examples are butabarbital, anabolic steroids, and acetaminophen with codeine, 17, 18*t*

Schedule IV, drugs with lower potential for addiction and abuse than Schedule III drugs; examples are chloral hydrate, phenobarbital, and diazepam, 17, 18*t*

Schedule V, drugs with low potential for addiction and abuse; example is low-strength codeine combined with other drugs to suppress coughing, 17, 18*t*

Schizophrenia spectrum and other psychotic disorders, classification of psychiatric disorders in DSM-5 characterized by distortions of reality such as delusions and hallucinations, 456

Schwann cell, 429*f*

Sciatic nerve, 435*f*

Sclera, tough protective outer layer of eyeball; commonly referred to as "white of eye," 474, 474*f*

Scleral, pertaining to sclera, 480

Scleral buckling, placing a band of silicone around outside of sclera to stabilize detaching retina, 489

Scleritis, inflammation of sclera, 484

Scleroderma, condition in which skin has lost its elasticity and become hardened, 68

Scleromalacia, softening of sclera, 482

Sclerotherapy, medical treatment for varicose veins; results in veins collapsing and stickings together, 171

Sclerotomy, to cut into the sclera, 489

Scoliosis, abnormal lateral curvature of spine, 112, 112*f*

Scrotum, sac that serves as container for testes; divided by septum, supports testicles and lies between legs and behind penis, 373–374, 373*f*

Sebaceous cyst, sac under skin filled with sebum or oil from sebaceous gland; can grow to large size and may need to be excised, 74

Sebaceous glands, also called *oil glands*; produce substance called *sebum* that lubricates skin surfaces and eyeball, 58, 59*f*, 61*f*, 62, 476

Seborrhea, oily discharge, 68

Sebum, thick, oily substance secreted by sebaceous glands that lubricates skin to prevent drying out, 62

Second-degree burn. *See* Burn

Secretion, third phase of urine production; additional waste products are added to filtrate as it passes through kidney tubules, 318–319, 318*f*

Sedative, produces relaxation without causing sleep, 450

Seizure, sudden, uncontrollable onset of symptoms, such as in an epileptic seizure, 439

Self-inoculation, infection that occurs when person becomes infected in different part of body by pathogen from another part of his or her own body, such as intestinal bacteria spreading to urethra, 207

Semen, contains sperm and fluids secreted by male reproductive system glands; leaves body through urethra, 373

Semen analysis, procedure used when performing fertility workup to determine if male is able to produce sperm; semen is collected by patient after abstaining from sexual intercourse for a period of three to five days; sperm in semen are analyzed for number, swimming strength, and shape; also used to determine if vasectomy has been successful; after a period of six weeks, no sperm should be present in sample from patient, 380

Semicircular canals, portion of labyrinth associated with balance and equilibrium, 494*f*, 495

Semiconscious, state of being aware of surroundings and responding to stimuli only part of time, 440

Semilunar valve, heart valves located between ventricles and great arteries leaving heart; pulmonary valve is located between right ventricle, and pulmonary artery; aortic valve is located between left ventricle and aorta, 151–152, 151*f*

Seminal vesicles, two male reproductive system glands located at base of bladder; secrete fluid that nourishes sperm into vas deferens; fluid plus sperm constitutes much of semen, 373, 373*f*, 374

Seminiferous tubules, network of coiled tubes that make up bulk of testes; sperm development takes place in walls of tubules and mature sperm are released into tubule in order to leave testes, 373–374, 403*f*

Sensorineural hearing loss, type of hearing loss in which sound is conducted normally through external and middle ear but there is a defect in inner ear or with cochlear nerve, resulting in inability to hear; hearing aid may help, 496

Sensory neurons, carry sensory information from sensory receptors to brain; also called *afferent neurons*, 433–434, 435*f*

Sensory receptors, nerve fibers located directly under skin surface; detect temperature, pain, touch, and pressure; messages for these sensations are conveyed to brain and spinal cord from nerve endings in skin, 58, 59*f*, 428

Sepsis. *See* Septicemia

Septal, pertaining to nasal septum, 239

Septicemia, having bacteria in bloodstream; commonly referred to as *sepsis* or *blood poisoning*, 193

Serous fluid, watery secretion of serous membranes, 234

Serum, clear, sticky fluid that remains after blood has clotted, 188

Thyromegaly, enlarged thyroid, 408

Thyrotoxicosis, condition that results from overproduction of thyroid glands; symptoms include rapid heart action, tremors, enlarged thyroid gland, exophthalmos, and weight loss, 411

Thyroxine (T4), hormone produced by thyroid gland; also known as T4 and requires iodine for production; regulates level of cell metabolism; the greater the level of hormone in the bloodstream, the higher the cell metabolism, 397t, 403–404

Tibia, also called *shin bone*; lower extremity bone, 91f, 98, 99f, 100, 101f, 101t

Tibial, pertaining to tibia or shin bone, 106

Tic douloureux. *See* Trigeminal neuralgia

Tidal volume (TV), amount of air that enters lungs in single inhalation or leaves lungs in single exhalation of quiet breathing, 235t

Tinea, fungal skin disease resulting in itching, scaling lesions, 75

Tinea capitis, fungal infection of scalp; commonly called *ringworm*, 75

Tinea pedis, fungal infection of foot; commonly called *athlete's foot*, 75

Tinnitus, ringing in ears, 499

Tissues, formed when cells of same type are grouped to perform one activity; for example, nerve cells combine to form nerve fibers; there are four types: nervous, muscle, epithelial, and connective
connective, 27f, 28–31, 30f
epithelial, 28, 30f
muscle, 28, 29, 30f, 122
nervous, 28, 30f, 31, 428

Tissue transglutaminase (tTG) **antibody test,** blood test for celiac disease, 293

T lymphocytes, type of lymphocyte involved with producing cells that physically attack and destroy pathogens, 205

Tongue, muscular organ in floor of mouth; works to move food around inside mouth and is also necessary for speech, 270–271, 271f, 272f

Tonic-clonic seizure, type of severe epileptic seizure characterized by loss of consciousness and convulsions; seizure alternates between strong continuous muscle spasms (tonic) and rhythmic muscle contraction and relaxation (clonic); also called *grand mal seizure*, 440

Tonometry, measurement of intraocular pressure of eye using tonometer to check for condition of glaucoma; generally part of normal eye exam for adults, 487

Tonsillar, pertaining to tonsils, 209

Tonsillectomy, surgical removal of tonsils, 215

Tonsillitis, inflammation of tonsils, 212

Tonsils, collections of lymphatic tissue located in pharynx to combat microorganisms entering body through nose or mouth; include pharyngeal tonsils, palatine tonsils, and lingual tonsils, 202, 205, 205f, 271f, 272f

Tooth cavity. *See* Dental caries

Topical, applied directly to skin or mucous membranes; distributed in ointment, cream, or lotion form; used to treat skin infections and eruptions, 45, 47f

Topical anesthesia, applied using either liquid or gel placed directly onto specific area; patient remains conscious; used on skin, cornea, and mucous membranes in dental work, 449

Torticollis, severe neck spasms pulling head to one side; commonly called *wryneck* or *crick in the neck*, 130

Total abdominal hysterectomy-bilateral salpingo-oophorectomy (TAH-BSO), removal of entire uterus, cervix, both ovaries, and both fallopian tubes, 368

Total calcium, blood test to measure total amount of calcium to assist in detecting parathyroid and bone disorders, 413

Total hip arthroplasty (THA), surgical reconstruction of hip by implanting prosthetic or artificial hip joint; also called *total hip replacement*, 117, 117f

Total hip replacement (THR). *See* Total hip arthroplasty

Total knee arthroplasty (TKA), surgical reconstruction of knee joint by implanting prosthetic knee joint; also called *total knee replacement*, 117

Total knee replacement (TKR). *See* Total knee arthroplasty

Total lung capacity (TLC), volume of air in lungs after maximal inhalation, 235t

Total parenteral nutrition (TPN), providing 100% of patient's nutrition intravenously; used when patient is unable to eat, 296

Toxemia. *See* Preeclampsia

Toxicity, extent or degree to which a substance is poisonous, 333

Toxic shock syndrome (TSS), rare and sometimes fatal staphylococcus infection that generally occurs in menstruating women; initial infection occurs in vagina and is associated with prolonged wearing of super-absorbent tampon; toxins secreted by bacteria then enter bloodstream, 361

Toxins, substances poisonous to body; many are filtered out of blood by kidney, 205

Trachea, also called *windpipe*; conducts air from larynx down to main bronchi in chest, 230, 232, 232f, 233f, 236f, 272f

Tracheal, pertaining to trachea, 106, 239

Tracheostenosis, narrowing and stenosis of lumen or opening into trachea, 244

Tracheostomy. *See* Tracheotomy

Tracheotomy, surgical procedure used to make opening in trachea to create airway; tracheostomy tube can be inserted to keep opening patent; also called *tracheostomy*, 253, 253f

Tracts, bundles of nerve fibers located within central nervous system, 428–429

Traction, process of pulling or drawing, usually with mechanical device; used in treating orthopedic (bone and joint) problems and injuries, 118

Tractotomy, precision cutting of a nerve tract in spinal cord to treat intractable pain or muscle spasms, 449

Trademark, pharmaceutical company's brand name for drug, 16

Transcutaneous electrical nerve stimulation (TENS), application of mild electrical current by device with electrodes placed on skin over painful area; relieves pain by interfering with nerve signal to brain on pain nerve, 449

and lumbar vertebrae, sacrum, and coccyx; also called *spinal column*, 95, 97–98, 98*f*, 98*t*, 111–113, 112*f*, 432

Vertebral region, spinal column region of body, 39*f*, 39*t*

Vertigo, dizziness caused by sensation that room is spinning, 499

Vesicle, small, fluid-filled raised spot on skin, 69, 69*f*

Vesicular, pertaining to seminal vesicle, 376

Vestibular, pertaining to vestibule, 498

Vestibular nerve, branch of vestibulocochlear nerve responsible for sending equilibrium information to brain, 494, 494*f*

Vestibule, inner ear structure off of which the cochlea, semicircular canals, utricle, and saccule open, 495

Vestibulocochlear nerve, eighth cranial nerve; responsible for hearing and balance, 434*t*, 494, 494*f*

Villi, finger-like projections from wall of small intestine; serve to increase surface area for nutrient absorption, 275–276, 277*f*

Viruses, group of infectious particles that cause disease, 205

Viscera, name for internal organs of body, such as lungs, stomach, and liver, 40

Visceral, pertaining to viscera or internal organs, 234

Visceral layer, inner pleural layer; adheres to surface of lung, 40

Visceral muscle. *See* Smooth muscle

Visceral pericardium, inner layer of pericardium surrounding heart, 150

Visceral peritoneum, inner layer of serous membrane sac encasing abdominopelvic viscera, 40, 150, 150*f*

Visceral pleura, inner layer of serous membrane sac encasing thoracic viscera, 40, 234

Vision, 477, 478*f*

Visual acuity (VA) **test,** measurement of sharpness of patient's vision; a Snellen chart is usually used for this test and patient identifies letters from distance of 20 feet, 487

Vital capacity (VC), total volume of air that can be exhaled after maximum inhalation; amount will be equal to sum of tidal volume, inspiratory reserve volume, and expiratory reserve volume, 235*t*

Vital signs (VS), respiration, pulse, temperature, skin color, blood pressure, and reaction of pupils; signs of condition of body functions, 236–237

Vitamin D therapy, maintaining high blood levels of calcium in association with vitamin D helps maintain bone density and treats osteomalacia, osteoporosis, and rickets, 118

Vitiligo, disappearance of pigment from skin in patches, causing a milk-white appearance; also called *leukoderma*, 75

Vitreous body, 474*f*

Vitreous humor, transparent jellylike substance inside eyeball, 475

Vocal cords, structures within larynx that vibrate to produce sound and speech, 232

Voiding, another term for urination, 316

Voiding cystourethrography (VCUG), X-ray taken to visualize urethra while patient is voiding after contrast dye has been placed in bladder, 329

Voluntary muscles, those that person can consciously choose to contract; skeletal muscles of arm and leg are examples, 122

Volvulus, condition in which bowel twists upon itself and causes painful obstruction that requires immediate surgery, 290, 290*f*

Vomer bone, facial bone, 95, 97, 97*f*, 97*t*

Voyeuristic disorder, paraphilic disorder characterized by receiving sexual gratification from observing others engaged in sexual acts, 456

Vulva, general term meaning external female genitalia; consists of Bartholin's glands, labia majora, labia minora, and clitoris, 348, 351

Vulvar, pertaining to vulva, 358

W

Walking pneumonia. *See Mycoplasma pneumonia*

Wall-eyed. *See* Exotropia

Warts. *See* Verruca

Wax emulsifiers, substances used to soften earwax to prevent buildup within external ear canal, 505

Wet gangrene, area of gangrene becoming infected by pus-producing bacteria, 75

Wheal, small, round raised area on skin that may be accompanied by itching, 69, 69*f*

Whiplash, cervical muscle and ligament sprain or strain, 113

White blood cell count (WBC), blood test to measure number of leukocytes in volume of blood; increase may indicate presence of infection or disease such as leukemia; decrease in WBCs is caused by X-ray therapy and chemotherapy, 196

White blood cell differential (diff), determines number of each variety of leukocytes in volume of blood, 196

White blood cells (WBCs), blood cells that provide protection against invasion of bacteria and other foreign material, 29*f*, 188

White matter, tissue in central nervous system; consists of myelinated nerve fibers, 428–429, 433

Whole blood, transfusion of a mixture of both plasma and formed elements, 197

Whooping cough. *See* Pertussis

Wilms' tumor, malignant kidney tumor found most often in children; also called *nephroblastoma*, 327

Windpipe. *See* Trachea

Wisdom teeth, 272, 273*f*

Womb. *See* Uterus

Word building, 11

Word root, foundation of medical term that provides basic meaning of word; in general, will indicate body system or part of body being discussed; word may have more than one word root, 2–3

Wryneck. *See* Torticollis